Management of Cardiovascular Disease in Women

Hanna Z. Mieszczanska • Gladys P. Velarde
Editors

Management of Cardiovascular Disease in Women

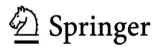 Springer

Editors
Hanna Z. Mieszczanska, MD
Division of Cardiology
University of Rochester Medical Center
Rochester, NY
USA

Gladys P. Velarde
Division of Cardiology
University of Florida College
of Medicine-Jacksonville
Jacksonville, FL
USA

ISBN 978-1-4471-5516-4   ISBN 978-1-4471-5517-1   (eBook)
DOI 10.1007/978-1-4471-5517-1
Springer London Heidelberg New York Dordrecht

Library of Congress Control Number: 2014931657

Printed on acid-free paper

Springer is part of Springer Science+Business Media (www.springer.com)

To my husband Richard, our children, Michael and Julia, and my mother, Maria, for your enduring patience, understanding, and support through the many long hours in the preparation of this book

Hanna Z. Mieszczanska

To the memory of my mother, Edmunda Emma Palacio, to whom I owe all that I am; and to my family with much love

Gladys P. Velarde

Preface

Recent decades have witnessed great progress in the treatment of cardiovascular disease (CVD). Due to improved therapies, preventive strategies and increased public awareness, CVD mortality has been on the decline over this span of time for both genders. Unfortunately, the decline has been less prominent for women. Once viewed as a man's disease, CVD remains the leading cause of mortality for women in the United States and is responsible for a third of all deaths of women worldwide and half of all deaths of women over 50 years of age in developing countries. In the United States, CVD far outdistances all other causes of death, including all forms of cancer combined. Since 1984, the total number of women who die of CVD every year is higher than the number of men. The statistics are sobering with about one female death in the United States every minute from CVD. That represents over 420,000 deaths per year according to the more recent statistics. Of these, more than one quarter of a million women will die this year from coronary heart disease (CHD) and about 64 % of women who die suddenly of CHD will have no prior symptoms. Despite a significant number of females with known CVD and increased awareness among women of heart disease as their major health threat, a substantial proportion of women (46 % as per most recent American Heart Association survey) remain unaware of their cardiovascular risk and continue to fail to recognize its significance. Among women in higher-risk groups, racial and ethnic minorities, this lack of awareness is more profound (over 60 % unaware) and has changed little in decades.

Poorly understood gender differences in pathobiologic mechanisms, clinical presentation, management and application of therapeutic and preventive strategies have contributed to this gap. A critically important factor has been the underrepresentation of women in CVD research to date. In fact, only one-third of CVD clinical trials report sex-specific results despite The Food and Drug Administration regulations requiring sex stratification data, as well as the National Institute of Health recommendations of increased inclusion of women in clinical trials.

This makes it difficult for researchers and clinicians to draw accurate conclusions about gender differences in mechanisms of disease, risks or benefits of a particular drug or device for the treatment of women with CVD. Furthermore, physicians and other healthcare providers continue to underestimate women's cardiovascular risk, in part because of utilization of suboptimal traditional risk assessment algorithms with consequent underutilization of preventive therapies for women.

Then what is so different about heart disease in women? Women *are* different physiologically and psychologically, and as a result their manifestations of cardiovascular problems may vary from men.

The development of CHD in women typically may lag 10–15 years behind that of men, but after menopause the atherosclerotic process appears to accelerate. In general, women with CHD tend to be older and sicker at presentation compared to men. Women often present with heart failure, are less likely to be diagnosed and treated efficiently and aggressively, and as a result of these challenges, generally have a worse medical prognosis than men following myocardial infarction or revascularization. Similarly, young women (<50 years of age) with CHD in particular are 1.5–2 times more likely to die within a year compared to their male counterparts following a myocardial infarction and coronary artery bypass surgery, respectively. The reason for this is still unknown. Although heart disease predominates at older ages, in the United States more than 18,500 women younger than age 65 die annually of CHD, 35 % of these women are younger than age 55 and a concerning increasing mortality trend seems to be evolving in women with CHD between the ages of 35 and 54. A rise rather than a decline in events, relative to men of this same age group, has been noted since 1997. Irrespective of age, women with CHD have more unfavorable early outcomes than men.

Several biological variables and pathophysiological mechanisms differ in women and remain poorly understood. Obvious differences such as vessel size and increased number of co-morbidities in the older female do not entirely explain the gender differences we see in terms of early adverse outcomes, frequency and type of angina, and heart failure presentation. In fact, paradoxical findings appear to juxtapose making the evaluation of ischemia and heart failure more challenging. The lower prevalence of obstructive coronary artery disease in women with angina relative to men as seen in coronary angiography, and the better left ventricular (LV) systolic function, as measured by LV ejection fraction in women relative to men as seen on echocardiography, are two of the most salient examples of gender differences in cardiovascular disease today. Despite the fact that women have less severe obstructive disease at angiography than men, they have a similar or higher burden of angina and consequent higher morbidity and mortality as previously noted. Nonetheless, it is the obstructive coronary atherosclerosis model, the "male model" of CHD that constitutes the basis for diagnostic and therapeutic strategies for both sexes. While this model is still valid for the majority of women afflicted with CAD, it is those that do not fit in this "obstructive CAD" model, the majority of whom are women, who remain a diagnostic and therapeutic challenge.

Congestive heart failure (CHF), often the end result of advanced ischemic heart disease but also the common resting ground of advanced hypertensive, diabetic and valvular heart disease, affects a significant number of women. Currently more than 2.6 million women are afflicted with CHF. For decades, only a small number of women have been included in major clinical research studies of CHF. This absence has contributed to an incomplete understanding of this condition in women. The exclusion of older participants and those with clinical HF and "preserved" LV ejection fraction (HFpEF), in most of the heart failure literature to date, has also magnified this problem as women make up the overwhelming majority of these two groups. The preponderance of diastolic dysfunction in older women with heart failure is poorly understood and has been poorly studied to date.

Other cardiomyopathies unique to women such as peripartum cardiomyopathy, chemotherapy induced cardiomyopathy, and stress induced or Takatsubo cardiomyopathy remain poorly understood and grossly ignored in clinical and translational research. No guidelines yet exist as of how to treat and prevent these conditions.

Diabetic women deserve special consideration given the alarming CV morbidity and mortality that affects this population. Undoubtedly, the obesity epidemic plays a significant role in the increased prevalence of diabetes and metabolic syndrome, especially in women of minority ethnic groups. The metabolic syndrome, especially in postmenopausal women, should also receive special attention with emphasis on early recognition (high triglycerides, low HDL, insulin resistance, abdominal obesity, and hypertension) and intervention due its strong association with diabetes and increased risk for CVD events. These recognizable and treatable risk factors, for reasons still not completely understood, appear to affect women more in terms of CV sequelae.

Additionally, important differences within women groups need to be recognized as women from minority ethnic groups have poorer CV outcomes than Caucasian women.

Among black women, CHD death rates are about 15 % greater and stroke rates 30 % greater than for white women. Statistics are not more favorable for Hispanic women whose rates lie somewhere in between black and white women when all Hispanics i.e. Caribbean, South American and Mexican Americans are included – data is limited in this more heterogeneous group as it is for Pacific Islanders and other emerging minorities in the United States.

Similarly, psychosocial factors, such as anxiety, depression, inadequate social and economic resources, care giver stress, marital stress, and adversities early in life are highly prevalent in women and have been linked to adverse cardiovascular outcomes in both genders but appear to affect women more. As a woman's role continues to evolve and our societies become more complex and faster-paced, women are more frequently juggling multiple roles, trying to balance the various demands of motherhood, professional careers, work and often as primary care givers for extended family members and aging parents. Combining all of these different responsibilities can be quite overwhelming to many.

Women, when affected by depression, have a harder time coping and are more likely to adopt unhealthy habits (poor diet, lack of exercise, no stress management techniques). Not surprisingly, women are diagnosed with depression twice as often compared with men and stress, depression and anxiety disorders are associated with higher cardiovascular risk among women compared with men. Proper discussion of these issues should take place during the evaluation of any women with symptoms of CVD, as stress may be contributing to some of the symptoms women present with, like palpitations or atypical chest pain.

In addition to traditional risk factors, women have some unique cardiac risk factors, including increased prevalence of autoimmune and inflammatory conditions, which predispose to accelerated atherosclerosis in these patients. Disorders such as gestational diabetes, hypertension, preeclampsia, or eclampsia may occur during pregnancy and significantly increase the risk of CV events later in life. Preeclampsia, for example, can double the risk for subsequent CVD, and gestational diabetes significantly increases the risk of future diabetes, and therefore CVD. Research into these complications of pregnancy is needed to improve pregnancy outcomes and guide efforts to improve risk factors and lower cardiovascular risk after pregnancy.

Despite the fact that women do not commonly experience heart disease in reproductive years, strategies for slowing the progression of CVD should begin during these years or earlier. This emphasizes the importance of a multidisciplinary approach where a variety of health care providers can intervene early to improve outcomes. Recognizing multiple risk factors can identify women at highest risk, even during the years that they are presumably protected by estrogen. Diet, exercise, weight control, smoking cessation and adequate blood pressure control can reduce risk as women age. Detailed, focused, individualized and advanced CV risk profile assessment may be necessary in certain cases where premature CVD is a dominant feature of first-degree relatives of women at young age.

Currently, several pathobiological mechanisms that appear different in the female heart, ranging from plaque adaptation, plaque vulnerability to ulceration and remodeling, thrombogenicity, atherogenicity of different lipoproteins, left ventricular remodeling to ischemic injury, emotional stress, arrythmogenicity, loading conditions and valvular dysfunction, to the role of inflammation, role of fluctuating hormones and their effect on the myocardium, endothelium, microvasculature, and autonomic regulation in the different stages of a woman's life, are under investigation. Gender-specific basic, translational and clinical research in these areas is paramount to a better understanding of cardiovascular gender differences

The purpose of this book is to provide a comprehensive overview of current knowledge of differences in cardiac problems in women including challenges and limitations of the available literature. Important and unique aspects to women's heart health such as pregnancy, the impact of emotional stress and other psychosocial issues that are specific to women are also tackled, thus providing a concise guide for cardiovascular care in women. This book is divided in four parts: Part I reviews epidemiology, classification, and discusses the most recent American College of Cardiology and American Heart Association (ACC/AHA) Effectiveness-based guidelines for the prevention of cardiovascular disease in women. Part II provides an extensive review and a guide to health care providers of diagnosis, evaluation and treatment of ischemic heart disease, congestive heart failure, valvular heart disease, arrhythmias, congenital heart disease, peripheral vascular disease, hypertension, metabolic syndrome and diabetes mellitus in women. Part III focuses on pregnancy and cardiovascular issues in women. Part IV, the final section, discusses special considerations in women including anticoagulation issues, hormone replacement therapy in postmenopausal women, integrative approaches to cardiac care, psychological and socioeconomic risk factors for CVD, and pharmacologic considerations specific to women.

We feel that it is imperative these topics be addressed not only by cardiologists, but by primary care providers, internists, and reproductive healthcare professionals who undoubtedly treat many different women in their practices. We believe that this manual will be useful to a wide range of practitioners who wish to learn more about the cardiovascular problems women face.

We would like to thank our contributors for an extensive review of the literature, their knowledge and expertise in preparing this book.

Jacksonville, FL, USA   Gladys Palacio-Velarde
Rochester, NY, USA   Hanna Z. Mieszczanska

Acknowledgements

This book is the result of many people's generous efforts. To our contributing authors and office staff at the University of Rochester and University of Florida campuses, and to Grant Weston and Liz Pope for their direction and advice, we extend our deepest gratitude.

Hanna Z. Mieszczanska
Gladys P. Velarde

Contents

Contributors

Alian Aguila, MD Division of Cardiology, University of Florida College of Medicine-Jacksonville, Jacksonville, FL, USA

Dominick J. Angiolillo, MD, PhD Division of Cardiology, University of Florida College of Medicine-Jacksonville, Jacksonville, FL, USA

Illena Antonetti, MD Department of Cardiovascular Disease, University of South Florida, Tampa, FL, USA

Khyati Baxi, MD Division of Cardiology, University of Florida College of Medicine-Jacksonville, Jacksonville, FL, USA

John D. Bisognano, MD, PhD Division of Cardiology, University of Rochester Medical Center, Rochester, NY, USA

Stephanie J. Carter, MD Division of Cardiology, University of Rochester Medical Center, Rochester, NY, USA

Leway Chen, MD, MPH Division of Cardiology, University of Rochester Medical Center, Rochester, NY, USA

Jung Rae Cho, MD Division of Cardiology, University of Florida College of Medicine-Jacksonville, Jacksonville, FL, USA

Rashaad A. Chothia, MD Division of Cardiology, University of Rochester Medical Center, Rochester, NY, USA

Naila Choudhary, MBBS Division of Cardiology, University of Rochester Medical Center, Rochester, NY, USA

Renee M. Dallasen, MD Department of Medicine and Department of Obstetrics and Gynecology, University of Rochester Medical Center, Rochester, NY, USA

Andrew Darlington, DO Division of Cardiology, University of Florida College of Medicine-Jacksonville, Jacksonville, FL, USA

Marci DeLosSantos, Pharm.D, BCPS (AQ Card) Department of Pharmacy, University of Florida Health – Jacksonville, Jacksonville, FL, USA

Katherine S. Dodd, DO, MPH Department of Medicine, University of Rochester Medical Center, Rochester, NY, USA

James Eichelberger, MD Division of Cardiology, University of Rochester Medical Center, Rochester, NY, USA

Lydia R. Engwenyu, MD Division of Cardiology, Department of Cardiovascular Medicine, University of Florida College of Medicine-Jacksonville, Jacksonville, FL, USA

Susan G. Fisher, MS, PhD Department of Clinical Sciences, Temple University School of Medicine, Philadelphia, PA, USA

Francesco Franchi, MD Division of Cardiology, University of Florida College of Medicine-Jacksonville, Jacksonville, FL, USA

John P. Gassler, MD Division of Cardiology, University of Rochester Medical Center, Rochester, NY, USA

Catherine Gracey, MD Department of Medicine, University of Rochester Medical Center, University of Rochester, Rochester, NY, USA

Jacinta Green, MD Division of Cardiology, University of Florida College of Medicine-Jacksonville, Jacksonville, FL, USA

Mimi Guarneri, MD, FACC UCSD School of Medicine, Scripps Center for Integrative Medicine, La Jolla, CA, USA

Luis A. Guzman, MD Division of Cardiology, Department of Cardiovascular Medicine, University of Florida College of Medicine-Jacksonville, Jacksonville, FL, USA

Diane M. Hartmann, MD Department of Medicine and Department of Obstetrics and Gynecology, University of Rochester Medical Center, Rochester, NY, USA

Wassim Jawad, MD Division of Cardiology, Department of Cardiovascular Medicine, University of Florida College of Medicine-Jacksonville, Jacksonville, FL, USA

Vijay Krishnamoorthy, MD Division of Cardiology, University of Rochester Medical Center, Rochester, NY, USA

Rachel Lee, MD Division of Cardiology, University of Florida College of Medicine-Jacksonville, Jacksonville, FL, USA

Division of Cardiology, University of Florida Health Science Center, Jacksonville, FL, USA

Rebecca Lewandowski, MD, PhD Division of Cardiology, Department of Medicine, University of Rochester Medical Center, Rochester, NY, USA

Joel A. Strom, MD, MEng Division of Cardiology, University of Florida College of Medicine-Jacksonville, Jacksonville, FL, USA

Hanna Z. Mieszczanska, MD Division of Cardiology, University of Rochester Medical Center, Rochester, NY, USA

Erica O. Miller, MD Department of Medicine, University of Rochester Medical Center, Rochester, NY, USA

Ana Muñiz-Lozano, MD Division of Cardiology, University of Florida College of Medicine-Jacksonville, Jacksonville, FL, USA

Janice Opladen, ACNP-BC Division of Cardiology, University of Rochester Medical Center, Rochester, NY, USA

Jason Pacos, MD Division of Cardiology, University of Rochester Medical Center, Rochester, NY, USA

Nicholas Paivanas, MD Department of Medicine, University of Rochester Medical Center, Rochester, NY, USA

Ambar Patel, MD Division of Cardiology, Department of Cardiovascular Medicine, University of Florida College of Medicine-Jacksonville, Jacksonville, FL, USA

Angelo Pedulla, MD Division of Cardiology, University of Rochester Medical Center, Rochester, NY, USA

Rebecca E. Pratt, MD Division of Pediatric Cardiology, University of Rochester Medical Center, Rochester, NY, USA

Malgorzata Relja, MD, DABPN Horizon Health Mental Health Center, Fredericton, Canada

Fabiana Rollini, MD Division of Cardiology, University of Florida College of Medicine-Jacksonville, Jacksonville, FL, USA

Saadia Sherazi, MD, MS Heart Research Follow up Program, University of Rochester Medical Center, Rochester, NY, USA

Sabu Thomas, MD Division of Cardiology, University of Rochester Medical Center, Rochester, NY, USA

Justin Tinsley, PharmD Department of Pharmacy, University of Florida Health – Jacksonville, Jacksonville, FL, USA

Christine Tompkins, MD Division of Cardiology, University of Rochester Medical Center, Rochester, NY, USA

Gladys P. Velarde, MD, FACC Division of Cardiology, University of Florida
Health Cardiology Center – Jacksonville, University of Florida College
of Medicine-Jacksonville, Jacksonville, FL, USA

Karolina M. Zareba, MD Division of Cardiology, University of Pittsburgh
Medical Center, Pittsburgh, PA, USA

Magdelena A. Zeglin-Sawczuk, MD Division of Cardiology,
University of Vermont College of Medicine, Burlington, VT, USA

Part I
Epidemiology, Classification, Guidelines

Chapter 1
Cardiovascular Disease in Women: Epidemiology of Cardiovascular Disease in Women- Sex Differences in Disease Incidence and Prevalence. Population Representation, Diversity, Disparities

Saadia Sherazi and Susan G. Fisher

Introduction

Cardiovascular disease (CVD) is the leading cause of death in both men and women in the United States and most other developed countries. While the magnitude of disease risk varies among individuals based on demographic as well as biopsychosocial factors, the entire U.S. population is vulnerable to CVD. Cardiovascular disease is associated with significant health and economic burden with estimated direct and indirect cost of $312.6 billion [1]. There are more women than men who die each year of CVD. In 2009, CVD claimed the lives of 401,495 (51.0 %) women and 386,436 (49.0 %) men [1]. Despite increases in awareness over the past decade, only 54 % of women recognize that heart disease is their number 1 killer [2]. The lifetime risk of a woman developing CVD by age 50 is estimated to be 39 % [3]. Although the number of men and women who die from CVD has decreased over the past several decades, this decline is less remarkable for women as shown in Fig. 1.1. Advances in medical treatment, application of evidence-based therapies for established CVD and the modification of coronary risk factors are major contributors to this decline in mortality. Nonetheless, since 1984, more women die from CVD annually than men; coronary deaths in women exceed deaths in women from all forms of cancer combined [4].

While the mortality disparity between women and men is decreasing, significant differences still exist among certain ethnic and racial groups [5]. Cardiovascular disease is a significant problem among minority women. It ranks as the number one

S. Sherazi, MD, MS
Heart Research Follow up Program, University of Rochester Medical Center, Rochester, NY, USA

S.G. Fisher, MS, PhD (✉)
Department of Clinical Sciences, Temple University School of Medicine, Philadelphia, PA, USA
e-mail: susan.fisher@tuhs.temple.edu

H.Z. Mieszczanska, G.P. Velarde (eds.),
Management of Cardiovascular Disease in Women,
DOI 10.1007/978-1-4471-5517-1_1, © Springer-Verlag London 2014

3

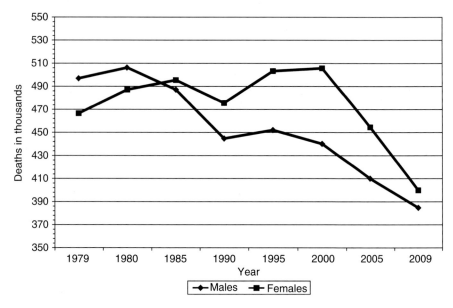

Fig. 1.1 Cardiovascular disease mortality trends for males and females (United States: 1979–2009). CVD excludes congenital cardiovascular defects (*International Classification of Diseases, 10th Revision* codes I00–I99). The overall comparability for cardiovascular disease between the *International Classification of Diseases, 9th Revision* (1979–1998) and *International Classification of Diseases, 10th Revision* (1999–2009) is 0.9962. No comparability ratios were applied (*Source*: National Center for Health Statistics [1])

cause of death for both African American and white women in the United States. Among Hispanic women, heart disease and cancer cause roughly the same number of deaths each year. For American Indian or Alaska Native and Asian or Pacific Islander women, heart disease is second only to cancer [6]. In 2009, six million, (one of every six) hospital stays were attributable to CVD (Agency for Healthcare Research and Quality, Nationwide Inpatient Sample) accounting for $71.2 billion in total inpatient hospital cost [1] (In 2003, 48.3 % of inpatient hospital stays for CVD was for women.). Although only 40 % of hospital stays for acute myocardial infarction (MI) and coronary artery disease (CAD) were for women, more than half of all stays for nonspecific chest pain, congestive heart failure, and stroke were for women. There was no difference between men and women in hospitalizations for cardiac dysrhythmias [7]. CVD is a major health problem in women that necessitates a strong emphasis on prevention to reduce the burden of CVD morbidity and mortality in our society. This chapter will discuss the epidemiology of CVD (incidence, prevalence and risk factors) in women, including coronary heart disease, congestive heart failure and stroke. We hope to highlight significant gender differences and provide greater appreciation of the influence of gender on cardiovascular risk and management.

Table 1.1 Prevalence of cardiovascular disease by race/ethnic background in men and women

Ethnic/racial background	Prevalence in 2010 in ≥20 years age (men) (%)	Prevalence in 2010 in ≥20 years age (women) (%)
NH White	36.6	32.4
NH Black	44.4	48.9
Mexican American	33.4	30.7

Abbreviations: NH Non-hispanic

Epidemiology of Cardiovascular Diseases

In the past, most epidemiological studies and major clinical trials which described the risk factors and natural disease history of CVD were conducted in racially homogenous cohorts (predominantly white). The generalizability of these findings to a more racially diverse population has been questioned. Current data support that the distribution of CVD risks and manifestations vary among ethnic/racial subgroups. CVD mortality and morbidity burden is tremendous, making it imperative to recognize these varied risks and disease presentations among diverse populations. It is most relevant in the U.S with rapidly changing demographics. Currently blacks make up 14 % of the total population and Hispanics account for 16 % of the total population. The number of Asians now residing in the U.S. is also increasing. Statistics from 2010 indicate that there are 42,900,000 (34.0 %) women and 40,700,000 (36.7 %) men who currently suffer from CVD in the U.S. [1]. As shown in Table 1.1 the prevalence of CVD varies by race/ethnic background. For both males and females the CVD prevalence rates are higher among Blacks than Whites. The risk of CVD increases among both males and females with age. Although there is a smaller proportion of females with CVD compared with males in those less than 60 years old and a similar proportion in those between 60 and 79 years, among the elderly (80 years and older) women have a higher prevalence of CVD as compared to men [1].

Coronary Artery Disease

Coronary artery disease (CAD) is one of the most common types of heart disease, killing more than 385,000 people annually including 176,255 (45.6 %) women. Overall CAD is less prevalent among women as compared with men 6,600,000 (5.1 %) and 8,800,000 (7.9 %) respectively. About 5.8 % of all white women, 7.6 % of black women, and 5.6 % of Mexican American women have CAD [8]. Most importantly almost two-thirds (64 %) of women who die suddenly of coronary heart disease have no previous symptoms [8]. Relatively younger women (women <50 years of age) are at highest risk for adverse outcomes related to myocardial infarction; with twofold higher risk of mortality when compared with men

(<50 years old) [9]. Women are reported to have higher frequency of angina, more office visits, more hospitalizations, increased myocardial infarction mortality, and increased heart failure compared to men [10].

Congestive Heart Failure

Over five million Americans are currently affected by congestive heart failure (CHF). While approximately 50 % of these are women, the prevalence rate is higher among men as compared with women 2,700,000 (2.5 %) and 2,400,000 (1.8 %) respectively [1]. CHF is associated with significant mortality and morbidity. Each year over 50,0000 individuals are newly diagnosed with CHF. Only slightly fewer are women (n = 320,000) than men (n = 350 000) [1]. Despite advances in medical treatments and improved prognosis CHF is associated with significant mortality, specifically 32,847 (58.2 %) women and 23,563 (41.8 %) men died due to CHF in 2009 (for all age groups). CHF is also a leading cause of hospital admissions, accounting for 522,000 hospital discharges in women and 501,000 in men. Though systolic heart failure is more prevalent in men, diastolic heart failure is much more prevalent in women and has higher mortality and morbidity in women [1].

Stroke

Stroke is a devastating, disabling illness with a huge impact on mortality, morbidity and quality of life. Stroke is associated with significantly higher mortality among women (n = 76,769; 59.6 %) when compared with men (n = 52,073; 40.4 %) [1]. This could be due to decreased diagnosis, and/or under-treatment of hypertension, hyperlipidemia, and atrial fibrillation. Over six million American 20 years of age or older currently suffer from stroke with a higher prevalence among women as compared with men. Data from 2010 indicate that among adults the prevalence of stroke for both sexes is 6,800,000 (2.8 % of US population), with higher prevalence among women 3,800,000 (3.0 %) when compared with men 3,000,000 (2.6 %) [1]. There is also a racial/ethnic variation in the prevalence of stroke within women with the highest prevalence among NH-AA (4.7 %), followed by NH-White females (2.9 %) and Mexican American females (1.4 %) [1].

Behavioral and Health Related Risk Factors

Men and women share similar CVD risk factors such as age, dyslipidemia, hypertension, smoking, obesity, diabetes and physical inactivity. Furthermore, women have additional risk factors, such as the use of contraceptives and the reduction of ovarian function with age. Although the classic risk factors for CVD are similar among women and men, differences exist in the importance and relative weighting of these risk factors. The Atherosclerosis Risk in Communities (ARIC) study examined more than 14,000 subjects, and demonstrated that >90 % of CVD events in blacks appeared to be explained by increased or borderline CVD risk factors as compared with 70 % of such events in white subjects. These findings suggest that higher CVD events in blacks result from increased risk factors thereby underscoring the importance of early detection and prevention of CVD risk factors [11]. A history of premature CVD in a family member has also been shown to increase the risk of CVD in both men [12] and women [13]. There has been an overall decline in death associated with CVD in women (23 % decrease since 2000) which is largely attributable to life style modification such as tobacco cessation, increased physical activity or use of medications to treat hypertension/high cholesterol [14]. Following is a brief discussion of key CVD risk factors with a specific focus on differences by gender, race and ethnicity:

Smoking

Smoking is a well established risk factor for developing sudden cardiac death, angina, myocardial infarction, peripheral vascular disease and stroke [15].

There are 81.7 % women who are current non-smokers as compared with 75.7 % of men who are reported to be non-smokers [1]. At younger ages (<50 years) smoking has more harmful effects in women than in men, with a larger negative impact of the total number of cigarettes smoked per day [16, 17]. A meta-analysis comparing pooled data of approximately 2.4 million smokers and nonsmokers found the relative risk ratio of smokers to nonsmokers for developing coronary heart disease was 25 % higher in women than in men [18].

The prevalence of smoking varies among women from different racial ethnic groups. In 2008–2010, Asian women (5.5 %) and Hispanic women (9.6 %) were less likely to be current cigarette smokers than non-Hispanic black women (17.6 %), non-Hispanic white women (20.9 %), and American Indian or Alaska Native women (20.7 %) [1].

The tobacco use has decreased in adults since year 2000, from 23.1 to 19.7 %, an overall decrease of 3.4 percentage points (3.2 percentage points among men and 3.6 percentage points among women) [14]. Smoking cessation has significant impact on the overall decline in the CVD mortality since 1950's and quitting smoking is associated with reduced risk of total mortality (pooled crude RR 0.64) [19].

Hypertension

There is higher number of men than women with high blood pressure until age 45–54 years. The numbers are similar for men and women with hypertension from ages 55–64, however, among those 65 years of age and older, women are much more likely than men to have hypertension [1]. The prevalence of HTN is highest among women from non-Hispanic blacks background (47 %) followed by non-Hispanic Whites (30.7 %) and Mexican Americans 28.8 %. The proportions for men are as follows: non-Hispanic whites, 33.4 % of men, non-Hispanic blacks, 42.6, Mexican Americans, 30.1 % [1]. Hypertension is one of the modifiable CVD risk factors that contribute towards most CVD deaths in women. There has been a significant decline in stroke related deaths in women since 1996 and improvement in the treatment for hypertension has been a major positive impact on stroke related mortality [20].

High Cholesterol

According to Adult Treatment Panel III, LDL <100 is considered optimal, while 100–129 near optimal, 130–159 borderline high, 160–189 high, and >190 very high. Total cholesterol of <200 is desirable, 200–239 borderline high, and >240 high. An HDL cholesterol <40 is considered low. Women tend to have lower total and LDL cholesterol as compared with men during their pre-menopause years. However, during menopause lipid profile changes lead to an increase in total cholesterol and LDL by 10 and 14 % respectively. The apolipoprotein (a) also increases by 4–8 % while HDL remains the same [21]. Over the past decade, treatment of high cholesterol improved in both primary and secondary prevention of CVD. In women age 45–65 years, the use of statins increased from 1.9 to 13.5 % and in women older than 65 the use increased from 3.5 to 32.8 % (2000–2010). Among men age 45–65 years, statin use increased from 2.5 to 16.8 % and in men older than 65 the use increased from 1.9 to 38.9 %. Despite increases in the statin use among women, a disparity of statin use persists between genders [14].

Obesity

Obesity is an independent risk factor for CVD, and is associated with significant mortality, morbidity and health cost. Obesity exists with other co-morbid conditions including diabetes mellitus, hypertension, coronary artery disease, sleep apnea and certain cancers.

Both obesity and diabetes are increasing at an alarming rate in women in the western societies. The rise in the rates of obesity and diabetes vary significantly by ethnic/racial backgrounds and socioeconomic status [22]. Overall, blacks have the highest prevalence of obesity in the United States followed by Hispanics, and then Whites. According to 2006–2008 statistics from the Centers for Disease Control (CDC), 21.8 % of NH-white women, 39.2 % of NH-black women, and 29.4 % of Hispanic women were obese (body mass index, $\geq$30 kg/m^2) [23]. The most dramatic rise in obesity rates is observed in women whose income is at 200 % of the poverty line

(3.6 % increases in obesity). The rise in obesity rate is 0.3 and 1.8 % in women with income just below and at 100–199 % of the poverty line [14]. At least three reasons may account for the racial and ethnic differences in obesity. First, racial and ethnic groups differ in behaviors that contribute to weight gain; secondly differences exist in individual attitudes and cultural norms related to body weight across racial/ethnic groups. Thirdly, at the population level there are clear ethnic/racial differences in access to affordable, healthful foods and safe locations to be physically active; this limited access may negatively impact diet and physical activity levels [23].

Diabetes Mellitus

Diabetes mellitus is considered a coronary artery equivalent. The prevalence of physician diagnosed cases of diabetes in adults >20 years of age was reported to be 19,700,000 (8.3 %) [1]. Out of these, 9,600,000 (8.7 %) were men and 10,100,000 (7.9 %) were women. Non-Hispanic black females account for 15.4 % of these cases, followed by 13.5 % among Non-Hispanic black men. This is followed by Mexican American women (12.0 %) and Mexican American men (11.4 %) [1]. The prevalence is lower among whites with men making up 7.2 % while women make up 6.2 % of the diabetic population [1]. In addition, black diabetics are more likely to suffer complications from diabetes, such as end-stage renal disease and lower extremity amputations.

Physical Inactivity

Physical inactivity is responsible for 12.2 % of the global burden of MI after accounting for other CVD risk factors such as cigarette smoking, DM, hypertension, abdominal obesity, lipid profile, and psychosocial factors [24]. Between National Health and Nutrition Examination (NHANES) 1988–1994 and NHANES 2001–2006, the non–age-adjusted proportion of adults who engaged in >12 sessions of physical activity per month declined from 57.0 to 43.3 % in men and from 49.0 to 43.3 % in women [25]. Physical inactivity is reported to be higher among women than men (33.2 % versus 29.9 %) [1]. However women are more likely to maintain a healthy weight than men (45.1 vs. 31.7 %). In a meta-analysis of longitudinal studies among women, relative risks (RRs) of incident CHD were 0.83 (95 % CI, 0.69–0.99), 0.77 (95 % CI, 0.64–0.92), 0.72 (95 % CI, 0.59–0.87), and 0.57 (95 % CI, 0.41–0.79) across increasing quintiles of physical activity compared with the lowest quintile [26].

In the Health Professionals Follow-Up Study, for every 3-h-per-week increase in vigorous-intensity activity, adjusted RR of MI was 0.78 (95 % CI, 0.61–0.98) for men. This 22 % reduction of risk can be explained in part by beneficial effects of physical activity on HDL cholesterol, vitamin D, apolipoprotein B, and HbA1c [27].

Summary and Conclusions

There could be several reasons for these observed differences in the cardiovascular care and outcomes. Factors leading towards higher CVD mortality among women are the differences in the risk factor profile among men and women. For example hypertension and diabetes are more prevalent among women, where as coronary artery disease is more prevalent among men. Although women have higher prevalence of angina when compared with men, they have lower prevalence of significant obstructive coronary artery disease. It is also noted in literature that among women who may be older, have higher risk factor burden yet have less significant obstructive CAD when compared with their male counterparts [10]. Despite less significant obstructive coronary artery disease women still face higher mortality and worse prognosis when compared with men.

Other factors include less representation of women particularly minority women in clinical trials with impact on the advances in treatment and management in the field of cardiovascular medicine for women. In typical CVD trial, 85 % of the study participants are men [28]. Women who do participate are predominantly postmenopausal.

Although overtime the enrollment of women in randomized clinical trials has increased, it continues to be low with regards to their relative representation in disease population. Overall the representation of women is reported to be highest among trials in hypertension (44 %), diabetes (40 %), and stroke (38 %) and lowest for heart failure (29 %), coronary artery disease (25 %), and hyperlipidemia (28 %). This is in contrast to the higher and rising prevalence of these diseases among women [29]. Therefore, we have typically relied on the sub-group and meta-analyses of clinical trials (which are underpowered to answer these questions) to better understand the influence of gender on outcomes such as mortality, morbidity and quality of life. For example, the results of Multicenter Automatic Defibrillator Implantation Trial with Cardiac Resynchronization Therapy (MADIT-CRT) showed that women obtain significantly greater reduction in death and heart failure with cardiac resynchronization therapy (CRT) than men [30]. CRT was also associated with greater echocardiographic evidence of cardiac remodelling in women than men. There were only 453 women (25 %) out of 1,820 study patients. Benefit from other life saving treatment in women might not be seen in other studies due to under representation of women in most of the major trials. Further trials with appropriate female representation are needed to better understand the epidemiology of CVD and treatment strategies.

References

1. Go AS, Mozaffarian D, Roger VL, Benjamin EJ, Berry JD, Borden WB, Bravata DM, Dai S, Ford ES, Fox CS, Franco S, Fullerton HJ, Gillespie C, Hailpern SM, Heit JA, Howard VJ, Huffman MD, Kissela BM, Kittner SJ, Lackland DT, Lichtman JH, Lisabeth LD, Magid D,

Marcus GM, Marelli A, Matchar DB, McGuire DK, Mohler ER, Moy CS, Mussolino ME, Nichol G, Paynter NP, Schreiner PJ, Sorlie PD, Stein J, Turan TN, Virani SS, Wong ND, Woo D, Turner MB, on behalf of the American Heart Association Statistics Committee and Stroke Statistics Subcommittee. Executive summary: heart disease and stroke statistics–2013 update: a report from the American Heart Association. Circulation. 2013;127:143–52.

2. Mosca L, Mochari-Greenberger H, Dolor RJ, Newby LK, Robb KJ. Twelve-year follow-up of American women's awareness of cardiovascular disease risk and barriers to heart health. Circ Cardiovasc Qual Outcomes. 2010;3:120–7.

3. D'Agostino RBS, Vasan RS, Pencina MJ, Wolf PA, Cobain M, Massaro JM, Kannel WB. General cardiovascular risk profile for use in primary care: the Framingham Heart Study. Circulation. 2008;117:743–53.

4. Wenger NK. Women and coronary heart disease: a century after Herrick: understudied, underdiagnosed, and undertreated. Circulation. 2012;126:604–11.

5. Mensah GA, Mokdad AH, Ford ES, Greenlund KJ, Croft JB. State of disparities in cardiovascular health in the United States. Circulation. 2005;111:1233–41.

6. Heron M. Deaths: leading causes for 2008. Natl Vital Stat Rep. 2012;60:1–94.

7. Elixhauser A, Jiang HJ. Hospitalizations for women with circulatory disease, 2003: statistical brief #5. In: Anonymous Healthcare Cost and Utilization Project (HCUP) statistical briefs, Rockville; 2006.

8. Roger VL, Go AS, Lloyd-Jones DM, Benjamin EJ, Berry JD, Borden WB, Bravata DM, Dai S, Ford ES, Fox CS, Fullerton HJ, Gillespie C, Hailpern SM, Heit JA, Howard VJ, Kissela BM, Kittner SJ, Lackland DT, Lichtman JH, Lisabeth LD, Makuc DM, Marcus GM, Marelli A, Matchar DB, Moy CS, Mozaffarian D, Mussolino ME, Nichol G, Paynter NP, Soliman EZ, Sorlie PD, Sotoodehnia N, Turan TN, Virani SS, Wong ND, Woo D, Turner MB, American Heart Association Statistics Committee and Stroke Statistics Subcommittee. Executive summary: heart disease and stroke statistics–2012 update: a report from the American Heart Association. Circulation. 2012;125:188–97.

9. Bairey Merz CN, Shaw LJ, Reis SE, Bittner V, Kelsey SF, Olson M, Johnson BD, Pepine CJ, Mankad S, Sharaf BL, Rogers WJ, Pohost GM, Lerman A, Quyyumi AA, Sopko G, WISE Investigators. Insights from the NHLBI-Sponsored Women's Ischemia Syndrome Evaluation (WISE) Study: Part II: gender differences in presentation, diagnosis, and outcome with regard to gender-based pathophysiology of atherosclerosis and macrovascular and microvascular coronary disease. J Am Coll Cardiol. 2006;47:S21–9.

10. Shaw LJ, Bairey Merz CN, Pepine CJ, Reis SE, Bittner V, Kelsey SF, Olson M, Johnson BD, Mankad S, Sharaf BL, Rogers WJ, Wessel TR, Arant CB, Pohost GM, Lerman A, Quyyumi AA, Sopko G, WISE Investigators. Insights from the NHLBI-sponsored Women's ischemia syndrome evaluation (WISE) study: part I: gender differences in traditional and novel risk factors, symptom evaluation, and gender-optimized diagnostic strategies. J Am Coll Cardiol. 2006;47:S4–20.

11. Hozawa A, Folsom AR, Sharrett AR, Chambless LE. Absolute and attributable risks of cardiovascular disease incidence in relation to optimal and borderline risk factors: comparison of African American with white subjects–Atherosclerosis Risk in Communities Study. Arch Intern Med. 2007;167:573–9.

12. Assmann G, Cullen P, Schulte H. Simple scoring scheme for calculating the risk of acute coronary events based on the 10-year follow-up of the prospective cardiovascular Munster (PROCAM) study. Circulation. 2002;105:310–5.

13. Ridker PM, Buring JE, Rifai N, Cook NR. Development and validation of improved algorithms for the assessment of global cardiovascular risk in women: the Reynolds Risk Score. JAMA. 2007;297:611–9.

14. Brown JR, O'Connor GT. Coronary heart disease and prevention in the United States. N Engl J Med. 2010;362:2150–3.

15. Ludvig J, Miner B, Eisenberg MJ. Smoking cessation in patients with coronary artery disease. Am Heart J. 2005;149:565–72.

16. Prescott E, Hippe M, Schnohr P, Hein HO, Vestbo J. Smoking and risk of myocardial infarction in women and men: longitudinal population study. BMJ. 1998;316:1043–7.
17. Grundtvig M, Hagen TP, German M, Reikvam A. Sex-based differences in premature first myocardial infarction caused by smoking: twice as many years lost by women as by men. Eur J Cardiovasc Prev Rehabil. 2009;16:174–9.
18. Huxley RR, Woodward M. Cigarette smoking as a risk factor for coronary heart disease in women compared with men: a systematic review and meta-analysis of prospective cohort studies. Lancet. 2011;378:1297–305.
19. Critchley JA, Capewell S. Mortality risk reduction associated with smoking cessation in patients with coronary heart disease: a systematic review. JAMA. 2003;290:86–97.
20. Lloyd-Jones D, Adams R, Carnethon M, De Simone G, Ferguson TB, Flegal K, Ford E, Furie K, Go A, Greenlund K, Haase N, Hailpern S, Ho M, Howard V, Kissela B, Kittner S, Lackland D, Lisabeth L, Marelli A, McDermott M, Meigs J, Mozaffarian D, Nichol G, O'Donnell C, Roger V, Rosamond W, Sacco R, Sorlie P, Stafford R, Steinberger J, Thom T, Wasserthiel-Smoller S, Wong N, Wylie-Rosett J, Hong Y, American Heart Association Statistics Committee and Stroke Statistics Subcommittee. Heart disease and stroke statistics–2009 update: a report from the American Heart Association Statistics Committee and Stroke Statistics Subcommittee. Circulation. 2009;119:480–6.
21. Maas AH, Appelman YE. Gender differences in coronary heart disease. Neth Heart J. 2010;18:598–603.
22. Coulter SA. Epidemiology of cardiovascular disease in women: risk, advances, and alarms. Tex Heart Inst J. 2011;38:145–7.
23. Centers for Disease Control and Prevention (CDC). Differences in prevalence of obesity among black, white, and Hispanic adults – United States, 2006–2008. MMWR Morb Mortal Wkly Rep. 2009;58:740–4.
24. Yusuf S, Hawken S, Ounpuu S, Dans T, Avezum A, Lanas F, McQueen M, Budaj A, Pais P, Varigos J, Lisheng L, INTERHEART Study Investigators. Effect of potentially modifiable risk factors associated with myocardial infarction in 52 countries (the INTERHEART study): case–control study. Lancet. 2004;364:937–52.
25. King DE, Mainous 3rd AG, Carnemolla M, Everett CJ. Adherence to healthy lifestyle habits in US adults, 1988–2006. Am J Med. 2009;122:528–34.
26. Schoenborn CA, Stommel M. Adherence to the 2008 adult physical activity guidelines and mortality risk. Am J Prev Med. 2011;40:514–21.
27. Chomistek AK, Chiuve SE, Jensen MK, Cook NR, Rimm EB. Vigorous physical activity, mediating biomarkers, and risk of myocardial infarction. Med Sci Sports Exerc. 2011;43:1884–90.
28. Dougherty AH. Gender balance in cardiovascular research: importance to women's health. Tex Heart Inst J. 2011;38:148–50.
29. Melloni C, Berger JS, Wang TY, Gunes F, Stebbins A, Pieper KS, Dolor RJ, Douglas PS, Mark DB, Newby LK. Representation of women in randomized clinical trials of cardiovascular disease prevention. Circ Cardiovasc Qual Outcomes. 2010;3:135–42.
30. Moss AJ, Hall WJ, Cannom DS, Klein H, Brown MW, Daubert JP, Estes 3rd NA, Foster E, Greenberg H, Higgins SL, Pfeffer MA, Solomon SD, Wilber D, Zareba W, MADIT-CRT Trial Investigators. Cardiac-resynchronization therapy for the prevention of heart-failure events. N Engl J Med. 2009;361:1329–38.

Chapter 2
Classification of Cardiovascular Disease Risk and Cardiovascular Disease Prevention in Women

Rebecca Lewandowski and Catherine Gracey

Overview

In 1948, the USA Public Health Service initiated the Framingham Heart Study to assess the epidemiology and risk factors for cardiovascular disease (CVD). It was the first such study of its kind—a well-constructed and longitudinally observed cohort. Men and women between the ages of 30 and 62 (5,209 individuals in total), free of CVD, were recruited from Framingham, MA beginning in 1948. Publications from the late 1950s and early 1960s associated with the Framingham Heart Study became some of the first publications to use of the term "risk factor." The term was thus broadly coined and accepted, used today as generalized patterns that suggest a predilection to developing heart disease. Analyses looked at patterns of elevated cholesterol, higher levels of blood pressure, and cigarette smoking and found that these identified elements combined to increase one's risk of developing coronary heart disease (CHD) over 6 years of follow up [1].

From these data from the Framingham Study, investigators were able to generate risk equations that linked common risk factors to CHD, stroke, and overall fatal and nonfatal cardiovascular disease. These equations and publications subsequently led to improved worldwide screening techniques that have served as the foundation for many of the clinical cardiovascular guidelines [2].

More recent publications from the Framingham Study have looked at the evolution of cardiovascular disease (CVD) over the last five decades in a general population sample of men and women. What continue to emerge from this study are the

R. Lewandowski, MD, PhD
Division of Cardiology, Department of Medicine,
University of Rochester Medical Center, University of Rochester, Rochester, NY, USA

C. Gracey, MD (✉)
Department of Medicine,
University of Rochester Medical Center, University of Rochester, Rochester, NY, USA
e-mail: catherine_gracey@urmc.rochester.edu

H.Z. Mieszczanska, G.P. Velarde (eds.),
Management of Cardiovascular Disease in Women,
DOI 10.1007/978-1-4471-5517-1_2, © Springer-Verlag London 2014

CVD differences between men and women: in prevalence, incidence, prognosis, and predisposing risk factors. For example, women tend to lag by 10–20 years behind men in CVD incidence. Women also tend to outlive men, and experience fewer atherosclerotic CVD events. Despite the differences, data from the Framingham cohort show that CVD has now become the leading cause of death in women, as well as men. Based on data from the Framingham study comparing the lifetime risk of coronary heart disease (CHD) with that of breast cancer, women are three times more likely to have a CHD event than breast cancer (24–32 % versus 7–12.5 % respectively). Conclusions to be drawn from this include the concept that CVD is a formidable health concern for women; one that warrants aggressive preventive measures for women of all ages. Epidemiology of hypertensive or atherosclerotic disease was not well-characterized prior to the Framingham study [3].

Both gender and age play a strong role in the lifetime risk of CHD. When compared side-by-side, the lifetime risk for CHD was lower for women in each age group when compared to men. And the overall lifetime risk for developing CHD is approximately 40 % in men, and 30 % in women. To put this in perspective, the overall lifetime risk that a woman develops breast cancer is much lower, at approximately 10 % (see Fig. 2.1) [4].

Despite the fact that CVD is the leading cause of mortality in women, women have largely been underrepresented in randomized control trials (RCT) that form the basis for our current standards of care. The 2007 guidelines for CVD prevention in women, for example, were based largely on RCT, which on average, were made up of 70 % male enrollment. This demonstrates an obvious disadvantage of sex-specific analyses, resulting in lack of public and professional awareness of female-specific coronary risk. Sex-specific knowledge gaps that currently exist include women's symptom presentation, optimal screening techniques, and diagnostic procedures. By default, through lack of representation, women are thus treated largely based on male-dominant RCTs. Women enrollment in RCTs does continue to increase (notably, from 9 %

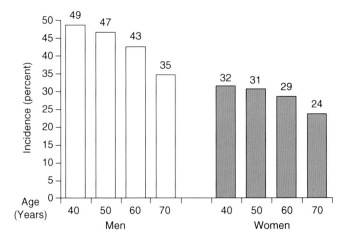

Fig. 2.1 The lifetime risk of hard coronary disease events, excluding angina pectoris (i.e., coronary insufficiency, myocardial infarction and coronary death) for men and women aged 40–60 years (Reprinted from Lloyd-Jones et al. [4], p. 80–92, with permission from Elsevier)

in 1970 to 41 % in 2006), but remains relatively low when compared to the overall prevalence of disease in women. And it is not just enrollment—A study by Melloni et al. showed that sex-specific results were discussed in only 31 % of primary trial publications. Ongoing efforts are needed to improve female representation so that sex-specific, evidenced-based recommendations may be determined [5].

In 1999, the American Heart Association (AHA) published the first women-specific clinical recommendations for the prevention of cardiovascular disease (CVD) [6]. Over the ensuing years, there has been significant progress in the awareness, treatment, and prevention of CVD in women. Part of that progress has been in the increasing awareness, on the part of both providers and patients, that heart disease is not exclusive to men. While there has been improvement, there are still a disproportionate number of women who do not identify CVD as their major health concern (despite the fact that over six million women in the US have known CVD). Sadly, women in the highest risk populations (women of racial and ethnic minorities) demonstrate the most persistent lack of awareness. Lack of awareness is not exclusive to the patient population—physicians and health care providers continue to underestimate cardiovascular risk in women. This erroneous calculation has been shown to correlate with suboptimal application of interventions for cardiovascular prevention. There has been increasing public awareness, however, with which there has been a 30 % decline in CVD-related mortality burden among women [7]. Indeed, the Nurses' Health study, a large study that included 85,941 women, looked at the trends in the incidence of coronary heart disease and changes in diet and lifestyle in women. Using the incidence of coronary disease in women over a 2-year period as a primary outcome, the study found that disease prevalence declined by 31 % with associated risk factor modification (including reduction in smoking, improvement in diet, and an increase in postmenopausal hormone use) [8, 9].

Public awareness efforts including the AHA "Go Red for Women" and the National Heart, Lung, and Blood Institute's "Heart Truth" campaigns have helped increase awareness that CVD is the leading cause of death among US women [10]. The 2011 AHA publication of "Effectiveness-Based Guidelines for the Prevention of Cardiovascular Disease in Women" advances understanding of the most clinically effective approaches to prevention and treatment [10]. The purpose of this chapter is to review the updated guidelines on the prevention of heart disease in women, including discussion of common risk factors, risk assessment of CVD in women, and interventions regarding lifestyle, major risk factors, and preventive medications, including the use of statins. Interventions which are not useful, or which may be harmful will also be discussed.

Definitions, Terms, and Classifications

Cardiovascular Disease (CVD)/Heart Disease (HD)

For the sake of this chapter, and as often found throughout the literature, "heart disease" and "cardiovascular disease" are often used interchangeably. Either term describes a broad range of diseases that affect the heart, including: heart rhythm problems (arrhythmias), diseases of the blood vessels, such as peripheral vascular disease, renal-vascular disease and coronary artery disease; heart infections; and congenital heart defects. Both terms also generally refer to conditions that involve narrowed or blocked blood vessels that can lead to a heart attack, chest pain (angina) or stroke. Conditions that affect the heart's muscle, heart valves or cardiac rhythm, and infections are also considered forms of heart disease [11].

Coronary Artery Disease (CAD)

when the major blood vessels that supply the heart with blood, oxygen and nutrients become damaged or diseased. Cholesterol-containing deposits (plaque) within the arteries are the main cause of coronary artery disease [12].

Relative Risk (RR)

Ratio of the likelihood of an event in persons with the risk factor versus in those without.

NCEP ATP3 Guidelines

The National Cholesterol Education Program Adult Treatment Panel III Guidelines, updated in 2004, are used to define cardiovascular risk and determine goals for lipids [13, 14].

Primary Prevention of Cardiovascular Disease: Effectiveness –Based Guidelines for the Prevention of Cardiovascular Disease in Women- 2011 Update

Risk Factors

The goal of primary prevention of cardiovascular disease is to deter the clinical presentation of symptomatic disease and prevent major cardiac adverse events in currently asymptomatic individuals [13]. To do this, one needs to prevent and optimize modifiable risk factors. "Risk factors" are just that-habits or traits that increase the risk of experiencing unwanted occurrences, such as cardiovascular disease. There have been nearly 200 risk factors and risky behaviors identified that increase a woman's risk of cardiovascular disease. While some, like genetics, are not modifiable, it is important to focus on those we can improve. Traditional major risk factors include hypertension, diabetes, dyslipidemia, male gender, cigarette smoking, age, and a family history of CVD [13, 14]. Male gender and family history are obviously not modifiable, but aggressive efforts to control other risk factors are critical in prevention of CVD. One large international case–control study—the INTERHEART study of acute myocardial infarction (AMI)—looked at risk estimates associated with traditional cardiovascular risk factors. They found that these risk factors are overall similar between men and women across various regions of the world; however, women had an increased risk associated with hypertension and diabetes. The study also showed that exercise and alcohol appeared to play a larger protective role in women than in men [8].

Age, Gender, and Hormones

The average age at which women develop CVD is roughly 10 years after the average age of men, in large part due to sex hormones. This has likely contributed to the misconception that women are less vulnerable to CVD. Sex hormones play a major role in the pathophysiology of cardiovascular disorders, and once post-menopausal females lose the protective benefits of estrogen, their risk of CVD is equal to that of men [15]. Estrogen is thought to play several roles in the pathophysiology and manifestations of heart disease in women. Estrogens are believed to be protective to coronary vessels by providing improved vascular tone. Experimental studies have shown that estrogens can adjust the response of vessels to various vasoactive substances, including angiotensin II, norepinephrine, and aldosterone, thereby preventing the same degree of vasoconstriction seen in men [16, 17]. Additionally, estrogen can increase the production or release of relaxing factors from the endothelium, thus improving endothelial function [18]. Estrogen can also improve a woman's lipid profile by reducing low-density lipoprotein cholesterol and increasing high-density cholesterol [19]. Women may have different clinical symptoms of ischemia because of two different mechanisms of estrogens: (1) they may directly alter pain perception in women, and (2) they may play a direct anti-anginal role by reducing the pain-producing effects of adenosine that cause the classic ischemic-like chest pain [20, 21]. In addition to the increased risk of CVD which comes with post-menopausal changes in sex hormone levels, increased age is also associated with a higher incidence of diabetes, hypertension, obesity, and other co-morbidities which also increase risk of CVD. Despite all of the previously noted benefits of estrogen for CVD prevention in women, not all estrogen is created equal. Specifically, exogenous estrogen in post-menopausal women has shown to be in fact even harmful. In fact, two studies in particular—the Heart and Estrogen/Progestin Replacement Study (HERS), and the Women's Health Initiative (WHI)—did not support the beneficial effects of hormone therapy in post-menopausal women (in either secondary or primary cardiovascular prevention). The WHI trial was actually terminated early after finding a small but significant increase in cardiovascular events and other adverse outcomes in the hormone therapy group [8, 22, 23].

Smoking

Tobacco use unfortunately continues to be the leading preventable risk factor for CHD in women, that has yet to be extinguished. Over the past 50 years, the risk of death from cigarette smoking continues to increase among women and the increased risk of death from all causes (lung cancer, COPD, any type of stroke, CVD, and all others) is now nearly identical for men and women, when compared to those who have not smoked [24]. Smoking has been associated with one-half of all coronary events in women. The meta-analysis by Rachel Huxley and Mark Woodward showed, that smoking confers a 25 % greater relative risk of coronary heart disease in women than in men [25]. The risk of death from ischemic heart disease in cigarette smokers is the same in men and women, almost three times higher than in those who have not smoked. A critical point to remember is that quitting smoking dramatically reduces mortality from all major smoking-related disease and it is never too late to quit. Early tobacco cessation is also important, as smoking cessation before 40 years of age reduces smoking-associated mortality by 90 % [26]. Another important point to recognize is that smokers on oral contraceptives are at even further increased risk of CHD. And while the prevalence of male smokers continues to be slightly higher than female smokers, there is smaller decline in tobacco use among women [27].

Hypertension

For both women and men, hypertension has been identified as a major cause of CVD [8]. With increasing age, there is progressive loss of arterial compliance, resulting in increasing overall prevalence of hypertension. Approximately 18 % of women are hypertensive prior to the age of 45, while nearly 80 % of elderly women are hypertensive (as compared to 25 % of men prior to the age of 45, and 72 % of men over 75) [7]. And in older women, the most common form of hypertension is actually isolated systolic hypertension. HTN is particularly prevalent among black women. Not only is there a disparity in the incidence of hypertension between men and women; there are also differences in the role that hemodynamic characteristics play in the pathology of hypertension and target end organ damage between men and women. In one study looking at 100 men and 100 women with similar rates of mild-to-moderate hypertension (also matched to equivalent age and race), hemodynamic differences were observed [28]. Men were on average found to have lower resting heart rates, longer left ventricular ejection fraction (LVEF) time, lower pulse pressures, and greater stress-induced rises in blood pressure and pulse pressure. Women on the other hand, were found to have lower total peripheral resistance, decreased blood volumes, and stress-responses related to hormonal status (the higher the estrogen activity, the less arterial pressure increased with mental stress) [28]. Also, in women taking oral contraceptives (especially those who are older, and with concomitant obesity), hypertension has been found to be two to three times more common than in women who are not on them [8].

Dyslipidemia

Another well-known cardiac risk factor, the contribution of dyslipidemia to CVD also differs between men and women. For both sexes, LDL-C is the major atherogenic lipoprotein [29]. Typically in the United States, the levels of LDL-C and triglycerides (TG's) are higher in men than in women. This holds true until women turn 55, at which point a shift occurs and women have higher levels. Regardless of the absolute level however, LDL-C remains the primary target for intervention in both sexes as noted in the NCEP guidelines. Despite higher levels of TGs in men, there is actually a stronger association between the TG level and CVD risk in women. This was demonstrated by a meta-analysis that showed that a 1 mmol/L (89 mg/dL) increase in TG levels was associated with a 32 % increased risk of CVD in men, versus a 76 % increased risk in women [29, 30]. HDL-C is the third important component of the lipid panel associated with increased CVD risk and several studies have shown that HDL-C is the most powerful predictor of CVD risk in women [29, 31–33]. Low levels of HDL-C have been shown to be a significant risk predictor in older women, but not in older men [34]. As will be later discussed, there are specific guidelines for lipid management in women to reduce risk.

Diabetes

CVD and diabetes are closely related, largely due to the effects of diabetes on vasculature. Diabetics are up to four times more likely to have CVD than non-diabetics [35]. One of the major mortality events in diabetics is CVD, and nearly two out of three diabetics will die from some sort of CVD. Men and women with diabetes often have subclinical vascular disease. And specifically in women, diabetes has been shown to confer greater prognostic information than any of the other traditional risk factors. It is thought of as a more devastating risk factor for women than men, often eliminating the other age- or hormone- protective cardiovascular disease advantages. Women with diabetes thus require intensive cardiovascular screening. This is also true in young women with gestational diabetes, who are prone to develop both subsequent diabetes mellitus and adverse coronary risk profiles [36].

Obesity

Obesity is increasingly frequent across all cultures and is recognized as a risk for cardiovascular disease. A report from Roger et al. in 2011 found that nearly two of every three US women >20 years of age is now overweight or obese [37]. The Nurses' Health Study, a prospective study by Manson et al., looked at 115,886 U.S. women between the ages of 30 and 55 who were free of diagnosed coronary disease, stroke, and cancer. They found a strong positive association between obesity and the occurrence of CVD (specifically in this study, non-fatal MI and fatal coronary disease) [38]. Obesity was categorized into five different groups based on body mass index

(BMI; weight in kilograms divided by the square of the height in meters): BMI <21, 21- <23, 23 to <25, 25 to <29, and ≥29. The risk of both non-fatal MI and fatal coronary disease was three times higher in the ≥29 group when compared to the leanest group, who had the lowest rates of coronary disease. Surprisingly, even women considered to be of "average weight" had a nearly 30 % higher risk of coronary events when compared to the leanest group [38]. There are several CHD risk factors affected by obesity, including hypertension, low HDL cholesterol, elevated triglycerides, diabetes mellitus, and elevated levels of inflammatory markers. Even relatively modest weight gain during the adult years is highly related to developing an increased risk factor burden. Nearly 23 % of CHD in men, and 15 % in women were obese in long-term analysis of Framingham data. Individuals with central obesity, largely because of concomitance of other risk factors or co-morbidities (very often present in obese women), have an increased risk of cardiovascular events [27, 39].

Metabolic Syndrome

Metabolic syndrome, which is defined by the presence of three or more risk factors described below (including central obesity), is more common in women with CHD when compared to men. The risk factors include increased abdominal obesity as defined by waist circumference (in men, greater than 40 in.; in women, greater than 35 in.), fasting blood triglycerides level greater than or equal to 150 mg/dL, low blood HDL cholesterol (in men, less than 40 bmg/dL; in women, less than 50 mg/dL), blood pressure greater than or equal to 130/85 mmHg, or fasting blood glucose greater than or equal to 110 mg/dL [27].

Psychosocial

Psychological stress also likely influences the onset and clinical course of CHD, which growing evidence suggests may be especially true for women. The previously mentioned INTERHEART study suggested that AMI was strongly associated with the combined exposure to psychosocial risk factors (including major life events, depression, perceived stress at home or work). Congruous with this, lower socioeconomic status (with increased psychosocial stressors and hardened lifestyle factors) has consistently been associated with increased cardiovascular morbidity and mortality. These psychosocial factors (well-documented to be more prevalent in women than in men), may also affect the adherence to, and ability to maintain a healthy lifestyle [40, 41].

Systemic Inflammatory Disease

The chronic inflammation associated with systemic inflammatory diseases is felt to accelerate the development of cardiovascular disease. Women with rheumatoid arthritis have a two to four times higher risk of myocardial infarction or new cardiovascular events compared with women who do not have rheumatoid arthritis and the mortality rate is 50 % higher for cardiovascular death in patients with rheumatoid arthritis compared to those without [42]. After controlling for common risk factors, patients with systemic lupus had a ten-fold higher relative risk for nonfatal myocardial infarction, 17 fold higher risk for death due to coronary heart disease, sevenfold higher risk for overall coronary heart disease, and an almost eightfold higher risk of stroke [43]. Studies have linked carotid atherosclerosis with disease duration in rheumatoid arthritis and systemic lupus [44, 45]. The increased risks associated with systemic collagen vascular inflammatory disease are not limited to women but these diseases predominantly affect women compared to men, making identification and management important. Aggressive control of the underlying inflammatory disease is recommended to decrease morbidity and mortality from cardiovascular disease [42, 43, 45–47]. Systemic collagen-vascular inflammatory disease is an independent risk factor for cardiovascular disease, as noted in the 2011 AHA guidelines, so presence of this condition should prompt further assessment of cardiovascular risk and risk factor modification [48–50].

Novel Risk Factors

Without dedicating the remainder of this chapter to the other 200+ risk factors associated with CVD, it is worthwhile to note that there has been interest in potential risk factors. The U.S. Preventive Services Task Force (USPSTF) published a review of "Emerging Risk Factors for CAD" [51], based on nine systematic reviews of novel risk factors recently receiving attention. The factors evaluated included C-Reactive Protein (CRP), coronary artery calcium score (as measured by electron-beam computed tomography), lipoprotein (a) level, homocysteine level, leukocyte level, fasting blood glucose, periodontal disease, ankle-brachial index, and carotid intima-media thickness. Based on the current evidence available, the review did not find the routine use of any of these nine aforementioned risk factors to be valuable for further risk stratification of intermediate-risk persons [41, 51]. That being said, CRP has been shown to be of some utility when incorporated into risk assessment scores, and particularly the Reynolds Risk Score. Specifically, a CRP level of >3.0 mg/L did reclassify approximately 5 % of intermediate-risk women in the Women's Health Study (however, it failed to reclassify any in the Cardiovascular Health Study), which suggests a small and inconsistent effect when CRP is used [8, 52].

AHA Guidelines

The updated 2011 AHA Guidelines addressed here include recommendations regarding: (1) the prevention of CVD in women, (2) interventions not useful/effective (and may be harmful) for the prevention of CVD in women, (3) a methodology for providers to assess CVD risk, and (4) and a classification system of the risk assessment.

Lifestyle Interventions

While lifestyle recommendations to decrease risk of cardiovascular disease may seem intuitive, they should not be overlooked or underestimated. Women who are in the "ideal cardiovascular health" group as defined in the AHA 2011 guidelines have a significantly decreased incidence of CVD compared to those with risk factors [10]. In addition, data from the Nurse's Health Study showed that women who adhered to lifestyle recommendations (similar to the ideal cardiovascular health group) had a relative risk reduction of about 80 % compared to those women not in this group [9]. Recommendations for optimization of modifiable risk factors (cigarette smoking, diet, physical activity, weight management) are as detailed in Table 2.1.

Major Risk Factor Interventions

Blood pressure is a major risk factor for cardiovascular disease and guidelines for women are those set by JNC 7 [53]. Optimal blood pressure goals are the same for both men and women; a goal of <120/80 mmHg should be achieved through lifestyle approaches including weight control, increased physical activity, alcohol moderation, sodium restriction, and increased consumption of fruits, vegetables, and low-fat dairy products (Class I; Level of Evidence B). When women remain hypertensive with blood pressure greater than 140/90 mmHg in the setting of other co-morbidities, (especially chronic kidney disease and diabetes mellitus) pharmacotherapy should be implemented. The drug regimen should be tailored towards specific vascular diseases. For example Table 2.2 identifies circumstances where individuals with certain co-morbidities would benefit from a specific drug class. Women with diabetes, for example, should likely be on an ACE inhibitor or ARB for both their hypertension and their diabetes, whereas women with any component of left ventricular failure would benefit from a beta-blocker and/or ACE inhibitor/ARB. Women in the "high-risk" group (those with acute coronary syndrome or MI) should be started on beta-blockers and/or ACE inhibitors/ARBs, with the addition of other drugs such as thiazides as needed to achieve goal blood pressure (Class I; Level of Evidence A). Note: In women who may become pregnant, ACE inhibitors should be used with caution, and are contraindicated in pregnancy.

Hyperlipidemia is also a major risk factor for cardiovascular disease. 3-Hydroxy-3-methylglutaryl-coenzyme A reductase inhibitors, or "statins", lower lipids by blocking cholesterol biosynthesis though they also have other downstream "pleiotropic effects" which reduce inflammation and clotting, likely adding to their clinical effect [54]. This class of medications will be discussed in more detail later in this chapter.

As a CHD equivalent [55], diabetes mellitus should be addressed in discussion of cardiovascular disease prevention. Women with diabetes mellitus may benefit from a goal HbA1c <7 % if this can be achieved without risk of hypoglycemia (Class IIa; Level of Evidence B).

Table 2.1 Recommendations for modifiable risk factors to achieve ideal

Risk factor	Recommendation	Level of evidence
Tobacco	Providers should advise all women not to smoke	Class I; Level of Evidence B
	Avoid environmental smoke.	
	For those women who do smoke:	
	Smoking cessation counseling should be provided at each encounter.	
	Nicotine replacement therapy and a formal smoking cessation program should be offered.	
Physical activity	Perform at least	Class I; Level of Evidence B
	150 min/week of moderate exercise,	
	75 min/week of vigorous exercise,	
	Or an equivalent combination of moderate- and vigorous-intensity aerobic physical activity.	
	Increasing moderate –intensity aerobic physical activity to 5 h/week, 2.5 h/week of vigorous –intensity aerobic physical activity, or an equivalent combination of both bestows additional cardiovascular benefits .	Class I; Level of Evidence B
	Muscle-strengthening activities that involve all major muscle groups should be performed on ≥2 days/week	Class I; Level of Evidence B
	Note: a comprehensive CVD risk-reduction regimen such as CV or stroke rehabilitation or a	Class I; Level of Evidence A
	physician-guided home- or community-based exercise training program should be recommended to women who have:	Class I; Level of Evidence B
	Suffered from a recent acute coronary syndrome or coronary revascularization, new-onset or chronic angina, recent cerebrovascular event, peripheral arterial disease.	
	Current/prior symptoms of heart failure and an LVEF ≤35 %	
Weight management	Weight loss guidance is vital	Class I; Level of Evidence B
	At least 60–90 min of moderate-intensity physical activity (e.g., brisk walking) on most, and preferably all, days of the week, should be performed	

(continued)

Table 2.1 (continued)

Risk factor	Recommendation	Level of evidence
Diet	Women consume a diet made up of:	Class I: Level of Evidence B
	Whole-grain, high-fiber foods,	Class IIb: Level of Evidence B
	Fish (especially oily fish) at least twice a week, and	
	Plentiful fruits and vegetables.	
	Women should avoid:	
	Trans-fatty acids	
	Limit intake of saturated fat, cholesterol, alcohol, sodium, and sugar	
	Women with hypercholesterolemia and/or hypertriglyceridemia may consider consumption of omega-3 fatty acids in the form of fish or in capsule form for primary and secondary prevention	
	Note: Dietary recommendations differ for pregnant women who should avoid fish due to concern for mercury contamination.	

Classification and Levels of Evidence:

Classification:

Class I Intervention is useful and effective

Class IIa Weight of evidence/opinion is in favor of usefulness/efficacy

Class IIb Usefulness/efficacy is less well established by evidence/opinion

Class III Procedure/test not helpful or treatment has no proven benefit; Procedure/test excess cost without benefit or harmful or treatment harmful to patients

Level of evidence:

A: Sufficient evidence from multiple randomized trials

B: Limited evidence from single randomized trial or other nonrandomized studies

C: Based on expert opinion, case studies, or standard of care

Adapted from Mosca et al. [10]

CVD indicated cardiovascular disease, *LVEF* left ventricular ejection fraction

Table 2.2 Preventive drug interventions

Pharmacologic agent	Dose	Designated population	Special considerations
Aspirin	75–325 mg	High risk women (women with HD; women with diabetes unless contraindicated)	If intolerant of aspirin therapy, would consider substituting with clopidogrel
Aspirin	81 or 100 mg every other day	At risk, or healthy women (women ≥65 year of age (81 mg daily or 100 mg every other day) if blood pressure is controlled and benefit for ischemic stroke and MI prevention is likely to outweigh risk of gastrointestinal bleeding and hemorrhagic stroke).	May be reasonable for women <65 year of age for ischemic stroke prevention (*Class IIb; Level of Evidence B*).
Warfarin	Titrated	For women with chronic or paroxysmal atrial fibrillation, warfarin should be used to maintain the INR at 2.0–3.0 unless they are considered to be at low risk for stroke (<1 %/year or high risk of bleeding).	Patients must adhere to strict blood work monitoring in order to titrate levels.
Dabigatran	150 mg taken orally, twice daily. Dosing should be adjusted for those with renal impairment.	Dabigatran is useful as an alternative to warfarin for the prevention of stroke and systemic thromboembolism in patients with paroxysmal to permanent AF and risk factors for stroke or systemic embolization.	Not to be used in women who have a prosthetic heart valve or hemodynamically significant valve disease, severe renal failure (creatinine clearance <15 mL/min), or advanced liver disease (impaired baseline clotting function) (*Class I; Level of Evidence B*).
Beta-blockers	Titrated	Should be used for up to 12 months (Class I; Level of Evidence A) or up to 3 years (Class I; Level of Evidence B) in all women after MI or ACS with normal left ventricular function unless contraindicated. Long-term β-blocker therapy should be used indefinitely tor women with left ventricular failure unless contraindications are present (*Class I; Level of Evidence A*).	Long-term β-blocker therapy may be considered in other women with coronary or vascular disease and normal left ventricular function (*Class IIb; Level of Evidence C*).

(continued)

Table 2.2 (continued)

Pharmacologic agent	Dose	Designated population	Special considerations
ACE inhibitors/ARBS	Titrated	Should be used (unless contraindicated) in women after MI and in those with clinical evidence of heart failure, LVEF ≤40 %, or diabetes mellitus (*Class I; Level of Evidence A*). In women after MI and in those with clinical evidence of heart failure, an LVEF ≤40 %, or diabetes mellitus who are intolerant of ACE inhibitors, ARBs should be used instead (*Class I; Level of Evidence B*).	ACE inhibitors are contraindicated in pregnancy and ought to be used with caution in women who may become pregnant.
Aldosterone Blockers	Titrated	Use of aldosterone blockade (eg. spirololactone) after MI is indicated in women who do not have significant hypotension, renal dysfunction, or hyperkaiemia who are already receiving therapeutic doses of an ACE inhibitor and β-blocker and have LVEF ≤40 % with symptomatic heart failure (*Class I; Level of Evidence B*).	

Adapted from Mosca et al. [10]

HD indicates heart disease, *MI* myocardial infarct, *INR* international normalized ratio, *AF* atrial fibrillation, *LVEF* left ventricular ejection fraction, *β-blocker* beta-blocker, *ACS* acute coronary syndrome, *ACE* angiotensin converting enzyme, *ARB* angiotensin receptor blocker

To summarize, several risk factors have been found to be more potent in women than in men, including:

1. Smoking has been associated with 50 % of all coronary events in women.
2. Diabetes appears to confer greater prognostic information in women than any of the other traditional cardiac risk factors
3. Metabolic syndrome/high triglycerides pose much higher risk for association with cardiovascular disease in women.
4. Several studies have shown that HDL-C is the most powerful predictor of CVD risk in women [29, 31–33].
5. The protective effects of exercise and alcohol appear to have somewhat larger effect in women than in men.

Additional medications used in the primary and secondary prevention of CVD are as noted in Table 2.2.

Interventions Not Useful/Effective and May Be Harmful for the Prevention of CVD in Women

In addition to recommendations for prevention, the 2011 AHA guidelines also provided Class III evidence guidance for interventions to avoid. The findings from the Framingham study of 2000 showed that menopausal therapy, including hormone therapy and selective estrogen-receptor modulators (SERMs), should not be used for the primary or secondary prevention of CVD (Class III, Level of Evidence A). In addition, neither the Women's Antioxidant Cardiovascular Study (WACS), nor the Women's Antioxidant and Folic Acid Cardiovascular Study (WAFACS) did not show nutritional supplements—including vitamins B, E, C, beta carotene, and folic acid supplements—to prevent the incidence or recurrence of CVD in women [49]. These data were published with the result of eliminating ineffective therapies from preventative regimens. The 2011 guidelines were updated to include the recommendation that nutritional supplements, including vitamins E, C, beta carotene, and folic acid (with or without B6 and B12 supplementation), should not be used for the primary or secondary prevention of CVD (Class III, Level of Evidence A).

Lastly, and perhaps most importantly, the routine use of aspirin for the prevention of CVD in healthy women <65 years of age is not recommended to prevent myocardial infarction (Class III, Level of Evidence B). Recommendations vary sharply between men and women. The Physicians' Health Study found that aspirin provided MI (but not stroke) protection in men; conversely, the Women's Health Study found aspirin to provide stroke benefit, but not MI protection in women [49, 56, 57].

Evaluation of Cardiovascular Risk (see Fig. 2.2)

Unfortunately, despite increasing awareness, major coronary events may be missed, as nearly half of major coronary events occur in asymptomatic individuals [58]. Efforts have thus been made to help clinicians accurately identify "at risk" individuals. Two well-known models exist to assess cardiovascular risk prediction: the Framingham-based risk assessment, and the Reynolds Risk score for CVD. The third National Cholesterol Education Program (NCEP) Adult Treatment Panel III (ATP-III) guidelines recommend that all adults should have their risk of coronary heart disease (CHD) event assessed in an office-based visit. The factors identified as "coronary risk factors" by the Framingham investigators include age, hypertension, smoking, diabetes, elevated total and LDL-cholesterol, and low HDL-cholesterol. Since 1966, these factors have been integrated into global risk scores for assessment of cardiovascular risk [59–61]. Based on risk factors, adults are characterized as having one of three levels of risk: low, intermediate, or high. Despite their accepted significance, it has been shown that nearly 20 % of all coronary events occur in the absence of these major risk factors [62]. Critiques of the Framingham risk assessment include the underestimation of both clinical [63] and subclinical [64–66] CHD risk in asymptomatic postmenopausal women. The Framingham risk score also does not include risk of stroke, angina, or coronary revascularization all of which are more prevalent in women as compared with men.

In 2007, in the setting of these Framingham risk score limitations, Ridker et al. developed a new model for the assessment of global cardiovascular risk in women— the Reynolds Risk Score. Recent comparative studies suggest that the Reynolds Risk Score is better calibrated than the Framingham-based model, particularly in the women with 5–10 % estimated 10-year risk as classified by the Framingham method [52]. The Reynolds Risk Score is determined by the following risk factors: age, systolic blood pressure, hemoglobin A1c if diabetic, current smoking, total and HDL-C, high sensitivity CRP (hsCRP), and parental history of myocardial infarction before age 60 years [67]. It has yet to be determined what preventative strategies (like statin therapy) may be implemented based on a woman's specific risk score, but future studies will likely guide therapy. Also, as noted previously, the utility of hsCRP are also debatable.

The formal algorithm for a woman's cardiovascular risk assessment, as proposed by AHA 2011 Guidelines (see Fig. 2.2) includes the Framingham risk assessment, and begins with a focused history. The algorithm categorizes women by level of risk, and guides providers to the appropriate recommendations as described in detail above. The first step is to ask pertinent questions regarding past medical, family, and pregnancy complication history. Women should also be screened for symptoms of CVD. History taking should be followed by standard physical exam (including blood pressure, body mass index, and waist size). Fasting lipoproteins and glucose should be obtained. This data would prove sufficient for Framingham risk

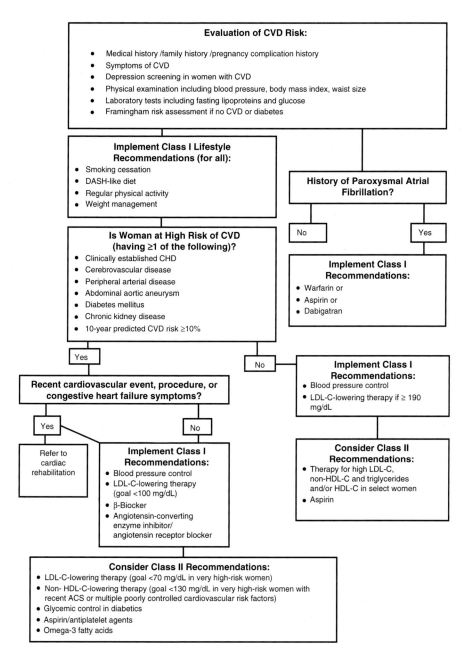

Fig. 2.2 Flow diagram for CVD preventive care in women. *CVD* indicates cardiovascular disease, *DASH* Dietary Approaches to Stop Hypertension, *CHD* coronary heart disease, *LDL-C* low-density lipoprotein cholesterol, *HDL-C* high-density lipoprotein cholesterol, and *ACS* acute coronary syndrome (Reprinted with permission Mosca et al. [10])

assessment (if no diabetes or CVD). If using the Reynolds Risk Score, hemoglobin A1c, hsCRP, and parental history of myocardial infarction before age 60 years should also be obtained.

All women should implement Class I lifestyle recommendations as outlined in detail Table 2.3 (smoking cessation, DASH-like diet, regular physical activity, and weight management).

If women have a history of paroxysmal atrial fibrillation, Class I anticoagulation recommendations should be implemented regarding warfarin, or aspirin, or dabigatran (see Chap. 10).

If a woman is considered to be at high risk of CVD (having ≥1 of the following: clinically established CHD, cerebrovascular disease, peripheral arterial disease, abdominal aortic aneurysm, diabetes mellitus, chronic kidney disease, or a Framingham 10-year predicted CVD risk ≥10 %), it should be determined if she has had a recent cardiovascular event, a recent cardiovascular procedure, or congestive heart failure symptoms. If she has had a recent CVD event, she should be referred to cardiac rehabilitation and class I recommendations implemented (blood pressure control, LDL-C-lowering therapy (goal <100 mg/dL), β-blocker, and angiotensin-converting enzyme inhibitor/angiotensin receptor blocker). If she has not had a

Table 2.3 Gender differences in traditional cardiac risk factors

	Men	Women
Risk factor threshold values		
Age threshold for ↑ disease risk	≥45 years	≥55 years
Family history of premature CHD	<55 years	<65 years
HDL cholesterol		<50 mg/dl
Population average values		
Lipids		
Total cholesterol	↑	↑ For women after age ~50 years
HDL cholesterol		↑
Prevalence rates		
Hypertension*	↑	
Smoking†	↑	
Coronary disease or outcome risk		
Triglycerides		↑
Diabetes mellitus		↑
Obesity (e.g., BMI ≥30 kg/m²)‡	↑	↑
Central obesity (>35 kg/m²*)		↑

Gaps narrow:
*In elderly
†Women lag in declining rates of smoking and noted increased prevalence of young female smokers
‡Obesity increasing in the last decade such that ~25 % of women are now obese with a body mass index (BMI)≥30 kg/m². Additionally, women generally engage in less leisure-time physical activity and exhibit a greater functional decline in their postmenopausal years
CHD coronary heart disease, *HDL* high-density lipoprotein.
Reprinted from Shaw et al. [105] with permission from Elsevier

recent CVD event, Class I recommendations for high risk women should be implemented. Class II recommendations may be considered, including omega-3 fatty acids, aspirin/antiplatelet agents, glycemic control in diabetics, and more aggressive lipid therapy.

Classification of CVD Risk in Women

The algorithm for evaluation of CVD risk (Fig. 2.2) helps providers assess disease state (which may range from healthy to having established or assumed cardiovascular disease). A new classification is that of women who meet criteria for "Ideal Cardiovascular Health." Please see Table 2.4 for a full description of these criteria, but in brief, this includes untreated total cholesterol, blood pressure, and fasting blood glucose all at goal, normal body mass index, abstinence from smoking, a healthy (DASH-like) diet, and physical activity at goal. If a woman achieves this classification, a report by Lloyd-Jones et al. showed an association with greater longevity, significant reductions in short-term, immediate-term, and lifetime risks for CVD events [68]. They were also found to have a greater quality of life in older ages, with lower associated Medicare costs [68]. This ideal cardiovascular health classification gives clear guidance to women and providers

Table 2.4 Classification of CVD risk in women

High risk (≥1 high-risk state)	At risk (≥1 major risk factor[s])	Ideal cardiovascular health (must have all of these)
Symptomatic CHD	Cigarette smoking Physical inactivity	No evidence of hypertension (BP <120/<80 mmHg untreated)
Symptomatic cerebrovascular disease	Obesity (especially central adiposity) Hypertension (SBP ≥120 mmHg, DBP ≥80 tnrn Hg, or treated hypertension)	Total cholesterol <200 mg/dL (untreated)
Symptomatic peripheral arterial disease	Elevated cholesterol (total cholesterol ≥200 mg/dL, HDL-C <50 mg/dL, or treated for dyslipidemia	Fasting blood glucose <100 mg/dL (untreated)
Abdominal aortic aneurysm	Poor diet	BMI <25 kg/m²
End-stage or chronic kidney disease	Systemic inflammatory/autoimmune collagen-vascular disease (e.g. lupus or rheumatoid arthritis)	Non-smoker
Diabetes mellitus	History of preeclampsia, gestational diabetes or pregnancy-induced hypertension	Adequate amount of physical activity
10-year predicted CVD risk ≥10 %	Poor exercise capacity on treadmill test Known advanced subclinical atherosclerosis (e.g. coronary calcification, carotid plaque)	Healthy diet, low in salt, alcohol, saturated fats and high in fruits and vegetables

Adapted from Mosca et al. [10]

regarding lifestyle goals. Conversely, presence of risk factors determines if a woman is "at risk" (at least one major risk factor like smoking history or hypertension), or "high risk" (at least one high-risk state like diabetes or chronic kidney disease).

Statins in Primary and Secondary Prevention of Cardiovascular Disease in Women

The class of medications known as statins are a critical tool in the primary and secondary prevention of cardiovascular disease. Statins have been shown to significantly decrease major cardiovascular events including myocardial infarction, need for cardiovascular revascularization, ischemic stroke, transient ischemic attacks, and mortality from cardiovascular disease. All-cause mortality has also been shown to be decreased in statin- treated patients [69–72]. Statins have a major effect on lipid levels, decreasing LDL levels by 18–55 %, increasing HDL 5–15 %, and decreasing triglycerides 7–30 %. In addition, they are felt to have "pleiotropic effects" which modify endothelial cell function, reduce inflammatory cell migration and inflammatory biomarkers, increase nitric oxide synthesis, enhance vascular smooth muscle relaxation, and inhibit platelet aggregation [54]. These anti-inflammatory and anti-thrombotic effects likely add to their clinical effectiveness.

Women have historically been underrepresented in trials of statins leading to insufficient information and questions regarding benefit of treatment, especially in primary prevention, and whether efficacy is the same as in men [73, 74]. A meta-analysis by Petretta suggested that "statins may not be as effective in women as in men without cardiovascular disease" however the authors went on to state that the studies may have been underpowered to observe differences, data was incomplete, and the duration of follow up may have been inadequate (an important point in primary prevention) [73]. More recent studies such as the Treating to New Targets (TNT), Heart Protection Study, and the Jupiter trial have demonstrated the benefits of lipid reduction with statins in decreases in the occurrence of endpoints of major cardiovascular events [75–77]. A recent meta-analysis by Kostis et al. of 140,000 patients, 40,000 of whom were women, demonstrated that statins are equally efficacious in men and women in both primary and secondary prevention of cardiovascular disease, stroke, and in decreasing all cause mortality [78]. They were also demonstrated to be equally efficacious across different levels of risk (low, medium, and high) between men and women. Lipids should be treated to goal based on level of cardiovascular risk without regard to gender.

Wenger et al. has emphasized that, as the population ages, the incidence of CVD will increase among women and that the great majority of persons over 80 years are women and are more likely to suffer cardiovascular events [75, 79]. During the perimenopausal to postmenopausal years, women experience a substantial increase in their LDL cholesterol and total cholesterol and a small decrease in total HDL cholesterol [80]. This is why the focus on risk factor modification and prevention in women should start early, in the premenopausal years.

Lipids have traditionally been undertreated in women compared with men [81, 82]. The increased awareness of the prevalence and risk of CVD in women will help providers and patients understand the need for appropriate treatment of modifiable risk factors, including dyslipidemia. Using risk stratification guidelines (such as the 2011 AHA Effectiveness based prevention guideline and the recently released 2013 ACC/AHA Guideline on the Treatment of Blood Cholesterol to Reduce Atherosclerotic Cardiovascular Risk in Adults) [83] and treating patients according to evidence based guidelines is critical in decreasing cardiovascular disease in all women [10, 83].

Practical Points in Diagnosis

The National Cholesterol Education Program Adult Treatment Panel III Guidelines, updated in 2004, have been used to define cardiovascular risk and determine goals for lipids [14, 70]. New guidelines on risk stratification and treatment of lipids were published in late 2013 and represent a paradigm shift in the treatment of lipids. Randomised controlled trial evidence showed that cardiovascular events were reduced using the maximum tolerated statin intensity rather than treating to a specific lipid goal (as in the prior guidelines), so the updated guidelines reflect this change [84].

The 2013 ACC/AHA guidelines divide patients into four categories in which the benefit of treatment clearly outweighs risk of therapy. These categories are:

1. Patients with clinical CVD.
2. Patients with LDL > 190 mg/dL.
3. Patients aged 40–75 years old with diabetes and LDL 70–189 mg/dL.
4. Patients aged 40–75 years old, with no CVD or diabetes, LDL 70–189 mg/dL, and 10 year global CVD risk > or equal to 7.5 %.

Patients with CVD who are under 75 years old should receive high intensity statin therapy while those who are 75 or older should receive moderate intensity statin therapy. Individuals older than 21 years old with an LDL greater than or equal to 190 mg/dL (group 2) should receive high intensity statin therapy given their high lifetime risk of developing cardiovascular disease. Patients aged 40–75 years old with diabetes (group 3) should have moderate intensity statin therapy although if they have a 10 year CVD risk of greater than or equal to 7.5 % they should be treated with high intensity statin therapy. Patients who are in group 4 (aged 40–75, no CVD or diabetes, LDL 70–189 and with a 10 year CVD risk greater than or equal to 7.5 %) should be offered moderate to high intensity statin therapy after discussion about benefits and potential risks of therapy (Table 2.5). Decisions regarding intensity of therapy should be made while considering the individual patient's other medical conditions, drug-drug interactions, and tolerance of medications.

Table 2.5 Statin therapy recommendation

Statin benefit group	Risk category	Recommendation for therapy
Clinical CVD	Age under 75	High intensity statin therapy
	Age 75 or older	Moderate intensity statin therapy
LDL ≥190	Age 21 or older	High intensity statin therapy
Diabetes, no clinical CVD, age 40–75, LDL 70–189	10 year global risk ≥7.5 %	High intensity statin therapy
	10 year global risk <7.5 %	Moderate intensity statin therapy
Age 40–75, LDL 70–189, no diabetes, no clinical CVD	10 year global risk ≥7.5 %	Moderate to high intensity statin therapy
	10 year global risk <7.5 %	Benefit of statin therapy not clear, decision should be made based on discussion with patient and consideration of additional risk factors

10 year global risk calculator can be found at: http://my.americanheart.org/cvriskcalculator
Clinical CVD includes coronary heart disease, stroke, peripheral arterial disease, *LDL* low density lipoprotein
Adapted from Stone et al. [83]

The 2013 ACC/AHA lipid guidelines note that some individuals may not be categorized into a risk group but may have higher risks because of underlying conditions which may raise their risk of cardiovascular disease.

The 2011 AHA guidelines included systemic autoimmune collagen-vascular disease (e.g., systemic lupus erythematosis or rheumatoid arthritis) as a risk factor for cardiovascular disease. Pregnancy complications including pre-eclampsia, gestational diabetes, and pregnancy induced hypertension are also conditions which place a woman in the "at risk" group (along with other traditional cardiac risk factors). Pregnancy may be considered a screening test for later in life CVD [85]. Coronary risk factor assessment and surveillance is warranted for such women, and a detailed history of pregnancy complications should be part of the routine cardiovascular risk assessment of all women. The degree of increased risk conferred by these conditions is not taken into account by risk calculators such as the Framingham 10 year CHD calculator or the global risk assessment calculator used in the 2013 ACC/AHA guidelines but they should be considered when evaluating overall risk. If a woman has multiple significant risk factors it may be prudent to consider her in a higher risk group and treat modifiable risk factors more aggressively.

The 2013 ACC/AHA guideline specifically states that there is no difference in approach based on gender. The assessment of 10 year CVD risk is done through "Pooled Cohort Equations", a risk calculator available at http.my.americanheart. org/cvriskcalculator. If a patient has a 10 year CVD risk of less than 7.5 % then the risk should be reviewed in 4–6 years.

High intensity statin regimens are those which are expected to decrease LDL level by greater than 50 % and include atorvastatin 40–80 mg daily or rosuvastatin 20–40 mg daily. Moderate intensity regimens should decrease LDL by 30–50 % and include atorvastatin 10–20 mg daily, rosuvastatin 5–10 mg daily, simvastatin 20–40 mg daily, pravastatin 40–80 mg daily, lovastatin 40 mg daily, or fluvastatin 40 mg twice daily. Once a patient has started statin therapy it is recommended that lipids be checked in 4–12 weeks to assess adherence to therapy rather than checking to see if a goal has been reached. Lipids can then be monitored every 3–12 months depending on the patient [83].

It is important to remember that for all patients, regardless of risk level, therapeutic lifestyle change (diet and exercise) are integral to risk reduction. Studies have shown that women (and men) who adhere to lifestyle guidelines regarding diet, exercise, weight control, and abstinence from smoking have a markedly decreased risk of cardiac events compared to those who do not [86, 87]. These lifestyle recommendations are also strongly endorsed in the 2011 AHA guidelines for the prevention of cardiovascular disease in women.

Practical Points in Treatment

Statins are very effective in lowering LDL cholesterol and are first line therapy in lipid management. There are various statins are available for prescription, all with demonstrated efficacy, but differing in cost, potency, and side effect profile. Statins also differ in how they are metabolized and whether they are more hydrophilic or lipophilic, thus affecting the side effect profile of the medication and potential drug-drug interactions.

While statins are generally very well tolerated, any medication can have side effects. It is important to be aware of the potential side effects of statins when prescribing and to inquire about adherence to therapy and possible side effects when following patients. This is especially critical when treating asymptomatic conditions such as hyperlipidemia as patients may potentially stop therapy when faced with a side effect if they do not fully understand the benefits of treatment [88]. Women are more prone to medication side effects because of gender differences in pharmacokinetics (secondary to hormonal effects; liver metabolism, and differences in body size, and fat and muscle composition). Women also tend to take more medications than men do, an issue which only increases as women age and develop more medical issues [89].

Typical statin adverse effects have been considered to be related to effects on liver and muscle. It is now felt that serious liver injury is quite rare and is idiosyncratic [90]. Routine monitoring of liver tests is not effective in detecting or preventing liver disease and is more likely to lead to discontinuation of a clinically indicated and important medication in response to unrelated abnormalities. Liver function should be checked prior to initiating a statin and then as clinically indicated thereafter.

Myalgias, described as muscle pain, weakness, or cramping may occur with the use of statins, with muscle pain being reported in randomized controlled trials in 1.5–3 % of participants [91]. The incidence in actual clinical practice is higher and is estimated at approximately 10 %. More serious effects of myopathy and rhabdomyolysis are much less common at between 5 and 11 and 1.6–3.4 per 100,000 person-years respectively [92]. Given the infrequency of serious muscle effects, it is not recommended that clinicians monitor muscle enzyme (creatinine kinase) levels routinely but to check if muscle symptoms occur. Certain groups of patients are at higher risk of myalgias, including those who have low body mass, or are female, elderly, physically active, have a family history of muscle pain, hypothyroidism, are on a high dose of a statin, or have an elevated creatinine kinase level at baseline (which could signify a subclinical myopathy) [91]. Muscle effects are felt to be dose related so decreasing the dose of a statin or changing to a lower dose of a more potent statin can ameliorate muscle symptoms. The lipophilic statins (simvastatin and atorvastatin) have a higher incidence of being associated with myalgias than do the hydrophilic statins (pravastatin, rosuvastatin, and fluvastatin) so changing to a different statin can also work to decrease muscle symptoms [91–93]. Rosuvastatin has a longer half life than other statins and has been tolerated and effective in meeting lipid goals when given every other day or even weekly though effect of this strategy on cardiovascular outcomes have not been studied [94, 95].

Cognitive effects have also been reported to occur with the use of statins. These symptoms are usually described as mental fogginess, or decreased memory or energy. While these effects have usually been described in observational studies, there has been a randomized controlled trial which showed a possible small effect in certain neuropsychological testing [96]. There is likely a higher risk of cognitive effects with the more lipophilic statins (atorvastatin and simvastatin) than the hydrophilic statins (pravastatin and rosuvastatin) [97]. There is also the suggestion that women may be more affected by cognitive symptoms of fatigue and decreased energy [98]. Cognitive symptoms were reversible with symptoms resolution within days to weeks of discontinuing the statin. If a patient develops cognitive side effects then holding the statin for 4–8 weeks before restarting with a less lipophilic statin would be a reasonable approach to this side effect.

A mildly increased risk of diabetes has been observed with the use of statins [99, 100]. The WOSCOPS study showed that there may have been a decreased risk of diabetes in participants treated with statins (relative risk of 0.7 with a confidence interval of 0.50–0.99) although it is important to note that this study only included men. Evaluation of results from other studies showed a possible slight increase in risk though with confidence intervals crossing one. The Jupiter trial (which included almost 40 % women) showed a slightly increased risk of diabetes (relative risk of 1.25 with a confidence interval of 1.05–1.49) [101]. Overall, a different meta-analysis showed an odds ratio of 1.09 (confidence interval of 1.02–1.17) [102]. The risk is small and appears to be a medication class effect and not associated with any individual statin. A meta-analysis found that the risk appears to be higher in women and in older participants [101, 102]. An observational study noted trends showing higher risk in women with lower BMI (less than 25) compared with higher (greater than 30), and possibly a higher risk in Asian women [103]. It is critical to remember that for a patient with established cardiovascular disease or at moderate to high risk for cardiovascular disease, the benefit of a statin outweighs the risk of diabetes and therapy should not be withheld based on the potential risk. For women at low risk of cardiovascular disease, the risks and benefits should be discussed and current guidelines reviewed.

Special Considerations

Statins are contraindicated in pregnant and lactating women, because they have not been tested in this population. They should be used with caution in decompensated liver disease. There are significant drug interactions between simvastatin or lovastatin and other drugs which share the same metabolic pathway; it is important to review current prescribing information and precautions. There is an increased risk of myopathy with concurrent use of statins and fibrates [93]. The risk of myopathy is higher in older patients, especially in women, in patients with multisystem disease taking multiple medications with potential for interactions. However, with appropriate care, statins can be used safely in these patients [104].

Summary

In summary, this chapter has focused on the primary prevention of cardiovascular disease. The AHA guidelines on the prevention of cardiovascular disease in women have evolved as new information is learned and will continue to be refined as new evidence becomes available. These guidelines offer accessible, practical recommendations that address lifestyle interventions, preventive and therapeutic pharmacotherapy, and cardiac risk assessment for CVD. Additionally, the 2011 guidelines address interventions *not* helpful, including hormone replacement therapy, in the prevention of CVD. There are currently two well-studied risk indices- the Framingham Risk Assessment and the Reynolds Risk Score, along with the new "Pooled Cohort Equations" as detailed in the 2013 ACC/AHA lipid guidelines [83], which can help providers identify at-risk women whose cardiac health may be optimized. Based on the risk assessment, preventative and therapeutic measures can be individualized for each patient.

The crucial role of lipid control in both primary and secondary prevention of cardiovascular disease in women was also discussed in this chapter. Using guidelines for risk stratification and encouraging therapeutic lifestyle changes and treatment of lipids through the judicious use of statins is key. While statins are generally very well tolerated, most side effects can be managed through medication and dosage adjustment.

These guidelines are informed by an increasing body of work specifically focused on cardiovascular disease prevention in women and on elucidating differences in the underlying pathophysiology of cardiovascular disease between genders.

References

1. Wilson PWF, et al. Prediction of coronary heart disease events part 1: the role of traditional risk factors. Circulation. 1998;97:1837–47.
2. Bitton A, Gaziano TA. The Framingham Heart Study's impact on global risk assessment. Prog Cardiovasc Dis. 2010;53:68–78.

3. Kannel WB. The Framingham Study: historical insight on the impact of cardiovascular risk factors in men versus women. J Gend Specif Med. 2002;5:27–37.
4. Lloyd-Jones DM, Larson MG, Beiser A, Levy D. Lifetime risk of developing coronary heart disease. Lancet. 1999;353:89–92.
5. Melloni C, et al. Representation of women in randomized clinical trials of cardiovascular disease prevention. Circ Cardiovasc Qual Outcomes. 2010;3:135–42.
6. Mosca L, et al. Guide to preventive cardiology for women. AHA/ACC scientific statement consensus panel statement. Circulation. 1999;99:2480–4.
7. Writing Group Members, et al. Heart disease and stroke statistics-2012 update: a report from the American Heart Association. Circulation. 2011;125:e2–220.
8. Vaccarino V, et al. Ischaemic heart disease in women: are there sex differences in pathophysiology and risk factors? Position paper from the working group on coronary pathophysiology and microcirculation of the European Society of Cardiology. Cardiovasc Res. 2011;90:9–17.
9. Stampfer MJ, et al. Postmenopausal estrogen therapy and cardiovascular disease. Ten-year follow-up from the nurses' health study. N Engl J Med. 1991;325:756–62.
10. Mosca L, et al. Effectiveness-based guidelines for the prevention of cardiovascular disease in women—2011 update a guideline from the American Heart Association. Circulation. 2011;123:1243–62.
11. Heart disease – MayoClinic.com at: http://www.mayoclinic.com/health/heart-disease/DS01120.
12. Coronary artery disease – MayoClinic.com at: http://www.mayoclinic.com/health/coronary-artery-disease/DS00064.
13. Grundy SM, et al. Primary prevention of coronary heart disease: guidance from Framingham: a statement for healthcare professionals from the AHA Task Force on Risk Reduction. American Heart Association. Circulation. 1998;97:1876–87.
14. National Cholesterol Education Program (NCEP) Expert Panel on Detection, Evaluation, and Treatment of High Blood Cholesterol in Adults (Adult Treatment Panel III). Third Report of the National Cholesterol Education Program (NCEP) Expert Panel on Detection, Evaluation, and Treatment of High Blood Cholesterol in Adults (Adult Treatment Panel III) final report. Circulation. 2002;106:3143–421.
15. Novella S, Dantas AP, Segarra G, Medina P, Hermenegildo C. Vascular aging in women: is estrogen the fountain of youth? Front Physiol. 2012;3:165.
16. Kneale BJ, Chowienczyk PJ, Brett SE, Coltart DJ, Ritter JM. Gender differences in sensitivity to adrenergic agonists of forearm resistance vasculature. J Am Coll Cardiol. 2000;36:1233–8.
17. Vitale C, Fini M, Speziale G, Chierchia S. Gender differences in the cardiovascular effects of sex hormones. Fundam Clin Pharmacol. 2010;24:675–85.
18. Roqué M, et al. Short-term effects of transdermal estrogen replacement therapy on coronary vascular reactivity in postmenopausal women with angina pectoris and normal results on coronary angiograms. J Am Coll Cardiol. 1998;31:139–43.
19. Matthews KA, et al. Are changes in cardiovascular disease risk factors in midlife women due to chronological aging or to the menopausal transition? J Am Coll Cardiol. 2009;54:2366–73.
20. Tousignant-Laflamme Y, Marchand S. Excitatory and inhibitory pain mechanisms during the menstrual cycle in healthy women. Pain. 2009;146:47–55.
21. Rosano GM, et al. 17-beta-estradiol therapy lessens angina in postmenopausal women with syndrome X. J Am Coll Cardiol. 1996;28:1500–5.
22. Speroff L. The heart and estrogen/progestin replacement study (HERS). Maturitas. 1998;31:9–14.
23. Rossouw JE, et al. Risks and benefits of estrogen plus progestin in healthy postmenopausal women: principal results from the Women's Health Initiative randomized controlled trial. JAMA. 2002;288:321–33.
24. Thun MJ, et al. 50-year trends in smoking-related mortality in the United States. N Engl J Med. 2013;368:351–64.
25. Huxley RR, Woodward M. Cigarette smoking as a risk factor for coronary heart disease in women compared with men: a systematic review and meta-analysis of prospective cohort studies. Lancet. 2011;378:1297–305.

26. Jha P, et al. 21st-century hazards of smoking and benefits of cessation in the United States. N Engl J Med. 2013;368:341–50.
27. Stramba-Badiale M, et al. Cardiovascular diseases in women: a statement from the policy conference of the European Society of Cardiology. Eur Heart J. 2006;27:994–1005.
28. Messerli FH, et al. Disparate cardiovascular findings in men and women with essential hypertension. Ann Intern Med. 1987;107:158–61.
29. Mosca L. Management of dyslipidemia in women in the post-hormone therapy era. J Gen Intern Med. 2005;20:297–305.
30. Hokanson JE, Austin MA. Plasma triglyceride level is a risk factor for cardiovascular disease independent of high-density lipoprotein cholesterol level: a meta-analysis of population-based prospective studies. J Cardiovasc Risk. 1996;3:213–9.
31. Bass KM, Newschaffer CJ, Klag MJ, Bush TL. Plasma lipoprotein levels as predictors of cardiovascular death in women. Arch Intern Med. 1993;153:2209–16.
32. Gordon T, Castelli WP, Hjortland MC, Kannel WB, Dawber TR. High density lipoprotein as a protective factor against coronary heart disease. The Framingham Study. Am J Med. 1977;62:707–14.
33. Boden WE. High-density lipoprotein cholesterol as an independent risk factor in cardiovascular disease: assessing the data from Framingham to the Veterans Affairs High–Density Lipoprotein Intervention Trial. Am J Cardiol. 2000;86:19L–22.
34. Manolio TA, et al. Cholesterol and heart disease in older persons and women. Review of an NHLBI workshop. Ann Epidemiol. 1992;2:161–76.
35. Booth GL, Kapral MK, Fung K, Tu JV. Relation between age and cardiovascular disease in men and women with diabetes compared with non-diabetic people: a population-based retrospective cohort study. Lancet. 2006;368:29–36.
36. Wenger NK. Should women have a different risk assessment from men for primary prevention of coronary heart disease? J Womens Health Gend Based Med. 1999;8:465–7.
37. Roger VL, et al. Heart disease and stroke statistics–2011 update: a report from the American Heart Association. Circulation. 2011;123:e18–209.
38. Manson JE, Stampfer MJ, Hennekens CH, Willett WC. Body weight and longevity. A reassessment. JAMA. 1987;257:353–8.
39. Wilson PW. Prediction of coronary heart disease events part 2: the contribution of lifestyle factors and new issues. Cardiol Rounds. 2004(8).
40. Tofler G. Psychosocial and other social factors in acute myocardial infarction. UpToDate 2013 At: http://www.uptodate.com/contents/psychosocial-and-other-social-factors-in-acute-myocardial-infarction?detectedLanguage=en&source=search_result&search=psychosocial+risk+factors+cardiovascular&selectedTitle=1%7E150&provider=noProvider.
41. Yusuf S, et al. Effect of potentially modifiable risk factors associated with myocardial infarction in 52 countries (the INTERHEART study): case–control study. Lancet. 2004;364:937–52.
42. Salmon JE, Roman MJ. Subclinical atherosclerosis in rheumatoid arthritis and systemic lupus erythematosus. Am J Med. 2008;121:S3–8.
43. Esdaile JM, et al. Traditional Framingham risk factors fail to fully account for accelerated atherosclerosis in systemic lupus erythematosus. Arthritis Rheum. 2001;44:2331–7.
44. Manzi S, et al. Age-specific incidence rates of myocardial infarction and angina in women with systemic lupus erythematosus: comparison with the Framingham Study. Am J Epidemiol. 1997;145:408–15.
45. Roman MJ, et al. Prevalence and correlates of accelerated atherosclerosis in systemic lupus erythematosus. N Engl J Med. 2003;349:2399–406.
46. Manzi S, Wasko MC. Inflammation-mediated rheumatic diseases and atherosclerosis. Ann Rheum Dis. 2000;59:321–5.
47. Roman MJ, et al. Arterial stiffness in chronic inflammatory diseases. Hypertension. 2005;46:194–9.
48. Asanuma Y, et al. Premature coronary-artery atherosclerosis in systemic lupus erythematosus. N Engl J Medicine. 2003;349:2407–15.
49. Wenger NK. Women and coronary heart disease: a century after Herrick: understudied, underdiagnosed, and undertreated. Circulation. 2012;126:604–11.

50. Hahn BH. Systemic lupus erythematosus and accelerated atherosclerosis. N Engl J Med. 2003;349:2379–80.
51. Helfand M, et al. Emerging risk factors for coronary heart disease: a summary of systematic reviews conducted for the U.S. Preventive Services Task Force. Ann Intern Med. 2009;151:496–507.
52. Cook NR, et al. Comparison of the Framingham and Reynolds Risk scores for global cardiovascular risk prediction in the multiethnic Women's Health Initiative. Circulation. 2012;125(1748–1756):S1–11.
53. Chobanian AV, et al. The seventh report of the Joint National Committee on prevention, detection, evaluation, and treatment of high blood pressure: the JNC 7 report. JAMA. 2003;289:2560–72.
54. Willey JZ, Elkind MSV. 3-Hydroxy-3-methylglutaryl-coenzyme A reductase inhibitors in the treatment of central nervous system diseases. Arch Neurol. 2010;67:1062–7.
55. Daniels LB, et al. Is diabetes mellitus a heart disease equivalent in women? Results from an international study of postmenopausal women in the Raloxifene Use for the Heart (RUTH) trial. Circ Cardiovasc Qual Outcomes. 2013;6:164–70.
56. Ridker PM, et al. A randomized trial of low-dose aspirin in the primary prevention of cardiovascular disease in women. N Engl J Med. 2005;352:1293–304.
57. Final report on the aspirin component of the ongoing Physicians' Health Study. Steering Committee of the Physicians' Health Study Research Group. N Engl J Med. 1989; 321:129–35.
58. Rosamond W, et al. Heart disease and stroke statistics–2007 update: a report from the American Heart Association Statistics Committee and Stroke Statistics Subcommittee. Circulation. 2007;115:e69–171.
59. Wilson PW, et al. Prediction of coronary heart disease using risk factor categories. Circulation. 1998;97:1837–47.
60. Expert Panel on Detection, Evaluation, And Treatment of High Blood Cholesterol In Adults. Executive summary of the third report of the National Cholesterol Education Program (NCEP) expert panel on detection, evaluation, and treatment of high blood cholesterol in adults (adult treatment panel III). JAMA. 2001;285:2486–97.
61. Wood D, et al. Prevention of coronary heart disease in clinical practice: recommendations of the Second Joint Task Force of European and other Societies on coronary prevention. Atherosclerosis. 1998;140:199–270.
62. Khot UN, et al. Prevalence of conventional risk factors in patients with coronary heart disease. JAMA. 2003;290:898–904.
63. Akosah KO, Schaper A, Cogbill C, Schoenfeld P. Preventing myocardial infarction in the young adult in the first place: how do the National Cholesterol Education Panel III guidelines perform? J Am Coll Cardiol. 2003;41:1475–9.
64. Nasir K, Michos ED, Blumenthal RS, Raggi P. Detection of high-risk young adults and women by coronary calcium and National Cholesterol Education Program Panel III Guidelines. J Am Coll Cardiol. 2005;46:1931–6.
65. Michos ED, et al. Framingham risk equation underestimates subclinical atherosclerosis risk in asymptomatic women. Atherosclerosis. 2006;184:201–6.
66. Michos ED, et al. Women with a low Framingham risk score and a family history of premature coronary heart disease have a high prevalence of subclinical coronary atherosclerosis. Am Heart J. 2005;150:1276–81.
67. Ridker PM, Buring JE, Rifai N, Cook NR. Development and validation of improved algorithms for the assessment of global cardiovascular risk in women: the Reynolds Risk Score. JAMA. 2007;297:611–9.
68. Lloyd-Jones DM, et al. Defining and setting national goals for cardiovascular health promotion and disease reduction the American Heart Association's Strategic Impact Goal through 2020 and beyond. Circulation. 2010;121:586–613.
69. O'Regan C, Wu P, Arora P, Perri D, Mills EJ. Statin therapy in stroke prevention: a meta-analysis involving 121,000 patients. Am J Med. 2008;121:24–33.

70. Grundy SM, et al. Implications of recent clinical trials for the National Cholesterol Education Program Adult Treatment Panel III guidelines. Circulation. 2004;110:227–39.
71. Taylor F, et al. Statins for the primary prevention of cardiovascular disease. Cochrane Database Syst Rev. (The Cochrane Collaboration and Taylor F, John Wiley & Sons, Ltd., 2013) at: http://summaries.cochrane.org/CD004816/statins-for-the-primary-prevention-of-cardiovascular-disease.
72. The effects of lowering LDL cholesterol with statin therapy in people at low risk of vascular disease: meta-analysis of individual data from 27 randomised trials: the Lancet at: http://www.thelancet.com/journals/lancet/article/PIIS0140-6736(12)60367-5/abstract.
73. Petretta M, Costanzo P, Perrone-Filardi P, Chiariello M. Impact of gender in primary prevention of coronary heart disease with statin therapy: a meta-analysis. Int J Cardiol. 2010;138: 25–31.
74. Walsh JME, Pignone M. Drug treatment of hyperlipidemia in women. JAMA. 2004;291:2243–52.
75. Wenger NK, Lewis SJ, Welty FK, Herrington DM, Bittner V. Beneficial effects of aggressive low-density lipoprotein cholesterol lowering in women with stable coronary heart disease in the Treating to New Targets (TNT) study. Heart. 2008;94:434–9.
76. Heart Protection Study Collaborative Group. MRC/BHF Heart Protection Study of cholesterol lowering with simvastatin in 20 536 high-risk individuals: a randomised placebocontrolled trial. Lancet. 2002;360:7–22.
77. Ridker PM, et al. Rosuvastatin to prevent vascular events in men and women with elevated C-reactive protein. N Engl J Med. 2008;359:2195–207.
78. Kostis WJ, Cheng JQ, Dobrzynski JM, Cabrera J, Kostis JB. Meta-analysis of statin effects in women versus men. J Am Coll Cardiol. 2012;59:572–82.
79. Wenger NK. Lipid abnormalities in women: data for risk, data for management. Cardiol Rev. 2006;14:276–80.
80. Matthews KA, Kuller LH, Sutton-Tyrrell K, Chang YF. Changes in cardiovascular risk factors during the perimenopause and postmenopause and carotid artery atherosclerosis in healthy women. Stroke. 2001;32:1104–11.
81. Wenger NK. Preventing cardiovascular disease in women: an update. Clin Cardiol. 2008;31:109–13.
82. Ansell BJ, et al. Reduced treatment success in lipid management among women with coronary heart disease or risk equivalents: results of a national survey. Am Heart J. 2006;152:976–81.
83. Stone NJ, et al. ACC/AHA Guideline on the Treatment of Blood Cholesterol to Reduce Atherosclerotic Cardiovascular Risk in Adults. A Report of the American College of Cardiology/American Heart Association Task Force on Practice Guidelines. J Am Coll Cardiol. 2013. doi:10.1016/j.jacc.2013.11.002.
84. Hayward RA, Krumholz HM. Three Reasons to Abandon Low-Density Lipoprotein Targets An Open Letter to the Adult Treatment Panel IV of the National Institutes of Health. Circ Cardiovasc Qual Outcomes. 2012;5:2–5.
85. Stampfer MJ, Hu FB, Manson JE, Rimm EB, Willett WC. Primary prevention of coronary heart disease in women through diet and lifestyle. N Engl J Med. 2000;343:16–22.
86. Stamler J, et al. Low risk-factor profile and long-term cardiovascular and noncardiovascular mortality and life expectancy: findings for 5 large cohorts of young adult and middle-aged men and women. JAMA. 1999;282:2012–8.
87. Roberts JM, Hubel CA. Pregnancy: a screening test for later life cardiovascular disease. Womens Health Issues. 2010;20:304–7.
88. Miller NH. Compliance with treatment regimens in chronic asymptomatic diseases. Am J Med. 1997;102:43–9.
89. Miller MA. Gender-based differences in the toxicity of pharmaceuticals–the Food and Drug Administration's perspective. Int J Toxicol. 2001;20:149–52.
90. Drug Safety and Availability > FDA Drug Safety Communication: important safety label changes to cholesterol-lowering statin drugs at: http://www.fda.gov/drugs/drugsafety/ucm293101.htm.

91. Jacobson TA. Toward'pain-free' toward statin prescribing: clinical algorithm for diagnosis and management of myalgia. Mayo Clin Proc. 2008;83:687–700.

92. Harper CR, Jacobson TA. The broad spectrum of statin myopathy: from myalgia to rhabdomyolysis. Curr Opin Lipidol. 2007;18:401–8.

93. Mancini GBJ, et al. Diagnosis, prevention, and management of statin adverse effects and intolerance: proceedings of a Canadian Working Group Consensus Conference. Can J Cardiol. 2011;27:635–62.

94. Backes JM, Moriarty PM, Ruisinger JF, Gibson CA. Effects of once weekly rosuvastatin among patients with a prior statin intolerance. Am J Cardiol. 2007;100:554–5.

95. Backes JM, et al. Effectiveness and tolerability of every-other-day rosuvastatin dosing in patients with prior statin intolerance. Ann Pharmacother. 2008;42:341–6.

96. Muldoon MF, Ryan CM, Sereika SM, Flory JD, Manuck SB. Randomized trial of the effects of simvastatin on cognitive functioning in hypercholesterolemic adults. Am J Med. 2004;117:823–9.

97. Rojas-Fernandez CH, Cameron J-CF. Is Statin-associated cognitive impairment clinically relevant? A narrative review and clinical recommendations. Ann Pharmacother. 2012;46:549–57.

98. Golomb BA, Evans M. Effects of statins on energy and fatigue with exertion: results from a randomized controlled trial. Arch Intern Med. 2012;172:1180–2.

99. Waters DD, et al. Predictors of new-onset diabetes in patients treated with atorvastatin: results from 3 large randomized clinical trials. J Am Coll Cardiol. 2011;57:1535–45.

100. Ridker PM, Pradhan A, MacFadyen JG, Libby P, Glynn RJ. Cardiovascular benefits and diabetes risks of Statin therapy in primary prevention: an analysis from the JUPITER trial. Lancet. 2012;380:565–71.

101. Rajpathak SN, et al. Statin therapy and risk of developing type 2 diabetes: a meta-analysis. Diabetes Care. 2009;32:1924–9.

102. Sattar N, et al. Statins and risk of incident diabetes: a collaborative meta-analysis of randomised statin trials. Lancet. 2010;375:735–42.

103. Culver AL, Ockene I. STatin use and risk of diabetes mellitus in postmenopausal women in the women's health initiative. Arch Intern Med. 2012;172:144–52.

104. Meagher EA. Addressing cardiovascular disease in women: focus on dyslipidemia. J Am Board Fam Pract. 2004;17:424–37.

105. Shaw L, et al. Insights From the NHLBI-Sponsored Women's Ischemia Syndrome Evaluation (WISE) Study: part I: gender differences in traditional and novel risk factors, symptom evaluation, and gender-optimized diagnostic strategies. J Am Coll Cardiol. 2006;47(3 Suppl):S4–S20.

Part II
Diagnosis, Evaluation and Treatment of Specific Conditions in Women

Chapter 3
Gender Differences in Clinical Manifestation and Pathophysiology of Ischemic Heart Disease- A Gender Paradox

Nicholas Paivanas, Janice Opladen, and Angelo Pedulla

Introduction

This chapter will cover the basic pathophysiology and symptom presentation of ischemic heart disease and will highlight the differences in heart disease between men and women. Heart disease affects millions of Americans and is the leading cause of death for both men and women in America [1]. Numerous risk factors for developing heart disease and the mechanisms by which a normal heart becomes a diseased heart have been previously identified. Coronary atherosclerosis leading to obstruction of the epicardial coronary arteries has been identified as the leading cause of heart disease. With this paradigm of coronary artery disease (CAD) in mind, clinicians typically evaluate and treat patients with angina with medications or interventions aimed at preventing or correcting obstructive CAD.

More recently, there have been observed differences in the incidence, prevalence, and burden of heart disease between men and women. This includes three striking observations: women have a higher prevalence of angina, a lower burden of obstructive CAD on angiography despite as many, if not more, traditional risk factors, and a worse prognosis for heart disease compared to men. All three of these observations are in the setting of a lower prevalence of obstructive CAD compared to men [2, 3]. Together, these observations have been termed the "gender paradox," which cannot be explained solely with the pathophysiology of obstructive CAD. This gender paradox has led to the postulate that ischemic heart disease is different in women and in men in its pathogenesis, symptoms and prognosis. To further the understanding of heart disease in women, the National Heart, Lung, and Blood Institute (NHLBI) created an initiative which resulted in the Women's Ischemic

N. Paivanas, MD (✉)
Department of Medicine, University of Rochester Medical Center, Rochester, NY, USA
e-mail: nicholas.paivanas@gmail.com

J. Opladen, ACNP-BC • A. Pedulla, MD
Division of Cardiology, University of Rochester Medical Center, Rochester, NY, USA

H.Z. Mieszczanska, G.P. Velarde (eds.),
Management of Cardiovascular Disease in Women,
DOI 10.1007/978-1-4471-5517-1_3, © Springer-Verlag London 2014

Symptom Evaluation (WISE) study [4, 5]. The NHLBI-WISE is a prospective cohort study designed to study gender differences in ischemic heart disease. It recruited women that were referred for diagnostic angiography for symptoms of ischemic heart disease. A total of 936 women were recruited and then followed over time. Numerous studies and sub-studies have been analyzed on data collected from this cohort, which has contributed vastly to our understanding of differences in ischemic heart disease between men and women.

In looking at the numbers of patients presenting to medical care with angina, a certain percentage will not have clinically significant obstruction of the coronary arteries. When comparing the sexes, women presenting with stable angina symptoms have been reported to have a significantly lower incidence of obstructive CAD than men (48 % vs. 67 %) with an impressive odds ratio of 0.37 for women compared to men [6, 7]. Evaluation of women with angina but without obstructive CAD on coronary angiography with phosphorus-31 nuclear magnetic resonance spectroscopy, a non-invasive imaging technique that measures aerobic and anaerobic metabolites to tell if a tissue is ischemic, interestingly revealed that 20 % will still have evidence of myocardial ischemia, suggesting microvascular disease involvement [8]. Clinically, this subset of women has worse cardiovascular outcomes compared to women without evidence of ischemia [3]. Consequently, the nomenclature of Ischemic Heart Disease (IHD) has been suggested as a better term than CAD in order to encompass these patients with poor outcomes from heart disease who do not exhibit obstructive CAD [8, 9].

A further concern with gender differences and heart disease is the difference in perception and reporting of myocardial ischemia. "Typical Angina" has been classified as symptoms of pain in the chest that are aggravated by exertion and relieved by rest or nitroglycerine. Chest pain that does not follow this pattern is termed either atypical angina or non-cardiac chest pain. Unfortunately, women have long been underrepresented in studies of heart disease. Studies of women with proven heart disease have revealed that women frequently describe their angina pain in ways that do not fall under the classification of "typical angina" [10].

Gender Differences in Clinical Manifestation of IHD

The presentation of IHD in women is frequently more complex and multifactorial than that in men. Due to the difference in presentation of ischemic heart disease in women, the diagnosis and treatment of ACS in women in the pre-hospital setting as well as emergency department may be sub-optimal, resulting in missed diagnoses, delays in treatments, and excess mortality [11, 12]. The following section will review typical angina and atypical angina and will then highlight some of the differences between symptoms typically reported by men and women.

Typical Angina Symptoms

Obtaining a clinical history has long been the most valuable tool in the clinician's diagnostic arsenal. Unfortunately, symptoms of cardiac ischemia vary between patients which can make clinical diagnosis challenging. In order to have a common language for evaluating patients, the terms typical angina, atypical angina, and non-anginal chest pain have been standardized in the literature [13]. Three clinical questions help to classify a patient's symptoms of chest discomfort: Is the discomfort sub-sternal? Is it precipitated by exertion? And, is there prompt relief with rest or nitroglycerine? If the patient's symptoms affirmatively follow all three of these clinical features, the symptoms are classified as "typical angina." Having two of the features classifies symptoms as "atypical angina," and having only one or none of the features classifies symptoms as "non-anginal." This system has been applied to a group of patients that underwent cardiac catheterization to determine how the symptoms correlated with presence or absence of obstructive CAD. The resulting data helped clinicians to assign a pre-test probability for obstructive CAD to patients based on age, sex, and classification of angina. Women were found to have a lower incidence of CAD compared to men of similar age and with similar angina classification with the notable exception of post-menopausal aged women with typical angina. While this classification of angina has proven to be hugely useful in the study, diagnosis and treatment of coronary disease, two limitations should be kept in mind when evaluating the history provided by women. The first is that it applies only to obstructive CAD that can be seen on angiography and was not developed to assess for microvascular disease. The second is that it places large emphasis on the symptom of chest pain. Other studies looking at prediction models for the prevalence of obstructive CAD in women based on symptom classification, age, and gender have found that women have significantly less obstructive CAD than would be predicted [14, 15].

Figure 3.1 reproduces the Diamond probability of coronary artery disease compared with actual observed coronary disease prevalence in symptomatic women from the National Heart, Lung, and Blood Institute Women's Ischemia Syndrome Evaluation (WISE) [14].

Symptoms Reported by Women

While both men and women will frequently report symptoms such as chest pain or pressure, symptoms reported by women also frequently fall into the classification of atypical angina or non-angina pain rather than typical angina. This can make it challenging for clinicians to accurately estimate their pretest probability of heart disease. It is important to have an appreciation for the variation in angina symptoms between men and women. Women are more likely to have angina at rest, during sleep, or with emotional or mental stress. They are also more likely to have symptoms such as neck and shoulder pain, nausea, vomiting, fatigue or dyspnea during an acute myocardial infarction [16].

Research on gender differences in symptoms has highlighted distinct differences in disease presentation. An observational study [17] of over one million patients with myocardial infarction demonstrated that while 70 % of men complained of chest pain, only 58 % of women complained of chest pain. Interestingly, this difference was most pronounced in younger women, and was not statistically significant in older women. While chest pain is certainly present in the majority of women with

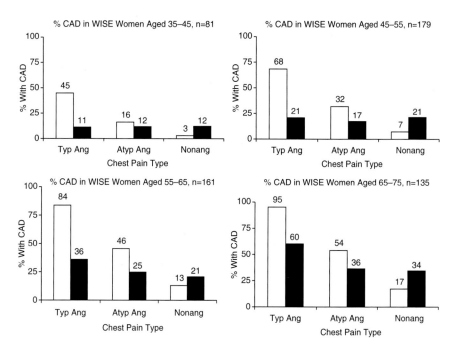

Fig. 3.1 From the National Heart, Lung, and Blood Institute Women's Ischemia Syndrome Evaluation (WISE), the Diamond probability of coronary artery disease (*open bars*) compared with actual observed coronary disease prevalence in symptomatic women (*solid bars*). *Atyp Ang* atypical angina, *Nonang* non-angina, *Typ Ang* typical angina (Reprinted from "Shaw et al. [14] with permission from Elsevier)

acute myocardial infarction, one study [18] demonstrated high rates of other symptoms including shortness of breath (58 %), weakness (55 %), and fatigue (43 %). Non-chest pain symptoms during the prodromal time leading up to a myocardial infarction were also frequently experienced. Notably, unusual fatigue (70 %), sleep disturbance (48 %), and shortness of breath (42 %) were more prevalent than chest discomfort (30 %). While actual symptom rates vary throughout the literature, the variety of non-chest pain symptoms in women remains impressive. A list of many of these common "atypical symptoms" is included in the Table 3.1 [10, 18–20].

Awareness of the variety and frequency of symptoms other than chest pain is important for patients so that they might seek medical attention in a timely manner. Early recognition and treatment of an acute coronary syndrome can clearly improve outcomes, but disturbingly a recent review of emergency medical services found that only 23 % of patients call 9-1-1 when experiencing an acute coronary syndrome [21]. It is also important for clinicians to recognize symptoms so that they can appropriately diagnose and treat women presenting with cardiac ischemia. While a history of typical angina symptoms is frequently associated with obstructive CAD in both men and women, a history of atypical angina in a woman with the aforementioned symptoms should also warrant careful consideration by the clinician. Even in the absence of obstructive CAD, advances in diagnostic technology are increasingly

Table 3.1 Variety of symptoms reported by women during ACS

Chest pain
Neck/jaw/tooth pain
Arm/shoulder/back pain
Cold sweat
Hot/flushed
Fatigue
Weakness
Cough
Heart racing/palpitations
Shortness of breath
Loss of appetite
Indigestion/nausea/vomiting
Arm numbness or burning
Dizziness/lightheadedness
Vision change
Headache

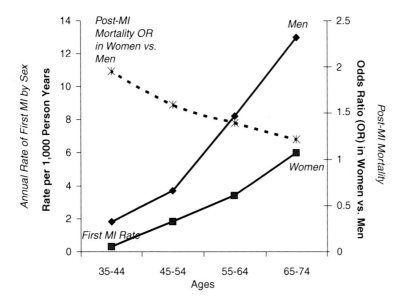

Fig. 3.2 Disparity between the lower incidence of myocardial infarction and worse outcomes in women compared to men (Reprinted from Merz. et al. [22] with permission from Elsevier)

identifying evidence of cardiac ischemia in symptomatic patients. This recognition of a pathophysiology for cardiac ischemia other than obstructive CAD could help to bridge the gap between lower rates of obstructive CAD in women with their high rate of poor cardiovascular outcomes. It is still unclear whether differences in the rates of underlying cardiac pathophysiology can help to explain some of the differences in symptoms experienced between the sexes.

Figure 3.2 reproduces the disparity between the lower incidence of myocardial infarction and worse outcomes in women compared to men [22].

Pathophysiology of Ischemic Heart Disease

As mentioned in the introduction, there is a gender paradox in that women appear to have less obstructive CAD and yet worse cardiovascular outcomes compared to men. In order to solve this gender paradox, multiple pathologies in addition to obstructive coronary disease have been suggested as contributing to IHD. These include obstructive CAD, plaque morphology, microvascular dysfunction, endothelial dysfunction, inflammatory conditions, and hormonal influence as displayed in Fig. 3.3.

Obstructive Coronary Artery Disease

The heart is a muscular organ that receives its blood supply from the coronary arteries originating at the aorta. These coronaries run along the epicardium before feeding deep into the myocardium. The majority of coronary artery disease in both men and women arises from obstructive disease of the epicardial portion of these coronary arteries. Without adequate blood flow from the coronary arteries, myocardial tissue becomes ischemic and loses its ability to efficiently contract and conduct electrical signals. These vital epicardial arteries branch out from the aorta in similar patterns in both men and women, but women commonly have smaller coronary artery diameter and less collateral arteries branching off of the major epicardial coronary arteries than do men [23]. Obstruction of the coronary arteries is most attributable to the chronic accumulation of lipids in arterial walls by the process of atherosclerosis. Obstructive atherosclerosis is more commonly seen in men than

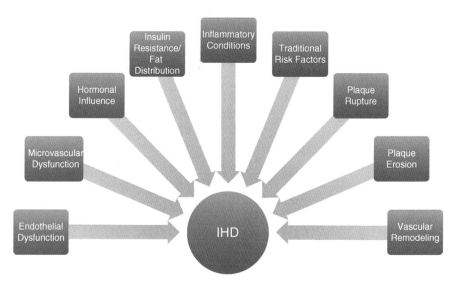

Fig. 3.3 Multiple factors contributing to Ischemic Heart Disease (IHD) in women

premenopausal women, but post menopausal women develop obstructive atherosclerosis at rates similar to those seen in men [24]. Major risk factors for the development of atherosclerosis include hyperlipidemia, hypertension, tobacco abuse, and diabetes mellitus. On a cellular level, in atherosclerosis, LDL deposited in the vessel walls triggers endothelial cells to signal monocytes. These monocytes differentiate into macrophages, which cross the endothelial wall and phagocytize the LDL particles. They then become lipid-laden foam cells that trigger smooth muscle cells to accumulate and develop a surrounding fibrous cap. With degradation caused by inflammatory cells, the fibrous cap can rupture, which uncovers the thrombogenic lipid core. This triggers thrombus generation, which can cause obstruction of blood flow through the artery and myocardial ischemia. Acute plaque rupture as well as plaque erosion and chronic narrowing from atherosclerosis can be seen on coronary angiography by injecting contrast dye and visualizing disruption in flow through the epicardial coronary arteries [25–28].

Plaque Erosion vs Plaque Rupture

Autopsies performed on women who died from sudden cardiac death reveal gender differences in plaque morphology. Lipid laden plaques with a necrotic core are more prevalent in men and, as discussed above, will typically rupture leading to sudden exposure of inflammatory cytokines and thrombus formation at the site of the plaque. Conversely, young women in particular have higher rates of plaques composed of smooth muscle and proteoglycan-rich matrix without a necrotic lipid laden core. In contrast to plaque rupture, these plaques without a necrotic core exhibit superficial erosion leading to thrombus formation. With plaque erosion, the core of the plaque remains intact and thrombi form after coming in contact with smooth muscle. Autopsies reveal thrombi at the site of plaque erosion as well as distal embolization of thrombi formed from plaque erosion [5, 29–32]. Importantly, these gender differences in plaque morphology tend to be most pronounced in younger pre-menopausal women whereas post-menopausal women generally have fewer differences in plaque morphology and incidence of obstructive CAD.

Remodeling

In response to atherosclerosis, coronary arteries undergo remodeling to preserve adequate blood flow. When plaques involve less than 40 % of the luminal area, "positive" or "outward" remodeling can lead to enlargement of the artery which preserves the intraluminal cross sectional area and blood flow [33]. Conversely, with "negative" or "inward" remodeling, the cross sectional area of the vessel is reduced and flow limitation is seen on coronary angiography. Whether a specific vessel will exhibit positive or negative remodeling continues to be an area of research, but some factors such as increased proteases from inflammatory cells seem to correlate with more positive remodeling [31]. Authors have suggested increased amounts of positive remodeling in women compared to negative remodeling in men as a way to reconcile the more diffuse atherosclerosis, increased endothelial dysfunction, and increased microvascular dysfunction seen in women with the decreased amount of luminal obstruction observed on coronary angiography compared to men [14, 29, 31, 34].

Microvascular Angina

In contrast to angina secondary to obstruction of the large epicardial coronary arteries, microvascular angina (previously referred to as cardiac syndrome X) is a term used to describe angina symptoms from ischemia originating in intramyocardial microvascular arteries. As mentioned in the introduction of this chapter, women with chest pain presenting for angiography more frequently lack obstructive coronary artery disease than men presenting for angiography [6–8], suggesting that there is a pathology other than obstructive coronary disease responsible for their symptoms. While the pathophysiology of microvascular angina is an ongoing topic of research, two of the major contributing factors appear to be endothelial-independent microvascular dysfunction and endothelial-dependent dysfunction [5]. This microvascular angina has been postulated to be more prevalent in women because of higher levels of inflammation and hormonal changes throughout women's lives. The higher prevalence of microvascular angina in women compared to men has led authors to address it primarily as a disease of women's hearts [35].

Microvascular Dysfunction

Microvascular dysfunction refers to disease in small coronary resistance vessels measuring 100–200 µm. It can encompass the abnormal coronary reactivity that is attributable to distal embolization from coronary plaque erosion, smaller arterial size, and positive remodeling [22, 29]. In the WISE study, one subset of 159 women with angina and non-obstructive CAD on coronary angiography underwent coronary flow reserve (CFR) testing. CFR was tested by injecting intracoronary adenosine and measuring the coronary velocity response. The CFR was found to be decreased in 47 % of these women, indicating disease of the microvasculature even in the absence of obstructive CAD [29]. Nuclear Magnetic Resonance Spectroscopy (NMRS) is a non-invasive imaging technique that uses a probe to detect different quantities of chemicals in a sample. Cardiac NMRS was also used in the WISE study to look for myocardial ischemia by measuring phosphocreatine/adenosine triphosphate ratio during handgrip exercise. Decrease in the phosphocreatine/adenosine triphosphate ratio in the heart signifies a shift from aerobic to anaerobic cellular metabolism, which indicates myocardial ischemia. In WISE, women with angina but no obstructive CAD, 20 % still showed evidence of myocardial ischemia on NMRS when performing handgrip exercise [8, 9, 36].

Retinal arteriolar narrowing is a noninvasive peripheral measure that can also be used to evaluate microvascular disease throughout the body [37]. In women with retinal arteriolar narrowing, there is an increased risk for development of IHD. In contrast, men with retinal arteriolar narrowing do not appear to have a significantly increased risk of developing IHD. Together, this combination of functional and pathological findings demonstrate that there are differences in the vasculature in men and women and suggests a significant role for the microvasculature in IHD. While obstructive CAD is established as the predominant pathology in men, microvascular disease appears to contribute disproportionately to the pathophysiology of heart disease in women.

Endothelial Dysfunction

Coronary endothelial function plays a role in regulating myocardial blood flow and can also be a predictor for future vascular disease. In the WISE study, investigators measured the change in coronary flow reserve in response to injections of acetylcholine (activating endothelial-dependent dilation), adenosine (non-endothelial-dependent microvascular dilation), and nitroglycerine (non-endothelial-dependent epicardial dilation) in women with angina but no obstructive CAD [38]. They identified that women with a poor response to acetylcholine had a higher rate of adverse IHD outcomes over a 4-year follow up. This suggests that endothelial dysfunction independently predicted and likely contributed to IHD. This warrants further research and may indicate a potentially new therapeutic target. In addition to invasive intracoronary injection of acetylcholine, brachial artery flow mediated dilation has been used as a peripheral measure of endothelial function and has also been correlated with increased IHD risk in women [5].

Risk Factors

Risk factors for microvascular dysfunction and endothelial dysfunction include many of the traditional risk factors associated with coronary atherosclerotic disease including obesity, dyslipidemia, hypertension, diabetes, and smoking. Increasing evidence also identifies psychological factors including stress and depression as having significant association with IHD and acute myocardial infarction [9, 39–42]. In women, and especially in post-menopausal women there is an increased clustering of many of the traditional risk factors for heart disease [5]. Additionally, vasculitis and general inflammatory auto-immune diseases such as lupus, rheumatoid arthritis, and thyroiditis have been associated with cardiac disease [14, 32]. Many autoimmune diseases, such as rheumatoid arthritis (RA) and systemic lupus erythematosus (SLE) have female predominance. Women with lupus in particular have been shown to have higher rates of cardiac disease beyond what would be estimated by their baseline traditional risk factors [43]. Accelerated atherosclerosis in patients with SLE and RA is associated with increased cardiovascular morbidity and mortality [44]. Inflammatory conditions are also more prevalent in women and general rates of inflammation as reflected by elevated C-reactive protein have been shown to be elevated in women [14]. The combination of risk factor clustering, higher rates of depression, higher rates of vasculitis, and higher rates of general inflammatory conditions could offer some explanation for the disproportionate burden of heart disease and specifically higher rates of microvascular and endothelial dysfunction in women.

Hormonal Influence

Women also have an element of endothelial dysfunction that appears to correlate with hormonal changes throughout their lives and the lack of positive estrogenic effects on blood vessels after menopause [5, 42]. Estrogen has been identified as a likely factor contributing to the lower risk of IHD in premenopausal women compared to age matched male controls. After menopause, the reduction in estrogen appears to be accompanied by a decrease in its protective effects and an increase in the risk of IHD. Estrogen in the female heart appears to have a number of beneficial effects, which notably include improved endothelial function and decreased flow resistance as well as improved vascular response to injury. Experimental evidence points to increases in nitric oxide production and up regulation of nitric oxide genes as a mechanism by which estrogen improves vasodilation. Estrogenic effects on Estrogen Receptors (ER) alpha and ER beta in the vasculature appear to play a major beneficial role in flow resistance and vascular response to injury.

Microvascular angina encompassing endothelial-independent microvascular dysfunction and endothelial-dependent dysfunction is more prevalent in women than men. NHLBI-WISE also demonstrated that it portends a poorer prognosis in women independent of whether macrovascular dysfunction is present [22]. Additionally, in women with endothelial dysfunction there is also a significant association with increased cardiovascular events [5, 45]. Through optimal blood pressure control and improvement in the degree of measured endothelial dysfunction, some researchers have shown improvement in rates of IHD events [45, 46]. This both supports the major role of endothelial dysfunction in IHD and highlights blood pressure control as a target for improving IHD outcomes in women.

Figure 3.4 shows one proposed model for the pathophysiology of ischemic heart disease in women [5].

Spontaneous Coronary Artery Dissection (SCAD)

Spontaneous Coronary Artery Dissection (SCAD) is a phenomenon that includes spontaneous dissection of the coronary intima or media and intramural hematoma formation. SCAD does not include dissections caused by plaque dissection in coronary atherosclerosis, or trauma to the vessel wall during angiography. Rather, the

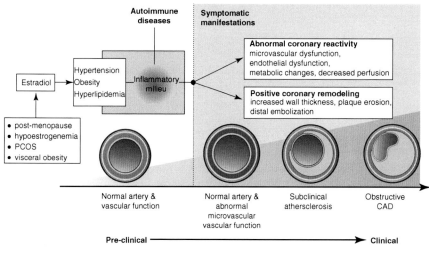

Progressive manifestations of ischemic heart disease

Fig. 3.4 One proposed model for the pathophysiology of ischemic heart disease in women (Reprinted from Shaw et al. [5] with permission from Elsevier)

current consensus is that SCAD is a separate entity that can occur in a heart without prior atherosclerotic disease [47–49]. SCAD continues to be an active area of research and has several unique features that make it especially applicable to a discussion of the female heart. The true prevalence of SCAD is not known, but has been estimated at 0.1–0.28 % of patients with ACS that undergo angiography or post-mortem examination. A recent cohort study estimated the overall annual incidence of SCAD as 0.26 per 100,000 persons. Despite this low overall incidence in the population, SCAD disproportionately affects women more than men (82 % vs. 18 %) and is associated strongly with peripartum status, which uniquely impacts the female heart.

Presentation of SCAD

On presentation, patients with SCAD commonly complain of chest pain and are often diagnosed with an acute coronary syndrome [47]. The presenting ACS diagnoses include 49 % STEMI, 44 % NSTEMI, and 7 % unstable angina. Ventricular tachycardia or fibrillation on presentation has also been recorded in 14 % of patients and multivessel coronary dissection in 23 %. The acute nature of SCAD and possible out of hospital mortality has led authors to believe that the presentation for a number of SCAD patients could be out of hospital sudden cardiac death. More widespread autopsy use in sudden cardiac death (especially in younger or peri-partum women) could reveal a greater incidence of SCAD in the population. Additionally, intraluminal hematoma formation without dissection is difficult to identify on angiography and could represent another area where SCAD is under diagnosed.

Diagnosis and Morphologic Characteristics of SCAD

There are several imaging techniques available that can diagnose SCAD including coronary angiography, intravascular ultrasound, and multidetector CT. The acute presentation of SCAD frequently leads patients to undergo coronary angiography. With contrast visualization, SCAD has been characterized as an: "involved lumen surrounded by a secondary, communicating lumen resembling a halo that fills and empties slowly; involved lumen longitudinally separated into two or three spaces by dissecting lines; or, coronary aneurysm that is seen to communicate, via a narrow neck, with the main lumen" [49]. Intramural hematoma can also develop and progress to obstruction of the coronary lumen, which can be visualized angiographically. Intravascular ultrasound further allows Doppler flow measurements to show flow into an intramural hematoma. Multidetector CT can noninvasively document SCAD and be used to follow change in the lesion(s) over time. Autopsy data, while limited in scope of practice, has helped to delineate the layers of coronary artery dissection.

The inciting factor and sequence of events for SCAD is not clear, and may vary from patient to patient. Spontaneous luminal dissection could result in hematoma formation or spontaneous hematoma formation could cause the dissection. Regardless of the inciting factor, both sequences of events can lead to extension and luminal obstruction that is clinically recognized as an acute coronary syndrome.

Figure 3.5 shows a coronary Angiogram of a 38 years old female presenting with chest pain and found to have a dissection/hematoma of the left coronary system (arrow).

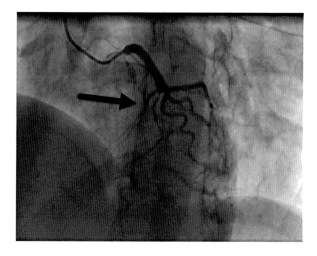

Fig. 3.5 Coronary Angiogram of a 38 years old female presenting with chest pain and found to have a dissection/hematoma of the left coronary system (*arrow*) (Image Courtesy of John Malzewski)

Predisposing Conditions for SCAD

Due to the low incidence, the total number of patients studied with SCAD is relatively small. Despite this, several interesting associations have been recognized including fibromuscular dysplasia, post-partum status, hormonal supplementation in women, and extreme physical activity in men [47]. SCAD has been indicated as the etiology of peripartum ACS in 16 % of patients. The change in hormonal status both in the post-partum patient and patient undergoing hormone supplementation might suggest that there is a role for alterations in the vasculature during these times which predisposes to SCAD. Fibromuscular dysplasia, which has been identified in 50 % of patients with SCAD, could be another predisposing factor which, under the right circumstances, can lead to SCAD. Extreme physical activity (more commonly seen in men than women with SCAD) could represent an inciting stress on an already predisposed vessel. While a single unifying genetic, hormonal, or environmental cause has not yet been identified in all patients with SCAD, it is not unreasonable to approach it as a combination of multiple underlying predisposing factors manifesting in the right environment.

Management and Prognosis of SCAD

Management of SCAD has not yet been studied with randomized controlled trials, and it would be very difficult to do so given the low incidence of the disease. Cohort studies and case reports give some data on outcomes with various interventions [47, 50], but because of their selection bias, have to be interpreted with caution. In a cohort of patients presenting with ACS and found to have SCAD on angiography, conservative management without intervention generally has resulted in the best outcomes with little acute in-hospital complications. Percutaneous coronary interventions are frequently much less successful in SCAD (65 % of patients) than in plaque mediated ACS and were frequently more complicated by failure to cross the lesion or propagation of the lesion leading to worse TIMI flow after the procedure. CABG has been seen as initially successful, but in one cohort 73 % of grafts that were placed were found to be occluded on follow up. While this data cannot definitively indicate a single best approach, it importantly highlights the high complication rate and risk of harm with interventions for SCAD compared with the same interventions when utilized for plaque mediated ACS.

Prognosis for patients after an initial SCAD event regardless of intervention appears to be better than that for other patients with ACS, with 1-year mortality estimated at 1.1 % and 10 years mortality estimated at 7.7 %. The recurrence rate however is high with 17 % at 4 years and 29 % at 10 years. Patients with SCAD reportedly have less hyperlipidemia, hypertension, tobacco abuse, and diabetes mellitus. However, due in part to the high rate of recurrence, the overall 10 years survival free from the combined endpoints of death, recurrent SCAD, myocardial infarction, or congestive heart failure is similar to other patients presenting with ACS [47].

Summary

Ischemic heart disease affects millions of American men and women. The gender paradox of increased ischemic heart disease burden in women despite decreased prevalence of obstructive CAD has led us to recognize that there is a variety of underlying pathophysiology that leads to ischemic heart disease. Obstruction in blood flow through the large epicardial coronary arteries through the process of atherosclerosis is recognized as the most common cause of ischemia in both male and female hearts. Dysfunction in the microvasculature through both endothelial independent microvascular disease and endothelial dependent disease is being increasingly recognized and is notable for its greater prevalence in the female heart. Hormonal, inflammatory, and anatomic differences between the genders likely impact the different prevalence of epicardial and microvascular disease between men and women and continue to be active areas of research. The prevalence of various symptoms of ischemic heart disease also differs between men and women. Many symptoms previously described as "atypical" are now understood to be part of the normal spectrum of IHD symptoms in women and should warrant appropriate evaluation for ischemic heart disease. The difference in underlying pathology between many male and female hearts may play a role in the difference in symptom presentation. Lastly, spontaneous coronary artery dissection, while an infrequent cause of acute coronary syndrome, is notable for its predilection for younger female hearts without traditional risk factors or presence of atherosclerosis. With research revealing more about the hormonal, inflammatory, and anatomic differences in male and female hearts, strategies for diagnosing and managing ischemic heart disease are increasingly tailored with respect to gender.

References

1. Mosca L, Hammond G, Mochari-Greenberger H, Towfighi A, Albert MA. Fifteen-year trends in awareness of heart disease in women: results of a 2012 American Heart Association national survey. Circulation. 2013;127:1254–63 .doi:10.1161/CIR.0b013e318287cf2f.
2. Bairey Merz CN. Women and ischemic heart disease paradox and pathophysiology. JACC Cardiovasc Imaging. 2011;4:74–7.
3. Gulati M, et al. Adverse cardiovascular outcomes in women with nonobstructive coronary artery disease. Arch Intern Med. 2009;169:843–50.
4. Pepine CJ. Ischemic heart disease in women. J Am Coll Cardiol. 2006;47:S1–3.
5. Shaw L, Bugiardini R, Bairey Merz CN. Women and ischemic heart disease: evolving knowledge. J Am Coll Cardiol. 2009;54:1561–75.
6. Shaw LJ, et al. Impact of ethnicity and gender differences on angiographic coronary artery disease prevalence and in-hospital mortality in the American College of Cardiology-National Cardiovascular Data Registry. Circulation. 2008;117:1787–801.
7. Merz CNB, et al. The Women's Ischemia Syndrome Evaluation (WISE) study: protocol design, methodology and feasibility report. J Am Coll Cardiol. 1999;33:1453–61.
8. Johnson BD, et al. Prognosis in women with myocardial ischemia in the absence of obstructive coronary disease: results from the National Institutes of Health-National Heart, Lung,

and Blood Institute-Sponsored Women's Ischemia Syndrome Evaluation (WISE). Circulation. 2004;109:2993–9.

9. Quyyumi A. A women and ischemic heart disease: pathophysiologic implications from the Women's Ischemia Syndrome Evaluation (WISE) Study and future research steps. J Am Coll Cardiol. 2006;47:S66–71.

10. Arslanian-Engoren C, et al. Symptoms of men and women presenting with acute coronary syndromes. Am J Cardiol. 2006;98:1177–81.

11. Pope JH, et al. Missed diagnoses of acute cardiac ischemia in the emergency department. N Engl J Med. 2000;342:1163–70.

12. Kudenchuk PJ, et al. Comparison of presentation, treatment, and outcome of acute myocardial infarction in Men versus women (the myocardial infarction triage and intervention registry). Am J Cardiol. 1996;78:9–14.

13. Diamond GA. A clinically relevant classification of chest discomfort. J Am Coll Cardiol. 1983;1:574–5.

14. Shaw LJ, et al. Insights from the NHLBI-Sponsored Women's Ischemia Syndrome Evaluation (WISE) Study: part I: gender differences in traditional and novel risk factors, symptom evaluation, and gender-optimized diagnostic strategies. J Am Coll Cardiol. 2006;47:S4–20.

15. Diamond GA, Forrester JS. Analysis of probability as an aid in the clinical diagnosis of coronary-artery disease. N Engl J Med. 1979;300:1350–8.

16. Douglas PS, Ginsburg G. The evaluation of chest pain in women. N Engl J Med. 1996;334:1311–5.

17. Canto JG, et al. Association of age and sex with myocardial infarction symptom presentation and in-hospital mortality. JAMA. 2013;307:813–22.

18. McSweeney JC, et al. Women's early warning symptoms of acute myocardial infarction. Circulation. 2003;108:2619–23.

19. Blomkalns A, Gibler WB, Newby LK. Evaluation of acute chest pain in women. Contemp Cardiol Coron Dis Women Evid Based Diagn Treat. 2004;227–42.

20. Miller CL. A review of symptoms of coronary artery disease in women. J Adv Nurs. 2002;39:17–23.

21. Newman JD, et al. Gender differences in calls to 9-1-1 during an acute coronary syndrome. Am J Cardiol. 2012. doi:10.1016/j.amjcard.2012.08.048.

22. Merz CNB, et al. Insights from the NHLBI-Sponsored Women's Ischemia Syndrome evaluation (WISE) Study: part II: gender differences in presentation, diagnosis, and outcome with regard to gender-based pathophysiology of atherosclerosis and macrovascular and microvascular cor. J Am Coll Cardiol. 2006;47:S21–9.

23. Abbasi S-H, Kassaian S-E. Women and coronary artery disease. Part I: basic considerations. J Tehran Heart Cent. 2011;6:109–16.

24. Maas AHEM, et al. Red alert for women's heart: the urgent need for more research and knowledge on cardiovascular disease in women: proceedings of the workshop held in Brussels on gender differences in cardiovascular disease, 29 September 2010. Eur Heart J. 2011;32:1362–8.

25. Libby P. Current concepts of the pathogenesis of the acute coronary syndromes. Circulation. 2001;104:365–72.

26. Libby P, Ridker PM, Hansson GK. Inflammation in atherosclerosis: from pathophysiology to practice. J Am Coll Cardiol. 2009;54:2129–38.

27. Pepine CJ, Nichols WW. The pathophysiology of chronic ischemic heart disease. Clin Cardiol. 2007;30:4–9.

28. Plank BG, Doling JM, Knight PA. Coronary artery disease. Man Outpatient Cardiol. 2012;79–216.

29. Reis SE, et al. Coronary microvascular dysfunction is highly prevalent in women with chest pain in the absence of coronary artery disease: results from the NHLBI WISE study. Am Heart J. 2001;141:735–41.

30. Burke AP, et al. Effect of risk factors on the mechanism of acute thrombosis and sudden coronary death in women. Circulation. 1998;97:2110–6.

31. Merz CNB, et al. Proceedings from the scientific symposium: sex differences in cardiovascular disease and implications for therapies. J Womens Health. 2010;19:1059–72.

32. Pepine CJ, et al. Some thoughts on the vasculopathy of women with ischemic heart disease. J Am Coll Cardiol. 2006;47:S30–5.
33. Glagov S, Weisenberg E, Zarins C, Stankunavicius R, Kolettis G. Compensatory enlargement of human atherosclerotic coronary arteries. N Engl J Med. 1987;316:1371–5.
34. Bellasi A, Raggi P, Merz CNB, Shaw LJ. New insights into ischemic heart disease in women. Cleve Clin J Med. 2007;74:585–94.
35. Marzilli M, et al. Obstructive coronary atherosclerosis and ischemic heart disease: an elusive link! J Am Coll Cardiol. 2012;60:951–6.
36. Han SH, et al. Sex differences in atheroma burden and endothelial function in patients with early coronary atherosclerosis. Eur Heart J. 2008;29:1359–69.
37. Wong TY, et al. Retinal arteriolar narrowing and risk of coronary heart disease in men and women: the Atherosclerosis Risk in Communities Study. JAMA. 2002;287:1153–9.
38. Von Mering GO, et al. Abnormal coronary vasomotion as a prognostic indicator of cardiovascular events in women: results from the National Heart, Lung, and Blood Institute-Sponsored Women's Ischemia Syndrome Evaluation (WISE). Circulation. 2004;109:722–5.
39. Quyyumi AA. Endothelial function in health and disease: new insights into the genesis of cardiovascular disease. Am J Med. 1998;105:32S–9.
40. Cai H, Harrison DG. Endothelial dysfunction in cardiovascular diseases: the role of oxidant stress. Circ Res. 2000;87:840–4.
41. Dzau VJ. Tissue angiotensin and pathobiology of vascular disease: a unifying hypothesis. Hypertension. 2001;37:1047–52.
42. Vaccarino V, et al. Ischaemic heart disease in women: are there sex differences in pathophysiology and risk factors? Position paper from the working group on coronary pathophysiology and microcirculation of the European Society of Cardiology. Cardiovasc Res. 2011;90:9–17.
43. Bessant R, et al. Risk of coronary heart disease and stroke in a large British cohort of patients with systemic lupus erythematosus. Rheumatology (Oxford). 2004;43:924–9.
44. Asanuma Y, et al. Premature coronary-artery atherosclerosis in systemic lupus erythematosus. N Engl J Med. 2003;349:2407–15.
45. Rossi R, Nuzzo A, Origliani G, Modena MG. Prognostic role of flow-mediated dilation and cardiac risk factors in post-menopausal women. J Am Coll Cardiol. 2008;51:997–1002.
46. Modena MG, Bonetti L, Coppi F, Bursi F, Rossi R. Prognostic role of reversible endothelial dysfunction in hypertensive postmenopausal women. J Am Coll Cardiol. 2002;40:505–10.
47. Tweet MS, et al. Clinical features, management, and prognosis of spontaneous coronary artery dissection. Circulation. 2012;126:579–88.
48. Fontanelli A, et al. Spontaneous dissections of coronary arteries and acute coronary syndromes: rationale and design of the DISCOVERY, a multicenter prospective registry with a case–control group. J Cardiovasc Med. 2009;10:94–9.
49. Angelini P. Spontaneous coronary artery dissection: where is the tear? Nature clinical practice. Cardiovasc Med. 2007;4:636–7.
50. Motreff P, et al. Management of spontaneous coronary artery dissection: review of the literature and discussion based on a series of 12 young women with acute coronary syndrome. Cardiology. 2010;115:10–8.

Chapter 4
Noninvasive Diagnosis of Coronary Artery Disease in Women

Karolina M. Zareba and Hanna Z. Mieszczanska

Introduction

Cardiovascular disease is the leading cause of mortality for women in the United States [1]. Annual population statistics continue to report a greater number of deaths from major cardiovascular diseases for women than men [2]. A recent update from the American Heart Association reported that a greater proportion of women die of sudden cardiac death than men [1]. When compared to men, more women have more heart failure and strokes after their first myocardial infarction. Approximately one third more women than men die in the hospital with an acute myocardial infarction. If they do leave the hospital, women die more often within 1 and 5 years of their first myocardial infarction as compared to men [1].

The evaluation of CAD in women presents a difficult and unique challenge for clinicians, due to their greater symptom burden, lower functional capacity, worse clinical outcome, and lower prevalence of obstructive CAD than men [3]. Table 4.1 lists the multiple factors affecting the accuracy of diagnostic testing in women [4]. However, the worse outcomes noted in women highlight the importance of non-invasive testing in early identification of women at risk of CAD.

Based on the Women's Ischemia Syndrome Evaluation (WISE) study, the assessment of CAD in women should not just focus on epicardial disease but also on abnormal coronary reactivity, microvascular dysfunction and distal microembolization. These factors not only contribute to higher rates of angina and ischemia in women, but also to their clinical outcome.

K.M. Zareba, MD
Division of Cardiology, University of Pittsburgh Medical Center, Pittsburgh, PA, USA
e-mail: kzarebamd@gmail.com

H.Z. Mieszczanska, MD (✉)
Division of Cardiology, University of Rochester Medical Center, Rochester, NY, USA
e-mail: hanna_mieszczanska@urmc.rochester.edu

H.Z. Mieszczanska, G.P. Velarde (eds.),
Management of Cardiovascular Disease in Women,
DOI 10.1007/978-1-4471-5517-1_4, © Springer-Verlag London 2014

Table 4.1 Factors affecting accuracy of diagnostic testing in women

Lower prevalence of coronary artery disease
Higher prevalence of non-ischaemic chest pain (microvascular abnormalities, mitral valve prolaps)
Less predictive symptomatology
Limited exercise tolerance due to older age at initial diagnosis
Different response to exercise than men
Limited exercise capacity (mostly due to older age)
Lower peak exercise values
Lesser increase in left ventricular ejection fraction
Increase in cardiac output by enhancing end-diastolic volume
Inappropriate catecholamine release
Hormonal influences of oestrongens mimicking digitalis-like false positive ECG response
Anatomical differences affecting stress test results
Female breast attenuation artefacts
Smaller coronary artery size
Smaller left ventricular chamber size
Higher prevalence of single vessel disease

Reprinted with permission from [4]

This chapter focuses on the noninvasive evaluation of CAD in women. Various classic and novel methods of establishing risk and diagnosing CAD are discussed along with specific benefits and pitfalls of each approach. A proposed approach is included at the end.

Noninvasive Diagnostic Testing

Noninvasive testing is used in the diagnosis and risk stratification of CAD to better identify patients who would benefit from medical therapy or revascularization procedures, as well as to exclude CAD. Although substantial research efforts have been made to improve the diagnosis and treatment strategies for women at risk, the detection of CAD in women can be problematic. A great challenge in diagnostic testing in women is selecting the appropriate test for the patient. Establishing pre-test probability is imperative to achieving optimal incremental value in post-test information. Thus selection of candidates for diagnostic testing is based on Bayesian theory, in which the post-test likelihood becomes a function of the patient's pre-test risk [5]. In low-risk women, the change from pre-test to post-test risk estimation is minimal. However, non-invasive testing is most useful in the intermediate-risk population, as it may shift women to lower-risk cohorts with negative test results, or higher-risk cohorts with abnormal results.

Early detection of ischemic heart disease is especially important in symptomatic women. As mentioned before, women with CAD experience worse outcomes than men, irrespective of age. These gender based differences exist as women tend to have more advanced disease, due to lack of early recognition and management. Accurately chosen noninvasive diagnostic tests can be useful in identifying women at the earliest stage of presentation so that appropriate therapeutic strategies can be implemented early on to improve the outcomes [4, 6, 7].

Establishing Risk

In the asymptomatic woman the goal of risk assessment is to identify those patients at increased risk of developing CAD. This can be achieved by various methods including patient history, risk factors, risk prediction scores, and biomarkers.

Various risk scores have been developed which incorporate numerous risk factors and attempt to stratify patients into low, intermediate or high risk categories. The Framingham risk score (FRS) is a global risk score which utilizes traditional risk factors for CAD including age, smoking, blood pressure, diabetes, and cholesterol values [8]. Women with low, intermediate, and high FRS have expected annual rates of CAD death or myocardial infarction of less than 0.6 % (low risk), 0.6–2.0 % (intermediate risk), and greater than 2 % (high risk), respectively. However, the FRS often underestimates risk in women [9]. In the Multi-Ethnic Study of Atherosclerosis, when excluding women with diabetes and those older than 79 years, 90 % of women were classified as "low risk" based on the FRS [10]. The use of coronary artery calcium scoring led to significant re-classification in this cohort.

The Reynolds risk score is a recently derived and validated gender-specific tool for predicting incident cardiovascular events (myocardial infarction, ischemic stroke, coronary revascularization, and cardiovascular death) [11]. The score includes age, systolic blood pressure, high-sensitivity C-reactive protein, total cholesterol, high density lipoprotein cholesterol (HDL), hemoglobin A1c, smoking status, and family history of premature myocardial infarction. When compared to the FRS, use of the Reynolds score resulted in risk reclassification in >40 % of intermediate FRS women.

The novel risk marker used in the Reynolds risk score, high-sensitivity C-reactive protein (hsCRP), has been shown to improve detection of CAD in women. Women on average have greater mean CRP measures from early age as compared to men [12]. It appears that this difference in CRP accounts for greater frequency of inflammatory mediated autoimmune diseases in women as compared to men, suggesting a possible role of inflammation in gender difference of CAD. Studies have shown that the relative risk of future cardiac events increases proportionally with increasing levels of hsCRP, thus accelerating risk [13, 14]. A position paper from the European Society of Cardiology noted that CRP is one of the best candidates for screening; however, evidence is lacking to recommend its routine use [15]. They noted that a CRP >3 mg/L reclassified only 5 % of intermediate risk women. Thus CRP has the greatest utility when is combined with the Reynolds risk score.

Several other risk factors are worth mentioning given the substantial gender-related variability in the prevalence and outcome associated with them. Hypertriglyceridemia is a potent independent risk factor for ischemic heart disease in women as compared to men [16]. In a meta-analysis of 17 studies hypertriglyceridemia increased the risk for coronary heart disease by 32 % in men and 76 % in women [17]. In a report from the WISE study, women with metabolic syndrome have an increased prevalence of subclinical disease and are at a two-fold higher relative risk for cardiac events as compared to women with a normal metabolic status [18].

Hormonal changes throughout a woman's lifetime also appear to play a key role in their risk for ischemic heart disease. Ovarian dysfunction, as seen in functional hypothalamic amenorrhea as well as polycystic ovarian syndrome, has been shown to be associated with premature atherosclerosis [19, 20]. A recent meta-analysis found that preeclampsia doubles the risk for subsequent ischemic heart disease [21]. Thus, obtaining a gynecological and obstetrical history can aid in further risk stratification.

An interesting new tool on the horizon is a gene expression score (GES) which was recently developed and validated as a reliable diagnostic approach in the assessment of non-diabetic patients, especially women, with suspected obstructive CAD [22]. The algorithm uses gender, age, and the expression level of 23 genes which then generates a score on a 1- to 40-point scale, where increasing scores indicate increasing likelihood of obstructive CAD. As compared to symptom or myocardial perfusion imaging diagnostic approaches, the GES performed similarly in women and men. The GES may be especially helpful in the assessment of obstructive CAD in non-diabetic women for whom the use of symptoms and functional testing has proven unreliable. In future decades further advances in genetically based risk stratification will allow for more tailored gender-based evaluation of CAD risk.

Evaluation of Atherosclerotic Burden

The noninvasive measurement of atherosclerotic burden is another great tool for evaluating women at risk of adverse ischemic events. An established tool used in clinical practice is the ankle brachial index. Studies have shown that in women, the prevalence of an ankle brachial index ≤0.90 increases with age (approximately <5 % for women <60 years of age, up to 10–35 % in women 60–80 years of age) and is more prevalent in Black and Hispanic women [23, 24]. The 10-year cardiovascular mortality for an ankle brachial index ≤0.90 even after adjusting for the Framingham Risk score was significantly elevated in women (HR 3.0, 95 % CI 2.0–4.4) and men (HR 2.9, 95 % CI 2.3–3.7) [25].

Novel imaging techniques have allowed further evaluation of subclinical CAD in women. The roles of carotid intima media thickness (IMT) as well as presence of focal plaques detected by ultrasonography have been extensively studied as subclinical atherosclerotic markers. In women a low risk carotid IMT was associated with a ~1 % 10 year coronary heart disease risk versus ~10 % for a high risk carotid IMT [26]. A higher carotid IMT predicted a relatively greater risk of coronary heart disease for women than men [27].

The measurement of coronary calcifications using coronary CT is another useful marker of atherosclerotic disease burden. Coronary artery calcium (CAC) measurements, with either electron beam tomography or multidetector CT, are calculated and translated into a mean Agatston score which further places patients in various risk categories. In one study of 220 women with a normal coronary arteriogram, none had detectable CAC thus yielding a negative predictive value of 100 % [28]. However, women with moderate (≥100) or high (≥400) CAC scores had greater prevalence of obstructive coronary disease in the same study. In a large cohort of over 10,000 asymptomatic patients (>4,000 women), the extent of CAC was an independent and incremental estimator of all-cause mortality [29]. For women, as compared to a CAC score of ≤10, the risk-adjusted relative risk ratios for all-cause mortality were elevated according to increasing CAC values: 2.5 for a CAC value of 11–100, 3.7 for CAC of 101–400, 6.3 for a CAC of 401–1,000, and 12.3 for a CAC of >1,000 ($p < 0.0001$). Importantly, in this large cohort, for a given CAC score mortality rates were 3–5 fold higher for women as compared to men – thus suggesting a need for gender-specific cutoff values. Calcified plaque burden parallels overall plaque burden as CAC is almost always present in cases of angiographically significant CAD, and thus demonstrates great sensitivity but low specificity since detection of calcification implies atherosclerosis, but it is not specific for luminal obstruction and does not reveal the hemodynamic significance of the stenosis [4]. However, the test has a high negative predictive value when no calcifications are identified.

Exercise Stress Testing

The exercise ECG is the oldest and most commonly used form of stress testing. Multiple studies have shown profound gender differences when using treadmill ECG testing. According to the ACC/AHA exercise testing guidelines, women should undergo exercise testing if they are at an intermediate pretest probability for CAD on the basis of symptoms and risk factors, have a normal ECG, and are capable of maximal exercise [30]. However, exercise ECG testing has diminished accuracy in women. In a meta-analysis of over 3,000 women undergoing exercise ECG studies, the sensitivity and specificity were 61 and 70 % respectively for detection of obstructive CAD [31]. In similar studies, the mean sensitivity and specificity in men were 72 and 77 %, respectively [30].

Several factors account for gender based differences in the accuracy of exercise ECG testing. Women tend to have lower CAD prevalence and a greater prevalence of single-vessel disease as compared to men, they tend to be older when they present, and women have decreased exercise tolerance – all factors contributing to a decreased ability of the test to induce ischemia and ST depression thus limiting accurate identification of women with CAD [7]. Women more often have resting ST-T wave changes and lower ECG voltage [32].

Several studies have shown that significant exertional ST segment depression in women did not differ between those surviving vs. those dying from cardiovascular death during a follow up period of 20 years [33, 34]. However, marked ST segment changes (≥2 mm ST depression, horizontal or downsloping) occurring at low workloads or persisting into recovery confirmed high risk status for women [32].

The use of the Duke treadmill score (DTS) has been shown to improve the accuracy of exercise ECG testing in women. The DTS is defined as exercise time – (5×ST deviation) – (4×chest pain [1 =nonlimiting, 2=limiting]). In a study of over 900 symptomatic women undergoing exercise ECG testing followed by coronary angiography, significant coronary stenoses (≥75 %) were present in 19, 35, and 89 % of low-, moderate-, and high risk women based on their DTS risk categories [35]. Another study of >5,000 asymptomatic women evaluated the association of the DTS and mortality [36]. They noted that after adjusting for the FRS, the risk of death decreased by 9 % for each unit increase in the DTS. Those women with a DTS <5 (moderate or high risk) had hazard ratios for death and cardiac death that were 2.2 and 2.5 times greater, respectively, than did those who had a DTS ≥5 (low risk), after adjusting for the FRS.

Functional capacity is a major predictor of adverse coronary events and all-cause mortality in both men and women. Women often have lower functional capacity as compared to men and have a greater functional decline with age [37]. Sedentary women are often incapable of performing greater than five metabolic equivalents (which are required to proceed to stage II of the aggressive Bruce protocol) due to excessive dyspnea and premature fatigue, thus leading to inadequate diagnostic information. In the abovementioned study of over 900 asymptomatic women, the investigators noted that the predictive value of the DTS was entirely due to the exercise component of the score. For each one metabolic equivalent increase in exercise capacity, the mortality was decreased by 17 % after adjusting for the FRS [36].

To better approximate performance during exercise ECG testing, it is important to estimate a woman's ability to perform activities of daily living as a guide to approximate peak metabolic equivalent levels. The Duke Activity Status Index (DASI) is a brief, self-administered, 12 item questionnaire which evaluates a subjects' ability to perform a variety of common activities of daily living, and was found to be a valid measure of functional capacity [38]. In the WISE study, two thirds of the cardiac events in women occurred in those with an estimated capacity of less than 4.7 DASI metabolic equivalents [39]. Women achieving less than 4.7 metabolic equivalents had a 3.7 fold increased risk of death or non-fatal myocardial infraction when compared to women reporting higher functional capacity. In the same study, each one metabolic equivalent increase in the DASI score was independently associated with an 8 % decrease in the risk of major adverse cardiovascular events. The current exercise testing guidelines support referral to pharmacologic stress testing with imaging in patients with submaximal exercise capacity [30].

The heart rate response further aids in risk stratification of women. The inability to reach 85 % of maximum age-predicted heart rate (HR) in women has been associated with a higher likelihood of CAD as well as with a decreased survival [40, 41]. Heart rate recovery in the first few minutes also improves risk assessment. In a study of 720 women undergoing exercise ECG testing and subsequent coronary angiography, 30 % had an abnormal HR recovery (defined as a decrease of HR

12 bpm or less in the first minute of recovery), which was independently predictive of death after adjustment for multiple covariates (HR 1.5, 95 % CI 1.2–1.9) [42]. Data on blood pressure response to exercise have been inconclusive in women.

Hormonal factors also play a role in exercise testing. Endogenous estrogen may have a digoxin-like effect thus promoting higher false positive exercise ECG rates in premenopausal women [3]. Angina and ischemia have been shown to vary by the menstrual cycle as well [43]. In the luteal/menstrual phase, where estradiol levels are low, a greater prevalence of ischemia and reduced time to ischemia onset have been noted. In postmenopausal women, hormone replacement therapy may result in false negative test results due to its vasodilatory properties [3].

Up until recently, there has been a lack of randomized controlled trials to guide diagnostic decisions in women thus resulting in variability of utilization patterns of various testing strategies. A recent randomized trial (What Is the Optimal Method for Ischemia Evaluation in Women [WOMEN] trial) of 824 symptomatic middle-aged (median = 62 years) women with suspected CAD evaluated the incremental value of myocardial perfusion imaging in clinical decision making over standard exercise ECG testing [44]. At 2 years of follow-up there was no difference in major adverse events (CAD death or hospitalization for acute coronary syndrome or heart failure) between both groups. Thus in low risk women, capable of exercise, the use of exercise ECG as the initial diagnostic strategy yielded similar outcomes to myocardial perfusion imaging but with significant diagnostic cost saving.

The exercise ECG is a commonly used form of stress testing; however, women who have an abnormal resting ECG, a decreased exercise capacity, or diabetes mellitus may need to undergo cardiac imaging with either exercise or pharmacologic stress.

Stress Echocardiography

Stress echocardiography is a useful tool not only for evaluation of stress induced ischemia but also for systolic and diastolic dysfunction, and the extent of ischemia and infarction. Assessment of valvular heart disease, or pericardial abnormalities can also help reveal an alternate explanation for symptoms of dyspnea or chest pain. Exercise echocardiography can be performed via a treadmill or bicycle, while for patients who cannot exercise, dobutamine is the most commonly used pharmacologic stress agent. Stress echocardiography has been shown to have high accuracy in detecting CAD in women.

Based on a compilation of meta-analyses on the diagnostic accuracy of stress echocardiography in women, the mean sensitivity was 84 % and mean specificity was 76 % [3]. When comparing exercise echocardiography to an exercise score (encompassing exercise ECG interpretation and exercise capacity and hemodynamics) in women, exercise echocardiography had higher sensitivity and specificity [45]. In a meta-analysis specifically comparing exercise ECG, exercise echocardiography, and exercise thallium for the diagnosis of angiographically confirmed

CAD in women, the investigators found that exercise echocardiography had the highest sensitivity and specificity of all three modalities [31]. Although stress echocardiography has somewhat lower sensitivity for detecting intermediate stenoses or single-vessel CAD, its high negative predictive value makes it particularly useful test to exclude ischemia in younger women [46]. Exercise echocardiography appears to have the best balance between accuracy and cost for the diagnosis of coronary artery disease in women as compared to exercise ECG [47].

Dobutamine stress echocardiography (DSE) has been found to have a mean sensitivity of 80 % and specificity of 84 % in a large meta-analysis, both higher than pharmacologic stress testing with adenosine or dipyridamole [48]. One study of 306 patients (96 women), found that the overall specificity and the regional accuracy of DSE was higher in women than in men [49].

Stress echocardiography has been shown to be useful for determining cardiovascular prognosis in women. One study showed that the results of exercise echocardiography have comparable implications in both men and women when evaluating outcomes of cardiac death and nonfatal myocardial infarction [50]. A large study examined the 5-year mortality in 4,234 women undergoing exercise or dobutamine stress echocardiography [51]. Risk-adjusted 5-year survival was 99.4, 97.6, and 95 % for exercising women with no, single, and multi-vessel ischemia. Significantly worse survival was noted for women undergoing dobutamine stress, where 5-year survival was 95, 89, and 86.6 % for those with no, single, and multi-vessel ischemia. A more recent study of over 8,000 patients (3,208 women) undergoing stress echocardiography (exercise, dobutamine, and dipyridamole) evaluated its prognostic value of suspected and known CAD [52]. In patients with known CAD, women had a higher event rate than men in the presence of ischemia. The annual event rate of death or nonfatal MI was 7.0 % in women and 5.8 % in men with CAD (p=0.08). The annual event rate was 2.4 % in women and 3.6 % in men with suspected CAD (p<0.0001).

Limitations to stress echocardiography include poor acoustic windows due to obesity or breast tissue as well as lung disease; however lack of radiation makes it an attractive option. In women, stress echocardiography with exercise or dobutamine is an effective and accurate noninvasive method of detecting ischemia and risk stratifying symptomatic women with intermediate to high pretest likelihood of CAD.

Myocardial Perfusion Imaging

Changes in myocardial perfusion are one of the first manifestations in the time course of the ischemic cascade, preceding wall motion abnormalities, ECG changes, and symptoms (Fig. 4.1). Myocardial perfusion imaging may thus provide a more precise measure of estimating CAD risk. Myocardial perfusion can be evaluated in women using single-photon emission computer tomography (SPECT), positron-emission tomography, or cardiac magnetic resonance (CMR).

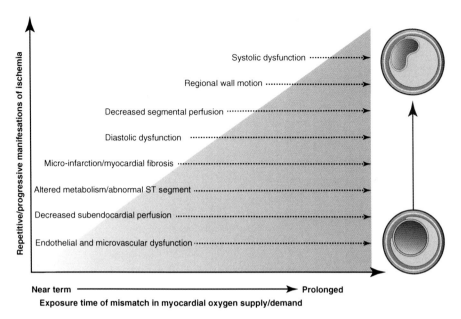

Fig. 4.1 Ischemic cascade (Reprinted with permission from [53])

Nuclear Myocardial Perfusion Imaging

The most commonly nuclear based myocardial perfusion imaging technique used today is single-photon emission computer tomography (SPECT) which can provide information on perfusion defects, global and regional ventricular function, and left ventricular volumes.

The average diagnostic accuracy based on several meta-analyses of stress SPECT imaging in women reveals a sensitivity of 81 % and specificity of 66 % [3]. In a study evaluating patients with known and suspected CAD, when correcting for selection bias, the sensitivity and specificity results did not differ significantly between men and women [54]. Another study comparing the diagnostic accuracy of thallium-201 (Tl-201) with gated technetium-99m (Tc-99m) sestamibi SPECT in women noted that the sensitivity for detecting CAD was similar for both tests [55]. However, specificity improved dramatically from 67 % for Tl-201 to 92 % for gated Tc-99 sestamibi SPECT. When focusing on symptomatic postmenopausal women undergoing exercise or pharmacologic stress ECG gated SPECT imaging, the sensitivity and specificity were both 88 % [56]. In men and women with left bundle-branch block, vasodilator pharmacologic stress SPECT imaging has been shown to be more accurate than exercise perfusion imaging in the identification of CAD [57].

Multiple large studies have demonstrated the powerful predictive value of myocardial perfusion imaging in women. In a study of 3,402 women and 5,009 men with symptoms, stress SPECT imaging had a similar prognostic ability regardless of gender [58]. For women without ischemia the 3 year survival rates were 99 % as compared to 85 % for those with ischemia of three vessel territories. A normal myocardial perfusion study demonstrated an annual cardiac event rate of <1 % in pooled data from more than 7,500 women [5]. The abovementioned study of postmenopausal women undergoing SPECT imaging also evaluated 5-year occurrence of hospitalization for acute coronary syndrome, myocardial infarction and new onset or worsening angina [56]. Cox survival analysis showed a 5-year cumulative event-free survival rate of 94 % for patients with normal test results, as compared to 48 % for those with abnormal SPECT scans. Dual-isotope myocardial perfusion imaging yields incremental prognostic value in both men and women; however, it is able to identify high risk women more accurately than high risk men [59].

Diabetic women are a special high risk group of patients for which myocardial perfusion imaging is especially beneficial in predicting outcomes. In a study of men and women with and without diabetes, the survival rates (both for death and death or myocardial infarction) for diabetic women were the lowest for any amount of ischemia as compared to all other groups [60]. Cardiac event rates were significantly higher among the 451 diabetic women than in the 1,635 nondiabetic women (8 % vs. 3.2 %, respectively; p < 0.01). Another study of over 5,000 patients (~50 % women) showed that dual isotope adenosine SPECT imaging provided incremental value over pre-scan data for the prediction of cardiac death in both genders [61]. Similarly, this study illustrated that diabetic women and patients with insulin-dependent diabetes had a significantly greater risk of cardiac death than other patients for any SPECT result.

A recent study evaluated the effect of gender on the prognostic information obtained from left ventricular volume indices and ejection fraction in a SPECT studies [62]. ECG-gated SPECT studies were evaluated for end-systolic and diastolic volume indices as well as ejection fraction in 891 patients (43 % women), and were used to predict hard cardiac events as well as the combined endpoint of all-cause mortality or non-fatal myocardial infarction. The investigators noted that women had smaller left ventricular volume indices and higher ejection fraction despite equivalent rates of hard cardiac events and the combined endpoint mentioned above. Thus, in women, the risk of subsequent events starts at smaller volume indices compared to men despite similar risk profiles.

There are several important limitations to SPECT imaging in women [32]. Women have smaller hearts raising the possibility that smaller areas of reduced myocardial perfusion may be missed as a result of limitation in spatial resolution. Breast tissue attenuation and obesity can interfere with image quality and cause false positive results. As SPECT flow is comparatively assessed across the myocardium, it can appear normal in the setting of global reductions in perfusion such as multi-vessel CAD, diffuse endothelial or microvascular disease, left ventricular hypertrophy, or cardiomyopathy [53]. Lastly, radiation exposure is of concern. The addition of ECG gating, attenuation correction protocols, and use of higher energy radioisotope technetium (which allowed lower dosing) have made SPECT imaging less problematic in women. Newer techniques such as ultrafast cardiac SPECT cameras with cadmium-zinc-telluride (CZT) -based detectors are faster, produce

Table 4.2 Comparison of diagnostic accuracy of commonly ordered tests

Author, year (Ref.)	Exercise electrocardiography		Stress echocardiography		Stress SPECT	
	Sensitivity (%)	Specificity (%)	Sensitivity (%)	Specificity (%)	Sensitivity (%)	Specificity (%)
Fleischmann et al., 1998 [94]	–	–	85	77	87	64
Kwok et al., 1999 [31]	61	70	86	79	78	64
Beattie et al., 2003 [95]	–	–	81	73	77	69
Average	61	70	84	76	81	66

Reprinted with permission from [3]

higher quality images as compared to conventional SPECT cameras, and may allow lower mean radiation dose and shorter imaging time [63]. Recent reports of stress SPECT imaging with only 4–5 mCi Tc-99m dose and a 12–16 min acquisition time in non-obese patients have been feasible, thus decreasing the patient's time in the imaging laboratory and decreasing the patient's radiation exposure [64]. Use of stress only protocol with this camera in patients with symptoms, presence of cardiac risk factors, but no prior history of CAD, can allow ultra-low dose of radiation (only 1–2 mSv), which may be especially useful in women.

Stress myocardial perfusion imaging is recommended for symptomatic women with intermediate to high pretest likelihood of CAD. Intermediate risk women, who have normal test results are unlikely to have CAD and usually do not need further testing. A normal SPECT in women has an excellent negative predictive value of 99 % and carries a very low event rate (<1 %) [65, 66].

Table 4.2 presents a comparison of diagnostic accuracy of commonly ordered tests.

Positron Emission Tomography

Myocardial perfusion imaging with the use of positron emission tomography (PET) is a novel tool which appears to be promising in women. Although gender based data is limited, diagnostic accuracy is very comparable in men and women, with a pooled mean sensitivity of 90 % and specificity of 89 % [67]. PET imaging has several advantages in women compared to SPECT, including superior spatial resolution, improved attenuation correction, and the additional data of blood flow [68]. This last advantage is particularly important in women as it permits quantification of regional and global myocardial blood flow to assess microvascular disease. In a study of 1,432 patients (~50 % women), vasodilator stress rubidium-82 PET myocardial perfusion imaging provided incremental prognostic value to historical and clinical variables as well as rest EF in predicting cardiac death or nonfatal myocardial infarction as well as all-cause death [69]. Of note, the effective radiation dose appears slightly greater for PET when compared to single isotope rest-stress SPECT imaging [70].

Cardiovascular Magnetic Resonance

Cardiac magnetic resonance (CMR) has developed progressively over the past few decades and, in its present form, provides a comprehensive cardiovascular assessment. It is the single imaging technology which can assess left and right ventricular function and mass, detailed anatomic evaluation of cardiac morphology and vasculature, as well as perfusion, viability, and metabolism. Myocardial cardiac perfusion images can be collected at rest and under stress (pharmacologic vasodilation with adenosine, or with dobutamine stress) during the first passage of gadolinium-based contrast agents. CMR has special advantages in women as it has excellent soft tissue characterization, three-dimensionality, superior temporal and spatial resolution, and the ability to quantify blood flow. CMR is free from ionizing radiation thereby avoiding radiation exposure to sensitive tissues, which can be especially important in women, as breast tissue is known to be sensitive to developing cancer as a result of radiation exposure.

Figure 4.2 shows a stress CMR in a woman with angina and triple vessel disease.

Recent studies have shown superior diagnostic accuracy of stress CMR in women. A report of 745 patients (204 women) undergoing dobutamine/atropine stress CMR and subsequent coronary angiography showed no gender-based differences in the detection of hemodynamically significant obstructive CAD, with a sensitivity of 85 % and specificity of 86 % in women [72]. Similar results have been found with adenosine first pass perfusion CMR in 256 symptomatic patients (77 females) at intermediate risk of CAD who underwent subsequent coronary angiography [73]. Adenosine first pass perfusion CMR in women had a sensitivity and specificity of 91 % for detecting significant CAD, superior to the results in men.

Stress CMR has been compared to other imaging modalities. The use of dobutamine CMR and DSE was evaluated in a study of 208 patients (61 women) undergoing both tests prior to coronary angiography [74]. The sensitivity and specificity was greatly increased with the use of dobutamine CMR as compared to DSE, and the sub-analysis in women yielded similar results. A recent pilot study compared the new technique of treadmill stress CMR with exercise SPECT in 43 patients

| DE-CMR | Stress-Perfusion | Rest-Perfusion | Coronary Angiogram |

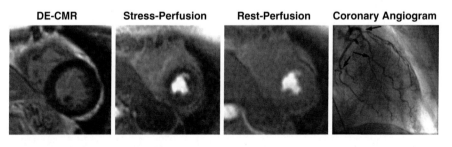

Fig. 4.2 Stress CMR in a woman with angina and triple vessel disease. There is no evidence of prior infarction on delayed-enhancement images; however, stress perfusion indicated defects in all three vascular territories. *DE-CMR* Delayed Enhancement CMR (Adapted with permission from [71])

(16 women) [75]. In this special combined protocol, patients underwent a rest technetium-99 SPECT and resting cine CMR and then proceeded to exercise on a modified CMR safe treadmill with ECG monitoring. At peak stress, technetium-99 was injected and the patient rapidly returned to the CMR scanner for post-exercise cine and perfusion imaging, and lastly was sent to complete the SPECT stress portion. In this small study, agreement between SPECT and CMR was moderate (kappa = 0.58) and the accuracy in eight patients who underwent coronary angiography was 7/8 for CMR and 5/8 for SPECT. A larger study comparing these two exercise stress modalities is currently underway.

The prognostic value of stress CMR has been demonstrated in several studies. A report of 461 patients (150 women) with known or suspected CAD, evaluated the prognostic value of a combined adenosine and dobutamine stress CMR assessed during a single session in predicting cardiac death or nonfatal myocardial infarction [76]. The 3-year event free survival was 99.2 % for patients with normal stress CMR scans and 83.5 % for those with abnormal results. Ischemia noted on stress CMR was an independent predictor of cardiac events and provided incremental value over clinical risk factors and resting wall motion abnormalities. Similar prognostic value has been shown for dobutamine/atropine CMR [77]. A recent study focusing on 266 women undergoing dobutamine CMR showed that inducible left ventricular wall motion abnormalities predicted cardiac death and myocardial infarction (HR 4.1, 95 % CI, 2.2–9.4) [78]

A very interesting report of 20 patients with syndrome X (16 women) and 10 matched controls (8 women) evaluated the use of adenosine stress CMR in detecting perfusion abnormalities in this patient population [79]. Syndrome X is characterized by atypical angina with abnormal exercise test results but normal coronaries; however, ischemia has not been implicated as the cause of chest pain in these patients. Adenosine administration provoked chest pain in 95 % of patients with syndrome X and CMR imaging demonstrated subendocardial hypoperfusion during these symptoms. This is especially interesting in women as they often have chest pain in the absence of obstructive CAD which may be attributed to microvascular angina. In the Coronary Artery Surgery Study, 50 % of women with chest pain referred for coronary angiography had minimal or no significant coronary stenoses, in contrast to 17 % of men [80]. In the WISE study, coronary microvascular dysfunction was also identified in half of the women with angina in the absence of obstructive epicardial disease [81]. The prognosis in these women is not benign as they have higher burden of persistent angina and potentially higher morbidity and mortality.

Stress CMR appears to be an excellent comprehensive imaging technique in evaluating CAD in women and has the ability to identify subendocardial ischemia, which may provide an etiology for women with persistent chest pain without obstructive CAD. However, CMR does have several limitations. Renal impairment is not a contraindication to gadolinium administration, however there is increased risk of nephrogenic systemic fibrosis in patients with severe renal failure. MRI incompatible hardware is a true contraindication; however, next generation devices (i.e. pacemakers) are now considered CMR safe.

Coronary CT Angiography

Coronary computer tomographic angiography (CTA) is an evolving noninvasive anatomic technique with high diagnostic accuracy for obstructive epicardial CAD [67]. It allows non-invasive visualization of coronary arteries and accurate detection of obstructive lesions as compared with invasive coronary angiography. In a study comparing the diagnostic accuracy of 64-slice coronary CTA in 51 women and 52 men, the sensitivity was 85 % and specificity was 99 % in both genders [82]. A recently published study of 230 patients (41 % women) undergoing both coronary CTA and invasive coronary angiography found that women tended to have more diffuse CAD, and at a 70 % stenosis threshold, the specificity of coronary CTA favored women when compared to men (94 % vs. 73 %, $P=0.001$) [83].

A recent large study (2,432 patients, 56 % female) evaluated the gender specific prognostic value of coronary CTA for predicting a composite endpoint of cardiac death and nonfatal myocardial infarction [84]. They noted that after age and gender stratification coronary CTA predicted events in women aged at least 60 years but not in women under 60 years old (coronary CTA predicted events in males of any age).

One important limitation to point out, particularly in younger women, is the increased radiation exposure, higher than that of conventional diagnostic coronary angiography. This is a factor which has to be taken into consideration in women with a potential increase in lifetime risk of cancer due to concentrated ionizing radiation to breast tissue [85]. Further studies are needed to reduce radiation exposure and evaluate the true prognostic value of coronary CTA in women across all age groups. However, coronary CTA allows accurate ruling out of obstructive CAD in women given that the negative predictive value exceeds 95 % – thus a normal study suggest an extremely low likelihood of obstructive stenoses in the epicardial arteries [82].

In conclusion, CTA represent an attractive method of excluding CAD in selected women with low to intermediate probability of disease, or for whom a false-positive stress test results are suspected [4].

Coronary Reactivity Testing

Women are disproportionally affected by vascular reactivity in the coronary circulation as well as other organ systems (examples include migraine headaches, Raynaulds phenomena) [53]. Vasospasm of the epicardial coronary arteries was thought to be the major contributor to angina in women; however, recent research identifies the microvascular coronary circulation as a culprit (Fig. 4.3). Studies show that men have greater atheroma burden and more diffuse epicardial endothelial dysfunction while women have more disease of the microcirculation [86, 87].

The WISE trial which focused on women evaluated coronary microvascular dysfunction in several studies. In a subset of 159 women with angina but no obstructive CAD, coronary microvascular dysfunction was evaluated by measuring coronary flow velocity reserve in response to intracoronary adenosine [81]. The investigators noted that approximately half of women with angina had coronary microvascular

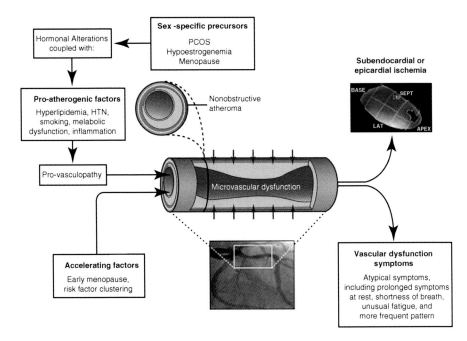

Fig. 4.3 Model of microvascular angina in women (Reprinted with permission from [53])

dysfunction, and this could not be predicted by standard CAD risk factors and hormone levels. Another WISE substudy evaluated cardiovascular outcomes in a similar patient population and noted that impaired coronary vasomotor response independently predicted adverse cardiac events regardless of CAD severity [88]. In a complication of 15 studies on coronary and peripheral testing for endothelial dysfunction, an abnormal result elevated the relative risk for major adverse cardiac events 10-fold [89]. Endothelial dysfunction appears to be an early sign of future CAD as shown in a study of women with sequential angiography after invasive endothelial function testing [90]. Figure 4.3 shows a model of microvascular angina in women.

Evaluation of endothelial dysfunction is important as it is reversible and thus associated with improved outcomes. In a study of 400 postmenopausal women with hypertension, improvement in flow mediated vasodilation (as measured by brachial artery ultrasonography) was seen with optimization of blood pressure and had a positive impact on prognosis [91]. Brachial artery size may be helpful to identify women with early atherosclerosis [92]. Another study evaluated the use of enhanced external counterpulsation (EECP) in patients with refractory angina by using reactive hyperemia-peripheral arterial tonometry. EECP enhanced peripheral endothelial function and led to symptomatic improvement [93].

In symptomatic women with positive stress test results and no evidence of obstructive disease on coronary angiography, further diagnostic testing may be warranted. Aside from invasive measures during coronary angiography, such as intravascular coronary ultrasound and intracoronary Doppler flow wire, noninvasive methods are now becoming available (i.e. brachial artery reactivity testing, digital reactive hyperemia peripheral artery tonometry, high frequency transthoracic Doppler harmonic echocardiography) and should be utilized.

Conclusions

Coronary artery disease has gender-specific differences in presentation as well as course and outcome. Despite a lower prevalence of obstructive CAD in women, the prevalence of symptoms and ischemia as well as mortality is higher in women. Multiple risk stratification and diagnostic strategies are available for the noninvasive evaluation of CAD in women. Obtaining a thorough history and exam, with special attention to atypical symptoms frequently experienced by women, can guide clinicians as to which strategy is best for each individual patient. Traditional risk factors along with novel risk scores and diagnostic tests to evaluate atherosclerotic burden can help identify women at risk. The diagnostic tests available for symptomatic women are expanding – with newer tests having greater diagnostic accuracy in women. In symptomatic women with suspected CAD, imaging with stress MPI or stress echocardiography can provide incremental value over clinical variables and exercise ECG. Novel methods for evaluating microvascular disease, including CMR and PET, and tests to detect endothelial dysfunction may yield further information for symptomatic women without obstructive CAD. Figure 4.4 summarizes the

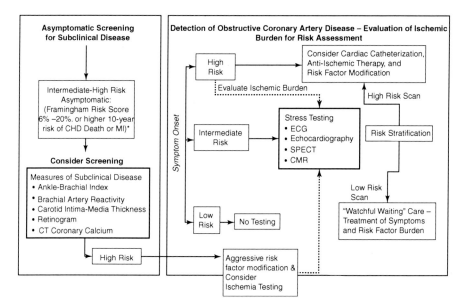

Fig. 4.4 Proposed mechanism for evaluating women for CAD (Reprinted with permission from [3])

proposed mechanism for evaluating women for the presence of CAD. Continued research is needed to better identify the optimal diagnostic and therapeutic approaches for women with CAD.

References

1. Go AS, et al. Heart disease and stroke statistics–2013 update: a report from the American Heart Association. Circulation. 2013;127(1):e6–245.
2. CDC. Center for Disease Control and Prevention – Deaths: final data for 2010. Available from: http://www.cdc.gov/nchs/data/dvs/deaths_2010_release.pdf. Accessed 20 Mar 2013.
3. Shaw LJ, et al. Insights from the NHLBI-Sponsored Women's Ischemia Syndrome Evaluation (WISE) Study: Part I: gender differences in traditional and novel risk factors, symptom evaluation, and gender-optimized diagnostic strategies. J Am Coll Cardiol. 2006;47(3 Suppl):S4–20.
4. Stangl V, et al. Current diagnostic concepts to detect coronary artery disease in women. Eur Heart J. 2008;29(6):707–17.
5. Shaw LJ, Iskandrian AE. Prognostic value of gated myocardial perfusion SPECT. J Nucl Cardiol. 2004;11(2):171–85.
6. Harrington RA. Women, acute ischemic heart disease, and antithrombotic therapy: challenges and opportunities. Circulation. 2007;115(22):2796–8.
7. Kohli P, Gulati M. Exercise stress testing in women: going back to the basics. Circulation. 2010;122(24):2570–80.
8. Califf RM, et al. 27th Bethesda Conference: matching the intensity of risk factor management with the hazard for coronary disease events. Task Force 5. Stratification of patients into high, medium and low risk subgroups for purposes of risk factor management. J Am Coll Cardiol. 1996;27(5):1007–19.
9. Michos ED, et al. Framingham risk equation underestimates subclinical atherosclerosis risk in asymptomatic women. Atherosclerosis. 2006;184(1):201–6.
10. Lakoski SG, et al. Coronary artery calcium scores and risk for cardiovascular events in women classified as "low risk" based on Framingham risk score: the multi-ethnic study of atherosclerosis (MESA). Arch Intern Med. 2007;167(22):2437–42.
11. Ridker PM, et al. Development and validation of improved algorithms for the assessment of global cardiovascular risk in women: the Reynolds Risk Score. JAMA. 2007;297(6):611–9.
12. Wong ND, et al. Distribution of C-reactive protein and its relation to risk factors and coronary heart disease risk estimation in the National Health and Nutrition Examination Survey (NHANES) III. Prev Cardiol. 2001;4(3):109–14.
13. Cook NR, Buring JE, Ridker PM. The effect of including C-reactive protein in cardiovascular risk prediction models for women. Ann Intern Med. 2006;145(1):21–9.
14. Ridker PM, et al. C-reactive protein, the metabolic syndrome, and risk of incident cardiovascular events: an 8-year follow-up of 14 719 initially healthy American women. Circulation. 2003;107(3):391–7.
15. Vaccarino V, et al. Ischaemic heart disease in women: are there sex differences in pathophysiology and risk factors? Position paper from the working group on coronary pathophysiology and microcirculation of the European Society of Cardiology. Cardiovasc Res. 2011;90(1):9–17.
16. Lerner DJ, Kannel WB. Patterns of coronary heart disease morbidity and mortality in the sexes: a 26-year follow-up of the Framingham population. Am Heart J. 1986;111(2):383–90.
17. Hokanson JE, Austin MA. Plasma triglyceride level is a risk factor for cardiovascular disease independent of high-density lipoprotein cholesterol level: a meta-analysis of population-based prospective studies. J Cardiovasc Risk. 1996;3(2):213–9.
18. Marroquin OC, et al. Metabolic syndrome modifies the cardiovascular risk associated with angiographic coronary artery disease in women: a report from the Women's Ischemia Syndrome Evaluation. Circulation. 2004;109(6):714–21.

19. Bairey Merz CN, et al. Hypoestrogenemia of hypothalamic origin and coronary artery disease in premenopausal women: a report from the NHLBI-sponsored WISE study. J Am Coll Cardiol. 2003;41(3):413–9.

20. Shaw LJ, et al. Postmenopausal women with a history of irregular menses and elevated androgen measurements at high risk for worsening cardiovascular event-free survival: results from the National Institutes of Health – National Heart, Lung, and Blood Institute sponsored Women's Ischemia Syndrome Evaluation. J Clin Endocrinol Metab. 2008;93(4):1276–84.

21. Bellamy L, et al. Pre-eclampsia and risk of cardiovascular disease and cancer in later life: systematic review and meta-analysis. BMJ. 2007;335(7627):974.

22. Lansky A, et al. A gender-specific blood-based gene expression score for assessing obstructive coronary artery disease in nondiabetic patients: results of the Personalized Risk Evaluation and Diagnosis in the Coronary Tree (PREDICT) trial. Am Heart J. 2012;164(3):320–6.

23. Allison MA, et al. Ethnic-specific prevalence of peripheral arterial disease in the United States. Am J Prev Med. 2007;32(4):328–33.

24. Ingelsson E, et al. Burden and prognostic importance of subclinical cardiovascular disease in overweight and obese individuals. Circulation. 2007;116(4):375–84.

25. Ankle Brachial Index Collaboration, et al. Ankle brachial index combined with Framingham Risk Score to predict cardiovascular events and mortality: a meta-analysis. JAMA. 2008;300(2):197–208.

26. Simon A, Chironi G, Levenson J. Comparative performance of subclinical atherosclerosis tests in predicting coronary heart disease in asymptomatic individuals. Eur Heart J. 2007;28(24): 2967–71.

27. Chambless LE, et al. Association of coronary heart disease incidence with carotid arterial wall thickness and major risk factors: the Atherosclerosis Risk in Communities (ARIC) Study, 1987–1993. Am J Epidemiol. 1997;146(6):483–94.

28. Haberl R, et al. Correlation of coronary calcification and angiographically documented stenoses in patients with suspected coronary artery disease: results of 1,764 patients. J Am Coll Cardiol. 2001;37(2):451–7.

29. Raggi P, et al. Gender-based differences in the prognostic value of coronary calcification. J Womens Health (Larchmt). 2004;13(3):273–83.

30. Gibbons RJ, et al. ACC/AHA 2002 guideline update for exercise testing: summary article: a report of the American College of Cardiology/American Heart Association Task Force on Practice Guidelines (Committee to Update the 1997 Exercise Testing Guidelines). Circulation. 2002;106(14):1883–92.

31. Kwok Y, et al. Meta-analysis of exercise testing to detect coronary artery disease in women. Am J Cardiol. 1999;83(5):660–6.

32. Mieres JH, et al. Role of noninvasive testing in the clinical evaluation of women with suspected coronary artery disease: consensus statement from the Cardiac Imaging Committee, Council on Clinical Cardiology, and the Cardiovascular Imaging and Intervention Committee, Council on Cardiovascular Radiology and Intervention, American Heart Association. Circulation. 2005;111(5):682–96.

33. Gulati M, et al. Exercise capacity and the risk of death in women: the St James Women Take Heart Project. Circulation. 2003;108(13):1554–9.

34. Mora S, et al. Ability of exercise testing to predict cardiovascular and all-cause death in asymptomatic women: a 20-year follow-up of the lipid research clinics prevalence study. JAMA. 2003;290(12):1600–7.

35. Alexander KP, et al. Value of exercise treadmill testing in women. J Am Coll Cardiol. 1998;32(6):1657–64.

36. Gulati M, et al. Prognostic value of the duke treadmill score in asymptomatic women. Am J Cardiol. 2005;96(3):369–75.

37. Poehlman ET. Menopause, energy expenditure, and body composition. Acta Obstet Gynecol Scand. 2002;81(7):603–11.

38. Hlatky MA, et al. A brief self-administered questionnaire to determine functional capacity (the Duke Activity Status Index). Am J Cardiol. 1989;64(10):651–4.

39. Shaw LJ, et al. The value of estimated functional capacity in estimating outcome: results from the NHBLI-Sponsored Women's Ischemia Syndrome Evaluation (WISE) Study. J Am Coll Cardiol. 2006;47(3 Suppl):S36–43.
40. Lauer MS, et al. Impaired chronotropic response to exercise stress testing as a predictor of mortality. JAMA. 1999;281(6):524–9.
41. Pratt CM, et al. Exercise testing in women with chest pain. Are there additional exercise characteristics that predict true positive test results? Chest. 1989;95(1):139–44.
42. Vivekananthan DP, et al. Heart rate recovery after exercise is a predictor of mortality, independent of the angiographic severity of coronary disease. J Am Coll Cardiol. 2003;42(5): 831–8.
43. Kawano H, et al. Menstrual cyclic variation of myocardial ischemia in premenopausal women with variant angina. Ann Intern Med. 2001;135(11):977–81.
44. Shaw LJ, et al. Comparative effectiveness of exercise electrocardiography with or without myocardial perfusion single photon emission computed tomography in women with suspected coronary artery disease: results from the What Is the Optimal Method for Ischemia Evaluation in Women (WOMEN) trial. Circulation. 2011;124(11):1239–49.
45. Williams MJ, et al. Comparison of exercise echocardiography with an exercise score to diagnose coronary artery disease in women. Am J Cardiol. 1994;74(5):435–8.
46. Gulati M, Shaw LJ, Bairey Merz CN. Myocardial ischemia in women: lessons from the NHLBI WISE study. Clin Cardiol. 2012;35(3):141–8.
47. Marwick TH, et al. Exercise echocardiography is an accurate and cost-efficient technique for detection of coronary artery disease in women. J Am Coll Cardiol. 1995;26(2):335–41.
48. Kim C, et al. Pharmacologic stress testing for coronary disease diagnosis: a meta-analysis. Am Heart J. 2001;142(6):934–44.
49. Elhendy A, et al. Gender differences in the accuracy of dobutamine stress echocardiography for the diagnosis of coronary artery disease. Am J Cardiol. 1997;80(11):1414–8.
50. Arruda-Olson AM, et al. Prognostic value of exercise echocardiography in 5,798 patients: is there a gender difference? J Am Coll Cardiol. 2002;39(4):625–31.
51. Shaw LJ, et al. Impact of gender on risk stratification by exercise and dobutamine stress echocardiography: long-term mortality in 4234 women and 6898 men. Eur Heart J. 2005;26(5):447–56.
52. Cortigiani L, et al. Impact of gender on risk stratification by stress echocardiography. Am J Med. 2009;122(3):301–9.
53. Shaw LJ, Bugiardini R, Merz CN. Women and ischemic heart disease: evolving knowledge. J Am Coll Cardiol. 2009;54(17):1561–75.
54. Santana-Boado C, et al. Diagnostic accuracy of technetium-99m-MIBI myocardial SPECT in women and men. J Nucl Med. 1998;39(5):751–5.
55. Taillefer R, et al. Comparative diagnostic accuracy of Tl-201 and Tc-99m sestamibi SPECT imaging (perfusion and ECG-gated SPECT) in detecting coronary artery disease in women. J Am Coll Cardiol. 1997;29(1):69–77.
56. Mieres JH, et al. Value of electrocardiographically gated single-photon emission computed tomographic myocardial perfusion scintigraphy in a cohort of symptomatic postmenopausal women. Am J Cardiol. 2007;99(8):1096–9.
57. Klocke FJ, et al. ACC/AHA/ASNC guidelines for the clinical use of cardiac radionuclide imaging–executive summary: a report of the American College of Cardiology/American Heart Association Task Force on Practice Guidelines (ACC/AHA/ASNC Committee to Revise the 1995 Guidelines for the Clinical Use of Cardiac Radionuclide Imaging). Circulation. 2003;108(11):1404–18.
58. Marwick TH, et al. The noninvasive prediction of cardiac mortality in men and women with known or suspected coronary artery disease. Economics of Noninvasive Diagnosis (END) Study Group. Am J Med. 1999;106(2):172–8.
59. Hachamovitch R, et al. Effective risk stratification using exercise myocardial perfusion SPECT in women: gender-related differences in prognostic nuclear testing. J Am Coll Cardiol. 1996;28(1):34–44.

60. Giri S, et al. Impact of diabetes on the risk stratification using stress single-photon emission computed tomography myocardial perfusion imaging in patients with symptoms suggestive of coronary artery disease. Circulation. 2002;105(1):32–40.
61. Berman DS, et al. Adenosine myocardial perfusion single-photon emission computed tomography in women compared with men. Impact of diabetes mellitus on incremental prognostic value and effect on patient management. J Am Coll Cardiol. 2003;41(7):1125–33.
62. Wexler O, et al. Effect of gender on cardiovascular risk stratification with ECG gated SPECT left ventricular volume indices and ejection fraction. J Nucl Cardiol. 2009;16(1):28–37.
63. Mouden M, et al. Impact of a new ultrafast CZT SPECT camera for myocardial perfusion imaging: fewer equivocal results and lower radiation dose. Eur J Nucl Med Mol Imaging. 2012;39(6):1048–55.
64. DePuey EG. Advances in SPECT camera software and hardware: currently available and new on the horizon. J Nucl Cardiol. 2012;19(3):551–81, quiz 585.
65. Hachamovitch R, et al. Exercise myocardial perfusion SPECT in patients without known coronary artery disease: incremental prognostic value and use in risk stratification. Circulation. 1996;93(5):905–14.
66. Metz LD, et al. The prognostic value of normal exercise myocardial perfusion imaging and exercise echocardiography: a meta-analysis. J Am Coll Cardiol. 2007;49(2):227–37.
67. Di Carli MF, Hachamovitch R. New technology for noninvasive evaluation of coronary artery disease. Circulation. 2007;115(11):1464–80.
68. Heller GV, Calnon D, Dorbala S. Recent advances in cardiac PET and PET/CT myocardial perfusion imaging. J Nucl Cardiol. 2009;16(6):962–9.
69. Dorbala S, et al. Incremental prognostic value of gated Rb-82 positron emission tomography myocardial perfusion imaging over clinical variables and rest LVEF. JACC Cardiovasc Imaging. 2009;2(7):846–54.
70. Einstein AJ, et al. Radiation dose to patients from cardiac diagnostic imaging. Circulation. 2007;116(11):1290–305.
71. Klem I, et al. Value of cardiovascular magnetic resonance stress perfusion testing for the detection of coronary artery disease in women. JACC Cardiovasc Imaging. 2008;1(4):436–45.
72. Gebker R, et al. Dobutamine stress magnetic resonance imaging for the detection of coronary artery disease in women. Heart. 2010;96(8):616–20.
73. Merkle N, et al. Diagnostic performance of magnetic resonance first pass perfusion imaging is equally potent in female compared to male patients with coronary artery disease. Clin Res Cardiol. 2010;99(1):21–8.
74. Nagel E, et al. Noninvasive diagnosis of ischemia-induced wall motion abnormalities with the use of high-dose dobutamine stress MRI: comparison with dobutamine stress echocardiography. Circulation. 1999;99(6):763–70.
75. Raman SV, et al. Real-time cine and myocardial perfusion with treadmill exercise stress cardiovascular magnetic resonance in patients referred for stress SPECT. J Cardiovasc Magn Reson. 2010;12:41.
76. Jahnke C, et al. Prognostic value of cardiac magnetic resonance stress tests: adenosine stress perfusion and dobutamine stress wall motion imaging. Circulation. 2007;115(13):1769–76.
77. Hundley WG, et al. Magnetic resonance imaging determination of cardiac prognosis. Circulation. 2002;106(18):2328–33.
78. Wallace EL, et al. Dobutamine cardiac magnetic resonance results predict cardiac prognosis in women with known or suspected ischemic heart disease. JACC Cardiovasc Imaging. 2009;2(3):299–307.
79. Panting JR, et al. Abnormal subendocardial perfusion in cardiac syndrome X detected by cardiovascular magnetic resonance imaging. N Engl J Med. 2002;346(25):1948–53.
80. Foussas SG, et al. Clinical characteristics and follow-up of patients with chest pain and normal coronary arteries. Angiology. 1998;49(5):349–54.
81. Reis SE, et al. Coronary microvascular dysfunction is highly prevalent in women with chest pain in the absence of coronary artery disease: results from the NHLBI WISE study. Am Heart J. 2001;141(5):735–41.

82. Pundziute G, et al. Gender influence on the diagnostic accuracy of 64-slice multislice computed tomography coronary angiography for detection of obstructive coronary artery disease. Heart. 2008;94(1):48–52.
83. Tsang JC, et al. Sex comparison of diagnostic accuracy of 64-multidetector row coronary computed tomographic angiography: results from the multicenter ACCURACY trial. J Cardiovasc Comput Tomogr. 2012;6(4):246–51.
84. Yiu KH, et al. Age- and gender-specific differences in the prognostic value of CT coronary angiography. Heart. 2012;98(3):232–7.
85. Einstein AJ, Henzlova MJ, Rajagopalan S. Estimating risk of cancer associated with radiation exposure from 64-slice computed tomography coronary angiography. JAMA. 2007;298(3):317–23.
86. Han SH, et al. Sex differences in atheroma burden and endothelial function in patients with early coronary atherosclerosis. Eur Heart J. 2008;29(11):1359–69.
87. Sun H, et al. Coronary microvascular spasm causes myocardial ischemia in patients with vasospastic angina. J Am Coll Cardiol. 2002;39(5):847–51.
88. von Mering GO, et al. Abnormal coronary vasomotion as a prognostic indicator of cardiovascular events in women: results from the National Heart, Lung, and Blood Institute-Sponsored Women's Ischemia Syndrome Evaluation (WISE). Circulation. 2004;109(6):722–5.
89. Bairey Merz CN, et al. Insights from the NHLBI-Sponsored Women's Ischemia Syndrome Evaluation (WISE) Study: Part II: gender differences in presentation, diagnosis, and outcome with regard to gender-based pathophysiology of atherosclerosis and macrovascular and microvascular coronary disease. J Am Coll Cardiol. 2006;47(3 Suppl):S21–9.
90. Bugiardini R, et al. Endothelial function predicts future development of coronary artery disease: a study of women with chest pain and normal coronary angiograms. Circulation. 2004;109(21):2518–23.
91. Modena MG, et al. Prognostic role of reversible endothelial dysfunction in hypertensive postmenopausal women. J Am Coll Cardiol. 2002;40(3):505–10.
92. Holubkov R, et al. Large brachial artery diameter is associated with angiographic coronary artery disease in women. Am Heart J. 2002;143(5):802–7.
93. Bonetti PO, et al. Enhanced external counterpulsation improves endothelial function in patients with symptomatic coronary artery disease. J Am Coll Cardiol. 2003;41(10):1761–8.
94. Fleischmann KE, Hunink MG, Kuntz KM, Douglas PS. Exercise echocardiography or exercise SPECT imaging? A meta-analysis of diagnostic test performance. JAMA. 1998;280(10):913–20.
95. Beattie WS, Abdelnaem E, Wijeysundera DN, Buckley DN. A meta-analytic comparison of preoperative stress echocardiography and nuclear scintigraphy imaging. Anesth Analg. 2006;102(1):8–16.

Chapter 5
Management of Stable Ischemic Heart Disease in Women

Rashaad A. Chothia and Jason Pacos

Introduction

Cardiovascular disease (CVD) remains the most common cause of death in women living in developed countries and outnumbers death from all forms of cancer combined [1]. Since 1984, the number of CVD deaths for females has exceeded those for males. With the advances in the diagnosis and treatment of coronary artery disease (CAD), there have been significant decreases in cardiovascular mortality seen in both sexes, with the major decline for women occurring after the year 2000 [2]. However, this reduction in mortality among women has remained less pronounced as compared with men [3]. The reason for this disparity may be gender differences in the pathophysiology of CAD or lower awareness of coronary disease in women leading to decreased implementation of evidence based care [4]. The Yentl syndrome (as described in 1991) pointed out the ubiquitous misrecognition of CVD as an affliction of men, with women seeming to require a higher burden of proof in order to receive appropriate diagnostic tests and therapeutic interventions [5]. There are recognized gender differences including a notable 10 year delay in the onset of ischemic heart disease (IHD) in women compared to men, that have been attributed to the protective effect of estrogen [6].

Stable angina is the most common manifestation of CVD, and is in fact, among women, the most common initial presentation of CAD, increasing in prevalence with advancing age [7]. It is a chronic medical condition with a low but appreciable incidence of acute coronary events, conferring increased mortality. Over the last 20 years, the National Institute of Health (NIH) and others have hastened to educate both the medical community as well as the public to recognize CVD risk in women.

R.A. Chothia, MD (✉) • J. Pacos, MD
Division of Cardiology,
University of Rochester Medical Center, Rochester, NY, USA
e-mail: rashaad_chothia@urmc.rochester.edu

H.Z. Mieszczanska, G.P. Velarde (eds.),
Management of Cardiovascular Disease in Women,
DOI 10.1007/978-1-4471-5517-1_5, © Springer-Verlag London 2014

In 1999, the American Heart Association (AHA) published the first consensus guideline for prevention of cardiovascular disease specifically in women [8]. The subsequent application of evidence-based therapy for prevention and treatment has resulted in increased gender equality and improved outcomes for women with IHD.

Stable ischemic heart disease (SIHD) encompasses a range of patients with underlying ischemic heart disease, which may include asymptomatic CAD, prior myocardial infarction (MI), or chronic angina. SIHD can vary from completely asymptomatic to severe ischemic symptoms with minimal activity. Stability in IHD is defined by the fact that symptoms are predictable and reproducible based on an expected level of exertion, and lingers relatively unchanged with respect to frequency and severity. Symptoms are typically brought on by exertion or emotional stress and relieved by rest or use of antianginal medications.

SIHD can be an initial presentation of CVD or residual symptoms after an acute ischemic event such as myocardial infarction. In contrast, unstable angina is an increase in frequency, intensity, or duration of ischemic symptoms that are part of the acute coronary syndromes (ACS), and have much worse short and long-term outcomes without urgent inpatient evaluation and treatment. The management of ACS is described elsewhere in the book. Currently, more than four million American women suffer symptoms of SIHD based on 2011 statistics from the American Heart Association, a number that is expected to grow [9].

Gender Specific Considerations in Stable Ischemic Heart Disease

Women with angina pectoris differ substantially from men with the same disease, tending to be older and sicker with more co-morbidities [10]. As described by Framingham data, women often present with chest pain as their first manifestation of ischemic heart disease in contrast to men who are more likely to present with acute myocardial infarction or sudden cardiac death [11]. This often makes the primary care provider the first medical professional with the opportunity to evaluate newly declared ischemic heart disease. Importantly, SIHD does not include acute coronary syndromes such as ST elevation myocardial infarction (STEMI), non-ST elevation myocardial infarction (NSTEMI), or intermediate/high risk unstable angina (UA). UA with low risk features, defined as patients <70 years old with new onset exertional angina lasting <20 min without ECG or cardiac marker abnormalities may also be considered SIHD [12] and selectively evaluated and treated as an outpatient. All newly diagnosed patients with stable ischemic heart disease should be referred to a cardiologist for evaluation of underlying ischemia and to decide if further testing or medical therapy is necessary. Clinicians should maintain close vigilance for any changing symptoms in their female patients with known SIHD in order to recognize early developments and prevent complications from uncontrolled ischemia.

Evaluation of Symptoms in Women

Obtaining a good history is most important for the clinical diagnosis of chronic stable angina. However, the description of "typical" angina symptoms is derived largely from observations made in mostly male populations. It is not clear whether symptoms in women can be judged by the same criteria used to diagnose coronary artery disease in men [10]. According to the National Institute for Health and Clinical Excellence (NICE) guidelines for stable angina, presentation of symptomatic coronary artery disease varies little between men and women. Typical exertion induced angina is the main complaint of both women and men with documented CAD. Diagnosis and management should be influenced by pre-test likelihood of disease and not only by gender [13]. Although women present frequently with similar symptoms as men, atypical chest pain and angina-equivalent symptoms such as dyspnea are more common in women. Women often manifest atypical symptoms of angina that can include fatigue, back pain, epigastric pain, palpitations, appetite loss, nausea, vomiting, and indigestion [14]. Women also complain more often of mental-stress induced angina, or angina at rest than men [15]. The burden of angina is higher in women as seen in a meta-analysis of 74 studies that included almost 25,000 cases of angina from 31 countries. Women were found to have a slightly higher prevalence of stable angina with a pooled sex ratio of 1.20 [16]. Unexpected presentations in women can cause the discounting of symptoms as non-ischemic with unintentional delays or missed diagnosis, and reduction in early evidence based therapies unless a high level of suspicion is maintained. This is made clear through multiple prospective investigations that evaluated patients with SIHD. When assessing patients with stable angina through the use of exercise stress testing and cardiac catheterization, investigators worldwide found a significant disparity in application of guideline recommendations between men and women [7, 17, 18]. In the Euro Heart survey of 3,779 patients of which 42 % were women with angina, the women were less likely at any time to have symptom triggered non-invasive exercise stress testing or invasive evaluations with cardiac catheterization, even if being evaluated by a cardiologist [19].

This trend is largely due to perceived coronary risk of women being less than that of men. Propagation of this concept is largely derived from the study of mostly male populations such as were enrolled in the Framingham Heart Study. These risk factors described in the 1960's defined male gender, age, hypertension, smoking, diabetes, and hyperlipidemia as major determinants of coronary heart disease [20], and led to the first models to evaluate risk of cardiovascular disease. Contemporary cohorts have since shown that classic coronary risk factors do not accurately represent risk in women. This has led to development of sex specific adjustments as well as addition of risk factors such as markers of inflammation and family history of early cardiovascular events that more accurately risk stratify the sexes [21, 22]. Hormonal status imparts additional risk as noted by postmenopausal women having increased prevalence of cardiovascular disease, though many gaps remain in understanding the pathophysiology involved [23]. Appropriate identification of women at high risk for development of coronary artery disease will increase the likelihood of making a correct diagnosis of IHD and preventing cardiac events.

An increased mortality in women after acute myocardial infarction (MI) has been documented for decades. Though applying a gender equal approach to therapy has made substantial improvements, women younger than 60 continue to have elevated risk of death after MI [24]. Women also have higher in-hospital mortality than men when presenting with initial symptoms of non-ACS chest pain, a finding that increases with age and with greater significance in white women [25].

The large population of women with symptomatic SIHD confers elevated morbidity with reduction in quality of life and ability to conduct previous activities of daily living. Women have more functional disability due to symptoms and present for more office visits and hospital admissions due to angina, estimated annually at 4 million visits for women versus 2.4 million for men [26]. Women have more complications of SIHD than men including acute MI, cardiovascular death, and congestive heart failure. Women also undergo more repeat ischemic evaluations with non-invasive and invasive testing adding to a ballooning health care expenditure [26–28]. This points towards the difficulties in diagnosing and managing SIHD in women and the need for improved recognition, symptom control, and use of evidence based therapy to prevent complications. Although the likelihood of obstructive coronary artery disease in women with chest pain is lower than in men, the incidence is still significant, and women should undergo the same evaluation as men do.

Mechanisms of Stable Ischemic Heart Disease in Women

Obstructive Coronary Artery Disease

The assumed etiology of SIHD in women and men stems from the concept that symptoms of angina pectoris are almost always related to intracoronary atherosclerosis with "significant stenosis" [10]. The buildup of intraluminal coronary plaque over time leads to hemodynamic obstruction with decreased flow. This in turn causes a mismatched delivery of oxygen with increased tissue demand during exertion or stress. This mechanism of epicardial artery obstruction is the leading cause of exertional angina symptoms in men, and many older women as the prevalence of obstructive CAD increases as women age equaling men around age 70 [26]. Overall, women report more symptoms of chest pain than men, though by coronary angiography, they are found to have a lower rate of obstructive CAD and better preservation of left ventricular function [25]. This disparity seen in women has led to investigation of an alternate mechanism for ischemic heart disease symptoms, and has garnered many insights into gender differences in the pathophysiology of SIHD.

SIHD Without Obstructive CAD

The Women's Ischemia Syndrome Evaluation (WISE) study evaluated women referred to angiography for chest pain evaluation, and surprisingly found up to 50 % of women with symptoms of typical or atypical angina had normal or non-obstructive epicardial arteries (<50 % stenosis) by cardiac catheterization compared to 17 % of men [28, 29]. Women were more often found to have diffuse non-obstructive CAD and elevated left ventricular end diastolic pressures, which may contribute to symptoms of angina [30]. Women are also known to have smaller epicardial coronary arteries than men even when corrected for body surface area [31]. Atherosclerosis in the walls of the epicardial arteries may play a different role in symptoms of ischemia for women than it does in men. Coronary intravascular ultrasound (IVUS) is an invasive modality that is used to evaluate atheroma present in the walls of coronary arteries. This atherosclerotic plaque is not seen through standard coronary angiography, which is more accurately described as "luminal angiography". IVUS can be utilized during heart catheterization using a catheter with an ultrasound transducer tip that is inserted directly into the coronary arteries. IVUS has shown in vivo that patients with non-obstructive CAD can have extensive extra luminal atheroma burden through the process of expansion of the internal elastic lamina known as positive remodeling [32]. Investigation with IVUS has led to the description of vulnerable or unstable plaques lacking the protective thick fibrous caps, and more likely to ulcerate or rupture causing ACS even without previously impinging significantly on the lumen of the epicardial arteries [33].

This concealed atherosclerosis was also seen by IVUS in women enrolled in the WISE study that presented with suspected ischemia, but without obstructive CAD seen during coronary angiography [34]. In a study of women presenting with acute MI but non-obstructive CAD, IVUS showed evidence of substantial atheroma buildup in the arterial wall that correlated with cardiac MRI findings of infarction [35]. The proposed mechanisms for these ischemic events include occult plaque rupture or ulceration with distal embolization of platelet debris as well as coronary vasospasm. In the absence of traditional intraluminal atherosclerosis visualized during cardiac catheterization, it may be challenging to diagnose the extent of atherosclerosis in the walls of the coronary arteries when tools such as IVUS are not used. The possible implications include missed diagnosis and lack of treatment for ischemic events caused by concealed CAD among women, as well as inappropriate reassurances that ischemic events were vasospastic or inflammatory (i.e. myocarditis). IVUS is unfortunately technically challenging and increases the time and risk of the diagnostic catheterization, which does tend to limit its use in SIHD evaluation.

Microvascular Angina

A more distinguishing feature largely in women has been found in the dysfunction of the coronary microvasculature. The coronary microvasculature is currently below the size threshold for visualization utilizing standard coronary angiography [36]. Coronary flow reserve is the auto-regulated ability to increase flow through these small coronary vascular beds in response to an increase in cardiac workload and metabolic requirements [36]. The normal coronary microvasculature dilates to allow increased blood flow and delivery of oxygen and nutrients to the cardiac tissue. If flow increase in the microvascular circulation is reduced by dysfunction of the small arteriolar vessels, regions of focal ischemia may occur in small areas scattered throughout the myocardium [37]. Coronary reactivity testing (CRT) is an invasive method performed through cardiac catheterization to directly measure the flow increase in response to a vasoactive drug challenge such as intracoronary adenosine that simulates increased cardiac demand. This vascular stress test allows a surrogate measurement of the function of the small resistance coronary arteries not visible by angiography and responsible for changes in coronary flow [38, 39]. In women with SIHD and non-obstructive or no coronary artery disease, abnormal CRT with attenuated coronary flow reserve has been seen in up to half of patients [39]. The loss of expected epicardial artery flow increase among these women without significant coronary obstruction is diagnostic for microvascular dysfunction [40]. Measurement of microvascular function using CRT is relatively safe though not routinely performed for reasons including a lack of standardized protocols, inexperience of many labs, and the increased time required during a diagnostic heart catheterization [41].

Microvascular dysfunction is implicated in what was initially designated cardiac syndrome X (CSX) in 1973 [42] and more recently termed microvascular angina (MVA). The classic definition of CSX or MVA is the triad of effort induced or persistent angina pectoris, a positive exercise stress test for myocardial ischemia, and angiographically normal coronary arteries [43, 44]. Microvascular dysfunction has been increasingly supported as the major mechanism for SIHD in the largely female group of symptomatic patients without obstructive coronary disease. The diagnosis of MVA as the cause of SIHD does of course require that other cardiac and non-cardiac causes of angina type chest pain have been ruled out [45]. The exact pathogenesis of MVA is not completely understood but is likely a multifactorial process including endothelial dysfunction, neuro-hormonal changes, inflammation, and abnormal nociception combined to cause the symptoms of SIHD seen in this female subgroup [46]. Systemic inflammatory markers including high-sensitivity C-reactive protein (hs-CRP), interleukins 6 and 18 (IL-6, IL-18), tumor necrosis factor α (TNF-α), and transforming growth factor (TGF)-β1 have been implicated in MVA but have not consistently been shown to correlate with decreased coronary flow reserve [47]. The current difficulty in confirming a diagnosis in this population requires the clinician to have a high index of suspicion to consider MVA in the appropriate symptomatic female patient and institute therapy for IHD aimed at risk reduction and prevention of future events.

Natural History and Prognosis

Our understanding of the progression and prognosis of SIHD in women is derived from the large population based cohorts that start with the Framingham Heart Study. In this first large cohort, mortality from angina was as high as seen in post-MI hospitalized patients. At 2 years of follow up, the rate of cardiac events in women with stable angina was found to be 6.2 % for non-fatal MI and 3.8 % for cardiac death

[48]. This data was collected prior to the use of cardioprotective medical therapy. Modern prospective randomized trials provide further insight to the prognosis of SIHD. The EUROPA trial between 1997 and 2000 randomized 12,218 low risk patients with SIHD to perindopril, an angiotensin converting enzyme inhibitor (ACE) or placebo [49]. The majority of patients were utilizing anti-platelet, beta-blocker, and lipid lowering therapies. The primary end point was non-fatal MI, cardiac arrest, and cardiac death with results showing an overall 20 % relative risk reduction with use of perindopril over 4.2 years mean follow up. In the 1779 females randomized, there was a primary event rate of 6.9 % in the treatment arm and 8.8 % with placebo that did not reach statistical significance. The main limitation with enrolling only 14.6 % of women in the sample leads to an inability to show statistical significant reduction in the primary end point for the female subgroup.

The previous belief that good outcomes are favored in women with angina and no significant coronary artery obstruction [50] has been disproved in recent large cohort trials. The WISE study showed that many women continue to suffer symptoms and signs of angina, and have a poor quality of life regardless of degree of CAD [30]. They also have a higher incidence of cardiovascular events and hospital readmissions than matched controls [51–54]. Adverse event rates in women with persistent chest pain and microvascular angina diagnosed by coronary reactivity testing during the WISE study were greater than twice that of women with matched risk factors and no history of ischemic symptoms. These previously considered low risk women had twice the rate of non-fatal MI, congestive heart failure, stroke, and cardiovascular death [53, 54]. The old paradigm of considering these women low-risk based on coronary angiography is no longer easily acceptable and management decisions should follow evidence-based guidelines for treatment of SIHD.

Recent prognostic data is found in the COURAGE trial, which randomized 2,287 patients with symptomatic SIHD and obstructive coronary artery disease to either guideline based medical therapy alone or medical therapy plus percutaneous coronary intervention (PCI) of obstructive lesions [55]. Only 15 % of these low to moderate risk patients enrolled were women. The authors showed no significant difference in primary outcomes between the two groups after a median follow up of 4.6 years with primary end points of non-fatal MI or cardiovascular death. The PCI group had a 13.2 % rate of non-fatal MI and 7.6 % rate for death, while the medical therapy group had 12.3 and 8.3 % respectively. The COURAGE data showed no difference in SIHD prognosis by utilizing guideline based medical therapy alone or combined with revascularization by PCI. There was not a subgroup analysis of women performed with a low rate of female enrollment. The disparity in female representation in large studies is beginning to change and will eventually lead to greater understanding of the gender similarities and differences in cardiovascular disease.

Diagnostic Testing and Risk Stratification

Determining when further testing is required to evaluate obstructive disease and risk-stratifying patients who may benefit from revascularization therapy is best achieved in consultation with a cardiologist. The primary care provider should vigilantly watch for symptoms of worsening ischemia at an early stage to allow timely referral for therapeutic intervention when indicated. Each patient's risk profile should be determined in order to determine those at high risk for cardiac events and those who would benefit from early revascularization instead of conservative medical therapy. Multiple clinical non-invasive and invasive tools are available to aid in the stratification of risk. Functional capacity remains a major indicator of cardiovascular risk, and validated clinical questionnaires can be utilized to quantify a patients symptoms and limitations in addition to obtaining a detailed history. The Women's Ischemia Syndrome Evaluation (WISE) [27], Seattle Angina Questionnaire (SAQ) [56], and Duke Activity Status Index (DASI) [57] are able to gather details on frequency and severity of angina and the level of physical activity being performed or obtainable. Utilizing validated questionnaires in the clinical setting can help in monitoring symptoms and alert the clinician to changes requiring further management.

The lesson from the COURAGE trial in patients with SIHD was that PCI did not reduce MI or death compared to medical therapy in low to intermediate risk patients with known obstructive CAD [55]. All patients with SIHD should therefore be optimally treated with guideline based medical therapy prior to consideration of revascularization. When symptoms are not adequately controlled with aggressive medical therapy, and the benefit of revascularization is deemed appropriate by the patient and the clinician, further diagnostic modalities are indicated. All providers should be mindful that a decision to proceed to non-invasive testing in women with SIHD should be considered in the context of the patients' willingness and the risk to benefit of ultimately undergoing revascularization. Frank discussion with the patient should be aimed at potential benefits of revascularization including angina relief, and to dispel misconceptions that coronary interventions in SIHD will prevent future myocardial infarcts.

The use of non-invasive modalities, such as exercise treadmill testing with or without the addition of an imaging modality including echocardiography or nuclear myocardial perfusion imaging, provide the clinician with the most diagnostic information. Exercise testing provides important data on functional capacity through exercise tolerance and symptom reproducibility. Imaging techniques help determine the extent of myocardium with ischemia present and aids in localizing anatomical regions that can be correlated with angiography to determine lesions likely responsible for anginal symptoms. Optimal selection of non-invasive modalities, including exercise and chemical stress testing for women, is detailed in a dedicated chapter along with a discussion on what constitutes a positive test.

If non-invasive testing suggests high-risk features as listed in Table 5.1, the next step is invasive coronary angiography to determine locations of lesions, severity of obstruction, and technical details to add to risk stratification and planning of a revascularization approach. Current ACCF/AHA guidelines state the indications for initial evaluation by coronary angiography for SIHD are limited to a few clinical situations: survivors of sudden cardiac death, new life threatening ventricular arrhythmias, and signs and symptoms of new acute heart failure [12].

Table 5.1 Noninvasive risk stratification: high risk findings (>3 % annual risk of death or MI)

1. Severe resting LV dysfunction (LVEF <35 %) not readily explained by noncoronary causes
2. Resting perfusion abnormalities ≥10 % of the myocardium in patients without prior history or evidence of MI
3. Stress ECG findings including ≥2 mm of ST-segment depression at low workload or persisting into recovery, exercise-induced ST-segment elevation, or exercise-induced VT/VF
4. Severe stress-induced LV dysfunction (peak exercise LVEF <45 % or drop in LVEF with stress ≥10 %)
5. Stress-induced perfusion abnormalities encumbering ≥10 % myocardium or stress segmental scores indicating multiple vascular territories with abnormalities
6. Stress-induced LV dilation
7. Inducible wall motion abnormality (involving >2 segments or 2 coronary beds)
8. Wall motion abnormality developing at low dose of dobutamine (≤10 mg/kg/min) or at a low heart rate (<120 beats/min)
9. CAC score >400 Agatston units
10. Multivessel obstructive CAD (≥70 % stenosis) or left main stenosis (≥50 % stenosis) on CCTA

Source: Reproduced with permission from ACCF/AHA Guidelines (Fihn et al. [12])
CCTA coronary computed tomography angiography, *LV* left ventricular, *LVEF* left ventricular ejection fraction, *MI* myocardial infarction, *VT/VF* ventricular tachycardia/ventricular fibrillation, *CAC* coronary artery calcium

Treatment of Women with Stable Ischemic Heart Disease

Women with signs and symptoms of myocardial ischemia irrespective of angiographic anatomy should be treated using optimal guideline based medical therapy [1]. Both genders with findings of non-obstructive coronary disease during cardiac catheterization were less likely to be prescribed secondary prevention medications at discharge as compared to those with obstructive CAD [58]. This represents a gap in optimal therapy for many more women who fall in this category and would likely benefit from proven therapies to prevent future cardiovascular events. Management of SIHD including medical therapy and revascularization procedures have also been shown to be utilized less in women than men when presenting with similar findings [7]. Guideline recommended therapy does not differ in regards to gender, and should be implemented equally. Therapeutic management for men and women with SIHD are aimed at two complimentary goals: first is controlling physiologic and metabolic markers of cardiovascular risk and hence prevention of cardiovascular events, second is therapy aimed at providing symptomatic relief and improving quality of life. Angina relief is particularly important for women who have a higher burden of symptoms with a greater reduction in functional status.

Cardiac Risk Factor Modification

Classic risk factors for development of ischemic heart disease are relevant for women as well as men as seen in the INTERHEART study, a worldwide case control study of close to 30,000 people in 52 countries. The study estimated that 90 % of the risk of MI is attributable to nine measureable risk factors: smoking, dyslipidemia, diabetes mellitus, hypertension, obesity, psychosocial stress, poor diet, lack of regular exercise, and alcohol consumption. Traditional risk factors are highly prevalent in women. However, certain risk factors place women at greater risk then men. There is a higher prevalence of obesity in women, especially extreme obesity with body mass index (BMI) ≥ 40 kg/m^2 [59]. Obesity infers greater risk of diabetes mellitus, hypertension, and is an independent risk factor for CVD, increasing mortality [60]. Women also have a higher prevalence of diabetes, and diabetic women have at least a three-fold greater risk of IHD than non-diabetics [61]. The risk of fatal IHD was shown to be 50 % higher in diabetic women as compared to men, in a meta-analysis of 37 prospective cohort studies [62]. Similarly, hypertensive women have a two to three fold increased risk of coronary events [63]. The metabolic syndrome consisting of the constellation of central obesity, glucose intolerance, hypertension, and dyslipidemia places women at the highest risk of developing IHD, to a greater extent than men with the metabolic syndrome, or either gender without the combination [64]. Female specific risk factors such as preeclampsia of pregnancy, doubles the risk of developing ischemic heart disease later in life [65]. Gestational diabetes and hormonal changes due to ovarian dysfunction [61], or the reductions in female specific hormones such as estrogen and progesterone that occur with menopause all increase a women's risk of developing cardiovascular disease. Importantly though, hormone therapy such as estrogen replacement is not recommended for primary or secondary prevention of CVD in women based on current guidelines [12].

The management of SIHD requires an intensification of lifestyle changes and risk factor reduction including aggressive lipid lowering directed at secondary prevention of future cardiac events. All cardiovascular risk factors should be modified in SIHD, and are recommended as Class I therapies (benefit outweighs risk) by the ACCF/AHA guidelines for SIHD [12]. Clinicians should aim to modify risk factors for primary and secondary prevention in women according to these guidelines which are described in more detail in the preceding dedicated chapter.

Life Style Modification

Patient education is key to successful lifestyle changes and risk factor modification. Dietary improvements reduce risk of cardiovascular events by decreasing the prevalence and severity of modifiable risks such as hypertension, dyslipidemia, and hyperglycemia. Smoking is the single most important preventable cause of IHD in women, especially in women younger than 50 years of age [66]. Smoking cessation and avoidance of second hand smoke improves endovascular function and reduces atherogenesis [67]. A retrospective look at patients with IHD comparing those who quit smoking to ongoing users found an estimated 36 % relative risk reduction in overall mortality [68]. Utilizing behavioral and pharmaceutical therapy in addition to the clinician's constant recommendation to quit smoking can significantly improve chances at success.

A weight loss approach with strong emphasis on limiting caloric intake, along with a diet low in saturated fats and cholesterol while high in fresh fruit, vegetables, and whole grains, should be the cornerstone of the clinician's dietary advice. The cardio-protective effects offered by daily consumption of fruits or vegetables, moderate consumption of alcohol three or more times per week, and moderate or strenuous physical exercise were stronger comparatively in women then men [69]. Setting patient goals based on weight and waist circumference allow self-monitored indicators that provide ongoing feedback and results, without clinic visits. The ACCF/AHA guidelines recommend reaching a BMI of 18.5–24.9 kg/m^2, and maintenance of a waist circumference less than 35 in. in women [12]. Many patients have difficulty in making drastic changes to their diet and benefit from a referral to a dietician.

Exercise regimens are an integral part of a successful weight loss and cardiac rehabilitation approach, which not only reduces the risk of future cardiac events but also helps in symptom control. Women tend to see greater benefit in adopting even a modest increase in regular physical activity. Benefits of exercise have been shown to improve female specific risk factors, particularly those associated with microvascular angina. Positive cardiovascular effects of exercise in women with SIHD are associated with beneficial changes in lipid levels, blood pressure, inflammation, endothelial function and autonomic regulation [70–72]. There is likely a dose–response relationship between exercise intensity and duration and the benefits seen in cardiovascular protection. The difficulty for most clinicians is the fact that a majority of women diagnosed with SIHD are older and partake in little to no daily physical activity at baseline.

There are differing guidelines for the amount and intensity of prescribed physical activity for prevention of cardiovascular disease development and reduction of future events. Current ACCF/AHA guidelines recommend 30–60 min of moderate-intensity aerobic activity preferably daily or at least five times a week [12]. The definition of moderate-intensity activity is what requires 3 to <6 MET (metabolic equivalent of task). Brisk walking is considered the minimal strenuous exercise qualifying as moderate-intensity. As walking is the most common leisure exercise among US adults, it is a good starting point, providing the pace is brisk. As a reference, 6 METs is obtained by reaching 5 min on a standard treadmill Bruce protocol, which is 2.5 mph at a 12 % grade. For most women with SIHD, the clinician can reasonably recommend starting an exercise regimen without the need for a medically supervised program.

Some patients, such as those with a history of multiple MI's, cardiac arrest, known severe functional impairment, or known residual exercise-induced ischemia on treadmill testing are considered to be at high risk of cardiac complications during exercise. This high-risk group should be referred for a medically supervised exercise program for 8–12 weeks to establish the appropriate prescription for a safe exercise regimen [12]. Specific patients who also should be referred for cardiac rehab include: post-MI, post-coronary revascularization either by (PCI) or surgically with coronary artery bypass grafting (CABG), valvular surgery, pacemaker or defibrillator implantation, cardiomyopathy, and compensated congestive heart failure. Cardiac rehab programs have a set protocol that increase intensity and duration of exercise while monitoring heart rate, blood pressure, and symptoms by physical therapists or exercise physiologists. Patients should continue participating in cardiac rehab until they are able to safely perform adequate exercise that is in line with their needs and health goals.

Medication Reducing Cardiovascular Risk
and Progression of Atherosclerosis

Antiplatelets

Aspirin is a cyclooxygenase inhibitor, which is indicated for lifelong secondary prevention in all patients with IHD. It provides benefit through prevention of platelet aggregation that leads to coronary thrombosis from plaque rupture. A reduction of 37 % in serious vascular events using aspirin therapy was found by meta-analysis of trials with nearly 3,000 patients with SIHD [73]. The optimal dose to obtain vascular protection and minimize risk of gastrointestinal side effects such as bleeding had been contentious, but was found in the same analysis to be as efficacious using 75–162 mg with less risk of bleeding compared to 325 mg. Providers should make an effort to reduce the dose to minimize risk of bleeding in patients who are using high dose aspirin for cardiovascular prevention. If intolerance or allergy to aspirin exists, substituting a thienopyridine such as clopidogrel which inhibits adenosine diphosphate (ADP) receptors, and provides anti-platelet effect with at least an equal risk reduction in recommended [74]. In patients who undergo PCI with intracoronary stent placement, use of both aspirin and an ADP receptor inhibitor is required for at least 1 month and up to 1 year depending on the type of stent, bare metal requiring less time than drug eluting. The use of dual anti-platelet therapy allows time for the stent to become covered by endothelial cells thereby eliminating direct contact of the metal with blood, and reducing the risk of acute stent thrombosis. At the end of the recommended time for dual anti-platelet therapy, reducing therapy to low dose aspirin alone is acceptable. Using both aspirin and clopidogrel long term for secondary prevention in SIHD was shown by the CHARISMA trial to have no significant benefit over aspirin alone [75]. However post-hoc analysis showed that high-risk groups including patients with recent MI, peripheral vascular disease, and ischemic stroke, did have less cardiovascular events with dual anti-platelet therapy. The use of long-term dual anti-platelet therapy may be beneficial in certain high-risk patients when preventive benefit outweighs the increased bleeding risk [12].

Angiotensin Converting Enzyme (ACE) Inhibitors and Angiotensin Receptor Blockers (ARB)

ACE's and ARB's are cardioprotective medications that provide positive effects in SIHD as well as anti-hypertensive action, prevention of nephropathy in diabetes, and beneficial effect in treatment of cardiomyopathy. These effects have been shown to significantly reduce cardiovascular events including MI and death in patients with reduced LVEF [76]. Initiation of ACE inhibitor therapy has also been shown to reduce mortality in the immediate post MI period [77]. ACE inhibitors may offer additional benefit in women based on the positive effects on vascular function and additional angina reduction [78]. An improvement in vascular function as measured by invasive coronary reactivity testing in women with MVA was shown in the WISE study after 16 weeks of therapy with the ACE inhibitor quinapril [79]. The response was strongest in women with the greatest baseline vascular dysfunction, and there was a statistical improvement in angina episodes also seen in the ACE inhibitor group compared to placebo. ACE inhibitors as a class are recommended for all patients with SIHD and either hypertension, diabetes mellitus, reduced LV function, or chronic kidney disease, unless contraindicated. ARB therapy has shown similar reductions in cardiovascular events though statistically less than ACE inhibitors making them a suitable replacement in SIHD for patients who are unable to tolerate ACE inhibitors [12]. Importantly, ACE inhibitors and ARB's are contraindicated during pregnancy. Before initiating these medications, younger pre-menopausal women should be asked about the possibility of being pregnant.

Anti-lipids

The use of HMG-CoA reductase inhibitor statin therapy in primary and secondary prevention of cardiovascular disease is well described and detailed in an earlier chapter of the book. In women with SIHD, data has shown lower is better even when compared to men. The data from the Pravastatin or Atorvastatin Evaluation and Infection Therapy-Thrombosis in Myocardial Infarction (PROVE IT-TIMI 22) trial found high dose statin therapy further reduced cardiovascular endpoints over standard dose therapy [80]. The reduction was enhanced more in women then men with established CVD. A low density lipoprotein (LDL) goal of <70 mg/dL was reached in 65 % percent of the women in the high dose group who obtained even greater risk reduction than men. The study found high dose statin therapy offered an additional 25 % relative risk reduction compared to standard dose therapy. Updated AHA guidelines recommend treatment of women with SIHD to a goal LDL cholesterol <100 mg/dL, and intensive LDL reduction in high-risk women preferably to <70 mg/dL [81]. It should be the primary lipid goal for clinicians to prevent progression of cardiovascular disease in women. There is also evidence proving statin therapy in addition to reducing atherosclerosis, improves vascular function by reducing vasoconstriction and increasing vasodilation through an endothelial mediated effect [82]. These endothelial, or pleiotropic effects may improve symptoms of angina mediated by inflammation and vascular dysfunction. Though more research is needed specifically in women, intensive statin therapy may have a larger role in prevention of cardiovascular events and in treatment of MVA.

Niacin, nicotinic acid, or vitamin B3 is a broad-spectrum lipid-regulating agent that has been used for decades prior to the statin era to reduce cardiovascular events. Niacin exerts its effects on both cholesterol metabolism and non-lipid mediated vascular protective effects [83]. The data for reduction in cardiovascular endpoints has been mixed with old pre-statin randomized controlled trials showing benefit in secondary prevention compared to placebo [84]. The AIM-HIGH trial randomized 3,414 patients, 14.8 % female with known CAD and on intensive statin therapy to extended release high dose niacin or placebo [85]. The trial concluded early after 3 years follow up when no significant difference was found in cardiovascular events, though

HDL was increased and triglycerides lowered significantly. Though the data remains mixed, current guidelines for SIHD recommend use of high dose niacin alone if intolerant to statins, or in combination with a statin to reach established lipid goals.

Anti-ischemic Therapies to Control Symptoms

Beta-Blockers

Based on ACCF/AHA guidelines for SIHD, beta-blockers are recommended as first line therapy for treatment of angina for both men and women [12]. They act through multiple mechanisms that reduce myocardial oxygen consumption. Reduction in heart rate (chronotropy) allows increased diastolic time, when filling of the myocardial vasculature occurs. A decrease in myocardial contraction (inotropy) and arterial afterload additionally lowers the workload imposed on the heart. In addition to angina relief, post-MI or ACS patients have a mortality benefit with use of beta blocking agents. Beta blockers should be utilized even in absence of angina for at least 3 years if left ventricular function is preserved, and indefinitely if LV function is 40 % or less [86]. Additional benefits have been noted in newer generation of beta-blockers. These effects can offer additional angina relief for individual patients. Carvedilol has vasodilatory effects and additional sympathetic alpha blockade that increases symptom relief in women with MVA [87]. Nebivolol has been shown to additionally improve endothelial function through antioxidant properties that reduce markers of inflammation [88]. A reasonable approach for the clinician managing angina symptoms is trialing alternate beta-blockers particularly in women with non-obstructive coronary artery disease who continue to have symptoms on recommended doses of initial beta-blocker choice.

Nitrates

Nitrates are an effective therapy for occasional and chronic angina symptom relief. Short and long-acting formulations of nitroglycerin rapidly cause direct vasodilatory effect on the epicardial arteries increasing oxygen delivery to the myocardium. Through decreasing preload, myocardial wall tension is lowered, in turn reducing ischemia and lowering blood pressure. The blood pressure lowering effect of nitrates can be dose limiting. Nitrate therapy has been shown to be effective in SIHD from both obstructive CAD and in women with microvascular angina. No clinical trial has directly evaluated the use of nitrates in patients with MVA, though an observational study of 99 patients with cardiac syndrome X found effective angina relief in 50 % of the patients [50]. Multiple formulations exist including sublingual dissolving tablets, mucosal sprays, topical pastes, and long-acting oral formulations of nitroglycerin such as isosorbide dinitrate and isosorbide mononitrate. Important caveats for the clinician using nitrate therapy include using the lowest dose that provides symptom control and educating patients to maintain nitrate free intervals of 10–14 h daily to prevent tolerance to the long-acting formulations. Long-acting preparations of nitrates do not cause tolerance to sublingual nitroglycerin, which should be also prescribed for immediate angina relief. The increasing need for quick acting nitroglycerin tablets or spray should key the clinician to worsening symptoms and the need for re-evaluation of the patients IHD. Directions should be given to all patients to present for immediate evaluation in an emergency room setting for angina symptoms not relieved after using 2–3 doses of short acting nitroglycerin. Patients should be reminded that sublingual nitroglycerin tablets lose potency within 6–12 months of opening the bottle and must be stored in the manufacturers container at all time.

Calcium Channel Blockers

Calcium channel blockers (CCBs), including the dihydropyridines: nifedipine and amlodipine, or the non-dihydropyridines: such as verapamil and diltiazem are the last major class of proven anti-anginal medications [89–91]. The effect of calcium channel blockade is a reduction in coronary vascular resistance with increased myocardial perfusion, coupled with decreased systemic arterial pressure. Negative inotropic and chronotropic response of the myocardium reduces oxygen demand and provides exertional angina relief [92]. Caution must be used with existing conduction defects due to sinus node depression and slowing of atrioventricular node conduction that can lead to bradycardia and heart block. This effect is more pronounced with the non-dihydropyridines diltiazem and verapamil and is augmented when used in combination with any beta-blocker. Use of the dihydropyridines amlodipine or nifedipine are least likely to cause excessive heart rate reductions or heart block, but can be limited by their strong effects on lowering blood pressure. Additionally in patients with reduced left ventricular ejection fraction and heart failure symptoms, calcium channel blockers should generally not be used due to worsening of cardiac contractility [93]. CCBs can be equally efficacious in treating angina in patients with intolerance to beta-blocker therapy, and is the recommended substitute. In select patients without conduction defects, combining calcium channel blockers with beta-blockers can provide additional symptom relief. In women with vaso-spastic angina, CCBs are the preferred therapy due to their direct coronary vasodilatory effects [87]. The drug interactions of calcium channel blockers (by utilizing cytochrome P450 metabolism) include amiodarone, digoxin, simvastatin, lithium, cyclosporine, and carbamazepine. Elderly women are more prone to drug interactions in general and clinicians should be aware of the possibilities and monitor them more carefully.

New Classes

Ranolazine is among the new antianginal drugs approved by the FDA in 2006 that work in an alternate manner compared to the standard therapy classes. Acting through inhibition of the late inward sodium current and decreasing the sodium dependent calcium current during ischemia, it reduces ventricular diastolic tension and myocardial oxygen consumption. Importantly, there is little to no effect on heart rate or blood pressure [12]. As shown in the CARISA and MERLIN TIMI-36 trials, ranolazine reduced the use of sublingual nitroglycerin and angina attacks in men and women [94, 95]. Women with MVA experienced a 29 % further decrease in angina symptoms as compared to men, and ranolazine may be particularly useful in treating women with SIHD without obstructive coronary artery disease [87]. Ranolazine has QTC prolonging effects that have not shown to be pro-arrhythmic alone, but should be used cautiously in combination with other QTC prolonging therapies including anti-arrhythmic drugs [12]. Ranolazine should not be used as initial therapy for angina, but can be useful as an adjunct to first line beta-blockers, CCBs, or both for the control of symptoms in women with SIHD from obstructive CAD, or microvascular disease.

A few drugs worth mentioning are currently not available in the USA, but approved and used in Europe and elsewhere for angina relief in both men and women. Ivabradine is an inhibitor of the "funny channel" (If) that is highly expressed in the sinoatrial node. Through inhibition of this mixed Na-K channel, Ivabradine lowers heart rate and offers similar negative chronotropic effects as beta blockers [87]. Nicorandil is a dual vasodilator with effect on both venous and arterial tone. It is a combined K-channel opener and a nitric oxide donor. The net effect is an increase in myocardial oxygen delivery and reduced demand [96]. Trimetazidine is a drug with antianginal properties not completely understood but thought to be secondary to inhibition of fatty acid oxidation. By altering the substrate for myocardial metabolism, it shifts energy production to glucose, which is more efficient in an environment with low oxygen delivery such as exercise-induced ischemia [97].

Therapy for Refractory Angina

Despite the multiple potential medical and surgical options, refractory angina is seen in growing numbers of patients with SIHD. The definition of refractory angina is symptoms of ischemia in a patient with multi-vessel CAD uncontrolled with medical therapy and not amenable to percutaneous or surgical intervention [12]. Alternative therapies are evidence based and accepted to improve quality of life.

Enhanced external counterpulsation (EECP) is the use of inflatable cuffs wrapped around the lower extremities that inflate sequentially from the calves up the thighs during diastole to augment diastolic pressure and coronary perfusion. They deflate immediately during systole reducing peripheral vascular resistance and improving cardiac output. Therapy is prescribed as hour-long sessions five times a week for 35 sessions, and has shown to decrease angina class and the number of anginal episodes, with women having equal response to men [98]. Contraindications to EECP are severe aortic regurgitation, decompensated heart failure, and severe peripheral vascular disease of the lower extremities.

Spinal cord stimulation involves placing a pulse generator subcutaneously with an electrical lead inserted in the spinal epidural space at the level of T1 or T2.

Stimuli are delivered in a continuous, cyclical, or intermittent mode with a resulting inhibition of pain transmission. Limited data has shown sustained improvement in angina symptoms with no major side effects [99].

Surgical interventions that can be considered include trans-myocardial revascu-larization (TMR) where multiple channels are formed by directing energy through the myocardium in order to denervate ischemic myocardium and stimulate microcir-culation. Thoracic sympathectomy to completely denervate the heart has been uti-lized alone or in conjunction with TMR for added effect. Referrals to centers offering heart transplant or implantation of ventricular assist devices (VAD) that reduce the workload on the ischemic heart may be considered in select qualifying patients.

Therapy Not Recommended for Treatment of SIHD

Current ACCF/AHA guidelines for SIHD have addressed some previously recom-mended therapies, which are now known to have no benefit in SIHD, or potential harm [12]. These include the use of estrogen therapy in postmenopausal women, supplemen-tation of vitamin C, vitamin E, or beta-carotene, and treatment of elevated homocyste-ine levels with folate, vitamin B6, or vitamin B12. The use of these therapies with the intent to reduce cardiovascular risk or improve clinical outcomes has a Class III recom-mendation (no proven benefit, possible harm) with level of evidence A (data from multiple high quality sources) and should not be used in treating SIHD in women.

Revascularization in SIHD

The decision process to select the appropriate patient with SIHD that will benefit from revascularization through either percutaneous coronary intervention (PCI) or coronary artery bypass grafting (CABG) has recently been the subject of intense investigation. The development of guidelines in 2011 by the American College of Cardiology Foundation/American Heart Association/ Society for Cardiovascular Angiography and Interventions (ACCF/AHA/SCAI) for PCI [100], and the revised appropriate use criteria (AUC) for coronary revascularization in 2012 [101] have laid the groundwork for evidence based clinical decisions making for revascular-ization in SIHD. A major point emphasized in the new guidelines is prioritizing the use of maximum medical therapy in all patients with SIHD. This includes ini-tiation and titration of antianginal therapy aimed at controlling symptoms using at least two classes of drugs as needed prior to consideration of revascularization (Fig. 5.1).

Though many patients with SIHD on optimal guideline based medical therapy will have significant risk reduction and symptom control, there remain two subsets that will benefit from a strategy involving revascularization. The first are the symp-tomatic patients who after optimizing medical therapy, and titration of antianginal drugs including at least two classes of medication continue to have limiting angina.

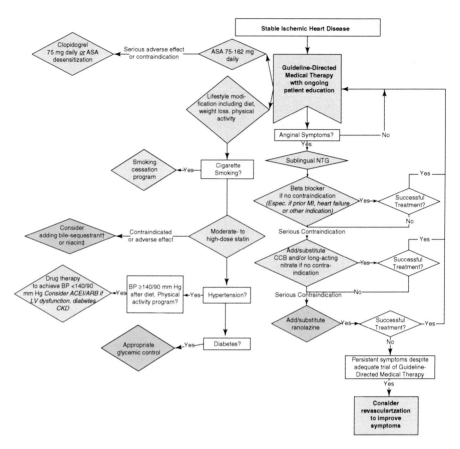

Fig. 5.1 Algorithm for guideline-directed medical therapy for patients with SIHD. †The use of bile acid sequestrant is relatively contraindicated when triglycerides are ≥200 mg/dL and is contraindicated when triglycerides are ≥500 mg/dL. ‡Dietary supplement niacin must not be used as a substitute for prescription niacin. *ACEI* angiotensin-converting enzyme inhibitor, *ARB* angiotensin-receptor blocker, *ASA* aspirin, *BP* blood pressure, *CCB* calcium channel blocker, *CKD* chronic kidney disease, *LV* left ventricular, *MI* myocardial infarction, *NTG* nitroglycerin (Adapted with permission from ACCF/AHA Guidelines (Fihn et al. [12]))

The second of the groups who benefit from revascularization are those with obstructive lesions with high likelihood of decreased survival. These patients are identified by stress testing with high-risk findings suggesting extensive areas of ischemic myocardium. This anatomically based group has evidence of obstructive disease either in all three vessels, or two vessels including the proximal left anterior descending (LAD) artery, or significant obstruction in the left main (LM) artery alone. Survivors of sudden cardiac death caused by a ventricular arrhythmia such as ventricular tachycardia or ventricular fibrillation should also have revascularization to prevent recurrence and improve survival [12] (Figs. 5.2 and 5.3).

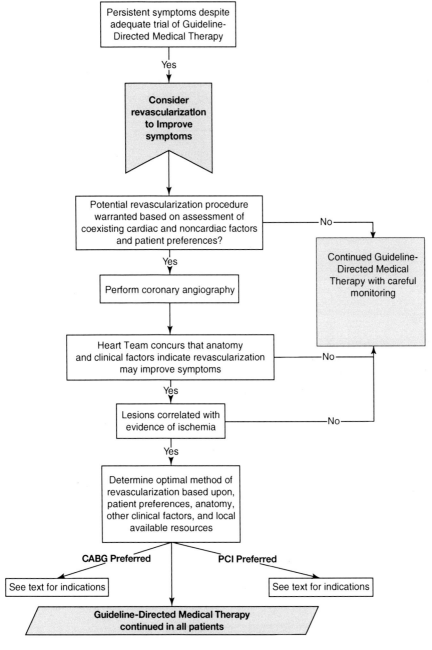

Fig. 5.2 Algorithm for revascularization to improve symptoms of patients with SIHD. *CABG* coronary artery bypass graft, *PCI* percutaneous coronary intervention (Adapted with permission from ACCF/AHA Guidelines (Fihn et al. [12]))

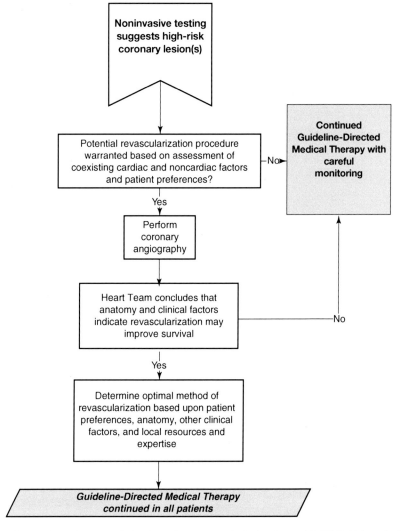

Fig. 5.3 Algorithm for revascularization to improve survival of patients with SIHD (Adapted with permission from ACCF/AHA Guidelines (Fihn et al. [12]))

Women have historically had worse outcomes from both post-PCI complications, and in-hospital mortality after PCI or CABG than their male counterparts [102–104]. There are several possible reasons for this disparity, including that women have more comorbidities such as diabetes mellitus, hypertension, chronic kidney disease, and left ventricular dysfunction. Women are also older in age at presentation, and have smaller blood vessels that can increase the risk of revascularization, though the risk has decreased in recent trials [105]. The decision to pursue revascularization in women with SIHD should be made using the same guideline based recommendations as in men.

Percutaneous Coronary Intervention (PCI)

In the past, women were under-represented in early PCI trials, and there was prior suggestion that women had worse outcomes than men with percutaneous revascularization. Recent studies have shown that revascularization with PCI for SIHD in women yields outcomes similar to men [105]. In the large PCI registry of 22,725 procedures between 2002 and 2003 from the Blue Cross Blue Shield of Michigan Cardiovascular Consortium (BMC2), gender differences were evaluated in relation to clinical outcomes [106]. The analysis showed there was no difference in mortality rates between women and men, with more than half of the procedures being done for SIHD rather than acute MI. Women tended to be older and had more comorbidities than men, were less often smokers and less likely to have had previous PCI or CABG. Women were more likely to have single-vessel disease (>70 %), and less likely to have multi-vessel disease compared to men. Women did have a significantly higher frequency of adverse outcomes after PCI. However, there was no difference in mortality or major cardiovascular events after adjusting for baseline characteristics, comorbidities, presentation, and lesion characteristics. Impaired kidney function and smaller size of women appeared to be largely responsible for the worse outcomes seen in females.

More recently, PCI was shown to be equally successful in both women and men. Whether in-hospital and long-term outcomes differ by gender remains unclear [4]. The National Cardiovascular Data Registry (NCDR) CathPCI Registry study of 426,996 patients ≥65 years of age (42.3 % women) undergoing coronary stenting from 2004 to 2008, found that women remain at higher risk of in-hospital mortality and other complications post-PCI [107], although women had a lower adjusted risk of death than men at 20.4 months of follow-up. Use of drug-eluting stents (DES) compared to bare metal stents (BMS) was associated with similarly improved long-term outcomes in both genders. Newer drug-coated stents using chemotherapeutic agents to further prevent restenosis have reduced the need for repeat interventions. Women, despite having a higher risk profile, were shown to have comparable benefits to men from PCI utilizing paclitaxel drug-eluting stents, as found in the "TAXUS Woman" Analysis study of more than 3,000 women [108]. The only exception was a slightly higher revascularization rate in the high-risk group of women. PCI remains a valuable method for revascularization that can be performed quickly, with equal or better long-term outcomes for women then men. The higher post-procedural risk of complications in women makes a more conservative approach to undergoing the procedure reasonable if symptoms and risk can be controlled medically [12].

Coronary Artery Bypass Grafting (CABG)

Surgical revascularization has been performed since the 1960's in order to create a new conduit for blood flow from the aorta to the coronary artery distal to blockages. Venous and arterial grafts are both utilized, though long term patency is greatly improved with arterial grafts, most commonly the left internal mammary artery (LIMA) [109].

Similarly to PCI, women have recently shown improvements in long-term outcomes following CABG, though peri-procedural morbidity and mortality remain higher in women than men. As in the previous studies, smaller body size in women, which is a surrogate for coronary artery size, largely accounted for the gender difference in outcomes [105]. The Bypass Angioplasty Revascularization Investigation 2 Diabetes (BARI 2D) trial randomized over 2,300 patients, 30 % of women with type 2 diabetes and SIHD, to medical therapy alone or a revascularization strategy deemed appropriate for CABG or PCI [110]. At 5 years, rates of survival did not differ significantly between the revascularization group and the medical therapy group. Overall, there was no significant difference in the rates of death and major cardiovascular events between patients undergoing CABG and those undergoing medical therapy. The study showed that in patients with diabetes and SIHD, intensive medical therapy was equally beneficial as an initial strategy compared to early revascularization by PCI or CABG. However, CABG was superior in diabetic patients with severe diffuse CAD undergoing revascularization. Gender-specific data is not yet available, but the BARI 2D findings reinforce the COURAGE data in a diabetic patient population specifically. More extensive discussion of surgical revascularization in women can be found in the chapter on cardiac surgery.

PCI Versus CABG

The decision to utilize PCI versus CABG is not always straightforward and is best determined by the heart team approach when either the LM is involved or lesions are complex. The heart team includes an interventional cardiologist, cardiac surgeon, and the primary cardiologist, who in discussion with the patient can plan a method for revascularization that offers the most benefit to the patient taking into account their preference. Scoring systems such as the SYNTAX score have been developed to guide decision-making. The SYNTAX trial, randomized 1,800 patients with complex CAD, either three-vessel disease or left main disease, to complete revascularization utilizing either PCI or CABG [111]. The primary results were in favor of CABG after 12 months of follow up with less major cardiovascular and cerebrovascular events. The study was important for its use of both newer methods of CABG and PCI with drug eluting stents (DES) representing a modern real world approach. The SYNTAX score was developed through post-hoc analysis of the CAD characteristics including lesion location, severity, and extend of coronary stenosis. Patients with low scores ≤22 were found to have no difference in outcomes at 3 years, while those with higher scores did worse with PCI [112]. Gender specific data analysis is absent in SYNTAX with women representing 21 % of the CABG arm, and 23.6 % in the PCI group. Current guidelines recommend approaching revascularization gender-neutrally. When done appropriately in non-straightforward cases, all relevant information is gathered which may include stress tests, viability studies, and the diagnostic angiogram. All options are discussed between the heart team and the patient prior to undergoing elective revascularization for SIHD.

All clinicians have the opportunity to help their patients utilize medical and life-style therapy to control symptoms of SIHD. Women with appropriate indications after optimization of guideline based medical therapy, should have revascularization options pursued by a cardiologist and in collaboration with a heart team to provide the best outcomes for the individual patient.

Summary

Ischemic heart disease (IHD) is the leading cause of mortality and morbidity in women. The cardiovascular risk of women tends to be underestimated with consequent underutilization of preventive therapies and appropriate guideline based IHD therapy for women [10]. This can be partially attributed to more frequent atypical anginal symptoms in females and difficulty in making the diagnosis of IHD. Obstructive coronary atherosclerosis, the male model of coronary artery disease, constitutes the basis for diagnosis and therapy for both genders. Because a large number of women with IHD present without obstructive CAD or are referred less often for coronary angiography, relatively fewer women will be treated. Noninvasive and invasive testing can be utilized in the evaluation of ischemic heart disease in women. With the advances in the treatment of coronary heart disease (CHD) and ischemic heart disease (IHD) in recent years, mortality from CAD has significantly improved. However, these reductions are smaller in women when compared to those seen in men.

Despite the fact that women with stable ischemic heart disease tend to have less obstructive coronary artery disease as compared to men, they tend to have a higher prevalence of symptoms, ischemia, and mortality. Microvascular angina is more prevalent in women and is not associated with a benign outcome. With the lack of standardized testing available, clinical diagnosis of ischemic symptoms is of primary importance. There is no gender difference in SIHD therapy based on current guidelines either for obstructive CAD or microvascular disease. The cornerstones of risk factor modification include exercise, lifestyle changes, dietary changes, weight reduction, and guideline based optimal medical therapy. Anti-anginal therapy including beta-blockers, calcium channel blockers, and nitrates remain mainstay of therapy in treating the symptomatic SIHD in women. Revascularization, either percutaneous or surgical, should be considered for medically refractory stable ischemic heart disease or in the presence of an acute coronary syndrome. With increasing awareness of IHD in women, clinicians and patients can start an early comprehensive approach utilizing lifestyle changes, medical therapy, and revascularization, which may help to close the gap between the genders.

References

1. Wenger NK. Women and coronary heart disease: a century after Herrick: understudied, under-diagnosed, and undertreated. Circulation. 2012;126(5):604–11.
2. Roger VL, et al. Heart disease and stroke statistics–2012 update: a report from the American Heart Association. Circulation. 2012;125(1):e2–220.
3. Bellasi A, et al. New insights into ischemic heart disease in women. Cleve Clin J Med. 2007;74(8):585–94.
4. Gupta A, et al. Most important outcomes research papers on cardiovascular disease in women. Circ Cardiovasc Qual Outcomes. 2013;6(1):e1–7.
5. Healy B. The Yentl syndrome. N Engl J Med. 1991;325(4):274–6.
6. Bairey Merz CN, et al. Proceedings from the scientific symposium: sex differences in cardiovascular disease and implications for therapies. J Womens Health (Larchmt). 2010;19(6):1059–72.
7. Daly C, et al. Gender differences in the management and clinical outcome of stable angina. Circulation. 2006;113(4):490–8.
8. Mosca L, et al. AHA/ACC scientific statement: consensus panel statement. Guide to preventive cardiology for women. American Heart Association/American College of Cardiology. J Am Coll Cardiol. 1999;33(6):1751–5.
9. Go AS, et al. Executive summary: heart disease and stroke statistics–2013 update: a report from the American Heart Association. Circulation. 2013;127(1):143–52.
10. Zuchi C, Tritto I, Ambrosio G. Angina pectoris in women: focus on microvascular disease. Int J Cardiol. 2013;163(2):132–40.
11. Lerner DJ, Kannel WB. Patterns of coronary heart disease morbidity and mortality in the sexes: a 26-year follow-up of the Framingham population. Am Heart J. 1986;111(2):383–90.
12. Fihn SD, et al. 2012 ACCF/AHA/ACP/AATS/PCNA/SCAI/STS guideline for the diagnosis and management of patients with stable ischemic heart disease: a report of the American College of Cardiology Foundation/American Heart Association task force on practice guidelines, and the American College of Physicians, American Association for Thoracic Surgery, Preventive Cardiovascular Nurses Association, Society for Cardiovascular Angiography and Interventions, and Society of Thoracic Surgeons. J Am Coll Cardiol. 2012;60(24):e44–164.
13. NHS-National Institute for Health and Clinical Excellence. Management of stable angina National Clinical Guideline Centre. 2011. http://www.nice.org.uk/guidance/CG126.
14. Milner KA, et al. Gender differences in symptom presentation associated with coronary heart disease. Am J Cardiol. 1999;84(4):396–9.
15. Pepine CJ. Angina pectoris in a contemporary population: characteristics and therapeutic implications. TIDES Investigators. Cardiovasc Drugs Ther. 1998;12 Suppl 3:211–6.
16. Hemingway H, et al. Prevalence of angina in women versus men: a systematic review and meta-analysis of international variations across 31 countries. Circulation. 2008;117(12):1526–36.
17. Steg PG, et al. Women and men with stable coronary artery disease have similar clinical outcomes: insights from the international prospective CLARIFY registry. Eur Heart J. 2012;33(22):2831–40.
18. Bugiardini R, et al. Factors influencing underutilization of evidence-based therapies in women. Eur Heart J. 2011;32(11):1337–44.
19. Daly CA, et al. The clinical characteristics and investigations planned in patients with stable angina presenting to cardiologists in Europe: from the Euro Heart Survey of Stable Angina. Eur Heart J. 2005;26(10):996–1010.
20. Dawber TR, Kannel WB. The Framingham study. An epidemiological approach to coronary heart disease. Circulation. 1966;34(4):553–5.
21. D'Agostino Sr RB, et al. General cardiovascular risk profile for use in primary care: the Framingham Heart Study. Circulation. 2008;117(6):743–53.
22. Ridker PM, et al. Development and validation of improved algorithms for the assessment of global cardiovascular risk in women: the Reynolds Risk Score. JAMA. 2007;297(6):611–9.

23. Vaccarino V, et al. Ischaemic heart disease in women: are there sex differences in pathophysiology and risk factors? Position paper from the working group on coronary pathophysiology and microcirculation of the European Society of Cardiology. Cardiovasc Res. 2011;90(1):9–17.
24. Vaccarino V, et al. Sex differences in mortality after acute myocardial infarction: changes from 1994 to 2006. Arch Intern Med. 2009;169(19):1767–74.
25. Shaw LJ, et al. Impact of ethnicity and gender differences on angiographic coronary artery disease prevalence and in-hospital mortality in the American College of Cardiology-National Cardiovascular Data Registry. Circulation. 2008;117(14):1787–801.
26. Shaw LJ, et al. Insights from the NHLBI-Sponsored Women's Ischemia Syndrome Evaluation (WISE) Study: part I: gender differences in traditional and novel risk factors, symptom evaluation, and gender-optimized diagnostic strategies. J Am Coll Cardiol. 2006;47(3 Suppl): S4–20.
27. Shaw LJ, et al. The economic burden of angina in women with suspected ischemic heart disease: results from the National Institutes of Health–National Heart, Lung, and Blood Institute–sponsored Women's Ischemia Syndrome Evaluation. Circulation. 2006;114(9):894–904.
28. Johnson BD, et al. Persistent chest pain predicts cardiovascular events in women without obstructive coronary artery disease: results from the NIH-NHLBI-sponsored Women's Ischaemia Syndrome Evaluation (WISE) study. Eur Heart J. 2006;27(12):1408–15.
29. Sharaf BL, et al. Detailed angiographic analysis of women with suspected ischemic chest pain (pilot phase data from the NHLBI-sponsored Women's Ischemia Syndrome Evaluation [WISE] Study Angiographic Core Laboratory). Am J Cardiol. 2001;87(8):937–41; A3.
30. Bairey Merz CN, et al. Insights from the NHLBI-Sponsored Women's Ischemia Syndrome Evaluation (WISE) Study: part II: gender differences in presentation, diagnosis, and outcome with regard to gender-based pathophysiology of atherosclerosis and macrovascular and microvascular coronary disease. J Am Coll Cardiol. 2006;47(3 Suppl):S21–9.
31. Sheifer SE, et al. Sex differences in coronary artery size assessed by intravascular ultrasound. Am Heart J. 2000;139(4):649–53.
32. Mintz GS, et al. Contribution of inadequate arterial remodeling to the development of focal coronary artery stenoses. An intravascular ultrasound study. Circulation. 1997;95(7):1791–8.
33. Schoenhagen P, et al. Arterial remodeling and coronary artery disease: the concept of "dilated" versus "obstructive" coronary atherosclerosis. J Am Coll Cardiol. 2001;38(2):297–306.
34. Khuddus MA, et al. An intravascular ultrasound analysis in women experiencing chest pain in the absence of obstructive coronary artery disease: a substudy from the National Heart, Lung and Blood Institute-Sponsored Women's Ischemia Syndrome Evaluation (WISE). J Interv Cardiol. 2010;23(6):511–9.
35. Reynolds HR, et al. Mechanisms of myocardial infarction in women without angiographically obstructive coronary artery disease. Circulation. 2011;124(13):1414–25.
36. Collins P. Coronary flow reserve. Br Heart J. 1993;69(4):279–81.
37. Maseri A, et al. Mechanisms of angina pectoris in syndrome X. J Am Coll Cardiol. 1991;17(2):499–506.
38. Cannon 3rd RO, Epstein SE. "Microvascular angina" as a cause of chest pain with angiographically normal coronary arteries. Am J Cardiol. 1988;61(15):1338–43.
39. Reis SE, et al. Coronary microvascular dysfunction is highly prevalent in women with chest pain in the absence of coronary artery disease: results from the NHLBI WISE study. Am Heart J. 2001;141(5):735–41.
40. Reis SE, et al. Coronary flow velocity response to adenosine characterizes coronary microvascular function in women with chest pain and no obstructive coronary disease. Results from the pilot phase of the Women's Ischemia Syndrome Evaluation (WISE) study. J Am Coll Cardiol. 1999;33(6):1469–75.
41. Wei J, et al. Safety of coronary reactivity testing in women with no obstructive coronary artery disease: results from the NHLBI-sponsored WISE (Women's Ischemia Syndrome Evaluation) study. JACC Cardiovasc Interv. 2012;5(6):646–53.
42. Kemp Jr HG, et al. The anginal syndrome associated with normal coronary arteriograms. Report of a six year experience. Am J Med. 1973;54(6):735–42.

43. Kothawade K, Bairey Merz CN. Microvascular coronary dysfunction in women: pathophysiology, diagnosis, and management. Curr Probl Cardiol. 2011;36(8):291–318.
44. Arthur HM, et al. Women, cardiac syndrome X, and microvascular heart disease. Can J Cardiol. 2012;28(2 Suppl):S42–9.
45. Kaski JC, et al. Transient myocardial ischemia during daily life in patients with syndrome X. Am J Cardiol. 1986;58(13):1242–7.
46. Nugent L, Mehta PK, Bairey Merz CN. Gender and microvascular angina. J Thromb Thrombolysis. 2011;31(1):37–46.
47. Marroquin OC, et al. Inflammation, endothelial cell activation, and coronary microvascular dysfunction in women with chest pain and no obstructive coronary artery disease. Am Heart J. 2005;150(1):109–15.
48. Kannel WB, Feinleib M. Natural history of angina pectoris in the Framingham study. Prognosis and survival. Am J Cardiol. 1972;29(2):154–63.
49. Fox KM, EURopean trial On reduction of cardiac events with Perindopril in stable coronary Artery disease Investigators. Efficacy of perindopril in reduction of cardiovascular events among patients with stable coronary artery disease: randomised, double-blind, placebo-controlled, multicentre trial (the EUROPA study). Lancet. 2003;362(9386):782–8.
50. Kaski JC, et al. Cardiac syndrome X: clinical characteristics and left ventricular function. Long-term follow-up study. J Am Coll Cardiol. 1995;25(4):807–14.
51. Humphries KH, et al. Angina with "normal" coronary arteries: sex differences in outcomes. Am Heart J. 2008;155(2):375–81.
52. Delcour KS, et al. Outcomes in patients with abnormal myocardial perfusion imaging and normal coronary angiogram. Angiology. 2009;60(3):318–21.
53. Gulati M, et al. Adverse cardiovascular outcomes in women with nonobstructive coronary artery disease: a report from the Women's Ischemia Syndrome Evaluation Study and the St James Women Take Heart Project. Arch Intern Med. 2009;169(9):843–50.
54. Pepine CJ, et al. Coronary microvascular reactivity to adenosine predicts adverse outcome in women evaluated for suspected ischemia results from the National Heart, Lung and Blood Institute WISE (Women's Ischemia Syndrome Evaluation) study. J Am Coll Cardiol. 2010;55(25):2825–32.
55. Boden WE, et al. Optimal medical therapy with or without PCI for stable coronary disease. N Engl J Med. 2007;356(15):1503–16.
56. Spertus JA, et al. Development and evaluation of the Seattle Angina Questionnaire: a new functional status measure for coronary artery disease. J Am Coll Cardiol. 1995;25(2):333–41.
57. Hlatky MA, et al. A brief self-administered questionnaire to determine functional capacity (the Duke Activity Status Index). Am J Cardiol. 1989;64(10):651–4.
58. Maddox TM, et al. Utilization of secondary prevention therapies in patients with nonobstructive coronary artery disease identified during cardiac catheterization: insights from the National Cardiovascular Data Registry Cath-PCI Registry. Circ Cardiovasc Qual Outcomes. 2010;3(6):632–41.
59. Ogden CL, et al. Prevalence of overweight and obesity in the United States, 1999–2004. JAMA. 2006;295(13):1549–55.
60. Poirier P, et al. Obesity and cardiovascular disease: pathophysiology, evaluation, and effect of weight loss: an update of the 1997 American Heart Association Scientific Statement on Obesity and Heart Disease from the Obesity Committee of the Council on Nutrition, Physical Activity, and Metabolism. Circulation. 2006;113(6):898–918.
61. Gulati M, Shaw LJ, Bairey Merz CN. Myocardial ischemia in women: lessons from the NHLBI WISE study. Clin Cardiol. 2012;35(3):141–8.
62. Huxley R, Barzi F, Woodward M. Excess risk of fatal coronary heart disease associated with diabetes in men and women: meta-analysis of 37 prospective cohort studies. BMJ. 2006;332(7533):73–8.
63. Wenger NK. Coronary heart disease: the female heart is vulnerable. Prog Cardiovasc Dis. 2003;46(3):199–229.

64. Gami AS, et al. Metabolic syndrome and risk of incident cardiovascular events and death: a systematic review and meta-analysis of longitudinal studies. J Am Coll Cardiol. 2007;49(4):403–14.
65. Bellamy L, et al. Pre-eclampsia and risk of cardiovascular disease and cancer in later life: systematic review and meta-analysis. BMJ. 2007;335(7627):974.
66. Satcher D, Thompson TG, Koplan JP. Women and smoking: a report of the Surgeon General. Nicotine Tob Res. 2002;4(1):7–20.
67. Barua RS, et al. Heavy and light cigarette smokers have similar dysfunction of endothelial vasoregulatory activity: an in vivo and in vitro correlation. J Am Coll Cardiol. 2002;39(11):1758–63.
68. Critchley JA, Capewell S. Mortality risk reduction associated with smoking cessation in patients with coronary heart disease: a systematic review. JAMA. 2003;290(1):86–97.
69. Yusuf S, et al. Effect of potentially modifiable risk factors associated with myocardial infarction in 52 countries (the INTERHEART study): case–control study. Lancet. 2004;364(9438):937–52.
70. Milani RV, Lavie CJ, Mehra MR. Reduction in C-reactive protein through cardiac rehabilitation and exercise training. J Am Coll Cardiol. 2004;43(6):1056–61.
71. Hambrecht R, et al. Regular physical activity improves endothelial function in patients with coronary artery disease by increasing phosphorylation of endothelial nitric oxide synthase. Circulation. 2003;107(25):3152–8.
72. Goldsmith RL, Bloomfield DM, Rosenwinkel ET. Exercise and autonomic function. Coron Artery Dis. 2000;11(2):129–35.
73. Antithrombotic Trialists Collaboration. Collaborative meta-analysis of randomised trials of antiplatelet therapy for prevention of death, myocardial infarction, and stroke in high risk patients. BMJ. 2002;324(7329):71–86.
74. CAPRIE Steering Committee. A randomised, blinded, trial of clopidogrel versus aspirin in patients at risk of ischaemic events (CAPRIE). CAPRIE Steering Committee. Lancet. 1996;348(9038):1329–39.
75. Bhatt DL, et al. Clopidogrel and aspirin versus aspirin alone for the prevention of atherothrombotic events. N Engl J Med. 2006;354(16):1706–17.
76. Pfeffer MA, et al. Effect of captopril on mortality and morbidity in patients with left ventricular dysfunction after myocardial infarction. Results of the survival and ventricular enlargement trial. The SAVE Investigators. N Engl J Med. 1992;327(10):669–77.
77. Indications for ACE inhibitors in the early treatment of acute myocardial infarction: systematic overview of individual data from 100,000 patients in randomized trials. ACE Inhibitor Myocardial Infarction Collaborative Group. Circulation. 1998;97(22):2202–12.
78. Chen JW, et al. Long-term angiotensin-converting enzyme inhibition reduces plasma asymmetric dimethylarginine and improves endothelial nitric oxide bioavailability and coronary microvascular function in patients with syndrome X. Am J Cardiol. 2002;90(9): 974–82.
79. Pauly DF, et al. In women with symptoms of cardiac ischemia, nonobstructive coronary arteries, and microvascular dysfunction, angiotensin-converting enzyme inhibition is associated with improved microvascular function: a double-blind randomized study from the National Heart, Lung and Blood Institute Women's Ischemia Syndrome Evaluation (WISE). Am Heart J. 2011;162(4):678–84.
80. Truong QA, et al. Benefit of intensive statin therapy in women: results from PROVE IT-TIMI 22. Circ Cardiovasc Qual Outcomes. 2011;4(3):328–36.
81. Mosca L, et al. Effectiveness-based guidelines for the prevention of cardiovascular disease in women–2011 update: a guideline from the american heart association. Circulation. 2011;123(11):1243–62.
82. Treasure CB, et al. Beneficial effects of cholesterol-lowering therapy on the coronary endothelium in patients with coronary artery disease. N Engl J Med. 1995;332(8):481–7.
83. Lavigne PM, Karas RH. The current state of niacin in cardiovascular disease prevention: a systematic review and meta-regression. J Am Coll Cardiol. 2013;61(4):440–6.

84. Group, C.D.P.R. Clofibrate and niacin in coronary heart disease. JAMA. 1975;231(4): 360–81.
85. AIM-HIGH Investigators, et al. Niacin in patients with low HDL cholesterol levels receiving intensive statin therapy. N Engl J Med. 2011;365(24):2255–67.
86. Kernis SJ, et al. Does beta-blocker therapy improve clinical outcomes of acute myocardial infarction after successful primary angioplasty? J Am Coll Cardiol. 2004;43(10):1773–9.
87. Sarbaziha R, et al. Therapy for stable angina in women. P T. 2012;37(7):400–4.
88. Kayaalti F, et al. Effects of nebivolol therapy on endothelial functions in cardiac syndrome X. Heart Vessels. 2010;25(2):92–6.
89. Ezekowitz MD, et al. Amlodipine in chronic stable angina: results of a multicenter double-blind crossover trial. Am Heart J. 1995;129(3):527–35.
90. Brogden RN, Benfield P. Verapamil: a review of its pharmacological properties and therapeutic use in coronary artery disease. Drugs. 1996;51(5):792–819.
91. Boman K, et al. Antianginal effect of conventional and controlled release diltiazem in stable angina pectoris. Eur J Clin Pharmacol. 1995;49(1–2):27–30.
92. Thadani U. Current medical management of chronic stable angina. J Cardiovasc Pharmacol Ther. 2004;9 Suppl 1:S11–29; quiz S98–9.
93. Hunt SA, et al. 2009 focused update incorporated into the ACC/AHA 2005 guidelines for the diagnosis and management of heart failure in adults a report of the American College of Cardiology Foundation/American Heart Association task force on practice guidelines developed in collaboration with the International Society for Heart and Lung Transplantation. J Am Coll Cardiol. 2009;53(15):e1–90.
94. Chaitman BR, et al. Effects of ranolazine with atenolol, amlodipine, or diltiazem on exercise tolerance and angina frequency in patients with severe chronic angina: a randomized controlled trial. JAMA. 2004;291(3):309–16.
95. Mehta PK, et al. Ranolazine improves angina in women with evidence of myocardial ischemia but no obstructive coronary artery disease. JACC Cardiovasc Imaging. 2011;4(5):514–22.
96. Frampton J, Buckley MM, Fitton A. Nicorandil. A review of its pharmacology and therapeutic efficacy in angina pectoris. Drugs. 1992;44(4):625–55.
97. Chaitman BR, Sano J. Novel therapeutic approaches to treating chronic angina in the setting of chronic ischemic heart disease. Clin Cardiol. 2007;30(2 Suppl 1):I25–30.
98. Arora RR, et al. The multicenter study of enhanced external counterpulsation (MUST-EECP): effect of EECP on exercise-induced myocardial ischemia and anginal episodes. J Am Coll Cardiol. 1999;33(7):1833–40.
99. Di Pede F, et al. Immediate and long-term clinical outcome after spinal cord stimulation for refractory stable angina pectoris. Am J Cardiol. 2003;91(8):951–5.
100. Levine GN, et al. 2011 ACCF/AHA/SCAI guideline for percutaneous coronary intervention. A report of the American College of Cardiology Foundation/American Heart Association task force on practice guidelines and the Society for Cardiovascular Angiography and Interventions. J Am Coll Cardiol. 2011;58(24):e44–122.
101. Patel MR, et al. ACCF/SCAI/STS/AATS/AHA/ASNC/HFSA/SCCT 2012 Appropriate use criteria for coronary revascularization focused update: a report of the American College of Cardiology Foundation Appropriate Use Criteria Task Force, Society for Cardiovascular Angiography and Interventions, Society of Thoracic Surgeons, American Association for Thoracic Surgery, American Heart Association, American Society of Nuclear Cardiology, and the Society of Cardiovascular Computed Tomography. J Am Coll Cardiol. 2012;59(9): 857–81.
102. Hannan EL, et al. Risk stratification of in-hospital mortality for coronary artery bypass graft surgery. J Am Coll Cardiol. 2006;47(3):661–8.
103. Singh M, et al. Correlates of procedural complications and a simple integer risk score for percutaneous coronary intervention. J Am Coll Cardiol. 2002;40(3):387–93.
104. Kim C, et al. A systematic review of gender differences in mortality after coronary artery bypass graft surgery and percutaneous coronary interventions. Clin Cardiol. 2007;30(10):491–5.

105. Lundberg G, King S. Coronary revascularization in women. Clin Cardiol. 2012;35(3): 156–9.
106. Duvernoy CS, et al. Gender differences in adverse outcomes after contemporary percutaneous coronary intervention: an analysis from the Blue Cross Blue Shield of Michigan Cardiovascular Consortium (BMC2) percutaneous coronary intervention registry. Am Heart J. 2010;159(4):677–683 e1.
107. Anderson ML, et al. Short- and long-term outcomes of coronary stenting in women versus men: results from the National Cardiovascular Data Registry Centers for Medicare & Medicaid services cohort. Circulation. 2012;126(18):2190–9.
108. Mikhail GW, et al. Influence of sex on long-term outcomes after percutaneous coronary intervention with the paclitaxel-eluting coronary stent: results of the "TAXUS Woman" analysis. JACC Cardiovasc Interv. 2010;3(12):1250–9.
109. Berger PB, et al. Frequency of early occlusion and stenosis in a left internal mammary artery to left anterior descending artery bypass graft after surgery through a median sternotomy on conventional bypass: benchmark for minimally invasive direct coronary artery bypass. Circulation. 1999;100(23):2353–8.
110. BARI 2D Study Group, et al. A randomized trial of therapies for type 2 diabetes and coronary artery disease. N Engl J Med. 2009;360(24):2503–15.
111. Serruys PW, et al. Percutaneous coronary intervention versus coronary-artery bypass grafting for severe coronary artery disease. N Engl J Med. 2009;360(10):961–72.
112. Kappetein AP, et al. Comparison of coronary bypass surgery with drug-eluting stenting for the treatment of left main and/or three-vessel disease: 3-year follow-up of the SYNTAX trial. Eur Heart J. 2011;32(17):2125–34.

Chapter 6
Invasive Therapy for Women Presenting with Acute Coronary Syndromes

Magdelena A. Zeglin-Sawczuk, Vijay Krishnamoorthy, and John P. Gassler

Introduction

More than 700,000 patients per year are discharged from U.S. hospitals with a diagnosis of acute coronary syndrome (ACS) [1]. The average age at presentation for a first myocardial infarction (MI) is 64.7 years for men and 72.2 years for women. The lifetime risk of developing coronary heart disease (CHD) after 40 years of age is 49 % for men and 32 % for women [2], while the incidence of CHD in women lags behind men by 10 years for total CHD and by 20 years for more serious clinical events such as MI and sudden death [3]. Although coronary artery disease (CAD) is the number one cause of mortality for both men and women in the United States [4, 5], it is underappreciated, especially by women in the at risk age range and the physicians taking care of them. In fact, female gender seems to confer unique qualities with respect to clinical presentation, pathophysiology and therapeutic options. Recently, a focus on raising awareness of these key differences in CAD presentation and therapies for women has occurred through public awareness campaigns (i.e. American Heart Association Go Red for Women).

The presentations experienced are significantly diverse with men more likely to present with sudden death or acute myocardial infarction, whereas women tend to develop atypical chest pain syndromes and angina pectoris [6, 7]. It is thought that the later presentation for women compared to men is potentially due to protective effect of estrogens (plaque stabilization, plaque rupture prevention) [8], but at the

M.A. Zeglin-Sawczuk, MD (✉)
Division of Cardiology, University of Vermont College of Medicine,
Burlington, VT, USA
e-mail: magdalena.zeglin-sawczuk@vtmednet.org

J.P. Gassler, MD • V. Krishnamoorthy, MD
Division of Cardiology, University of Rochester Medical Center,
601 Elmwood Ave, 679-C, Rochester, NY 14642, USA
e-mail: john_gassler@urmc.rochester.edu

H.Z. Mieszczanska, G.P. Velarde (eds.),   113
Management of Cardiovascular Disease in Women,
DOI 10.1007/978-1-4471-5517-1_6, © Springer-Verlag London 2014

same time, women with acute coronary syndromes (ACS) carry higher risk profile at the time of presentation since they tend to be older, have more co-morbid conditions, such as diabetes mellitus (DM) and hypertension, and more often present with heart failure when compared to men [4, 7, 9].

Pathophysiology

Previous studies have suggested that the pathophysiology of ACS in women and men may also differ. Men are more likely to have ruptured plaques [10, 11], whereas women more often present with plaque erosions [12, 13]. This observation may potentially explain the longer periods of angina upon presentation in women rather than sudden onset of chest pain in men. The results of the PROSPECT trial (Providing Regional Observations to Study Predictors of Events in the Coronary Tree) demonstrated that women with ACS have less extensive CAD by angiography [4, 9], lower rates of plaque rupture, smaller necrotic cores and less calcium, but similar overall plaque burden. Additionally, generally smaller lumen diameters in women's coronary arteries were confirmed by intravascular ultrasound (IVUS), along with significantly smaller total fibrous plaque volume. These high risk features may explain similar rates of adverse cardiovascular events such as sudden cardiac death and myocardial infarction (MI) at 3 years, despite less extensive CAD in women [4]. Thin capped fibroatheroma (TCFA) appear to identify more vulnerable plaque in women compared to man and seem to be the strongest histological predictor of major adverse cardiac events (MACE) [4].

Given the lower likelihood of obstructive CAD at the time of angiography in women who present with a history consistent with ACS, it is hypothesized that there may be a greater burden of microvascular disease and abnormal vasodilatory reserve leading to subendocardial ischemia, or coronary spasm that mimics ACS secondary to epicardial vessel obstructive CAD [14].

ACS/NSTEMI

Despite the high cardiovascular morbidity and mortality in women presenting with ACS and the established benefits of percutaneous coronary intervention (PCI) in reducing fatal and non- fatal ischemic complications in high risk acute coronary syndrome patients, only about one third of annual PCI procedures for ACS are performed in women. Women experience greater time delays in undergoing diagnostic angiography and PCI and undergo diagnostic coronary angiography less frequently than men [15]. Some of these differences in practice may partially be explained by the female patient's risk profile at presentation including advance age and increased potential risk for adverse procedural outcomes.

Gender differences in the management of ACS have been described in both observational and randomized clinical studies [16–19]. As noted above, women are less likely to undergo diagnostic coronary angiography and revascularization for ACS [17]. Controversy exists with respect to the benefit of revascularization treatment in women in the setting of ACS. A subgroup analysis of the FRISC 2 trial (Fragmin and Revascularization during Instability in Coronary artery disease) and RITA 3 trial (Third Randomized Intervention Trial of Unstable Angina) demonstrated that an early revascularization strategy in women might be associated with an increased risk of death and MI when compared to a more conservative strategy [20, 21]. In contrast, the results of the TACTICS- TIMI 18 trial (Treat angina with Aggrastat and determine Cost of Therapy with an Invasive or Conservative Strategy- Thrombolysis in Myocardial Infarction-18) demonstrated an equal benefit from early revascularization in men and women, with the highest benefit in women at highest risk (defined as presence of elevated cardiac biomarkers) [22]. A meta-analysis of randomized clinical trials (RCT) by O'Donoghue, et al., comparing an early invasive strategy with conservative therapy in patients with unstable angina/ non-ST segment elevation myocardial infarction (UA/NSTEMI) found that invasive strategy has a comparable benefit in men and high risk women (high risk again defined as elevated biomarkers or ST segment deviation on EKG) for reducing the composite end point of death, MI, or re-hospitalization with ACS. In contrast, low risk women (without biomarker elevation) had a non-significantly higher risk of death or MI compared with those treated conservatively [14].

The OASIS 5 invasive sub study demonstrated no difference in the primary outcome between routine invasive and selective invasive strategies in women, but suggested a higher mortality in the routine invasive group [23]. Finally, data from SWEDEHEART study (Swedish Web- System for Enhancement and Development of Evidence- Based Care in Heart Disease Evaluated According to Recommended Therapies) demonstrated a similar mortality benefit in both genders presenting with UA/NSTEMI treated with an early invasive strategy, without a gender interaction: women (RR = 0.46, 95 % CI 0.38–0.55) and men (RR = 0.45, 95 % CI 0.40–0.52) [24].

In summary, based on evidence presented above, high risk patients of either gender benefit from an early invasive strategy, and have better outcomes with early revascularization than conservative therapy. Alternatively, low risk patients, especially women (defined as TIMI risk score <3, no ST segment deviation, and negative biomarkers) should be treated conservatively [14, 16]. This is reflected in the ACC/AHA guidelines update [16] (Table 6.1, Fig. 6.1).

STEMI (ST Elevation Myocardial Infarction)

STEMI comprises 25–40 % of ACS presentations in observational studies. According to the most recent National Registry of Myocardial Infarction 4 (NRMI-4), that number is around 29 % of ACS presentations [25, 26]. Significant improvements in the understanding the pathophysiology of atherosclerosis, especially the mechanism of acute myocardial infarction and intervening with appropriate therapies has resulted in not only a decreased incidence of recurrent STEMI, but also improved mortality rates, both in-hospital (5–6 %) and at 1-year (7–18 %) [27, 28].

Table 6.1 Early invasive vs. conservative therapy for patients with UA/ NSTEMI adapted from ACC/AHA guidelines

Preferred strategy	Patient characteristics
Early Invasive	Recurrent angina or ischemia at rest or with low-level activities despite intensive medical therapy
	Elevated cardiac biomarkers (TnT or TnI)
	New ST-segment depression
	Signs or symptoms of HF
	New or worsening mitral regurgitation
	High-risk findings from noninvasive testing
	Hemodynamic instability
	Sustained ventricular tachycardia
	PCI within 6 months
	Prior CABG
	High-risk score (e.g., TIMI, GRACE)
	Mild to moderate renal dysfunction
	Diabetes mellitus
	Reduced LV function (LVEF <40 %)
Conservative	Low-risk score (e.g., TIMI, GRACE)
	Patient or physician preference in the absence of high-risk features

With permission from Jneid et al. [16]

Approximately 20–30 % of patients presenting with STEMI are women [29, 30]. In earlier STEMI trials women were significantly underrepresented. This is thought to be due to the basic pathophysiologic difference in ACS presentation between men and women. Women presented more often with NSTEMI as they tended to have more atherosclerotic plaque erosion whereas men had plaque rupture and vessel occlusion [8, 31]. However the proportion of women, especially younger women, has increased in the STEMI population. This proportionate increase in women seems to be related to an increase in risk factors such as smoking and obesity in these studies suggesting possible change in plaque pathophysiology and, therefore, plaque instability. Also, women tend to have increased mortality after a STEMI compared to men despite receiving optimal or similar therapy to men [29, 32]. Women also seem to have higher incidence of complications from the therapy administered including more bleeding from antiplatelet and lytic therapy, more vascular complications, and also increased rates of renal failure [32–35]. Thus the increase in the incidence of STEMI in women combined with the higher mortality despite optimal therapy, and higher complication rates with invasive and non-invasive therapy make them a unique group requiring special consideration and more dedicated research.

The treatment of STEMI includes the acute phase and long term management phase. The acute management includes pre-hospital management, reperfusion strategies, and the management of the hospitalization including the complications of the MI and the reperfusion strategy selected.

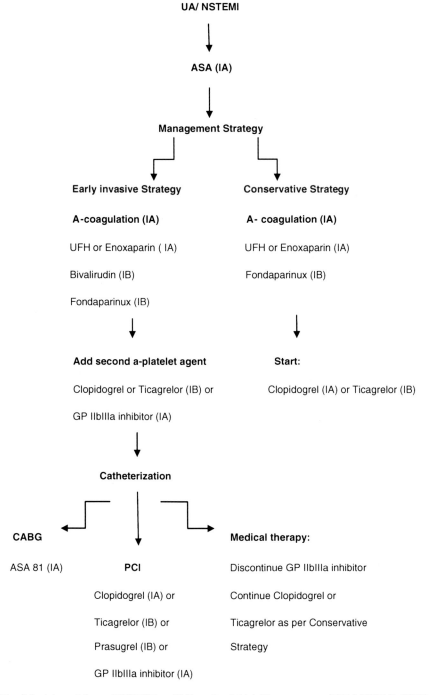

Fig. 6.1 Adapted from ACC/AHA guidelines for Initial Management of UA/NSTEMI (2012) (With permission from Jneid et al. [16])

Pre-hospital Management

Initial studies raised the concern, which was probably justified during that time period that women were not getting standard of care management for their STEMI presentations. In the CRUSADE (Can Rapid Risk Stratification of Unstable Angina Patients Suppress Adverse Outcomes with Early Implementation of the ACC/AHA Guidelines) registry female gender was a strong independent predictor of a failure to receive reperfusion therapy among patients who had no contraindications [36]. Women included in the NCDR (National Cardiovascular Data Registry) ACTION Registry–GWTG (Get With The Guidelines) presented later after symptom onset, had longer door-to-fibrinolysis or door-to-balloon (or device) (D2B) times, and did not receive aspirin or beta blockers within 24 h of presentation as often [36]. However, a recent assessment of the effects of a statewide program for treatment of STEMI suggests significant improvements in treatment times that were similar for whites and blacks and for women and men [37]. Recognizing the problem has been the real challenge in pre-hospital management of STEMI in women. Women tend to present with atypical symptoms delaying the initial diagnosis [38]. However, once the diagnosis has been established the morbidity and mortality are driven by the patient's co-morbidities rather than by sub-optimal treatment. There are still regional differences in symptom recognition to ECG time and also symptom onset to hospital time as demonstrated by multiple studies [39, 40]. Thus, there is a need for more campaigns to educate women and health care workers to recognize atypical symptoms for angina, and obtain a timely ECG as soon as it is recognized.

Once EMS suspects a possible ACS on a call the patient is asked to chew 324 mg (four 81 mg tablets) of aspirin to help hasten the onset of systemic action. Nitroglycerin in the appropriate clinical setting may help with some symptom relief, but has not demonstrated any mortality benefit in trials. Also, caution should be exercised with inferior STEMI patients as right ventricular involvement of the infarction could potentially cause significant hypotension with nitroglycerin. Oxygen therapy is routinely administered and has no proven harm and opioids seem to relieve anxiety and pain. Activation of the STEMI alarm at hospitals that perform primary PCI by the EMS personnel from the field has resulted in shorter door to balloon times resulting in better outcomes [41].

ED and Hospital Management

Once in the emergency room, the focus shifts to choosing the appropriate reperfusion strategy [42]. If primary PCI is available, it should be performed in the shortest time possible. The ACC/AHA guidelines recommend that reperfusion (the door to balloon time) be achieved in <60 min from time of arrival to the ED. If primary PCI is not available and the nearest primary PCI center is >120 min away, then the ACC/AHA Class 1 recommendation is to consider thrombolytic therapy if no contraindications exist. If thrombolytic therapy is the reperfusion strategy of choice for the patient, it should be accomplished within 30 min of arrival to the ED. Dual anti-platelet therapy should be initiated as soon as possible. Currently, there are three drug options are available for patient's undergoing urgent PCI: clopidogrel, prasugrel, and ticagrelor. No published literature exists on gender specific differences in the type of thrombolytic therapy or anti-platelet agents.

PCI: Invasive reperfusion therapy has no significant gender related issues per se. In general, women tend to have more diffuse disease in significantly smaller vessels making them less than ideal for PCI. Women tend to be older than men at the time of presentation, with more comorbidities and, therefore, they tend to have more complex lesions. For these reasons the procedural success rate in women in various studies is lower than that of men [42]. Also, patients with failed PCI attempts have a higher short term and long term mortality, in some studies up to 20 and 50 %, respectively [43]. The evidence suggests that MACE is reduced with placement of a stent when compared to balloon angioplasty alone in STEMI. Even though they have smaller caliber vessels and a higher incidence of DM requiring smaller stents, both risk factors for in-stent restenosis, women tend to have a lower incidence of restenosis compared to men [44]. The drug eluting stents seem to perform equally well in women and men [45]. Thus, it appears that choice of stent should not be guided by gender differences.

Early Invasive Therapy: Adjunctive Pharmacotherapy

Antiplatelet Therapy

Aspirin

Acetylic Acid (ASA) irreversibly blocks cyclo-oxygenase and the synthesis of arachadonic acid- derived thromboxane A2- a strong promoter of platelet aggregation. ASA significantly inhibits platelet function within 60 min of administration [46]. ASA therapy reduces cardiovascular mortality, which is well established. ASA (four 81 mg tablets) should be administered as soon as possible after presentation with acute coronary syndrome and continued indefinitely [16]. The ISIS-2 trial (International Study of Infarct Survival- 2) demonstrated that reduction in mortality with ASA vs. placebo in acute MI was lower in women (16 %) when compared to men (22 %), although the difference was not statistically significant [47]. Further analyses revealed no clear outcome benefit of ASA in doses greater than 100 mg/day compared with lower doses in women, despite previously reported higher platelet reactivity, and resulted in higher incidence of bleeding [48–51].

P2Y12 Receptor Inhibitors

Thienopyridines: Clopidogrel and prasugrel, selectively and irreversibly inhibit the P2Y12 ADP platelet receptor, which plays a critical role in platelet activation and aggregation. Both agents work synergistically with ASA in providing greater platelet inhibition than either agent alone [46].

The prodrug, clopidogrel, is inactive in vitro, and is metabolized by a cytochrome P450-3A4 to become the active metabolite. The standard 300 mg loading dose of clopidogrel requires up to 6 h for maximal antiplatelet effect, whereas a 600 mg dose achieves that goal in about 2 h. Full platelet inhibition is achieved within 2–3 days of therapy onset with a daily dose of clopidogrel 75 mg following a loading dose. Platelet function recovers in 5–7 days after discontinuation of the drug [46]. The pivotal trial for Clopidogrel, the CURE trial (Clopidogrel in Unstable angina to prevent Recurrent Events), evaluated 12,562 patients with UA/NSTEMI who were randomized to clopidogrel or placebo, and demonstrated a 20 % relative risk reduction in the composite primary end point of death, MI, stroke at 1 year, at the cost of 1 % increased risk of major bleeding. Similar benefits were observed in women (RR 0.77, 95 % CI 0.52–1.15) and men (RR 0.65, 95 % CI 0.48–0.87) [49, 52]. A significant limitation of the trial was the non- routine use of an early invasive strategy at the time of study as only 44 % of patients underwent cardiac catheterization at the time of index hospitalization. A 9.6 % rate of major bleeding was observed among patients who received clopidogrel within 5 days of CABG [49, 52]. Accordingly the ACC/AHA guidelines recommend that clopidogrel should be discontinued 5–7 days before CABG unless the urgency of CABG outweighs the risk of bleeding (class 1 indication) [16, 42].

Prasugrel is a novel thienopyridine and prodrug and, like clopidogrel, requires conversion to an active metabolite before binding to the platelet P2Y12 receptor to confer antiplatelet activity. Prasugrel inhibits ADP–induced platelet aggregation more rapidly, more consistently, and to a greater extent than does clopidogrel in patients with coronary artery disease, undergoing PCI [53]. The TRITON- TIMI 38 trial (Trial to Assess Improvement in Therapeutic Outcomes by Optimizing Platelet Inhibition with Prasugrel- Thrombolysis in Myocardial Infarction 38) was a landmark trial that studied prasugrel (60 mg loading dose, followed by 10 mg/day) in patients with ACS (74 % with UA/NSTEMI) compared to standard dose Clopidogrel (300 mg followed by 75 mg/day) in 13,600 patients [53]. The prasugrel loading dose was administered before, during or within 1 h after PCI but only after coronary anatomy had been defined. Prasugrel was associated with 2.2 % absolute risk reduction and a 19 % relative risk reduction with respect to the primary end point (a composite of cardiovascular death, MI, stroke). Data from a landmark analysis demonstrated that prasugrel was superior to clopidogrel within hours of administration, which is consistent with its more rapid onset of action. The rates of stent thrombosis were significantly reduced when compared to clopidogrel, from 2.4 to 1.1 % (p<0.001) by prasugrel. However, prasugrel was associated with significant increase in the rate of bleeding complications (2.4 % for prasugrel compared to 1.8 % for clopidogrel, HR 1.32, 95 % CI1.03–1.68, p=0.03), including the rates of fatal bleeding, and CABG- related bleeding [53].

A post hoc analysis suggested three groups of ACS patients who did not have net clinical benefit (defined as the rate of death, MI, stroke or non- CABG related bleeding) from prasugrel. Patients with history of stroke or TIA had net harm from prasugrel therapy and patients age ≥75 years or with a body weight of <60 kg had no net benefit from prasugrel therapy. In both treatment groups patients with at least one of these risk factors had higher rates of bleeding than those without them [53]. While there are not gender specific data available for prasugrel, female patients tend to be older and generally weigh less, often falling into one of the relative contraindication categories.

Ticagrelor is a novel non-thienopyridine, reversible P2Y12 antagonist, which does not require metabolic activation in vivo, has a rapid onset of action, greater inhibition of platelet aggregation and significantly faster reduction in effect at drug termination when compared to clopidogrel. The pivotal trial for ticagrelor, the PLATO trial (Study of Platelet Inhibition and Patient Outcomes) enrolled 18,624 patients with ACS (16.7 % with UA, 42.7 % with NSTEMI) and randomized them to receive a standard dosing regimen of clopidogrel (300 mg loading dose followed by 75 mg/day) or ticagrelor (180 mg loading dose, followed by 90 mg twice daily) [54]. The composite endpoint of cardiovascular death, MI or stroke as well as the primary safety end point of major bleeding event was compared between the groups. Ticagrelor was associated with 2 % ARR (HR 0.84, 95 % CI 0.770.92, p=0.0003) of the primary endpoint in patients with NSTEMI. The benefits of ticagrelor were present at 30 days of therapy and persisted for up to 360 days, and were similar across invasive or conservative strategies. Notably Ticagrelor was associated with 1.4 % ARR in all- cause mortality and lower rates of definite stent thrombosis without an increase in the risk of bleeding, including CABG- related bleeding [54].

The pivotal trials for prasugrel and ticagrelor demonstrated relatively smaller reductions in the primary endpoint in women compared to men, however, neither of the studies clearly defined a significant interaction between gender and treatment assignment nor were they powered to analyze treatment interactions between subgroups [55].

GP IIb/IIIa Inhibitors

Abciximab, tirofiban, eptifibatide block the platelet GP IIb/IIIa receptor mediated final common pathway of platelet aggregation by preventing binding of fibrinogen [46]. Their efficacy has been well established during PCI procedures in patients with UA/NSTEMI, particularly among high risk patients, such as those with elevated cardiac biomarkers and diabetes mellitus [56, 57].

Although treatment with GP IIb/IIIa antagonists was associated with a significant reduction in death or MI at 30 days in men, women had worse outcomes with such therapy [55, 56]. This difference can potentially be explained in part by clinical characteristics of the patients. Women enrolled in those trials tended to be older, had more extensive MI's and had more co-morbid conditions. When risk was further stratified by troponin level no gender differences were seen [55]. More recent trials have not demonstrated significant differences in outcomes stratified by gender, potentially due to concomitant use of clopidogrel [55, 58].

Anticoagulant Therapy

Unfractionated Heparin (UFH) is an indirect thrombin inhibitor, which complexes with antithrombin (AT), converting this circulating cofactor from a slow to rapid inactivator of thrombin, factor Xa, and to a lesser extent, factors XIIa, XIa and IXa [46]. The anticoagulant response to a standard dose of UFH varies widely among patients, which makes it necessary to monitor the response in each patient, using the activated clotting time (ACT) and to titrate the dose to the individual patient anticoagulation level. In women UFH has been commonly used in combination with ASA for medical treatment of UA/NSTEMI as well as in early invasive strategy with PCI [15].

A weight adjusted dosing regimen is standard for all patients with a goal ACT: 250–350 s [15]. Lower doses of heparin and therefore lower ACTs should be considered in women and elderly patients, especially when used in combination with GP IIb/IIIa inhibitors during PCI [59]. It has also been recognized that prolonged therapy with UHF has been associated with increased risk of bleeding without adding benefit and therefore, no additional heparin is recommended after completion of the PCI procedure [59].

Low Molecular Weight Heparin (LMWH)

Enoxaparin and Dalteparin are low molecular weight heparins, which are fragments of UFH produced by a controlled enzymatic depolymerization process. Similar to unfractionated heparin they work by binding to antithrombin 3, causing a conformational change that accelerates the interaction of AT with thrombin and factor Xa [46]. Compared to UFH, LMWH's anti- Xa activity predominates over its anti-thrombin activity. In addition it has better bioavailability, is more conveniently administered by subcutaneous injections, produces more predictable dose response, causes less platelet activation and results in less heparin induced thrombocytopenia (HIT) [59]. The efficacy and safety of the a commonly used LMWH, enoxaparin, was studied in patients with UA/NSTEMI undergoing PCI in 2 trials. The A-Z Trial (Aggrastat to Zocor phases) enrolled 3,987 patients, 29 % of which were women, and the SYNERGY trial (Superior Yield of the New Strategy of Enoxaparin, Revascularization, and Glycoprotein IIb/IIIa Inhibitors) enrolled 9,978 patients of which 34 % were women. Both studies met their non- inferiority endpoints, demonstrating no significant reduction in benefit of enoxaparin when compared to UFH in either women or men undergoing PCI for ACS. No significant difference in the rate of major bleeding was found between two agents [60, 61].

Direct Thrombin Inhibitors

Bivalirudin is a synthetic direct thrombin inhibitor with a short half-life. It acts on both circulating and clot-bound thrombin, with much higher thrombin specificity when compared to UFH and no platelet activation effect. It has been extensively studied in patients with ACS undergoing PCI. In a meta-analysis of 8,497 patients undergoing elective or urgent PCI for ACS, comparing direct thrombin inhibitors to UFH, there was a significant reduction in death or MI (4.6 % vs 6.6 %, RRR 0.68, 95 % CI 0.57–0.83, p < 0.001) and lower rates of bleeding complications [62]. In the REPLACE 2 trial (Randomized Evaluation in Percutaneous Coronary Intervention Linking Angiomax to Reduced Clinical Events) bivalirudin with provisional or bailout use of GB IIb/IIIa inhibitor was compared to planned use of UFH with GP IIb/IIIa inhibitors in 6,010 patients (26 % women) undergoing PCI looking at ischemic and bleeding outcomes. In that trial female gender was an independent predictor of death and bleeding complications [63]. Among women treated with bivalirudin or heparin there was no difference in the individual or composite ischemic end points, but bivalirudin was associated with a significant reduction in major bleeding at 30 days that persisted out to 6 months (34.1 % with UFH vs 19.7 % with bivalirudin, p < 0.001) [63].

The landmark ACUITY trial confirmed the reduced bleeding event rates with Bivalirudin and its non- inferiority with respect to ischemic outcomes in patients with UA/NSTEMI undergoing PCI [64]. In this trial 13,819 patients (4,157 were women, 30.1 %) were enrolled, and randomized into three different treatment arms: heparin (UFH or enoxaparin) +/− GPI, or bivalirudin plus GPI, or bivalirudin alone. Major bleeding (not related to CABG), composite ischemia (death, MI, revascularization), and net clinical outcome (composite ischemia or bleeding) were compared. Women had similar 30 days composite ischemic event rates as men (7 %vs 8 %, p = 0.07), but greater 30 day rates of major bleeding (8 % vs 3 %, p < 0.001) and net clinical outcomes (13 % vs 10 %, p < 0.001). One year ischemic outcomes and mortality were similar in both genders [64].

At 30 days women treated with bivalirudin as compared to GPI + UFH had significantly less major bleeding events (5 % vs 10 %, p < 0.001) and the same rate of composite ischemia (7 % vs 6 %, p = 0.15). There was no difference found in 1 year composite ischemia and mortality endpoints in women with respect to treatment with bivalirudin vs UFH + GPI. In summary, bivalirudin monotherapy compared to GPI- based strategy in women resulted in significantly reduced bleeding rates, but similar 1 year composite ischemia and mortality rates [64, 65].

The medical management of acute coronary syndromes is outlined in the AHA/ACC guidelines as noted in Table 6.2.

Outcomes by Device

Bare Metal Stents and Drug Eluting Stents

In clinical trials, the outcomes with bare metal stenting in women are similar to men in regards to in- hospital mortality and target lesion revascularization [66]. In a real world experience of patient and lesion subsets, mortality rates are similar or higher

Table 6.2 Summary of ACC/AHA guidelines for the management of Patients with Unstable Angina/N-ST Elevation Myocardial Infarction (2007, 2011, 2012)

Anti- ischemic therapy

Class I indications:

Bedrest and Telemetry

Oxygen (maintain saturation >90 %)

Nitrates (sl nitroglycerin x3, oral/topical, iv for ongoing ischemia, heart failure, hypertension)

Oral Beta Blockers: should be initiated in first 24 h if no contraindications exist

ACE inhibitors: should be initiated in first 24 h for heart failure or EF <40 %

ARB: for patients who cannot tolerate ACE inhibitors

Statin

Class IIa indications:

Iv Beta Blockers if no contraindications exist (see below)

ACE inhibitors in all patients with ACS

Class III (what should not be given)

Nitrates if BP <90 mmHg or RV infarction

Nitrates within 24 h of Sildenafil or 48 h of Tadalafil use

Immediate release dihydropyridine CCB in the absence of Beta Blocker therapy

Iv ACE inhibitors

Iv Beta Blockers in patients with: acute heart failure, low output state or cardiogenic shock, PR interval >0.24 s, 2nd or 3rd degree heart block, active asthma, or reactive airway disease

NSAID's and Cox-2 inhibitors

Anti-platelet therapy

Class I indications

ASA (162–325 mg), non-enteric coated[a, b]

Clopidogrel for patients with ASA allergy/intolerance (300–600 mg loading dose followed by 75 mg maintance dose) ot Ticagrelor

GI prophylaxis should be given to patients with history of GI bleeding

The use of dual a-platelet therapy or GP IIb/IIIa should be evaluated based on whether and invasive or conservative strategy is used

Patients with UA/NSTEMI in whom invasive strategy is selected should receive dual a-platelet therapy on presentation (Class1A); in addition to ASA, choice of 2nd a- platelet agent should include one of the following:

Before PCI:

Clopidogrel (loading dose 300–600 mg, followed by 75 mg daily for minimum 12 months) or Ticagrelor or

An iv GP IIb/IIIa inhibitor, preferably iv eptifibatide or tirofiban

At the time of PCI:

Clopidogrel if not started before PCI (600 mg should be given as early as possible before or at the time of PCI, or

Prasugrel (60 mg loading dose should be given promptly and no later than 1 h of PCI, followed by 10 mg daily for minimum 12 months) or

Ticagrelor (180 mg loading dose, followed by 90 mg twice daily for minimum 12 months) or Iv GP IIb/IIIa inhibitor

Anticoagulant therapy: relative choice depends on invasive vs conservative strategy

Class I indications

Unfractionated Heparin or

Table 6.2 (continued)

Enoxaparin or
Bivalirudin or
Fondaparinux

With permission from Jneid et al. [16]

[a]Recommended loading dose ASA: 162–325 mg, followed by 325 mg for 1 month after PCI, and 81–162 mg daily(Class IA)

[b]It is reasonable to use 81 mg of daily ASA after PCI in preference to higher maintenance doses (Class IIa B)

in women after stenting because of other confounding risk factors rather than female gender [63]. An analysis by Onuma, et al. which compared bare metal stents (BMS) with drug eluting stents (DES) in women showed no difference in 3- year outcomes between the genders, despite worse baseline clinical characteristics in women [67]. In patients treated throughout the BMS and DES eras, there were no differences by gender in all- cause mortality, MI or target lesion revascularization (TLR) at 3 years. Higher procedural complexity was observed in the DES era. At 3 years MACE and revascularization rates in women were significantly lower with DES than BMS (HR for TLR 0.52, 95 % CI 0.36–0.75, HR for MACE 0.63, 95 % CI 0.48–0.83) [64]. Another study by Fath- Ordoubadi et al., demonstrated equal efficacy and safety of DES in both genders [68]. Multivariate analysis in this study, which evaluated age, hypertension, diabetes mellitus, and number of diseased vessels, demonstrated that gender was not a predictor for adverse outcomes [68].

Gender-based differences in long-term clinical and angiographic outcomes after coronary revascularization with DES were also analyzed in a recent study by Stefanini, et al. [69]. After adjustment for baseline differences, women and men had a similar risk of cardiac death or MI (odds ratio [OR]: 1.13, 95 % confidence interval [CI]: 0.82–1.56, p=0.44), cardiac death (OR: 1.04, 95 % CI: 0.61–1.80, p=0.87), and MI (OR: 1.07, 95 % CI: 0.75–1.53, p=0.71) at 2 years. Similarly, the risk of target lesion revascularization (OR: 1.09, 95 % CI: 0.77–1.54, p=0.62), target vessel revascularization (OR: 0.88, 95 % CI: 0.63–1.22, p=0.43), and definite or probable stent thrombosis (OR: 0.73, 95 % CI: 0.38–1.38, p=0.33) were comparable for women and men. Follow-up angiography demonstrated no differences in terms of in-stent late loss (0.18±0.54 mm vs. 0.20±0.99 mm, p=0.76) and in-segment binary restenosis (8.5 % vs. 8.5 %, p=0.76) [69].

Female Gender and Adverse Outcomes After PCI

Many discrepancies have been reported regarding the prognosis and differences in adverse outcomes in women compared to men undergoing PCI. Registries and randomized trials analyzing early and late major adverse cardiovascular ischemic events have reported increased [70–72], neutral [73–75] and, even lower risk [76, 77] outcomes for women as compared to men. It has been suggested that women with ACS at younger age had higher mortality compared with men at the same age [4, 6, 78, 79]. After adjustment for several risk factors female gender remained a risk factor for in-hospital mortality in ACS for patients aged 51–60 [80]. An analysis by Duvernoy et al., demonstrated that women had a higher frequency of adverse outcomes after PCI, including in- hospital death, vascular complications, stroke, and MACE after adjusting for clinical and procedural characteristics. The relationship of increased risk of death and MACE was no longer present after adjusting for renal function and lower body surface area [81], suggesting an important impact of impaired kidney function and smaller size of female patients on long- term prognosis. Another analysis by Pendyala, et al., revealed a significant difference between the genders in independent correlates of mortality and MACE, and different impact of traditional prognostic correlates in women and men [82]. Women tend to have similar or lower rates of restenosis when compared to men despite smaller vessel sizes and higher prevalence of DM [71, 83, 84], factors usually associated with higher restenosis and revascularization rates. The reasons for these findings are unclear.

Bleeding Risk and Vascular Complications

Data from several sources suggest that gender-related differences exist in bleeding complications in ACS patients. In a multivariate analysis by Subherval et al., female gender was identified as an independent predictor of major in-hospital bleeding (OR 1.31, 95 % CI 1.23–1.39) in patients with ACS [83]. In the CRUSADE (Can Rapid risk stratification of Unstable angina patients Suppress Adverse outcomes with Early implementation of the ACC/AHA guidelines) registry, women who underwent PCI for UA/NSTEMI, had a much higher risk of major in-hospital bleeding compared to men (14.1 % vs 5.9 %, $p < 0.001$) [84].

Women undergoing PCI tend to have more access- related bleeding. In contrast, men tend to have GI bleeding after an MI. Possible explanations for this finding include smaller blood vessels in women and specific vascular reactivity [55]. In the same registry, a significant interaction was found between gender, GP IIb/IIIa inhibitor use and bleeding risk ($p = 0.014$). The increased risk of bleeding due to use of GPIIb/IIIa or anticoagulant agents like UFH or enoxaparin, may be related to excessive dosing of those agents (15 % of major bleeding events observed were due to excess drug doses) [64, 83, 84]. After adjusting for age, weight, and renal function, women remained at higher risk for excessive dosing and major bleeding events, as the authors found that excessive dosing of antithrombotic agents occurred in 72 % of women compared to 27 % of men [85, 86]. However, the ISAR- REACT and ACUITY trials [85, 86] provide data to suggest that bleeding complications remain higher among women compared to men even when they receive appropriate doses of antithrombotic agents.

Bleeding and vascular complications related to PCI result in significant morbidity and mortality [87–90] and given the higher bleeding event rates in women with ACS, this phenomenon has major prognostic implications. Bleeding events carry substantial risk of future ischemic events due to strong inflammatory response as well as high incidence of discontinuation of dual anti-platelet therapy after PCI [55].

Female gender predicts vascular complications depending on the vascular access site. In patients undergoing PCI through a femoral access risk for groin bleeding, retroperitoneal bleeds, psuedoaneurysm formation, and AV fistula formation exist. These complications persist despite significant improvement in antithrombotic therapy, use of smaller size sheaths, use of closure devices, and fluoroscopy guidance for femoral access [90, 91].

The ACC-NCDR Registry showed that female gender predicts vascular complications during both diagnostic and interventional cardiac procedures (RR 2.18, $p < 0.001$). Women had an increased risk of death as well (RR 2.59, $p < 0.001$) compared to men [91]. A subsequent study by the same group from 2007 showed persistent risk of vascular complications in women, when compared to men, despite overall improvement in rates of vascular complications in women [92]. Data from large multicenter registry of patients undergoing PCI demonstrate that women with bleeding and vascular complications tend to be older, have lower body mass index, and presented more frequently with renal failure and congestive heart failure. The linear relationship between risk of bleeding/vascular complications and age in women from this study identified elderly women as one of the highest risk groups [90].

In the same registry, women with bleeding or vascular complications had nearly a three- fold increased incidence of stroke, MI and all-cause mortality compared with women without bleeding/vascular complication. After controlling for clinical characteristics, the presence of bleeding/vascular complications remained a strong independent predictor of major adverse cardiac event (OR 1.84, 95 % CI 1.31–2.62, $p = 0.001$) including a 75 % increased risk of death, MI or stroke during the index hospitalization [90].

While studies from the past decade demonstrate a significant improvement in rates of bleeding and vascular complications in women undergoing PCI, they continue to have at least a two-fold increased risk of bleeding and vascular complications compared to men [90].

Arterial Access in Women: Radial Versus Femoral Artery

As outlined above female gender has been consistently identified as a risk factor for hemorrhagic complications in the setting of non- ST- elevation ACS, STEMI and elective PCI. Implementing several strategies may reduce the risk of bleeding [93]; such as the use of bivalirudin [64], appropriate dosing of anti- thrombotic agents [94], improved access techniques, utilization of vascular closure devices, use of smaller size sheaths, fluoroscopic guidance for femoral access, and the radial access to the arterial system [93, 95]. Clinical data suggest that the arteriotomy site may be responsible for the majority of bleeding complications during PCI [95] therefore the radial approach effectively reduces or eliminates access-site bleeding. Randomized trials show that a transradial approach reduced the bleeding risk by up to 70 %

compared to the transfemoral arterial access [95, 96]. Despite this significant safety profile, data from NCDR shows that women are less likely to undergo transradial PCI compared to men [97]. The transradial approach can be more challenging in women due to smaller caliber radial arteries, smaller body habitus, increased tortuosity and higher potential for spasm [93, 98]. Women more often experience local access-site complications after transradial approach, such as more frequent forearm hematomas than men [99]. Radial access can lead to higher rates of procedural failure when compared to femoral access, which might be augmented in women due to these anatomic differences and greater propensity to spasm [96].

More studies need to examine the optimal choice of arterial access in women undergoing PCI. An ongoing randomized, controlled trial, the SAFE PCI trial, is comparing the radial and femoral approach in women undergoing PCI and should provide some answers for this clinical dilemma.

Bleeding Avoidance Strategies (BAS)

There are no randomized controlled trials on different bleeding avoidance strategies (BAS) in women undergoing PCI, but there is emerging data nonetheless. BAS include vascular closure devices, use of bivalirudin as the anticoagulant, radial approach, and combinations of these three. The National Cardiovascular Data Registry's (NCDR) Cath PCI data from July 2009 to March 2011 was analyzed and recently published [100]. The incidence of bleeding following PCI was 7.8 % in women and 3.7 % in men. The use of any BAS differed slightly between women and men (75.4 % vs.75.7 %, p=0.01). Also, in women bivalirudin was used more often and radial approach and vascular closure devices were less often used. Despite suboptimal use of BAS, there was significant reduction in bleeding events with BAS (6.3 % absolute risk reduction). When both the radial approach and bivalirudin were used, an absolute reduction of 9.5 % (69 % reduction in bleeding events) was noted. Since blood transfusion is linked to mortality, an effort to increase awareness to avoid unnecessary blood transfusion is required [101]. In the event of a bleeding complication, conservative management initially is important. The ACC/AHA guidelines recommend waiting to transfuse a patient until their hemoglobin falls below 8 g% especially if the patient is clinically tolerating the blood loss, and the bleeding has been stopped.

Vascular Complications

The small caliber of women's peripheral vessels and tortuosity affects the caliber of sheath placed for angiography and PCI as well as increasing the potential for limb ischemia if an intra-aortic balloon pump (IABP) is required for hemodynamic support. For the same reasons vascular complications are more common in women. From 1994 to 1998, a national database reported twice as many complications in women with regard to stroke (0.4 % vs 0.2 %, P<.001) and vascular complications (5.4 % vs 2.7 %, P<.001) [102]. These increased risks persist even in more recent studies such as in the American College of Cardiology-National Cardiovascular Data Registry (ACC-NCDR) analyses from 2004 to 2006. The vascular complications were mostly related to access site issues including femoral pseudoaneurysm, retroperitoneal hemorrhage, and access site bleeding [103].

Cardiogenic Shock

In the SHOCK trial there was no effect of gender on the incidence and survival of cardiogenic shock in women when adjusted for other risk factors [104]. Cardiac power output (CPO), calculated as the mean arterial pressure times the cardiac output/451, has since emerged as the strongest predictor of mortality in cardiogenic shock and in the SHOCK trial women had significantly lower CPO suggesting a physiologic difference in the female myocardium and need for different therapeutic strategies to manage cardiogenic shock in women [105].

Mechanical Complications

In the SHOCK Registry women were noted to have a significantly higher incidence of mechanical complications including ventricular septal rupture and severe acute mitral regurgitation. Women as a group were 4.6 years older and had a higher incidence of hypertension, diabetes and a lower cardiac index. When adjusted for the comorbidities and complications, gender by itself was not an independent risk factor for death. The mortality of this cohort however was high at 61 % [105].

Renal Insufficiency

In ACS patients a higher prevalence of renal insufficiency has been noted in women. Women tend to have lower serum creatinine levels for similar renal function compared to men resulting in underestimation of the problem. Since post-PCI renal failure also correlates with short and long term mortality more attention should be focused on contrast use, peri-procedural hydration, and monitoring of renal function in women. The prognostic impact of a reduced GFR in women is similar to that in men thereby diminishing the effects of gender on mortality [106].

Mortality After ACS

Our understanding of the gender difference in mortality in ACS population is still evolving. On first glance, it appeared that women had higher incidence of morbidity and mortality (short term and long term) from ACS [107]. However, women also had increased incidence of comorbidities (like DM, history of heart failure, prior stroke), smaller coronary arteries, smaller peripheral vasculature leading to reduced use of therapies such as intra-aortic balloon pumps as well as higher rates of bleeding and vascular complications. Women also had an increased incidence of mortality from surgical revascularization [108]. Therefore, it is still unclear if female gender is an independent risk factor. The results in published literature are diverse and depend not only on the type of ACS population studied (UAP vs. NSTEMI vs. STEMI) but also on type of study (Randomized Controlled Trial or Observational Registry data) thereby making it difficult to draw a definite conclusion [109].

Several large trials have helped in the analysis of the effect of these comorbidities including angiographic burden of disease on patient mortality [109]. There is significant heterogeneity in the angiographic burden of disease in women included in various types of ACS trials which correlates with mortality and accounts for gender differences. More women with unstable angina tend to have non-obstructive CAD and thereby have better prognosis than men in this category. Women with acute myocardial infarction, however, have a prognosis similar to men. In women with myocardial infarction, when adjusted for co morbidities especially the angiographic burden of disease, their overall prognosis is similar to men. This is true across all age groups [107].

Even contemporary era studies in the STEMI population continue to suggest a worse prognosis in women, especially young women (less than 55 years of age) [110, 111] (Fig. 6.2). This is a significant finding as premenopausal women generally have been considered to have hormonal protection against coronary artery disease development. The exact reason for this increased mortality is still not clear. A more aggressive nature of disease seems to be contributing but cannot entirely explain the gender differences in outcomes. This higher mortality persists even long term with women having a 50 % higher mortality than men 2 years after sustaining an AMI [112]. The Variation in Recovery: Role of Gender on Outcomes of Young AMI Patients (VIRGO) study has been undertaken in the United States to understand the various factors including clinical, genetic, and socioeconomic status and their influence on these poor outcomes in women [113].

Conclusion

Women make up a significant proportion of patient's presenting with acute coronary syndromes in 2013. Unfortunately, there is often still a delay in the time to therapy related to an underappreciation of the symptoms and the actual risks of ACS, both by the health care providers and the patients themselves. This delay, along with the other clinical differences described, including older age, smaller size, and commorbidities, often lead to more complex procedures.

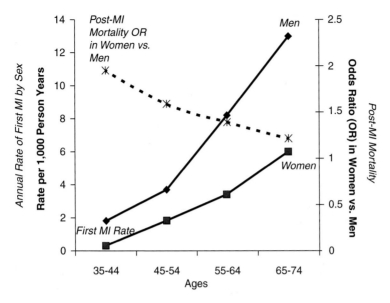

Fig. 6.2 (With permission from Bairey Merz [111])

In general, and as indicated in the most recent ACC/AHA guidelines presented, moderate to high risk female patients should be treated similarly to their male counterparts. The differences in potential complications between the genders do reach a significantly high level to warrant withholding treatment that is clearly defined as reducing morbidity and mortality across the spectrum of presentations. Low risk female patients, however, are best served by further non-invasive risk stratification before undertaking any invasive assessment, when factoring in the risk benefit ratio. All of the therapies that are appropriate for men are also appropriate for women, though the physician caring for these patients needs to be cognizant of the risks, especially bleeding, and actively try to mitigate the excess risk by any and all means, including appropriate dosing of medications and radial access where possible.

Gender equality extends to ACS therapy, even though the genders are not exactly the same. As we go forward with individualized medicine, more research needs to be performed to define if there are gender based differences above and beyond those that we are already aware of that warrant significant differences in therapy in this important patient population.

References

1. Go AS, Mozaffarian D, Roger VL, et al. Heart disease and stroke statistics–2013 update: a report from the American Heart Association. Circulation. 2013;127:e6–245.
2. Lloyd-Jones DM, Larson MG, Beiser A, Levy D. Lifetime risk of developing coronary heart disease. Lancet. 1999;353:89–92.
3. Thom TJ, Kannel WB, Silbershatz H, D'Agostino Sr RB. Cardiovascular diseases in the United States and prevention approaches. In: Fuster V, Alexander RW, O'Rourke RA, editors. Hurst's the heart. 10th ed. New York: McGraw-Hill; 2001. p. 3–7.

4. Lansky AJ, Ng V, Maehera A, et al. Gender and the extent of atherosclerosis, plaque composition, and clinical outcomes in acute coronary syndromes. JACC Cardiovasc Imaging. 2012;5:S62–72.
5. Heron M. Deaths: leading causes for 2004. National vital statistics report, vol. 46(5). Hyatsville: National Center for Health Statistics; 2007.
6. Heer T, Schiele R, Schneider S, et al. Gender differences in acute myocardial infarction in the era of reperfusion (the MITRA registry). Am J Cardiol. 2002;89:511–7.
7. Hochman JS, Tamis JE, Thompson TD, et al. Global Use of strategies to Open Occluded Coronary Arteries in Acute Coronary Syndromes IIb Investigators. Sex, clinical presentation and outcome in patients with acute coronary syndrome. N Engl J Med. 1999;341:226–32.
8. Lerner DJ, Kannel WB. Patterns of coronary heart disease morbidity and mortality in the sexes: a 26- year follow-up of the Framingham population. Am Heart J. 1986;111:383–90.
9. Claassen M, Sybrandy KC, Appelman YE, Asselbergs FW. Gender gap in acute coronary heart disease: myth or reality? World J Cardiol. 2012;4(2):36–47.
10. Cheruvu PK, Fin AV, Gardner C, et al. Frequency and distribution of thin cap fibroatheroma and ruptured plaques in human coronary arteries: a pathologic study. J Am Coll Cardiol. 2007;50:940–9.
11. Gurfinkel E, Vigliano C, Janavel JV, et al. Presence of vulnerable coronary plaques in middle-aged individuals who suffered a brain death. Eur Heart J. 2009;30:2845–53.
12. Farb A, Burke AP, Tang AL, et al. Coronary plaque erosion without rupture into a lipid core: a frequent cause of coronary thrombosis in sudden coronary death. Circulation. 1996;93:1354–63.
13. Kramer MC, Rittersma SZ, de winter RJ, et al. Relationship of thrombus healing to underlying plaque morphology in sudden coronary death. J Am Coll Cardiol. 2010;55:122–32.
14. O'Donoghue M, Boden WE, Braunwald E, et al. Early invasive vs conservative treatment strategies in women and Men with unstable angina and non- ST- segment elevation myocardial infarction. A Meta- analysis. JAMA. 2008;300(1):71–80.
15. Lansky AJ, Hochman JS, Ward PA, et al. AHA scientific statement. Percutaneous coronary intervention and adjunctive pharmacotherapy in women. Circulation. 2005;111:940–53.
16. Jneid H, Anderson JL, Wright SR, et al. 2012 ACCF/AHA focused update of the guideline for the management if patients with unstable angina/non-ST- elevation myocardial infarction (updating the 2007 guideline and replacing the 2011 focused update). Circulation. 2012;126:875–910.
17. Hvelplund A, Galatius S, Madsen M, et al. Women with acute coronary syndrome are less invasively examined and subsequently less treated that men. Eur Heart J. 2010;31:684–90.
18. Doyle F, De La Harpe D, McGee H, et al. Gender differences in the presentation and management if acute coronary syndromes: a national sample of 1365 admissions. Eur J Cardiovasc Prev Rehabil. 2005;12:376–9.
19. Alfredsson J, Stenestrand U, Wallentin L, et al. Gender differences in management and outcome in non- ST- elevation acute coronary syndrome. Heart. 2007;93:1357–62.
20. Invasive compared with non-invasive treatment in unstable coronary artery disease: FRISC II prospective randomized multicenter study. Lancet. 1999;354:708–15.
21. Fox KAA, Poole- Wilson PA, Henderson RA, et al. Interventional versus conservative treatment for patients with unstable angina or non- ST elevation myocardial infarction: the British Heart Foundation RITA 3 Randomized Trial. Lancet. 2002;360:743.
22. Glaser R, Herrman HC, Murphy SA, et al. Benefit of an early invasive management strategy in women with acute coronary syndromes. JAMA. 2002;288:3124–9.
23. Swahn E, Alfredsson J, Afzal R, et al. Early invasive compared with selective invasive strategy in women with non- ST-elevation acute coronary syndrome: a substudy of the OASIS 5 trial and meta-analysis of previous randomized trials. Eur Heart J. 2012;1:51–60.
24. Alfredsson J, Lindback J, Wallentin L, Swahn E. Similar outcome with invasive strategy in men and women with non- ST- elevation acute coronary syndrome. From the Swedish Web-System for Enhancement and Development of Evidence- Based Care in Heart Disease

Evaluated According to Recommended Therapies (SWEDEHEART). Eur Heart J. 2011;32:3128–36.

25. Roe MT, Parsons LS, Pollack Jr CV, Canto JG, Barron HV, Every NR, Rogers WJ, Peterson ED, National Registry of Myocardial Infarction Investigators. Quality of care by classification of myocardial infarction:treatment patterns for ST-segment elevation vs non-ST-segment elevation myocardial infarction. Arch Intern Med. 2005;165:1630–6.

26. Mandelzweig L, Battler A, Boyko V, Bueno H, Danchin N, Filippatos G, Gitt A, Hasdai D, Hasin Y, Marrugat J, Van de Werf F, Wallentin L, Behar S, Euro Heart Survey Investigators. The second Euro Heart Survey on acute coronary syndromes: characteristics, treatment, and outcome of patients with ACS in Europe and the Mediterranean Basin in 2004. Eur Heart J. 2006;27:2285–93.

27. Fox KA, Steg PG, Eagle KA, Goodman SG, Anderson Jr FA, Granger CB, Flather MD, Budaj A, Quill A, Gore JM, GRACE Investigators. Decline in rates of death and heart failure in acute coronary syndromes, 1999-2006. JAMA. 2007;29:1892–900.

28. Yeh RW, Sidney S, Chandra M, Sorel M, Selby JV, Go AS. Population trends in the incidence and outcomes of acute myocardial infarction. N Engl J Med. 2010;362:2155–65.

29. Benamer H, Tafflet M, Bataille S, et al. Female gender is an independent predictor of in-hospital mortality after STEMI in the era of primary PCI: insights from the greater Paris area PCI Registry. CARDIO-ARHIF Registry Investigators. EuroIntervention. 2011;6(9):1073–9.

30. Jackson EA, Moscucci M, Smith DE, et al. The association of sex with outcomes among patients undergoing primary percutaneous coronary intervention for ST elevation myocardial infarction in the contemporary era: insights from the Blue Cross Blue Shield of Michigan Cardiovascular Consortium (BMC2). Am Heart J. 2011;161:106–112.e1.

31. Burke AP, Farb A, Malcom GT, et al. Effect of risk factors on the mechanism of acute thrombosis and sudden coronary death in women. Circulation. 1998;97:2110–6.

32. Wijnbergen I, Tijssen J, van 't Veer M, Michels R, Pijls NH. Gender differences in long-term outcome after primary percutaneous intervention for ST-segment elevation myocardial infarction. Catheter Cardiovasc Interv. 2013;82:379–84.

33. Mrdovic I, Savic L, Milika A, et al. Sex-related analysis of short- and long-term clinical outcomes and bleeding among patients treated with primary percutaneous coronary intervention: an evaluation of the RISK-PCI data. Can J Cardiol. 2013;29:1097–103.

34. Gevaert SA, De Bacquer D, Evrard P, et al. Renal dysfunction in STEMI-patients undergoing primary angioplasty: higher prevalence but equal prognostic impact in female patients; an observational cohort study from the Belgian STEMI registry. BMC Nephrol. 2013;14:62.

35. Anderson ML, Peterson ED, Brennan JM, et al. Short- and long-term outcomes of coronary stenting in women versus men results from the National Cardiovascular Data Registry Centers for Medicare & Medicaid services cohort. Circulation. 2012;126:2190–9.

36. Gharacholou SM, Alexander KP, Chen AY, et al. Implications and reasons for the lack of use of reperfusion therapy in patients with ST-segment elevation myocardial infarction: findings from the CRUSADE initiative. Am Heart J. 2010;159:757–63.

37. Glickman SW, Granger CB, Ou F-S, et al. Impact of a statewide ST-segment-elevation myocardial infarction regionalization program on treatment times for women, minorities, and the elderly. Circ Cardiovasc Qual Outcomes. 2010;3:514–21.

38. Gulati M, Shaw LJ, Merz B. Myocardial ischemia in women – lessons from the NHLBI WISE study. Clin Cardiol. 2012;35(3):141–8.

39. Aguilar SA, Patel M, Castillo E, et al. Gender differences in scene time, transport time, and total scene to hospital arrival time determined by the use of a prehospital electrocardiogram in patients with complaint of chest pain. J Emerg Med. 2012;43(2):291–7.

40. Dreyer RP, Beltrame JF, Tavella R, Air T, Hoffmann B, et al. Evaluation of gender differences in door-to-balloon time in ST-elevation myocardial infarction. Heart Lung Circ. 2013;22(10):861–9.

41. Mathews R, Peterson ED, Li S, et al. Use of emergency medical service transport among patients with ST-segment-elevation myocardial infarction: findings from the National

Cardiovascular Data Registry Acute Coronary Treatment Intervention Outcomes Network Registry-Get with the Guidelines. Circulation. 2011;124:154–63.
42. O'Gara PT, Kushner FG, Ascheim DD, et al. ACCF/AHA guideline for the management of ST-elevation myocardial infarction. A report of the American College of Cardiology Foundation/American Heart Association Task Force on Practice Guidelines. J Am Coll Cardiol. 2013;61(4):e78–140.
43. Barbash IM, Ben-Dor I, Torguson R, Maluenda G, et al. Clinical predictors for failure of percutaneous coronary intervention in ST-elevation myocardial infarction. J Interv Cardiol. 2012;25(2):111–7.
44. Presbitero P, Belli G, Zavalloni D, Rossi ML, et al. "Gender paradox" in outcome after percutaneous coronary intervention with paclitaxel eluting stents. EuroIntervention. 2008;4(3):345–50.
45. Stefanini GG, Kalesan B, Pilgrim T, et al. Impact of gender on clinical and angiographic outcomes among patients undergoing revascularization with drug-eluting stents. JACC Cardiovasc Interv. 2012;5(3):301–10.
46. Baim D. Grossman's cardiac catheterization, angiography, and intervention. Philadelphia: Lippincott Williams & Wilkins; 2006.
47. ISIS-2 Collaborative Group Randomized Trial of intravenous streptokinase, oral aspirin, both or neither among 17,187 cases of suspected acute myocardial infarction: ISIS-2. Lancet. 1988;2: 349–60.
48. Quinn MJ, Aronow HD, Califf RM, et al. Aspirin dose and six-month outcome after an acute coronary syndrome. J Am Coll Cardiol. 2004;43:972–8.
49. Peters RJ, Mehta SR, Fox KA, Clopidogrel in Unstable angina to prevent Recurrent Events (CURE) Trial Investigators, et al. Effects of aspirin dose when used alone or in combination with clopidogrel in patients with acute coronary syndromes: observations from the Clopidogrel in Unstable angina to prevent Recurrent Events(CURE) study. Circulation. 2003;108:1682–7.
50. Steinhubl SR, Bhatt DL, Brennan DM, CHARISMA investigators, et al. Aspirin to prevent cardiovascular disease: the association of aspirin dose and clopidogrel with thrombosis and bleeding. Ann Intern Med. 2009;150:379–86.
51. Mehta SR, Tanguay JF, Eikeboom JW, et al. Double dose versus standard- dose clopidogrel and high- dose versus low- dose aspirin in individuals undergoing percutaneous coronary intervention for acute coronary syndromes (CURRENT- OASIS 7): a randomized factorial trial. Lancet. 2010;376:1243.
52. Mehta SR, Yusuf S, Peters RJ, et al. Clopidogrel in Unstable angina to prevent Recurrent Events trial (CURE) Investigators. Effects of Pretreatment with clopidogrel and aspirin followed by long- term therapy in patients undergoing percutaneous coronary intervention: the PCI- CURE study. Lancet. 2001;358:527–33.
53. Wiviott SD, Braunwald E, McCabe CH, et al. Prasugrel versus clopdogrel in patients with acute coronary syndromes. N Engl J Med. 2007;357:2011–5.
54. Allentin L, Becker RC, Budaj A, et al. Ticagrelor versus Clopidogrel in patients with acute coronary syndromes. N Engl J Med. 2009;361:1045–57.
55. Wang TY, Angiolillo DJ, Cushman M, et al. Platelet biology and response to antiplatelet therapy in women. J Am Coll Cardiol. 2012;59:891–900.
56. Boersma E, Harrington RA, Moliterno DJ, et al. Platelet glycoprotein IIb/IIIa inhibitors in acute coronary syndromes: a meta-analysis of all major randomized clinical trials. Lancet. 2002;359:189–98.
57. Bhatt DL, Lincoff AM, Califf RM, et al. The benefit of abciximab in percutaneous coronary revascularization is not device- specific. Am J Cardiol. 2000;85:1060–4.
58. Giugliano RP, White JA, Bode C, EARLY –ACS Investigators, et al. Early versus delayed, provisional eptifibatide in acute coronary syndromes. N Engl J Med. 2009;360:2176–90.
59. Lincoff AM, Tcheng JE, Califf RM, et al. Standard versus low- dose weight- adjusted heparin in patients treated with the platelet glycoprotein IIb/IIIa receptor antibody fragment abciximab

(c7E Fab) during percutaneous coronary revascularization. PROLOG Investigators. Am J Cardiol. 1997;79:286–91.

60. Blazing PA, De Lemos JA, White H, A-Z Investigators, et al. Safety and efficacy enoxaparin vs unfractionated heparin in patients with non- ST-elevation acute coronary syndromes who receive tirofiban and aspirin: a randomized controlled trial. JAMA. 2004;292:55–64.

61. Ferguson JJ, Califf RM, Antman EM, SYNERGY Trial Investigators, et al. Enoxaparin versus unfractionated heparin in high- risk patients with non- ST- segment acute coronary syndromes managed with an intended early invasive strategy: primary results of the SYNERGY randomized trial. JAMA. 2004;292:45–54.

62. Direct Thrombin Inhibitor Trialists' Collaborative Group. Direct thrombin inhibitors in acute coronary syndromes: principal results of meta- analysis based on individual patients' data. Lancet. 2002;359:294–302.

63. Lincoff AM, Kleiman N, Kereiakes D, REPLACE- 2 Investigators, et al. Long-term efficacy of bivalirudin and provisional glycoprotein IIb/IIIa blockade vs heparin and planned glycoprotein IIb/IIIa blockade during percutaneous coronary intervention: REPLACE- 2 trial. JAMA. 2004;292:696–703.

64. Lansky AJ, Mehran R, Cristea E, et al. Impact of gender and antithrombin strategy on early and late clinical outcomes in patients with Non- ST-elevation Acute Coronary Syndromes (from the ACUITY trial). Am J Cardiol. 2009;103:1196–203.

65. Stone GW, McLaurin BT, Cox DA, Investigators ACUITY, et al. Bivalirudin for patients with acute coronary syndromes. N Engl J Med. 2006;355:2203–16.

66. Chauhan MS, Ho KK, Baim DS, et al. Effect of gender on in-hospital and one- year outcomes after contemporary coronary artery stenting. Am J Cardiol. 2005;95:101–4.

67. Onuma Y, Kukreja N, Daeman J, et al. Impact of sex on 3-year outcome after percutaneous coronary intervention using bare- metal and drug- eluting stents in previously untreated coronary artery disease. J Am Coll Cardiol Intv. 2009;2:603–10.

68. Fath- Ordoubadi F, Barac Y, Abergel E, et al. Gender impact on prognosis of acute coronary syndrome patients treated with drug- eluting stents. Am J Cardiol. 2012;110:636–42.

69. Stefanini GG, Kalesan B, Pilgrim T, et al. Impact of sex on clinical and angiographic outcomes among patients undergoing revascularization with drug- eluting stents. J Am Coll Cardiol. 2012;5:301–10.

70. Mehilli J, Kastrati A, Dirschinger J, et al. Differences in prognostic factors and outcomes between women and men undergoing coronary artery stenting. JAMA. 2000;284:1799–805.

71. Lansky AJ, Pietras C, Costa RA, et al. Gender differences in outcomes after primary angioplasty versus primary stenting with and without abciximab for acute myocardial infarction: results of the Controlled Abciximab and Device Investigation to Lower Late Angioplasty Complications (CADILLAC) trial. Circulation. 2005;111:1611–8.

72. Ndrepepa G, Mehilli J, Bollwein H, et al. Sex-associated differences in clinical outcomes after coronary stenting in patients with diabetes mellitus. Am J Med. 2004;117:830–6.

73. Onuma Y, Kukreja N, Daemen J, et al. Impact of sex on 3-year outcome after percutaneous coronary intervention using bare-metal and drug-eluting stents in previously untreated coronary artery disease: insights from the RESEARCH (Rapamycin-Eluting Stent Evaluated at Rotterdam Cardiology Hospital) and T-SEARCH (Taxus-Stent Evaluated at Rotterdam Cardiology Hospital) Registries. JACC Cardiovasc Interv. 2009;2:603–10.

74. Lansky AJ, Costa RA, Mooney M, et al. Gender-based outcomes after paclitaxel-eluting stent implantation in patients with coronary artery disease. J Am Coll Cardiol. 2005;45:1180–5.

75. Singh M, Rihal CS, Gersh BJ, et al. Mortality differences between men and women after percutaneous coronary interventions. A 25-year, single-center experience. J Am Coll Cardiol. 2008;51:2313–20.

76. Mehilli J, Kastrati A, Bollwein H, et al. Gender and restenosis after coronary artery stenting. Eur Heart J. 2003;24:1523–30.

77. Nakatani D, Ako J, Tremmel JA, et al. Sex differences in neointimal hyperplasia following endeavor zotarolimus-eluting stent implantation. Am J Cardiol. 2011;108:912–7.

78. Berger JS, Brown DL. Gender- age interraction in early mortality following pimary angioplasty for acute myoocardial infarction. Am J Cardiol. 2006;98:1140–3.
79. Srinivas VS, Garg S, Negassa A, et al. Persistent sex difference in hospital outcome following percutaneous coronary intervention: results from the New York State reporting system. J Invasive Cardiol. 2007;19(6):265–8.
80. Radovanovic D, Erne P, Urban P, et al. Gender differences in management and outcomes in patients with acute coronary syndromes: results on 20.290 patients from the AMIS Plus Registry. Heart. 2007;93:1369–75.
81. Duvernoy C, Smith DE, Manohar P, et al. Gender differences in adverse outcomes after contemporary percutaneous coronary intervention: an analysis from the Blue Cross Blue Shield of Michigan Cardiovascular Consortium (BMC2) Percutaneous Coronary Intervention Registry. Am Heart J. 2010;159(4):677–83.
82. Pendyala LK, Torguson R, Loh JP, et al. Comparison of adverse outcomes after contemporary percutaneous coronary intervention in women versus men with acute coronary syndrome. Am J Cardiol. 2013;111(8):1092–8.
83. Subherwal S, Bach RG, Chen AY, et al. Baseline risk of major bleeding in non- ST- elevation myocardial infarction: the CRUSADE (Can Rapid risk stratification of Unstable angina patients Suppress Adverse outcomes with Early implementation of the ACC/AHA guidelines) bleeding score. Circulation. 2009;119:1873–82.
84. Alexander KP, Chen AY, Lewby LK, et al. Sex differences in major bleeding with glycoprotein IIb/IIIa inhibitors: results from the CRUSADE (Can Rapid risk stratification of Unstable angina patients Suppress Adverse outcomes with Early implementation of the ACC/AHA guidelines) initiative. Circulation. 2006;114:1380–7.
85. Kastrati A, Mehilli J, Schuhlen H, et al. Intracoronary Stenting and Anti- Thrombotic Regimen- Rapid Early Action for Coronary Treatment Study Investigators. A clinical trial of abciximab in elective percutaneous coronary intervention after pretreatment with clopidogrel. N Engl J Med. 2004;350:232–8.
86. Manoukian SV, Feit F, Mehran T, et al. Impact of major bleeding o 30- day mortality and clinical outcomes in patients with acute coronary syndromes: an analysis from the ACUITY trial. J Am Coll Cardiol. 2007;49:1362–8.
87. Dropped G, Berger PB, Hehilli J, et al. Periprocedural bleeding and 1- year outcome after percutaneous coronary interventions: appropriateness of including bleeding as a component of a quadruple end point. J Am Coll Cardiol. 2008;51:690–7.
88. Dauerman HL, Applegate RJ, Cohen DJ. Vascular closure devices: the second decade. J Am Coll Cardiol. 2007;50:1617–26.
89. Eikelboom JW, Mehta SR, Anad SS, et al. Adverse impact of bleeding on prognosis in patients with acute coronary syndromes. Circulation. 2006;114:774–82.
90. Ahmed B, Piper WD, Dauerman HL, et al. Significantly improved vascular complications among women undergoing percutaneous coronary intervention. A report from the Northern New England percutaneous coronary intervention registry. Circ Cardiovasc Interv. 2009;2:423–9.
91. Tavris DR, Gallauresi BA, Lin BJ, et al. Risk of local adverse events following cardiac catheterization by hemostasis device use and gender. J Invasive Cardiol. 2004;16:459–64.
92. Tavris DR, Gallauresi BA, Dey S, et al. Risk of local adverse events by gender following cardiac catheterization. Pharmacoepidemiol Drug Saf. 2007;16:125–31.
93. Rao SV, Krrucoff MW. Transradial PCI in women: problem solved or clinical equipoise? J Invasive Cardiol. 2011;23:4.
94. Alexander KP, Chen AY, Roe MT, et al. Excess dosing of antiplatelet and antithrombotic agents in the treatment of non- ST- elevation acute coronary syndromes. JAMA. 2005;294:3108–16.
95. Jolly SS, Amlani S, Hamon M, et al. Radial versus femoral access for coronary angiography or intervention and the impact on major bleeding and ischemic events: a systemic review and meta- analysis of randomized trials. Am Heart J. 2009;157:132–40.
96. Rao SV, Cohen MG, Kandzari DE, et al. The transradial approach to percutaneous coronary intervention: historical perspective, current concepts, and future directions. J Am Coll Cardiol. 2010;55:2187–95.

97. Rao SV, Ou FS, Wang TY, et al. Trends in the prevalence and outcomes of radial and femoral approaches to percutaneous coronary intervention: a report from the national cardiovascular data registry. J Am Coll Cardiol Intv. 2008;1:379–86.

98. Saito S, Ikei H, Hosokawa G, Tanaka S. Influence of the ratio between radial artery inner diameter and sheath outer diameter on radial artery flow after transradial coronary intervention. Catheter Cardiovasc Interv. 1999;46:173–8.

99. Tizon- Marcos H, Bertrand OF, Rodes- Cabau J, et al. Impact of female gender and transradial coronary stenting with maximal antiplatelet therapy on bleeding and ischemic outcomes. Am Heart J. 2009;157:740–5.

100. Daugherty SL, Thompson LE, Kim S, et al. Patterns of Use and comparative effectiveness of bleeding avoidance strategies in Men and women following percutaneous coronary interventions: an observational study from the National Cardiovascular Data Registry®. J Am Coll Cardiol. 2013. doi:10.1016/j.jacc.2013.02.030.

101. Adnan K. Chhatriwalla, Amit P. Amin, Kevin F. Kennedy, et al.; for NCDR Registry. Association between bleeding events and in-hospital mortality after percutaneous coronary intervention. JAMA. 2013;309(10):1022–9.

102. Peterson ED, Lansky AJ, Kramer J, et al. Effect of gender on the outcomes of contemporary percutaneous coronary intervention. Am J Cardiol. 2001;88:359–64.

103. Akhter N, Milford-Beland S, Roe MT, Piana RN, Kao J, Shroff A. Gender differences among patients with acute coronary syndromes undergoing percutaneous coronary intervention in the American College of Cardiology-National Cardiovascular Data Registry (ACC-NCDR). Am Heart J. 2009;157(1):141–8.

104. Wong SC, Sleeper LA, Monrad ES et al.; SHOCK Investigators. Absence of gender differences in clinical outcomes in patients with cardiogenic shock complicating acute myocardial infarction. A report from the SHOCK Trial Registry. J Am Coll Cardiol. 2001;38(5):1395–401.

105. Fincke R, Hochman JS, Lowe AM, et al.; SHOCK Investigators. Cardiac power is the strongest hemodynamic correlate of mortality in cardiogenic shock: a report from the SHOCK trial registry. J Am Coll Cardiol. 2004;44(2):340–8.

106. Sederholm Lawesson S, Tödt T, Alfredsson J, et al. Gender difference in prevalence and prognostic impact of renal insufficiency in patients with ST-elevation myocardial infarction treated with primary percutaneous coronary intervention. Heart. 2011;97(4):308–14.

107. Vaccarino V. Ischemic heart disease in women: many questions, Few facts. Circ Cardiovasc Qual Outcomes. 2010;3:111–5.

108. Hernández Antolín RA, Rodríguez Hernández JE. Effect of sex on revascularization strategy. Rev Esp Cardiol. 2006;59(5):487–501.

109. Berger JS, et al. Sex differences in mortality following acute coronary syndromes. JAMA. 2009;302(8):874–82.

110. Vaccarino V, Parsons L, Every NR, Barron HV, Krumholz HM. Sex-based differences in early mortality after myocardial infarction. National Registry of Myocardial Infarction 2 Participants. N Engl J Med. 1999;341:217–25.

111. Bairey Merz CN, Shaw LJ, Reis SE, Bittner V, et al. Insights from the NHLBI-Sponsored Women's Ischemia Syndrome Evaluation (WISE) Study: part II: gender differences in presentation, diagnosis, and outcome with regard to gender-based pathophysiology of atherosclerosis and macrovascular and microvascular coronary disease. J Am Coll Cardiol. 2006;47(3 Suppl):S21–9.

112. Vaccarino V, Parsons L, Peterson ED, Rogers WJ, Kiefe CI, Canto J. Sex differences in mortality after acute myocardial infarction: changes from 1994 to 2006. Arch Intern Med. 2009;169:1767–74.

113. Lichtman JH, Lorenze NP, D'Onofrio G. Variation in recovery: role of gender on outcomes of young AMI patients (VIRGO) study design. Circ Cardiovasc Qual Outcomes. 2010;3: 684–93.

Bibliography

Berger JS, et al. Sex differences in mortality following acute coronary syndromes. JAMA. 2009;302(8):874–82.

Lundberg G, King S. Coronary revascularization in women. Clin Cardiol. 2012;35(3):156–9.

Merz CNB. The Yentl syndrome is alive and well. Eur Heart J. 2011;32(11):1313–5.

Naik N, et al. Interventional management of ACS in women: STEMI and NSTEMI. Interv Cardiol Clin. 2012;1:173–82.

Steingart RM. Sex differences in the management of coronary artery disease. N Engl J Med. 1991;325:226–30.

Stock EO. Cardiovascular disease in women. Curr Probl Cardiol. 2012;37:450–526.

Chapter 7
Coronary Artery Bypass Graft, Valvular, and Advanced Heart Failure Surgeries in Women

Naila Choudhary and Leway Chen

Cardiovascular disease (CVD) is the leading cause of mortality in men and women. An estimated 83.6 million American adults (>1 in 3) have one or more types of cardiovascular diseases. In 2010, an estimated 7.6 million inpatient cardiovascular operations and procedures were performed in the United States; 4.4 million were performed on men, and 3.2 million were performed on women [1]. In clinical trials on cardiovascular diseases, women are generally under-represented, raising potential concerns for bias. In clinical trials used to support 2007 American Heart Association (AHA) guidelines for CVD prevention in women, women represented only one third of patients despite similar prevalence of disease in men and women. Only 31 % of primary trial publications specifically reported results in women. Representation of women was lowest among trials for heart failure (29 %) and CAD (25 %) [2].

Various studies have demonstrated gender related differences in survival after different cardiac procedures. Some studies attribute this difference to baseline dissimilarities in risk factors for men and women, while others emphasize that gender itself plays a distinct role and is an independent predictor of morbidity and mortality. In this chapter, we have reviewed literature to understand unique gender related characteristics as they pertain to different cardiac surgeries, with special emphasis on coronary artery bypass graft, cardiac valve surgeries and advanced heart failure surgeries.

N. Choudhary, MBBS (✉) • L. Chen, MD, MPH
Division of Cardiology, University of Rochester Medical Center, Rochester, NY, USA
e-mail: naila.choudhary@gmail.com

H.Z. Mieszczanska, G.P. Velarde (eds.),
Management of Cardiovascular Disease in Women,
DOI 10.1007/978-1-4471-5517-1_7, © Springer-Verlag London 2014

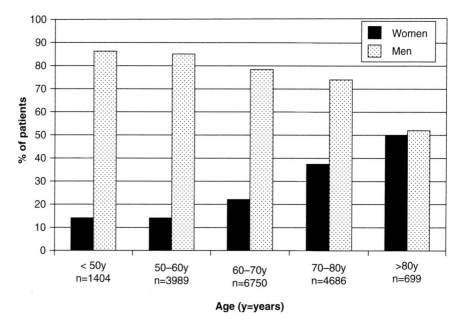

Fig. 7.1 Percentage of women and men in the different age groups undergoing coronary artery bypass grafting (Reprinted from [5]; with permission from Elsevier)

Coronary Artery Bypass Grafting (CABG)

Although female prevalence of CVD is similar to that of male, females suffering from coronary artery disease (CAD) are less likely to undergo coronary revascularization procedures in comparison to males. In the Survival and Ventricular Enlargement (SAVE) study [3], Steingart and coworkers noted that almost 50 % women had angina limiting their physical activity as opposed to 31 % men; however, only 15 % women compared with 27 % men underwent cardiac catheterization. Similarly, despite inadequate symptom relief on medical therapy, women were referred for CABG less frequently than men (6 % vs.12 %).

Coronary artery disease is generally less common in younger women; however mortality rate for women less than 50 years of age after myocardial infarction (MI) was reportedly more than twice that for men of the same age; [4, 5] Figs. 7.1 and 7.2. In recent years, though MI mortality persistently higher in younger women, women had experienced significant improvements in mortality than did younger men after MI. This could be related to improvement in risk profile on presentation over the years or improvement in gender related referral bias for treatment [6].

Influence of Gender on CABG Mortality

CABG has been shown to improve survival in patients with multi-vessel coronary artery disease and left main coronary artery disease [7, 8]. The association of gender

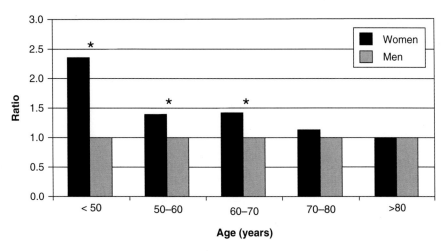

Fig. 7.2 Relative mortality of women compared with men in the different age groups. *p <0.05 (Reprinted from [5]; with permission from Elsevier)

with mortality and morbidity after CABG has been debated by many studies for more than 20 years. The results of studies analyzing role of female gender as an independent risk factor for long-term survival after coronary artery bypass surgery has been variable and controversial (Table 7.1) [9–13]. In a report of 8,907 CABG patients, women were found to have lower long term survival in comparison to men, but patient related risk factors and not gender itself was found to be associated with poor outcomes [9]. In contrast, report from Bypass Angioplasty Revascularization Investigation (BARI) suggested that men and women had similar post-CABG survival at 5 years. However women had higher risk profile and after adjusting for multiple risk factors, female sex was an independent predictor of improved survival at 5 years [10]. Yet some other reports indicated the female gender was associated with decreased likelihood of survival long term. Weintraub et al. reported that 20-year survival after CABG was 37 % in men and 29 % in women [11].

Gender Related Pre-operative Surgical Risk Factors for CABG

Certain pre-operative risk factors have been found to be unique characteristics of either sex. A number of researchers have concluded that this difference in pre-existing risk factors may directly or indirectly influence short and long term outcomes. The European System for Cardiac Operative Risk Evaluation (Euro-SCORE) is a well-validated scoring system to help predict mortality from cardiac surgery based on certain risk factors [14]. In this risk stratification, female gender is an independent risk factor for worse outcomes after cardiac surgery.

In general, male CABG patients have lower left ventricular ejection fraction, significant smoking history and history of prior myocardial infarction [13, 15, 16]. Female CABG patients on the other hand, generally present at an older age compared to their male counterparts. This could be related to protective effects of female

Table 7.1 Summary of studies evaluating long-term survival in men and women post-CABG

First author and reference #	Year published	No. of patients	Men N (%)	Women N (%)	Survival in relation to gender
SH Rahimtoola [9]	1993	8,907	6,927 (78 %)	1,979 (22 %)	Gender was not an independent predictor of poor survival
AK Jacobs [10]	1998	1,829	1,340 (73 %)	489 (27 %)	Female sex – an independent predictor of improved 5-year survival
D Abramov [12]	2000	4,823	3,891 (81 %)	932 (19 %)	Women – late survival increased compared to men
WS Weintraub [11]	2003	3,939	3,312 (84 %)	627(16 %)	Female gender-associated with poor likelihood of long term survival
SE Woods [13]	2003	5,324	3,582 (67 %)	1,742 (33 %)	Gender – not an independent predictor of mortality

sex hormones in reproductive age group. Older age at presentation and its association with co-morbid conditions may contribute to increased surgical risk and poor outcomes in women. Women have higher incidence of peripheral vascular disease, hypertension, diabetes mellitus, chronic renal insufficiency and congestive heart failure [13, 15, 16]. Women are more likely than men to undergo emergent cardiac surgery and present with cardiogenic shock [17]. Emergent cardiac surgery in women may be a reflection of referral bias for women presenting at more advanced stage of coronary artery disease with associated hemodynamic instability which may negatively impact survival.

Female patients have generally smaller body mass index and body surface area (BSA) in comparison to their male counterparts. Most reports conclude that smaller BSA in female CABG patients is not a significant risk factor for operative mortality [15, 18]. A retrospective analysis by Rannuci and colleagues from Italy found that female gender and small body surface area were associated with severe intraoperative hemodilution and subsequent need of blood transfusions. They commented that larger BSA in women is likely related to obesity and hence associated with prolonged intensive care unit (ICU) length of stay. Men with small BSA were reported to have longer ICU stay likely resulting from hemodilution associated with smaller BSA and its associated complications [18]. Anemia is a well-identified predictor of poor outcomes in patients with coronary artery disease and in general population. Post-operative anemia after CABG surgery may persist for months and has been found to be associated with impaired outcomes. Westesbrink et al. reported that for every 1 mg/dL decrease in Hb, there was a 13 % increase in cardiovascular events and a 22 % increase in all-cause mortality in CABG patients [19]. Women tend to have more anemia pre and post-operatively and are more likely to receive blood transfusions which put them at further increased risk of complications and poor outcomes compared to men [19–21].

Gender Related Surgical Risk Factors for CABG

The use of internal mammary artery (IMA) for bypass grafting has been shown to be associated with improved short and long term survival in patients undergoing CABG. Despite this fact, many studies have reported significantly less use of IMA conduit in women [15, 22, 23]. Study of 541,368 coronary artery bypass graft surgery procedures reported by 745 hospitals in the STS National Cardiac Database from 2002 through 2005 revealed that IMAs were used less frequently in women than men (odds ratio for at least one IMA: 0.62; 95 % confidence interval: 0.61–0.63, odds ratio for bilateral IMA: 0.65; 95 % confidence interval: 0.63–0.68) [23]. Some authors relate this disparity to smaller BSA in women while others found that the difference persists even after the adjustment for BSA [24].

Off pump CABG in comparison to conventional CABG on cardiopulmonary bypass was thought to be associated with improved outcomes and less complications in post-operative period in terms of need of blood transfusion, neurological complications and major adverse cardiac events. However, two major clinical trials published recently (CORONARY: CABG Off or On pump Revascularization Study, and GOPCABE: German Off-Pump Coronary Artery Bypass Grafting in Elderly Patients) reported no significant difference between off pump and on pump CABG group in outcomes of death, myocardial infarction and stroke [25, 26]. However, there were reportedly fewer transfusion and more incomplete revascularization in off pump CABG group. In the pre-specified sub-group analysis of CORONARY trial, no significant interaction was found between operative techniques and gender for primary end-points [25].

Association of Gender with Post-CABG Complications

Current data on gender and its influence on complication after CABG are variable. Women have been found to report more post-operative angina than men [10, 12], which may be related to underutilization of IMA conduits, less complete revascularization and smaller coronary size in women, and gender differences in pre-operative risk profile. However, women were found to less likely require percutaneous or surgical re-intervention [12]. Post- CABG neurological complications contribute to significant morbidity in this population; however data remains inconclusive about its association with gender. Some studies report significantly higher neurological morbidity in women [27, 28], others find no relationship with either sex [22], and yet there are also reports of worse neurological outcome in men [7]. Most studies have found no association of gender with post-operative risk of infections despite existing differences in baseline clinical characteristics [13, 22, 29]. Women tend to have longer hospital stay, ICU length of stay and more days on mechanical ventilation and more commonly require intra-aortic balloon counter-pulsation, vasopressors and dialysis [12, 22, 30].

Cardiac Valve Surgeries

In addition to reports on association of gender with CABG outcomes, there has been increased interest by many authors to understand its relationship to cardiac valvular surgeries and combined CABG and valve surgeries. Combined CABG and valve surgeries have increased mortality and morbidity than CABG alone or primary valve surgery alone. The role of gender as an independent risk factor for patients undergoing combined valve and CABG surgery remains unclear. Some authors report that female gender is associated with worse outcomes in terms of long term survival while others found no association [31, 32]. Women were reported to have more risk factors in comparison to men, which is similar to the findings of studies reporting influence of gender on CABG outcomes. The pre-operative risk factors should be strongly considered when analyzing outcomes after combined surgeries.

Mitral and Aortic Valve Disease in Men and Women Undergoing Valve Surgery

For mitral valve disease, women undergo mitral valve replacement more often compared to men who undergo mitral valve repair more frequently. This may be related to differences in etiology of mitral valve disease in men and women. Women are more likely to have mitral valve stenosis, mixed mitral valve disease and rheumatic valve disease compared to men who more likely have myxomatous mitral valve disease [31, 32]. This difference in surgical procedure may be reason for observed differences in gender-related outcome in some studies [31].

Women have been found to be referred for aortic valve replacement at an older age compared to men [33]. This could be related to delayed referral or development of symptoms at more advanced stage of disease in women. In addition, incidence of bicuspid aortic valves is two to three folds higher in men than women, which could explain younger age at presentation for aortic valve replacement in men. Aortic valve pathology has been reported to be different in male and female patients undergoing aortic valve replacement. Women undergo surgery more often for aortic stenosis and less often for aortic regurgitation than men [33, 34].

Re-operation following valve replacement surgery particularly with structural failure of tissue prosthesis is a common occurrence. Couple of studies report that women tend to have longer time period free of first redo operation particularly following aortic valve replacement [33, 35]. The exact mechanism remains unclear and could be related to hormonal differences or late calcification in women or a reflection of late referral in women.

Pregnancy and Valvular Surgeries

Hemodynamics changes, increase in blood volume, anemia and increase in cardiac output, are well known to occur in pregnancy and may worsen the existing valvular disease. Pregnant women with prosthetic heart valves are at increased risk of poor cardiovascular outcomes. In addition, mechanical prosthesis presents a particular challenge in women of child bearing age due to need of rigorous maintenance of anticoagulation. Pregnant women with mechanical valves are at highly increased risk of thromboembolism, on the other hand, anticoagulants also increase the risk of maternal and fetal hemorrhage and can be teratogenic (warfarin). Recently published guidelines by American College of Chest Physicians recommend use of unfractionated heparin (UFH) or low molecular weight heparin (LMWH) throughout pregnancy, or use of UFH/LMWH until 13th week of pregnancy with substitution by vitamin K antagonist (VKA) close to delivery in these situations. Women with older generation valve in mitral position or high risk for thromboembolism may be continued on VKA with substitution with UFH/LMWH closer to delivery [36].

Bioprosthetic valves seem to be more compatible with pregnancy as they do not require anticoagulation and its associated risk. However, there are some reports that suggest rapid deterioration of bioprosthesis with pregnancy requiring re-operation [37, 38]. More early miscarriages and pregnancy termination has been reported in women with valvular prosthesis compared to control [38]. In brief, the choice of valve should be considered carefully in young women undergoing valve replacement surgeries and pre-conception counseling plays a vital role.

Advanced Heart Failure Surgeries

According to National Health and Nutrition Examinations Surveys 2007–2010 data, an estimated 5.1 million (2.1 %) Americans ≥20 years of age have heart failure. Of these 5.1 million heart failure population, 2.7 million are male and 2.4 million are females. It is projected that by 2030, the prevalence of heart failure will increase by 25 % of 2013 estimates [1, 39]. Although survival after diagnosis of heart failure has improved over time; such improvement is less evident in women and elderly as shown by data from the Olmsted County Study. Heart failure mortality remains high and nearly 50 % of heart failure population dies within 5 years of diagnosis [40]. According to the data published by National Hospital Discharge Survey; from 2000 to 2010, the rate of CHF hospitalization for males under age 65 increased significantly while the rate for females aged 65 and over decreased significantly [41].

The benefits of heart failure therapies have been supported by evidence derived from multiple large multicenter randomized trials. Heart transplantation remains the gold standard therapy and has been proven to improve survival in select patients with advanced end-stage heart failure. However, with limited availability of donor organs, longer waiting time or ineligibility of recipient due to number of reasons, this option might always not be considerable. In such situations, implantation of ventricular assist devices (VAD), as bridge to transplant, bridge to recovery or as a destination therapy, have been shown to improve survival and quality of life.

Heart Transplantation

According to data published in 2012 by the registry of the International Society of Heart and Lung Transplantation (ISHLT)-the largest existing data registry for heart transplant outcomes worldwide, the median survival of heart transplant recipient is 10 years for those surviving first year post-transplant. In such patients, the likelihood of survival is 63 % at 10 years and 27 % at 20 years [42]. The median survival continues to improve over the last three decades and is likely related to improvement in immunosuppression and post-transplant care in general. According to ISHLT 2012 report [42], the proportion of female recipients has increased from 19.3 % (1992–2000) to 22.3 % (2001–2005) to 23.7 % (2006-June 2011); p-value = <0.0001. The proportion of female donors has decreased from 31.6 % (1992–2000) to 31 % (2001–2005) to 30.6 % (2006-June 2011); p-value = 0.0545.

Donor and Recipient Sex Match/Mismatch

Donor and recipient gender plays an important role in long term survival after cardiac allograft transplantation. In an ISHLT report of 60, 584 adult heart transplant recipients, male recipients of female allografts had a 10 % increase in adjusted mortality compared to male recipients of male allograft, however female recipients of female allografts had a 10 % decrease in adjusted mortality compared to female recipients of male allografts (p <0.0001) [43]. Similarly, data from United Network for Organ Sharing (UNOS) on all first United States heart transplantation showed that male recipients of female allograft have 15 % increase in mortality compared to male recipients of male allograft. However, UNOS data suggested no significant increase in mortality in women receiving opposite sex donor organs [44]. These observations seem to be related to genetic, biological, hormonal or immunological differences in men and women. Women's prior pregnancies and resultant allosensitization could likely play a role. At present, gender itself is not a criterion for allocation of donor organs to recipients.

Role of Gender in Analysis of Risk Factors for Heart Transplant

Sex related differences have also been demonstrated in baseline recipient characteristics, risk factors and potential post-transplant complications. Male recipients are generally older, heavier, have increased serum creatinine and higher incidence of ischemic cardiomyopathy [43, 45, 46]. Female recipients on the other hand, have generally higher level of panel reactive antibody (PRA), increased pulmonary vascular resistance and higher incidence of dilated cardiomyopathy [43, 44, 47]. Patients receiving heart transplant for non-ischemic cardiomyopathy have been reported to have better survival compared to patients who receive allograft for ischemic cardiomyopathy [42].

Limitation of exercise capacity varies with severity of heart failure. Peak oxygen consumption (peak VO2) provides an objective assessment of functional capacity and is an important prognostic marker in the evaluation of advanced heart failure patients. It is used frequently in clinical practice to determine need and candidacy for advanced heart failure therapies. Peak VO2 less than 14 ml/kg/min in patients not on beta-blockers and less than 10 ml/kg/min in patients on beta-blockers has been found to be associated with poor prognosis [48, 49]. Elmariah et al. reported that women had a significantly lower peak VO2 than men and despite lower peak VO2 women had better survival at all levels of exercise capacity [50]. It raises the concern of poor prognostic efficacy of this test in women leading potentially to premature transplantation. The lower peak VO2 in women is thought to be related to less muscle mass, lower baseline metabolic rate, and lower hemoglobin levels in women compared to men. A lower threshold value for peak VO2 in female heart failure patients may be considered in future.

Post-transplant Complications and Gender

Outcomes after heart transplant have been influenced by development of graft-related complication, the most important being cardiac allograft vasculopathy (CAV), acute graft failure and allograft rejection. Data from Spanish National Heart Transplantation Registry demonstrated higher incidence of acute graft failure in women [47]. Data has been contradictory in regards to association of gender on the incidence of CAV. ISHLT registry reported lower relative risk of development of CAV in female donor gender and female recipient gender in comparison to other donor-recipient gender combinations [42].

However, at the Berlin Heart Center [51], allografts from premenopausal female to male transplant more frequently developed endothelial disease (p-value=0.021) and stenotic microvasculopathy (p-value=0.024). These findings suggest the possible vasculoprotective and immunologic role of sex hormones and their receptors in the pathophysiology of transplant vasculopathy.

Ventricular Assist Devices

VADs has been shown to improve mortality and morbidity in heart failure patients who are either not a candidate for heart transplant or are too sick to wait for donor. The design of VADs have evolved over the years from earlier generation large size

Table 7.2 Summarizes the bench mark trials of ventricular assist devices

First author reference #	Study	Study design	Patient assignment	Enrollment period	Women	Men	1-year survival	2-year survival
EA Rose [54]	REMATCH	Randomized, non-blinded	OMM vs. LVAD (1:1)	1998–2001	26 (20 %)	103	25 % in OMM 52 % in LVAD	8 % in OMM 23 % in LVAD
MS Slaughter [55]	HeartMate II	Randomized, non-blinded	CF-LVAD vs. PF-LVAD (2:1)	2005–2007	31 (15 %)	169	68 % in CF-LVAD 55 % in PF-LVAD	58 % in CF-LVAD 24 % in PF-LVAD

Under-representation of women is evident

OMM optimal medical management, *CF-LVAD* continuous flow left ventricular assist device, *PF-LVAD* pulsatile flow left ventricular assist device volume displacement pulsatile flow pumps to newer generation smaller rotary pump providing continuous flow. The earlier generations of VADs were thought to be under-utilized in women due to anatomical constraints of large pulsatile pump in anatomically smaller body size of women. However, with the newer smaller size of LVAD, the under-utilization in women is still persistent which may likely be secondary to significant gender differences in diagnostic approach and treatment for end-stage heart failure (Table 7.2). In mechanical circulatory support (MCS) population, VAD implantation in females is generally under emergency circumstances [52]. Hsich et al. published report on 1936 LVAD patients, of which 26 % women were listed to be in critical cardiogenic shock compared to 19 % men (p-value=0.01) [53].

Survival in Men and Women After VAD

Survival in women who undergo VAD has been evaluated by few studies. Some authors report equal survival in men and women undergoing VAD [56], while others report superior survival in men compared to women [57] which in turn was evidently related to higher risk profile in women indicating a more advanced stage of heart failure at the time of VAD implantation. INTERMACS (Interagency Registry for Mechanically Assisted Circulatory Support) is a national registry for patients implanted with MCS device and is maintained at University of Alabama. Analysis of their data revealed no significant sex difference in mortality with either a pulsatile- or a continuous-flow left ventricular assist devices (LVAD) for the 1,936 patients (21 % female) [53].

Comparison of Adverse Events and Bridge to Transplant After VAD by Gender

The survival on LVAD is limited by number of complications post-LVAD including bleeding, infectious risk, thrombosis and so forth. Few studies looked into the association of gender with these adverse events after LVAD implantation but the results remains controversial. A published data report from INTERMACS registry demonstrated no significant sex differences in time to first bleed, infection, or device malfunction [53]. However, women, compared with men, had a shorter time to first neurological event that was statistically significant. Bogaeve et al. found lower rate of device related infection in women, similar rate of ischemic stroke between men and women but a trend towards higher rates of hemorrhagic strokes in women [56].

When VAD are implanted as bridge to transplant, there are reports of significantly lower rate of heart transplantation in women [53, 56]. Given the retrospective nature of these studies, it is assumed to be related to sensitization in women with pregnancies or issues related to BSA matching between donor and recipient heart. To better understand, gender related differences in outcomes in this particular population, there remains the need of large prospective trial to address specific issues.

Conclusion

Despite the similar prevalence of coronary artery of disease in men and women, women are less likely to undergo revascularization. In women who undergo CABG, the incidence of post-operative angina and incomplete revascularization remains high. The mortality in younger women undergoing CABG is also higher than men. Many factors influencing mortality and morbidity in men and women have been studied and pre-operative risk profile along with other factors seems to drive this difference. Surgical techniques also deserve important consideration particularly those that have been shown to impact outcomes such as use of internal mammary artery for bypass grafting. Despite various advances in availability of health care, delayed referral leading to presentation at more advanced stage of disease and requiring emergent surgery in women remains evident.

Similar to CABG, women undergoing valve surgery or combined valve and coronary revascularization surgery have far more risk factors than men, which negatively impact short and long term outcomes. In addition, there are differences between men and women in etiology of valve disease and should be considered when interpreting the results of various studies. The choice of valve is of particular importance in women of child bearing age. Pregnant women with prosthetic valves are at increased risk of poor cardiovascular outcomes, moreover bioprostheticvalves are more likely to undergo deterioration with hemodynamic stress of pregnancy. Potential teratogenic effects of certain anticoagulation agents should be carefully discussed with patients.

Similar to any cardiac surgery, women are less likely to undergo heart transplantation than men with advanced heart failure; however the number of female allograft recipients has been increasing over the years. Donor-recipient gender mismatch seems to negatively affect outcomes particularly in male recipients of female donor heart. However, given the limited availability of organs, long waiting times and several other factors, donor/recipient gender is not a considerable factor in the current organ allocation system. Prior pregnancies leading to allosensitization in women undergoing evaluation for heart transplant may negatively affect their candidacy.

VADs are also implanted less frequently in women with advanced heart failure. Although body surface area is important, it does not seem to be a limiting factor with newer generation VADs. Women undergo emergent VAD implantation more frequently than men indicating more advanced stage of disease, higher risk profile and referral bias. In bridge to transplant patients, women are less likely to receive heart transplantation than men.

In summary, several studies have analyzed the association of gender with life-saving cardiac surgeries. The results of studies are variable and in some cases contradictory to each other, likely a reflection of dissimilarities in study designs and/or heterogeneity in sample population. Women have been underrepresented in most clinical trials. The need of large prospective study with equal enrollment of both sexes is evident. Women tend to have worse risk profile than men indicating more advanced stage of disease or probably late referral for therapeutic considerations. The anatomical, pathophysiological and hormonal differences in both sexes should also be considered when analyzing outcomes and complications

References

1. Go AS, Mozaffarian D, et al. Heart disease and stroke statistics—2013 update. A report from the American Heart Association. Circulation. 2013;127:e6–245.
2. Melloni C, Berger JS, Wang TY, Gunes F, Stebbins A, Pieper KS, Dolor RJ, Douglas PS, Mark DB, Newby LK. Representation of women in randomized clinical trials of cardiovascular disease prevention. Circ Cardiovasc Qual Outcomes. 2010;3(2):135–42.
3. Steingart RM, Packer M, Hamm P, Coglianese ME, Gersh B, Geltman EM, Sollano J, Katz S, Moyé L, Basta LL, et al. Sex differences in the management of coronary artery disease. Survival and Ventricular Enlargement Investigators. N Engl J Med. 1991;325(4):226–30.
4. Vaccarino V, Parsons L, Every NR, Barron HV, Krumholz HM. Sex-based differences in early mortality after myocardial infarction. National Registry of Myocardial Infarction 2 Participants. N Engl J Med. 1999;341(4):217–25.
5. Regitz-Zagrosek V, Lehmkuhl E, Hocher B, Goesmann D, Lehmkuhl HB, Hausmann H, Hetzer R. Gender as a risk factor in young, not in old, women undergoing coronary artery bypass grafting. J Am Coll Cardiol. 2004;44(12):2413–4.
6. Vaccarino V, Parsons L, Peterson ED, Rogers WJ, Kiefe CI, Canto J. Sex differences in mortality after acute myocardial infarction: changes from 1994 to 2006. Arch Intern Med. 2009;169(19):1767–74.
7. Davies SW, O'Neal WT, Sawyer RG, Efird JT, Ferguson T. A comparison of the long term survival of 306,868 patients with multivessel coronary artery disease undergoing CABG and PCI: a meta-analysis of retrospective studies. J Am Coll Cardiol. 2013;61(10_S). doi:10.1016/S0735-1097(13)61214-0
8. Sá MP, Soares AM, Lustosa PC, Martins WN, Browne F, Ferraz PE, Vasconcelos FP, Lima RC. Meta-analysis of 5,674 patients treated with percutaneous coronary intervention and drug-eluting stents or coronary artery bypass graft surgery for unprotected left main coronary artery stenosis. Eur J Cardiothorac Surg. 2013;43(1):73–80.
9. Rahimtoola SH, Bennett AJ, Grunkemeier GL, Block P, Starr A. Survival at 15 to 18 years after coronary bypass surgery for angina in women. Circulation. 1993;88(5 Pt 2):II71–1178.
10. Jacobs AK, Kelsey SF, Brooks MM, Faxon DP, Chaitman BR, Bittner V, Mock MB, Weiner BH, Dean L, Winston C, Drew L, Sopko G. Better outcome for women compared with men undergoing coronary revascularization: a report from the Bypass Angioplasty Revascularization Investigation (BARI). Circulation. 1998;98:1279–85.
11. Weintraub WS, Clements Jr SD, Crisco LV, Guyton RA, Craver JM, Jones EL, Hatcher Jr CR. Twenty-year survival after coronary artery surgery: an institutional perspective from Emory University. Circulation. 2003;107(9):1271–7.
12. Abramov D, Tamariz MG, Sever JY, Christakis GT, Bhatnagar G, Heenan AL, Goldman BS, Fremes SE. The influence of gender on the outcome of coronary artery bypass surgery. Ann Thorac Surg. 2000;70:800–5.
13. Woods SE, Noble G, Smith JM, Hasselfeld K. The influence of gender in patients undergoing coronary artery bypass graft surgery: an eight-year prospective hospitalized cohort study. J Am Coll Surg. 2003;196:428–34.
14. Nashef SA, Roques F, Michel P, Gauducheau E, Lemeshow S, Salamon R. European system for cardiac operative risk evaluation (EuroSCORE). Eur J Cardiothorac Surg. 1999;16(1):9–13.

15. Edwards FH, Carey JS, Grover FL, Bero JW, Hartz RS. Impact of gender on coronary bypass operative mortality. Ann Thorac Surg. 1998;66:125–31.
16. Ennker IC, Albert A, Pietrowski D, Bauer K, Ennker J, Florath I. Impact of gender on outcome after coronary artery bypass surgery. Asian Cardiovasc Thorac Ann. 2009;17:253–8.
17. Blankstein R, Ward RP, Arnsdorf M, Jones B, Lou YB, Pine M. Female gender is an independent predictor of operative mortality after coronary artery bypass graft surgery: contemporary analysis of 31 Midwestern hospitals. Circulation. 2005;112(9 Suppl):I323–1327.
18. Ranucci M, Pazzaglia A, Bianchini C, Bozzetti G, Isgrò G. Body size, gender, and transfusions as determinants of outcome after coronary operations. Ann Thorac Surg. 2008;85:481–7.
19. Westenbrink BD, Kleijn L, de Boer RA, Tijssen JG, Warnica WJ, Baillot R, Rouleau JL, van Gilst WH. Sustained postoperative anaemia is associated with an impaired outcome after coronary artery bypass graft surgery: insights from the IMAGINE trial. Heart. 2011;97(19):1590–6.
20. Rogers MA, Blumberg N, Saint SK, Kim C, Nallamothu BK, Langa KM. Allogeneic blood transfusions explain increased mortality in women after coronary artery bypass graft surgery. Am Heart J. 2006;152(6):1028–34.
21. van Straten AH, Hamad MA, van Zundert AJ, Martens EJ, Schönberger JP, de Wolf AM. Preoperative hemoglobin level as a predictor of survival after coronary artery bypass grafting: a comparison with the matched general population. Circulation. 2009;120(2):118–25.
22. Aldea GS, Gaudiani JM, Shapira OM, Jacobs AK, Weinberg J, Cupples AL, Lazar HL, Shemin RJ. Effect of gender on postoperative outcomes and hospital stays after coronary artery bypass grafting. Ann Thorac Surg. 1999;67:1097–103.
23. Tabata M, Grab JD, Khalpey Z, Edwards FH, O'Brien SM, Cohn LH, Bolman III RM. Prevalence and variability of internal mammary artery graft use in contemporary multivessel coronary artery bypass graft surgery: analysis of the Society of Thoracic Surgeons National Cardiac Database. Circulation. 2009;120:935–40.
24. O'Connor GT, Morton JR, Diehl MJ, Olmstead EM, Coffin LH, Levy DG, Maloney CT, Plume SK, Nugent W, Malenka DJ. Differences between men and women in hospital mortality associated with coronary artery bypass graft surgery. The Northern New England Cardiovascular Disease Study Group. Circulation. 1993;88:2104–10.
25. Lamy A, Devereaux PJ, Prabhakaran D, Taggart DP, Hu S, Paolasso E, Straka Z, Piegas LS, Akar AR, Jain AR, Noiseux N, Padmanabhan C, Bahamondes JC, Novick RJ, Vaijyanath P, Reddy SK, Tao L, Olavegogeascoechea PA, Airan B, Sulling TA, Whitlock RP, Ou Y, Pogue J, Chrolavicius S, Yusuf S. Effects of off-pump and on-pump coronary-artery bypass grafting at 1 year. N Engl J Med. 2013;368(13):1179–88.
26. Diegeler A, Börgermann J, Kappert U, Breuer M, Böning A, Ursulescu A, Rastan A, Holzhey D, Treede H, Rie FC, Veeckmann P, Asfoor A, Reents W, Zacher M, Hilker M. Off-pump versus on-pump coronary-artery bypass grafting in elderly patients. N Engl J Med. 2013;368(13):1189–98.
27. Vaccarino V, Abramson JL, Veledar E, Weintraub WS. Sex differences in hospital mortality after coronary artery bypass surgery: evidence for a higher mortality in younger women. Circulation. 2002;105:1176–81.
28. Hogue Jr CW, Barzilai B, Pieper KS, Coombs LP, DeLong ER, Kouchoukos NT, Dávila-Román VG. Sex differences in neurological outcomes and mortality after cardiac surgery: a Society of Thoracic Surgery National Database Report. Circulation. 2001;103:2133–7.
29. Koch CG, Khandwala F, Nussmeier N, Blackstone EH. Gender and outcomes after coronary artery bypass grafting: a propensity-matched comparison. J Thorac Cardiovasc Surg. 2003;126:2032–43.
30. Butterworth J, James R, Prielipp R, Cerese J, Livingston J, Burnett D. Female gender associates with increased duration of intubation and length of stay after coronary artery surgery. CABG Clinical Benchmarking Database Participants. Anesthesiology. 2000;92(2):414–24.
31. Ibrahim MF, Paparella D, Ivanov J, Buchanan MR, Brister SJ. Gender-related differences in morbidity and mortality during combined valve and coronary surgery. J Thorac Cardiovasc Surg. 2003;126:959–64.

32. TmDoenst JI, Borger MA, David TE, Brister SJ. Sex-specific long-term outcomes after combined valve and coronary artery surgery. Ann Thorac Surg. 2006;81:1632–6.
33. Kulik A, Lam BK, Rubens FD, Hendry PJ, Masters RG, Goldstein W, Be'dard P, Mesana TG, Ruel M. Gender differences in the long-term outcomes after valve replacement surgery. Heart. 2009;95:318–26.
34. Hamed O, Persson PJ, Engel AM, McDonough S, Smith JM. Gender differences in outcomes following aortic valve replacement surgery. Int J Surg. 2009;7:214–7.
35. Weerasinghe A, Edwards MB, Taylor KM. First redo heart valve replacement: a 10-year analysis. Circulation. 1999;99:655–8.
36. Guyatt GH, Akl EA, Crowther M, Gutterman DD, Schünemann HJ. Antithrombotic therapy and prevention of thrombosis, 9th edition: American College of Chest Physicians evidence-based clinical practice guidelines. Chest. 2012;141(2 Suppl):7S–47.
37. Sbarouni E, Oakley CM. Outcome of pregnancy in women with valve prostheses. Br Heart J. 1994;71:196–201.
38. Sillesen M, Hjortdal V, Vejlstrup N, Sørensen K. Pregnancy with prosthetic heart valves — 30 years nationwide experience in Denmark. Eur J Cardiothorac Surg. 2011;40:448–54.
39. Heidenreich PA, Trogdon JG, et al. Forecasting the future of cardiovascular disease in the United States: a policy statement from the American Heart Association. Circulation. 2011;123:933–44.
40. Roger VL, Weston SA, et al. Trends in heart failure incidence and survival in a community-based population. JAMA. 2004;292(3):344–50.
41. Hall MJ, Levant S, DeFrances CJ. Hospitalization for congestive heart failure: United States, 2000–2010. NCHS data brief, no 108. Hyattsville: National Center for Health Statistics; 2012.
42. Stehlik J, Edwards LB, Kucheryavaya AY, Benden C, Christie JD, Dipchand AI, Dobbels F, Kirk R, Rahmel AO, Hertz MI. The registry of the International Society for Heart and Lung Transplantation: 29th official adult heart transplant report–2012. J Heart Lung Transplant. 2012;31(10):1052–64.
43. Khush KK, Kubo JT, Desai M. Influence of donor and recipient sex mismatch on heart transplant outcomes: analysis of the International Society for Heart and Lung Transplantation Registry. J Heart Lung Transplant. 2012;31(5):459–66.
44. Weiss ES, Allen JG, Patel ND, Russell SD, Baumgartner WA, Shah AS, Conte JV. The impact of donor-recipient sex matching on survival after orthotopic heart transplantation: analysis of 18,000 transplants in the modern era. Circ Heart Fail. 2009;2:401–8.
45. Eifert S, Kofler S, Nickel T, Horster S, Bigdeli AK, Beiras-Fernandez A, Meiser B, Kaczmarek I. Gender-based analysis of outcome after heart transplantation. Exp Clin Transplant. 2012;10(4):368–74.
46. Regitz-Zagrosek V, Petrov G, Lehmkuhl E, Smits JM, Babitsch B, Brunhuber C, Jurmann B, Stein J, Schubert C, Merz NB, Lehmkuhl HB, Hetzer R. Heart transplantation in women with dilated cardiomyopathy. Transplantation. 2010;89:236–44.
47. L Almenar, on behalf of Spanish Heart Transplant Teams. Influence of sex on heart transplantation mortality: data from the Spanish National Heart Transplantation Registry. Rev Esp Cardiol Supl. 2008;8:49D–54D.
48. Mancini DM, Eisen H, Kussmaul W, Mull R, Edmunds Jr LH, Wilson JR. Value of peak exercise oxygen consumption for optimal timing of cardiac transplantation in ambulatory patients with heart failure. Circulation. 1991;83(3):778–86.
49. Lund LH, Aaronson KD, Mancini DM. Predicting survival in ambulatory patients with severe heart failure on beta-blocker therapy. Am J Cardiol. 2003;92:1350–4.
50. Elmariah S, Goldberg LR, Allen MT, Kao A. Effects of gender on peak oxygen consumption and the timing of cardiac transplantation. J Am Coll Cardiol. 2006;47:2237–42.
51. Hiemann NE, Knosalla C, Wellnhofer E, Lehmkuhl HB, Hetzer R, Meyer R. Beneficial effect of female gender on long-term survival after heart transplantation. Transplantation. 2008;86:348–56.

52. Potapov E, Schweiger M, Lehmkuhl E, Vierecke J, Stepanenko AS, Weng G, Pasic M, Huebler M, Regitz-Zagrosek V, Hietzer R, Krabatsch T. Gender differences during mechanical circulatory support. ASAIO J. 2012;58:320–5.
53. Hsich EM, Naftel DC, Myers SL, Gorodeski EZ, Grady KL, Schmuhl D, Ulisney KL, Young JB. Should women receive left ventricular assist device support? Findings from INTERMACS. Circ Heart Fail. 2012;5:234–40.
54. Rose EA, Gelijns AC, Moskowitz AJ, Heitjan DF, Stevenson LW, Dembitsky W, Long JW, Ascheim DD, Tierney AR, Levitan RG, Watson JT, Ronan NS, Shapiro PA, Lazar RM, Miller LW, Gupta L, Frazier OH, Desvigne-Nickens P, Oz MC, Poirier VL, Meier P. Long-term mechanical left ventricular assistance for end-stage heart failure. N Engl J Med. 2001;345:1435–43.
55. Slaughter MS, Rogers JG, Milano CA, Russell SD, Conte JV, Feldman D, Sun B, Tatooles AJ, Delgado III RM, Long JW, Wozniak TC, Ghumman W, Farrar DJ, Frazier OH. Advanced heart failure treated with continuous-flow left ventricular assist device. N Engl J Med. 2009;361(23):2241–51.
56. Bogaev RC, Pamboukian SV, Moore SA, Chen L, John R, Boyle AJ, Sundareswaran KS, Farrar DJ, Frazier OH. Comparison of outcomes in women versus men using a continuous-flow left ventricular assist device as a bridge to transplantation. J Heart Lung Transplant. 2011;30:515–22.
57. Morgan JA, Weinberg AD, Hollingsworth KW, Flannery MR, Oz MC, Naka Y. Effect of gender on bridging to transplantation and post transplantation survival in patients with left ventricular assist devices. J Thorac Cardiovasc Surg. 2004;127:1193–5.

Chapter 8
Heart Failure and Pulmonary Hypertension in Women

Andrew Darlington, Jacinta Green, and Gladys P. Velarde

Heart failure is characterized as a syndrome caused by cardiac dysfunction, leading to neurohormonal and circulatory abnormalities, resulting in the characteristic signs/symptoms of fluid retention, shortness of breath, and fatigue, particularly on exertion [1]. The worldwide prevalence and incidence continues to rise over time and is rapidly approaching epidemic proportions. In the United States alone, there are an estimated six million people living with heart failure and 670,000 new cases diagnosed each year, of which 320,000 of these are women [2]. This has led to an annual expenditure approaching nearly 39 billion dollars [2, 3].

HFrEF and HFpEF

The heart failure population can be further characterized by identifying those patients with reduced ejection fraction (HFrEF) and those with preserved ejection fraction (HFpEF) (Table 8.1) Prior population-based studies have demonstrated that each contribute roughly 50 % to that of the overall heart failure population [4, 5]. There appears to be a gender-discrepancy in regards to the prevalence of HFpEF with females greatly outnumbering their male counterparts [6]. The reason for this divergence is not clearly understood but several proposed mechanisms may partly explain this difference. First, women are more likely than men to develop concentric left ventricular remodeling as a result of chronic pressure overload states such as systemic arterial hypertension [7]. The presence of concentric left ventricular remodeling contributes to a greater degree of diastolic dysfunction and depressed

A. Darlington, DO • J. Green, MD • G.P. Velarde, MD, FACC (✉)
Division of Cardiology, University of Florida College of Medicine-Jacksonville,
ACC Building 5th floor 655 West 8th Street, Jacksonville, FL 32209, USA
e-mail: gladys.velarde@jax.ufl.edu

H.Z. Mieszczanska, G.P. Velarde (eds.),
Management of Cardiovascular Disease in Women,
DOI 10.1007/978-1-4471-5517-1_8, © Springer-Verlag London 2014

Table 8.1 Definitions of HFrEF and HFpEF

Classification	EF	Description
I. Heart failure with reduced ejection fraction (**HFrEF**)	≤40	Alo referred to as systolic HF
		Efficacious therapies well demonstrated to date.
II. Heart failure with preserved ejection fraction (**HFpEF**)	≥50	Also referred to as diastolic HF.
		Diagnosis of exclusion
		Efficacious therapies have not yet been identified
(a) HFpEF, borderline	41–49	Intermediate group.
		Treatment and outcomes similar to HFpEF
(b) HFpEF, improved	>40	Subset of HFpEF patients where EF improved or recovered.
		May be distinct group
		Needs to be characterized better

Adapted from [10]

EF Ejection fraction, *HF* heart failure, *HFpEF* heart failure with preserved ejection fraction, *HFrEF* heart failure with reduced ejection fraction

Table 8.2 ACC/AHA Guidelines Staging System

Stage	Description
A	Patients at high risk for developing heart failure who have no structural heart disease or symptoms of heart failure.
B	Patients who have not yet developed symptoms of heart failure but have structural heart disease.
C	Patients with a history of symptoms of heart failure with associated underlying structural heart disease.
D	Patients with end stage heart failure requiring advanced treatments.

Adapted from [10]

ventricular reserve during stress [8]. Ventricular-arterial stiffening, which plays an important role in the pathophysiology of HFPEF, is seen to a greater extent in women than in men. In addition, the age-related increase in ventricular stiffness appears to be further enhanced in females as opposed to males [9].

In 2005, the American College of Cardiology/American Heart Association (ACC/AHA) introduced a new staging system for heart failure [44]. This staging system remains unchanged in the recently released 2013 ACC/AHA guidelines (Table 8.2) [10]. The purpose was to highlight that heart failure is a progressive syndrome with a spectrum ranging from asymptomatic patients with risk factors to end-stage disease. The first two stages (A and B) comprise asymptomatic patients and may account for over 50 % of the population, based on this new classification system [10]. Stage A includes only patients with risk factors for the development of heart failure such as diabetes, hypertension, obesity and coronary artery disease. Emphasis has been placed on early recognition of risk factors and targeted, aggressive treatment in order to prevent progression to the more advanced disease stages. Stage B includes patients with evidence of structural heart disease such as left ventricular systolic dysfunction or left ventricular hypertrophy but without symptoms related to heart failure. Early appropriate therapy such as the use of beta-blockers

Table 8.3 New York Heart Association Classification

Class	Description
I	Patients with cardiac disease but without symptoms[a] or limitations in physical activity.
II	Patients with cardiac disease resulting in mild symptoms and slight limitations in ordinary activity.
III	Patients with cardiac disease resulting in symptoms with less than ordinary activity.
IV	Patients with cardiac disease resulting in the inability to carry out any physical activity without symptoms. There are symptoms at rest.

Adapted from The Criteria Committee of the New York Heart Association [90]
[a]Symptoms include fatigue, palpitations, dyspnea, or angina pain

and ACE inhibitors in patients with asymptomatic low ejection fraction reduces mortality and delays the development of symptomatic disease [10]. Patients with evidence of structural heart disease and current or prior symptoms of heart failure are classified as Stage C. The vast majority of clinical trials have targeted this stage, including pharmacological agents and device therapies. Finally, Stage D classification includes patients who have advanced end stage heart failure and may require specialized interventions, including inotropic therapy, heart transplantation and left ventricular assist device placement. Current estimates suggest that there are approximately 100,000–250,000 patients in the United States with Stage D heart failure who may be eligible for these therapies [10]. The New York Heart Association (NYHA) has created a functional classification system for describing the severity of symptoms including NYHA Class I–IV (Table 8.3).

When evaluating women for their likelihood of developing heart failure it is important to know the risk factors for heart failure as they relate specifically to gender. Coronary artery disease (CAD), the most prevalent risk factor for the development of heart failure is more common in males than in females [11]. However, females suffer from a higher prevalence of both hypertension and diabetes compared to males and their presence appears to confer a higher risk for developing heart failure [12, 13] (Fig. 8.1).

The presence of obesity also increases the risk for heart failure in females more so than in males [13]. The Framingham study suggests that overall prognosis in women is significantly better than in men after the onset of heart failure [14]. This may be due to the fact that women have less ischemic cardiomyopathy, and survival might be related to sex differences in etiology. However, due to the longer lifespan of women compared to men as well as the increased incidence of heart failure in older females compared to males, the overall total number of heart failure-related deaths may be higher in women [14].

It is important to recognize that heart failure is a clinical syndrome that largely relies on history and physical exam for an accurate diagnosis. The symptoms of both HFREF and HFPEF are similar between men and women and in general, patients with heart failure will present in one of three ways. These include (1) decreased exercise tolerance, typically with complaints of dyspnea on exertion or fatigue (2) fluid retention and weight gain manifesting as leg and/or abdominal swelling and (3) asymptomatic or with symptoms of another cardiac or non-cardiac

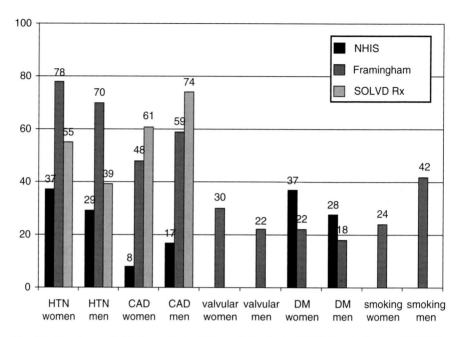

Fig. 8.1 Prevalence of risk factors in the HF population in the NHIS, Framingham and SOLVD studies (Reproduced with permission from Lund and Mancini [88])

disorder such as an arrhythmia, pulmonary or systemic thromboembolic event [10]. Physical exam findings of increased jugular venous pressure and the presence of the hepato-jugular reflex correspond to elevated pulmonary capillary wedge pressures and are highly sensitive findings in heart failure [15]. During the cardiovascular exam the presence of an S3 represents a poor prognostic indicator [15]. Patients may also have an S4, which may indicate diastolic dysfunction. The presence of any of a variety of murmurs may indicate possible valvular disease. Lung exam findings of rales and dullness at the lung bases are consistent with pulmonary edema and/or pleural effusion. Of note, the presence of these pulmonary physical exam findings lack diagnostic sensitivity in chronic heart failure [15]. Additional findings consistent with more advanced, low output heart failure include cold and pale extremities, altered sensorium and decreased urine output.

Laboratory investigation should include a basic metabolic panel to assess for potential abnormalities in serum creatinine, blood urea nitrogen and sodium, all of which serve as negative prognostic markers in heart failure [16, 17]. Anemia noted on a complete blood count (CBC) is also a well-known negative prognostic marker [18]. The clinical use of natriuretic peptides (BNP and proBNP) in heart failure are potentially numerous and have both diagnostic and prognostic utility [19]. The recent 2013 AHA/ACC heart failure guidelines identify the use of natriuretic peptides as useful elements to achieved optimal dosing of guided directed medical therapy in selected patients, while acknowledging that their usefulness of serial measurement to reduce outcomes is not well established [10]. Thus their use is strictly as an adjunct to that of the history and physical exam. In females, natriuretic peptide levels are typically elevated when compared to men [20]. In addition, when compared with HFrEF, natriuretic peptide levels are lower in HFpEF, a population in which females outnumber males [21]. A chest x-ray can provide quick visualization of heart and lung to determine if there is cardiomegaly, pulmonary edema, pulmonary vascular congestion, and pleural effusions. ECG which can show evidence of myocardial ischemia, injury, or infarction, atrial enlargement, left ventricular hypertrophy (LVH), or low voltage. Echocardiography is the gold standard imaging study for the evaluation of heart failure and can be used to determine the presence of systolic and diastolic function as well as hypertrophy, valvular and pericardial disease. As previously noted, females tend to present with concentric hypertrophy more than males, who have a higher prevalence of eccentric hypertrophy [7]. Concentric LVH and left atrial enlargement are characteristic structural changes noted on echo study in HFPEF and among the very elderly, over 80 % of women were found to display LVH [22].

Therapy of HF in Women

Management of HF with Reduced Ejection Fraction (HFrEF)

Current evidence is inconclusive as to whether or not clinical differences exist between men and women with HFREF using standard heart failure treatment. This is due to the overall low percentage of females enrolled in these studies and the small amount of gender specific data recovered from these studies. Recommendations for the treatment of women with heart failure have been made by the Heart Failure Society of America whose conclusions derived from this limited database are simply that the management of HFREF should remain similar for both women and men. The following section will therefore summarize what we currently know in regards to the management of HFREF and HFPEF and how this may be approached in the female population.

Angiotensin converting enzyme inhibitors (ACE-I) are an established first line therapy for chronic HFREF and the mechanism of their benefit is likely secondary to decreasing the maladaptive neurohormonal response by the renin angiotensin aldosterone system in the syndrome of heart failure. ACE-I have been shown to decrease short-term mortality by 40 % in patients with advanced heart failure [23] and by 16 % in patients with less advanced disease [24]. ACE-I also decrease mortality in patients with reduced left ventricular dysfunction with or without a prior myocardial infarction, even in the absence of symptoms [25, 26]. Similarly, clinical studies on ACE-I suggest comparable effects in women and men with heart failure.

Angiotensin II receptor blockers (ARBs) are accepted as a potential alternative to ACE-I, especially in patients who are intolerant to ACE-I secondary to cough [27]. ARBs are non-inferior to ACE-I in the management of post-MI patients complicated by symptomatic heart failure [28]. Subsequent analysis of several heart failure trials have found a similar significant reduction in mortality and HF hospitalizations in women as compared to men [29]. The recommendations for ARBs are similar for men and women and are recommended for those intolerant to ACE-I.

Beta-blockers are also an accepted first line therapy for symptomatic heart failure patients. The mechanism of benefit from beta-blockers in heart failure is thought to involve inhibition of the long-term deleterious effects of the sympathetic nervous system. In patients with HFREF, beta-blockers have been found to significantly decrease mortality and heart failure re-hospitalizations [30–32]. Review of the beta-blocker data on women with symptomatic HFrEF suggests that both genders receive similar benefit from the use beta-blockers [33]. Given this evidence, recommendations are to use beta- blockers for both men and women with heart failure.

Data from the African-American Heart Failure Trial (A-HeFT) demonstrated a reduction in mortality of 43 % using hydralazine and isosorbide dinitrate in addition to standard therapy, including ACE-I and beta blockers [34]. The A-HeFT trial included 40 % women, more than previous trials, and found similar improvement in heart failure outcomes including primary composite score, first heart failure hospitalization, and event-free survival in both men and women [35].

Sustained activation of aldosterone appears to play an important role in the pathophysiology of heart failure with elevated circulating levels of aldosterone enhancing sodium retention. In addition, deleterious effects on the vasculature and myocardium have been documented [36]. There is a general lack of sex-specific data from prospective trials on the benefits of aldosterone antagonists for women with left ventricular systolic dysfunction and symptoms of heart failure. However, adequate numbers of women were included in two large randomized, controlled trials of these agents and subgroup analyses were shown to demonstrate benefit in women [37, 38]. Similar to prior HF guidelines, the most recent 2013 ACC/AHA guidelines offer safeguards of creatinine levels needing to be ≤ 2.0 mg/dL in women (vs. 2.5 mg/dL in men) [10].

Digoxin therapy, though demonstrated to decrease heart failure hospitalizations, has not been shown to improve survival [39]. Retrospective analysis of the Digitalis Investigation Group (DIG) trial suggested an increased risk of death from any cause among women, but not men, with heart failure and reduced left ventricular ejection fraction [40]. However, further analysis of the same trial reported no excess mortality in either women or men when serum digoxin concentrations were between 0.5 and 0.9 mg/ml [41]. Digoxin levels are higher in women compared to men at any given dose likely due to decreased lean body mass and renal function.

Management of HF with Preserved Ejection Fraction (HFpEF)

HFpEF is associated with increased morbidity and mortality similar to that seen in the population with reduced ejection fraction [4, 5]. This is especially concerning for women, since females are more likely to have HFpEF than their male counterparts [6]. Unlike the clinical trial data in the HFrEF population, women have been well represented in the clinical trials of HFpEF. Among the few prospective studies

Table 8.4 Recommendations for treating patients with heart failure and preserved left ventricular ejection fraction

Class I guidelines
Physicians should control hypertension in accordance with published guidelines (Level of Evidence B)
Physicians should use diuretics to control pulmonary congestion and peripheral edema (Level of Evidence C)
Class IIa guidelines
Coronary revascularization is reasonable in patients with CAD in whom ischemia is having adverse effect on cardiac function despite GDMT (Level of Evidence C)
Physicians should manage atrial fibrillation according to guidelines to improve symptoms of HF (Level of Evidence C)
Beta blockers, ACE inhibitors, and Angiotensin II receptor blockers should be used for BP control (Level of Evidence C)
Class IIb guidelines
Angiotensin II receptor blockers may be useful in decreasing hospitalizations (Level of Evidence B)
Class III guidelines
Nutritional supplementation is not recommended in HFpEF (Level of evidence C)

Adapted from [10]

CAD coronary artery disease, *ACE* angiotensin converting enzymes, *GDMT* guideline-directed medical therapy, *HF* heart failure, *HFpEF* heart failure with preserved ejection fraction

of HFpEF, the percentage of females ranged from 61 to 76 % of the overall study populations [3, 42, 43]. Several professional societies have published guidelines that specifically address HFpEF [1, 44]. However, none of these guidelines, including the most recent 2013 ACC/AHA HF guidelines recently released [10] can be considered evidence-based, as there are currently no proven heart failure-specific therapies for which to use in this population, unlike those with reduced left ventricular ejection fraction. Society recommendations are generally similar and include the use of long-term diuretic therapy, when appropriate, to control or prevent edema along with ACE-I, ARBs and beta-blockers to treat hypertension (Table 8.4). Low sodium diet, without specific dietary sodium restriction (previously advocated on 2005 ACC/AHA guidelines), and fluid restriction recommendations are similar to that of the HFrEF population. Evaluation for ischemic heart disease and inducible myocardial ischemia, when applicable is also recommended [1, 44].

Cardiac resynchronization therapy with defibrillator (CRT-D) is an approved treatment for patients with advanced stages of heart failure in the setting of a widened QRS, and this therapy is associated with a reduction in symptoms, improvement in functional capacity, and a decrease in hospitalization and mortality [45]. Data suggests that women seem to benefit more from CRT-ICD therapy than men. As a result of CRT-D therapy, women have decreased cardiac volumes with improvements in LVEF compared to males [46]. In addition, a sub-study of the MADIT-CRT Trial demonstrated that women may have a significantly greater benefit from device therapy than men with regards to overall mortality and cardiac-related outcomes [47]. The reason for this seemingly sex-related benefit is unclear but may relate to the higher proportion of studied males with ischemic cardiomyopathy and non-left bundle branch block morphology on ECG, both indicators of poor response to CRT-D [47].

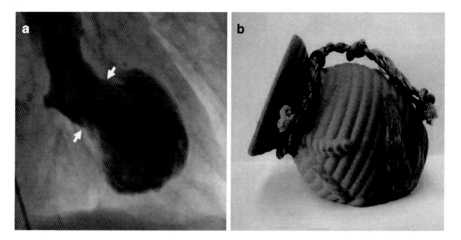

Fig. 8.2 (a) Ventriculogram of the heart during the contraction phase from a patient with takotsubo's cardiomyopathy. Note the distinctive shape with a narrow neck (*arrows*) and ballooned lower portion, which contracts abnormally. (b) The Japanese takotsubo (ceramic pot used to trap octopus) has a shape that closely resembles that of the heart on the left. (Reproduced with permission from Sharkey [89])

Takotsubo's Cardiomyopathy

Takotsubo's cardiomyopathy (TC), also referred to as the apical ballooning or broken heart syndrome is a rare disorder first described in the early 1990s by the Japanese. They reported on a unique, reversible cardiomyopathy that appeared to be precipitated by acute stress [48]. They discovered that these subjects were usually postmenopausal women who often developed signs and symptoms of an acute coronary syndrome (ACS) proximate to a strong emotional stressor. This presentation was associated with a transient apical and/or mid-ventricular wall motion abnormality resembling an octopus trap [48] (Fig. 8.2).

Subsequent angiography typically displayed a lack of obstructive coronary artery disease (CAD).

The precise pathophysiologic mechanism of TC is unknown. Pharmacologically induced coronary artery spasm has been documented in a number of TC cases [49]. However, the actual significance of these clinical findings remain unclear at the present time. The presence of a catecholamine surge has accrued perhaps the most evidence in favor of a mechanism for this cardiomyopathy [50]. TC typically occurs proximate to either a physical or emotional stressor, states characterized by high circulating catecholamines. Finally, animal studies have shown that the administration of both alpha and beta blocker therapy prevents the development of this form of cardiomyopathy [51].

To date, it is largely unknown why TC predominates in women but several theories have been proposed to explain this finding. One possibility may be related to gender differences in myocardial sensitivity to catecholamine toxicity with subsequent intra-myocyte calcium overload [52]. Another is that females typically have a smaller left ventricular cavity size which may predispose them to left ventricular

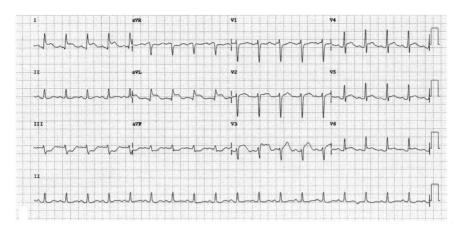

Fig. 8.3 Electrocardiogram of a patient with takotsubo's cardiomyopathy demonstrating ST segment elevation in the anterior precordial and high lateral limb leads with recipricol changes in the inferior limb leads. (Reproduced with permission from Sharkey [89])

outflow tract obstruction and increased intra-ventricular pressure gradients. This may in turn cause an oxygen mismatch in the apex resulting in ballooning [53].

As mentioned previously, those presenting with TC are most commonly postmenopausal women [48]. In a systematic review, women accounted for 82–100 % of patients with an average age of 62–75 years, although cases have been described in individuals as young as 10 and as old as 91 years of age [54]. Typically, a prior strong emotional or physical stressor predates presentation though in some no precipitating event is identified [48]. Clinical presentation usually involves acute dyspnea and chest pressure or tightness not dissimilar to that of a patient with an acute coronary syndrome. ECG abnormalities are a mainstay and include ST elevation, pathologic appearing Q waves, QT prolongation and deep, symmetrical T wave inversions [54] (Fig. 8.3).

These findings, when combined with cardiac biomarker elevations that are commonly seen make it very difficult on initial evaluation to distinguish TC from that of an ST elevation myocardial infarction. Furthermore, it has been estimated that as many as 6 % of women presenting with an apparent ACS may actually have TC [55]. The hallmark echocardiographic findings consist of apical and/or midventricular wall motion abnormalities that do not correlate with the distribution of a single major epicardial coronary distribution with hyperkinesis of the basal myocardial segments [54]. Variants have been reported in young females presenting with stress cardiomyopathy after an acute emotional or physical stress demonstrating isolated basal hypokinesis only [55] (Fig. 8.4)

Emergent cardiac catheterization most commonly reveals a lack of obstructive coronary artery disease that could account for the observed regional wall motion abnormalities.

Currently there is a lack of available clinical trial data in TC with which to guide therapy so management is typically performed on an empiric basis. Fortunately, due to the reversible nature of TC, supportive care will usually suffice. In rare instances,

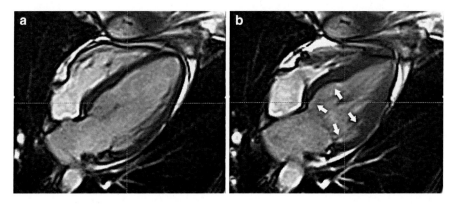

Fig. 8.4 Cardiac magnetic resonance imaging demonstrating in (**a**) diastole and (**b**) systole. The unusual pattern of basal akinesis (*arrows*) with preserved mid and apical function. The so-called "reverse takotsubo pattern". (Reproduced with permission from Sharkey [89])

hemodynamic compromise leading to cardiogenic shock occurs, requiring the assistance of intravenous inotropes and even mechanical support by means of an intra-aortic balloon pump. Anticoagulation should be considered, at least during the initial hospital course to prevent the formation of left ventricular thrombus and subsequent thromboembolism, which is a common cause of mortality in these patients. Given the role that catecholamines may play in the pathophysiology of TC, long-term beta-blocker therapy to prevent recurrence has been suggested though no clear and consistent data exists to support its use [54].

TC is an uncommon disorder that predominates in women where several hypotheses, including myocardial dysfunction mediated through catecholamine-induced damage through regional variation in number or sensitivity of myocardial adrenergic receptors from base to apex and their variable response to stress and hormonal influences to the presence of altered coronary arterial regulation similar to coronary spasm have been proposed. It is likely that the pathogenesis of TTC is multifactorial and the exact pathophysiologic mechanism remains elusive.

Pulmonary Hypertension

Pulmonary Hypertension (PH) is a heterogeneous group of disorders that has been defined as a resting mean pulmonary artery pressure of ≥25 mmHg by right heart catheterization [56]. A strong female predominance of several types of PH have been well demonstrated over time yet the specific mechanism(s) that drive this predilection are currently unclear. This section will review the classification, diagnosis and treatment of PH with a focused emphasis on women.

The most recent clinical classification was created in 2008 and has divided PH into five main groups characterized by widely different pathologic features [56]. Group I PH, otherwise known as pulmonary artery hypertension (PAH) will be the major emphasis of this section. It is a rare condition, characterized by a prevalence of 15–50 patients per million [57]. PAH encompasses idiopathic PAH, HIV, connective tissue disease-related PH and PH mediated by various drugs and toxins. PAH is characterized by medial hypertrophy as well as intimal proliferative and fibrotic changes (concentric, eccentric). The pulmonary veins are classically unaffected and by definition the pulmonary capillary wedge pressure remains under 15 mmHg [56]. The prognostic outlook of this population is dismal with historical data suggesting a median survival of only 2.8 years in those with a diagnosis of idiopathic PAH [58].

The other major causes of PH (Groups II-V) include left heart disease (Group II), which involves advanced stages of heart failure and left-sided valve disease [56]. PH is commonly related to a passive backflow of pressure that is completely reversible upon relief of the left sided pathology [59]. However, in more advanced cases the degree of PH is out of proportion to the level of pressure generated by left heart pathology. This form of reactive PH may still be reversible after treatment with vasodilator therapy but can also lead to a fixed form of pulmonary artery hypertension, characterized by structural arterial remodeling [59]. Group III PH, is characterized by various lung disorders causing hypoxemia, such as chronic obstructive pulmonary disease (COPD), obstructive sleep apnea (OSA) or interstitial lung disease (ILD) [56]. Hypoxia induces medial hypertrophy and vasoconstriction of the pulmonary arterial vasculature, leading to increases in pulmonary arterial pressures. Group IV PH, identified as chronic thromboembolic disease is typically caused by single or recurrent pulmonary emboli. This leads to progressive vascular remodeling with symptoms of dyspnea, fatigue, hypoxemia and eventual right heart failure. Pulmonary thromboendarterectomy is recommended in select patients with PH that persists despite appropriate anticoagulation [60]. Group V PH corresponds to various clinical disorders like sarcoidosis, histiocytosis X and chronic anemias such as sickle cell. The underlying mechanisms are not clearly elucidated at the present time with treatment is typically directed towards the underlying disease process.

Cardiovascular findings on physical examination consistent with pulmonary hypertension and right ventricular pressure overload include: a large a wave in the jugular venous pulse, a second heart sound with a loud pulmonic component, and a fourth heart sound of right ventricular origin [61]. Late in the course, signs of right ventricular failure (e.g., hepatomegaly, peripheral edema, ascites) may be present. Patients with severe pulmonary hypertension may also have prominent v waves in the jugular venous pulse as a result of tricuspid regurgitation, a third heart sound of right ventricular origin and a high-pitched diastolic murmur of pulmonic regurgitation. Cyanosis is a late finding and unless the patient has associated lung disease, is usually attributable to a markedly reduced cardiac output, with systemic vasoconstriction and ventilation-perfusion mismatch in the lung [61].

There are several essential testing modalities that assist not only in the diagnosis of PH but also guide potential therapy. Doppler echocardiography has become the preferred screening test for PH. Doppler echo assessment of pulmonary artery pressure is feasible through its ability to estimate right ventricular systolic pressures obtained by measuring peak velocity of the tricuspid regurgitant jet and applying the Bernoulli formula [61]. Echo also provides the additional advantage of evaluating left-sided ventricular function and valves. However, right heart catheterization remains the gold standard and is required for the definitive diagnosis and characterizing the severity of PH [61]. A chest radiograph may show enlargement of the main pulmonary artery and its major branches. The right ventricle and atrium may also be enlarged. The electrocardiogram (ECG) in patients with PAH may exhibit right atrial enlargement and right ventricular hypertrophy. T wave inversions in the anterior precordial leads represent repolarization abnormalities associated with right ventricular hypertrophy. A perfusion lung scan is a highly sensitive test for the diagnosis of chronic pulmonary thromboembolism and is thus recommended for all patients who present with pulmonary hypertension [61]. Contrast enhanced chest computed tomography (CT) scans are also helpful in diagnosing chronic thromboembolic pulmonary disease. High-resolution CT may also assist in the diagnosis of interstitial lung disease as a cause for PH [61].

The discussion on therapeutic approaches to PH pertains to treatment specific to PAH (Group 1) patients. Of note, none of the large scale trials showed that one sex benefited more than the other from a particular therapy [3, 62]. Data on the use of these drugs in the other PH groups is scant and largely inconclusive. High dose calcium channel blockers appear to have a role in improving both morbidity and mortality in roughly 20 % of those with PAH who have a significant response to vasodilatory testing during right heart catheterization [64]. Prostacyclins (epoprostenol, iloprost, treprostinil) are a common therapy used in the treatment of PAH. Prostacyclin, produced by the vascular endothelium has potent vasodilatory and anti-proliferative effects. Positive benefits have been noted with prostacyclins in relation to exercise tolerance, hemodynamics and even survival [65]. Delivery is by intravenous, inhalation or subcutaneous routes. Serious complications typically relate to problems related to the drug delivery systems such as infection and pump malfunction. Sildenafil, a phosphodiesterase type 5 inhibitor, acts by promoting sustained levels of cyclic GMP which is a selective pulmonary vasodilator. Noted benefit in exercise capacity and hemodynamic profiles has been seen in those with PAH [66]. Endothelin-1 exerts mitogenic and vasoconstrictive effects on the pulmonary vasculature and is active in patients with PAH. Both selective (Ambrisentan) and non-selective (Bosentan) endothelin antagonists are approved for use in PAH and have been shown to improve exercise capacity and time to clinical worsening [63, 67]. Of note, these drugs are pregnancy category X (i.e. known teratogens).

Various forms of PAH including idiopathic and heritable forms as well as connective-tissue disease associated PAH have shown a clear female predominance [68, 69]. Registry data has shown a nearly 10:1 female-male ratio of scleroderma-associated PAH [70]. Several hypotheses exist to potentially explain the large discrepancy between females and males with PAH. Estrogen has been proposed as a detrimental compound to both the pulmonary vasculature and the right ventricle however animal study has refuted this by demonstrating the favorable effects of estrogen on the pulmonary vasculature [71]. Whether or not this discrepancy is related to differences in estrogen metabolism, other unidentified sex hormones or differences between animal and human models of disease is currently unknown. A second potential mechanism for the female predominance in PAH is lower testosterone levels in females. Testosterone may be beneficial for the pulmonary vasculature and right ventricle as there is ample laboratory testing that testosterone acts as a pulmonary vasodilator acutely [72]. A third proposed mechanism relates to the increased environmental exposure of females to various environmental agents, including anorexigens and estrogenic medications [73]. Unfortunately, current data on this topic is very limited and therefore does not allow any meaningful conclusions to be drawn on the role of these agents in the development of PAH.

Interestingly, despite the female predominance seen in PAH, the overall mortality rates are actually lower than in males [74, 75]. The gender discrepancy in observed mortality may be driven by differences in right ventricular function. Right ventricular function is closely linked with overall mortality in the PH population [76] and data has shown that male sex is associated with lower right ventricular ejection fraction compared to female counterparts [76].

Due to several obligatory hemodynamic changes that occur during gestation, including increased cardiac output [77], pregnancy represents a particularly dangerous state for pregnant women with PAH. High pulmonary vascular resistance typically seen in patients with PAH limits this blood supply to the feto-placental unit. As a result, maternal mortality though improved due to availability of current PAH therapy is still unacceptably high [78]. As a result of this risk, general recommendations typically include pregnancy avoidance altogether. This can be safely performed by means of sterilization.

Through research endeavors, great strides have been made in the field of PH, particularly in the identification of various mechanisms leading to the development of this disease state. This has lead to the development of several drug therapies, which have improved functional capacity and lowered mortality. Further research is clearly needed to better characterize the mechanism(s) behind the female predominance of PH.

Breast Cancer Therapy and Cardiomyopathy

It is estimated that 1 out of 8 women in the US will develop invasive breast cancer and most of these women will require chemotherapy [79]. Therefore, understanding chemotherapy associated cardiomyopathy from common chemotherapeutic agents used in the management of breast cancer is of great interest. Anthracyclines such as doxorubicin and daunorubicin are common chemotherapeutic agents that are likely to be toxic to myocytes and cause cardiomyopathy. Anthracyclines are used in the treatment of solid tumors, including breast cancers. Doxorubicin's toxic effects on cardiac function are typically dosage dependent with exposure >550 mg/m^2 having a 7.5 % risk of developing cardiomyopathy and >700 mg/m^2 having a 20 % risk. Because of these dose dependent effects, most oncologists now limit the maximum cumulative dose to <450 mg/m^2 for doxorubicin [80]. Patients who develop cardiomyopathy typically develop LV dysfunction and heart failure within the first year of completing therapy, however it can occur many years after the initial exposure [81]. Therefore, patients who will start treatment with an anthracycline should undergo a baseline echocardiogram to determine LV function prior to initial dose with follow up echocardiograms to assess for deterioration in LV function as the cumulative dosage approaches 450 mg/m^2.

Another common cardiotoxic chemotherapeutic agent used for the treatment of breast cancer is trastuzumab. An antibody directed against human epidermal growth factor receptor 2 (HER2) encoded by the proto-oncogene ERBB2, trastuzumab is used in the treatment of metastatic breast cancer. Trastuzumab has been studied and found to have an increased risk of up to 7 % of left ventricular dysfunction. This risk is increased to 27 % when used with anthracycline [82]. In contrast to anthracycline-induced cardiac toxicity, trastuzumab-induced cardiac injury is largely reversible after treatment discontinuation [83].

Chest-wall radiotherapy in patients with breast cancer can put women at increased risk of radiation-induced cardiotoxicity. At high-dose and volumes, radiation therapy decreases breast cancer deaths at the expense of increased cardiovascular mortality [84]. The pericardium is the most commonly affected cardiac structure as a result of radiotherapy. Patients may present with an underlying pericardial effusion either with or without accompanying symptoms [85]. More concerning are those presenting with significant signs and symptoms of severe heart failure related to constrictive pericarditis [85]. New technology, dosage adjustments, and strategies designed to avoid irradiation of the heart and great vessels are needed to continue improve overall survival in patients receiving radiation therapy.

Peripartum Cardiomyopathy

Peripartum Cardiomyopathy (PPCM) is a unique condition of unknown cause. It is reported in 1:300 to 1:4,000 live births [86] and is defined as LV dysfunction during the last trimester of pregnancy or the early puerperium. Risks for PPCM include advanced maternal age, multiparity, multifetal pregnancy, African American descent, preeclampsia, gestational hypertension and long term tocolysis [87]. Its etiology remains unknown but most theories involve hemodynamic and immunologic causes. This important cardiomyopathy, its treatment, prognosis and sequelae will be covered extensively in the pregnancy chapter.

Conclusion

The prevalence of Congestive Heart Failure (CHF) is rapidly expanding throughout the world and will continue to do so in the future as both the general population ages and the overall incidence of distinct risk factors for heart failure such as hypertension, obesity and diabetes continue to climb. Of importance, women make up nearly half of all new cases of CHF occurring annually. However, despite the large number of women suffering from CHF, particularly those with preserved ejection fraction, pulmonary hypertension and cardiomyopathies largely unique to the female gender such as breast cancer-related cardiomyopathy, peripartum cardiomyopathy and Takotsubo's cardiomyopathy (TCM), the mechanism(s) behind this female predominance are poorly characterized and clinical trials continue to lag behind. Thus, the focus of this chapter is to provide an overview of congestive heart failure, pulmonary hypertension and several cardiomyopathies unique to the female population and to highlight the overall impact that these disease processes have on female gender. Moving forward, we need to stress the importance of continued dedicated research in the field with a particular emphasis on the female population.

Acknowledgments
Alan Miller, MD
Professor of Medicine University of Florida College of Medicine – Jacksonville, Jacksonville, Florida, US

References

1. Lindenfeld J, Albert NM, Boehmer JP, et al. HFSA 2010 comprehensive heart failure practice guidelines. J Card Fail. 2010;16(6):1–194.
2. Lloyd-Jones DM. Cardiovascular risk prediction: basic concepts, current status, and future directions. Circulation. 2010;15:1768–77.
3. Lee WC, Chavez YE, Baker T, et al. Economic burden of heart failure: a summary of recent literature. Heart Lung. 2004;6:362–71.
4. Owan TE, Hodge DO, Herges RM, et al. Trends in prevalence and outcome of heart failure with preserved ejection fraction. N Engl J Med. 2006;3:251–9.
5. Bhatia RS, Tu JV, Lee DS, et al. Outcome of heart failure with preserved ejection fraction in a population-based study. N Engl J Med. 2006;3:260–9.
6. Lee DS, Gona P, Vasan RS, et al. Relation of disease pathogenesis and risk factors to heart failure with preserved or reduced ejection fraction: insights from the framingham heart study of the national heart, lung, and blood institute. Circulation. 2009;24:3070–7.
7. Piro M, Della Bona R, Abbate A, et al. Sex-related differences in remodeling. J Am Coll Cardiol. 2010;11:1057–65.
8. Borlaug BA, Lam CS, Roger VL, Rodeheffer RJ, Redfield MM. Contractility and ventricular systolic stiffening in hypertensive heart disease insights into the pathogenesis of heart failure with preserved ejection fraction. J Am Coll Cardiol. 2009;5:410–8.
9. Redfield MM, Jacobsen SJ, Borlaug BA, et al. Age and gender-related ventricular-vascular stiffening: a community-based study. Circulation. 2005;15:2254–62.
10. College of Cardiology Foundation/American Heart Association Task Force on Practice. 2013 ACCF/AHA Guideline for the Management of Heart Failure: a report of the American College of Cardiology Foundation/American Heart Association Task Force on practice guidelines. Circulation. 2013;128(16):240–327.
11. Ghali JK, Krause-Steinrauf HJ, Adams KF, et al. Gender differences in advanced heart failure: insights from the BEST study. J Am Coll Cardiol. 2003;12:2128–34.
12. Levy D, Larson MG, Vasan RS, et al. The progression from hypertension to congestive heart failure. JAMA. 1996;20:1557–62.
13. Peterson LR, Herrero P, Schechtman KB, et al. Effect of obesity and insulin resistance on myocardial substrate metabolism and efficiency in young women. Circulation. 2004; 18:2191–6.
14. Ho KK, Anderson KM, Kannel WB, et al. Survival after the onset of congestive heart failure in Framingham Heart Study subjects. Circulation. 1993;1:107–15.

15. Drazner MH, Rame JE, Stevenson LW, et al. Prognostic importance of elevated jugular venous pressure and a third heart sound in patients with heart failure. N Engl J Med. 2001;8: 574–81.
16. Smith GL, Lichtman JH, Bracken M, et al. Renal impairment and outcomes in heart failure: systematic review and meta-analysis. J Am Coll Cardiol. 2006;10:1987–96.
17. Lee WH, Packer M. Prognostic importance of serum sodium concentration and its modification by converting-enzyme inhibition in patients with severe chronic heart failure. Circulation. 1986;73:257–67.
18. Tang WH, Tong W, Jain A, et al. Evaluation and long-term prognosis of new-onset, transient, and persistent anemia in ambulatory patients with chronic heart failure. J Am Coll Cardiol. 2008;5:569–76.
19. McCullough PA, Nowak RM, McCord J, et al. B-type natriuretic peptide and clinical judgment in emergency diagnosis of heart failure: analysis from Breathing Not Properly (BNP) Multinational Study. Circulation. 2002;4:416–22.
20. Cauliez B, Berthe MC, Lavoinne A. Brain natriuretic peptide: physiological, biological and clinical aspects. Ann Biol Clin (Paris). 2005;1:15–25.
21. O'Donoghue M, Chen A, Baggish AL, et al. The effects of ejection fraction on N-terminal ProBNP and BNP levels in patients with acute CHF: analysis from the ProBNP Investigation of Dyspnea in the Emergency Department (PRIDE) study. J Card Fail. 2005;5:S9–14.
22. Koster NK, Reddy YM, Schima SM, et al. Gender-specific echocardiographic findings in nonagenarians with cardiovascular disease. Am J Cardiol. 2010;2:273–6.
23. Swedberg K, Kjekshus J. Effects of enalapril on mortality in severe congestive heart failure: results of the Cooperative North Scandinavian Enalapril Survival Study (CONSENSUS). Am J Cardiol. 1988;2:60A–6.
24. Effect of enalapril on survival in patients with reduced left ventricular ejection fractions and congestive heart failure. The SOLVD Investigators. N Engl J Med. 1991;5:293–302.
25. Pfeffer MA, Braunwald E, Moye LA, et al. Effect of captopril on mortality and morbidity in patients with left ventricular dysfunction after myocardial infarction. N Engl J Med. 1992;10:669–77.
26. Effect of enalapril on mortality and the development of heart failure in asymptomatic patients with reduced left ventricular ejection fractions. The SOLVD Investigators. N Engl J Med. 1992;327(10):685–91.
27. Granger CB, McMurray JJ, Yusuf S, CHARM Investigators and Committees, et al. Effects of candesartan in patients with chronic heart failure and reduced left-ventricular systolic function intolerant to angiotensin-converting-enzyme inhibitors: the CHARM-Alternative trial. Lancet. 2003;362:772–6.
28. Pfeffer MA, McMurray JJ, Velazquez EJ, Valsartan in Acute Myocardial Infarction Trial Investigators, et al. Valsartan, captopril, or both in myocardial infarction complicated by heart failure, left ventricular dysfunction, or both. N Engl J Med. 2003;49:1893–906.
29. Majahalme SK, Baruch L, Aknay N, et al. Comparison of treatment benefit and outcome in women versus men with chronic heart failure (from the Valsartan Heart Failure Trial). Am J Cardiol. 2005;95:529–32.
30. The Cardiac Insufficiency Bisoprolol Study II (CIBIS-II): a randomized trial. CIBIS II Investigators and Committees. Lancet. 1999;353:9–13.
31. Effect of metoprolol CR/XL in chronic heart failure: Metoprolol CR/XL Randomised Intervention Trial in Congestive Heart Failure (MERIT-HF). MERIT-HF Study Group. Lancet. 1999;353:2001–7.
32. Packer M, Coats AJ, Fowler MB, et al. Effect of carvedilol on survival in severe chronic heart failure. N Engl J Med. 2001;344:1651–8.
33. Ghali JK, Piña IL, Gottlieb SS, Deedwania PC, Wikstrand JC. MERIT-HF Study Group. Metoprolol CR/XL in female patients with heart failure: analysis of the experience in Metoprolol Extended-Release Randomized Intervention Trial in Heart Failure (MERIT-HF). Circulation. 2002;13:1585–91.

34. Taylor AL, Ziesche S, Yancy C, African-American Heart Failure Trial Investigators, et al. Combination of isosorbide dinitrate and hydralazine in blacks with heart failure. N Engl J Med. 2004;20:2049–57.
35. Taylor AL, Lindenfeld J, Ziesche S, A-HeFT Investigators, et al. Outcomes by gender in the African-American Heart Failure Trial. J Am Coll Cardiol. 2006;11:2263–7.
36. Young MJ, Funder JW. Mineralocorticoid receptors and pathophysiological roles for aldosterone in the cardiovascular system. J Hypertens. 2002;20:1465–8.
37. Pitt B, Zannad F, Remme WJ. The effect of spironolactone on morbidity and mortality in patients with severe heart failure. Randomized Aldactone Evaluation Study Investigators. N Engl J Med. 1999;341:709–17.
38. Pitt B, Remme W, Zannad F, et al. Eplerenone, a selective aldosterone blocker, in patients with left ventricular dysfunction after myocardial infarction. N Engl J Med. 2003;348:1309–21.
39. The Digitalis Investigation Group. The effect of digoxin on mortality and morbidity in patients with heart failure. N Engl J Med. 1997;336:525–33.
40. Rathore SS, Wang Y, Krumholz HM. Sex-based differences in the effect of digoxin for the treatment of heart failure. N Engl J Med. 2002;347:1403–11.
41. Adams KF, Patterson JH, Gattis WA, et al. Relationship of serum digoxin concentration to mortality and morbidity in women in the digitalis investigation group trial: a retrospective analysis. J Am Coll Cardiol. 2005;46:497–504.
42. Smith GL, Masoudi FA, Vaccarino V, et al. Outcomes in heart failure patients with preserved ejection fraction: mortality, readmission, and functional decline. J Am Coll Cardiol. 2003;41:1510–8.
43. Philbin EF, Rocco Jr TA, Lindenmuth NW, et al. Systolic versus diastolic heart failure in community practice: clinical features, outcomes, and the use of angiotensin-converting enzyme inhibitors. Am J Med. 2000;109:605–13.
44. ACC/AHA 2005 guideline update for the diagnosis and management of chronic heart failure in the adult. A report of the American College of Cardiology/American Heart Association Task Force on practice guidelines (Writing Committee to Update the 2001 Guidelines for the Evaluation and Management of Heart Failure). Circulation. 2005;112:e154–e235.
45. Epstein AE, DiMarco JP, Ellenbogen KA, et al. ACC/AHA/HRS 2008 guidelines for device-based therapy of cardiac rhythm abnormal- ities: a report of the American College of Cardiology/American Heart Association Task Force on Practice Guidelines (Writing Committee to Revise the ACC/AHA/NASPE 2002 Guideline Update for Implantation of Cardiac Pacemakers and Antiarrhythmia Devices). J Am Coll Cardiol. 2008;51:e1–62.
46. Bristow MR, Saxon LA, Boehmer J, et al. Cardiac-resynchronization therapy with or without an implantable defibrillator in advanced chronic heart failure. N Engl J Med. 2004;350:2140–50.
47. Arshad A, Moss AJ, Foster E, et al. Cardiac resynchronization therapy is More effective in women than in men. The MADIT-CRT (Multicenter Automatic Defibrillator Implantation Trial with Cardiac Resynchronization Therapy) trial. J Am Coll Cardiol. 2011;57:813–20.
48. Tsuchihashi K, Ueshima K, Uchida T, Angina Pectoris Myocardial Infarction Investigations Japan, et al. Transient left ventricular apical ballooning without coronary artery stenosis: a novel heart syndrome mimicking acute myocardial infarction. J Am Coll Cardiol. 2001;38:11–8.
49. Dote K, Sato H, Uchindo A, et al. Myocardial stunning due to multivessel spasms: a review of 5 cases. J Cardiol. 1991;21:203–14.
50. Wittstein IS, Thiemann DR, Lima JAC, et al. Neurohumoral features of myocardial stunning due to sudden emotional stress. N Engl J Med. 2005;352:539–48.
51. Ueyama T, Kasamatsu K, Hano T, et al. Emotional stress induces transient left ventricular hypocontraction in the rat via activation of cardiac adrenoceptors: a possible animal model of "tako-tsubo" cardiomyopathy. Circ J. 2002;7:712–3.
52. Kneale BJ, Chowienczyk PJ, Brett SE, Coltart DJ, Ritter JM. Gender differences in sensitivity to adrenergic agonists of forearm resistance vasculature. J Am Coll Cardiol. 2000;36:1233–8.

53. Movahed MR, Donohue D. Review: transient left ventricular apical ballooning, broken heart syndrome, ampulla cardiomyopathy, atypical apical ballooning, or Tako-Tsubo cardiomyopathy. Cardiovasc Revasc Med. 2007;4:289–92.
54. Bybee KA, Kara T, Prasad A, et al. Transient left ventricular apical ballooning: a syndrome that mimics ST-segment elevation myocardial infarction. Ann Intern Med. 2004;141:858–65.
55. Shimizu M, Kato Y, Masai H, et al. Recurrent episodes of Takotsubo-like transient apical ballooning occurring in different regions: a case report. J Cardiol. 2006;48:101–7.
56. Simonneau G, Robbins IM, Beghetti M. Updated clinical classification of pulmonary hypertension. J Am Coll Cardiol. 2009;54:S43–54.
57. Humbert M, Sitbon O, Chaouat A, et al. Pulmonary arterial hypertension in France: results from a national registry. Am J Respir Crit Care Med. 2006;173:1023–30.
58. D'Alonzo GE, Borst RJ, Bergofsky EH, et al. Survival in patients with primary pulmonary hypertension. Results from a national prospective registry. Ann Intern Med. 1991;115:343–9.
59. Guazzi M, Borlaug BA. Pulmonary hypertension due to left heart disease. Circulation. 2012;126:975–90.
60. Piazza G, Goldhaber SZ. Chronic thromboembolic pulmonary hypertension. N Engl J Med. 2011;364:351–60.
61. Galie N, Hoeper MM, Humbert M, et al. Guidelines for the diagnosis and treatment of pulmonary hypertension. The Task Force for the Diagnosis and Treatment of Pulmonary Hypertension of the European Society of Cardiology (ESC) and the European Respiratory Society (ERS), endorsed by the International Society of Heart and Lung Transplantation (ISHLT). Eur Heart J. 2009;30:2493–537.
62. Galie N, Ghofrani HA, Torbicki A, et al. Sildenafil citrate therapy for pulmonary arterial hypertension. N Engl J Med. 2005;353(20):2148–57.
63. Rubin LJ, Badesch DB, Barst RJ, et al. Bosentan therapy for pulmonary arterial hypertension. N Engl J Med. 2002;12:896–903.
64. Sitbon O, Humbert M, Jaïs X, et al. Long term response to calcium channel blockers in idiopathic pulmonary arterial hypertension. Circulation. 2005;23:3105–11.
65. Gomberg-Maitland M, Olschewski H. Prostacyclin therapies for the treatment of pulmonary arterial hypertension. Eur Respir J. 2008;4:891–901.
66. Nagendran J, Archer SL, Soliman D, et al. Phosphodiesterase type 5 is highly expressed in the hypertrophied human right ventricle and acute inhibition of phosphodiesterase type 5 improves contractility. Circulation. 2007;3:238–48.
67. Galie N, Badesch D, Oudiz R, et al. Ambrisentan therapy for pulmonary arterial hypertension. J Am Coll Cardiol. 2005;3:529–35.
68. Loyd JE, Butler MG, Foroud TM, et al. Genetic anticipation and abnormal gender ratio at birth in familial primary pulmonary hypertension. Am J Respir Crit Care Med. 1995;1:93–7.
69. Austin ED, Cogan JD, West JD, et al. Alterations in estrogen metabolism: implications for higher penetrance of FPAH in females. Eur Respir J. 2009;5:1093–9.
70. Chung L, Liu J, Parsons L, et al. Characterization of connective tissue disease associated pulmonary arterial hypertension from the REVEAL registry: identifying systemic sclerosis as a unique phenotype. Chest. 2010;6:1383–94.
71. Moore LG, McMurtry IF, Reeves JT, et al. Effects of sex hormones on cardiovascular and hematologic responses to chronic hypoxia in rats. Proc Soc Exp Biol Med. 1978;4:658–62.
72. Jones RD, English KM, Pugh PJ, et al. Pulmonary vasodilatory action of testosterone: evidence of a calcium antagonistic action. J Cardiovasc Pharmacol. 2002;6:814–23.
73. Wagner JD, Kaplan JR, Burkman RT, et al. Reproductive hormones and cardiovascular disease: mechanism of action and clinical implications. Obstet Gynecol Clin North Am. 2002;3:475–93.
74. Humbert M, Sitbon O, Yaici A, et al. Survival in incident and prevalent cohorts of patients with pulmonary arterial hypertension. Eur Respir J. 2010;3:549–55.
75. Benza RL, Miller DP, Gomberg-Maitland M, et al. Predicting survival in pulmonary arterial hypertension. Insights from the Registry to Evaluate Early and Long-Term Pulmonary Arterial Hypertension Disease Management (REVEAL). Circulation. 2010;2:164–72.

76. Kawut SM, Al-Naamani N, Agerstrand C, et al. Determinants of right ventricular ejection fraction in pulmonary arterial hypertension. Chest. 2009;3:752–9.
77. Carbillon L, Uzan M, Uzan S. Pregnancy, vascular tone, and maternal hemodynamics: a crucial adaptation. Obstet Gynecol Surv. 2000;55:574–81.
78. Bedard E, Dimopoulos K, Gatzoulis MA, et al. Has there been any progress made on pregnancy outcomes among women with pulmonary arterial hypertension? Eur Heart J. 2009;3:256–65.
79. Howlader N, Noone AM, Krapcho M, et. al.,editors. SEER cancer statistics review, 1975–2009 (Vintage 2009 populations), National Cancer Institute. Bethesda. 2012. Retrieved Sept 7 2012.
80. Swain SM, Whaley FS, Ewer MS. Congestive heart failure in patients treated with doxorubicin: a retrospective analysis of three trials. Cancer. 2003;97:2869–79.
81. Jensen BV, Skovsgaard T, Nielsen SL. Functional monitoring of anthracycline cardiotoxicity: a prospective, blinded, long-term observational study of outcome in 120 patients. Ann Oncol. 2002;5:699–709.
82. Tan-Chiu E, Yothers G, Romond E, et al. Assessment of cardiac dysfunction in a randomized trial comparing doxorubicin and cyclophosphamide followed by paclitaxel, with or without trastuzumab as adjuvant therapy in node-positive, human epidermal growth factor receptor 2-overexpressing breast cancer: NSABP B-31. J Clin Oncol. 2005;23:7811–9.
83. Seidman A, Hudis C, Pierri MK, et al. Cardiac dysfunction in the traztuzumab clinical trials experience. J Clin Oncol. 2002;5:1215–21.
84. Rutqvist LE, Rose C, Cavallin-Stahl E. A systematic overview of radiation therapy effects in breast cancer. Acta Oncol. 2003;42:532–45.
85. Stewart JR, Fajardo LF, Gillette SM, et al. Radiation injury to the heart. Int J Radiat Oncol Biol Phys. 1995;31:1205–11.
86. Elkayam U, Tummala PP, Rao K, et al. Maternal and fetal outcomes of subsequent pregnancies in women with peripartum cardiomyopathy. N Engl J Med. 2001;344:1567–71.
87. Demakis JG, Rahimtoola SH, et al. Natural course of peripartum cardiomyopathy. Circulation. 1971;44:1053–61.
88. Lund A, Mancini D. Heart failure in women. Med Clin N Am. 2004;88:1321–45.
89. Sharkey SW. Takotsubo cardiomyopathy: natural history. Heart Fail Clin. 2013;9:123–36.
90. The Criteria Committee of the New York Heart Association. Diseases of the heart and blood vessels: nomenclature and criteria for diagnosis. 6th ed. Boston: Little Brown; 1964.

Chapter 9
Valvular Heart Disease in Women

Alian Aguila, Wassim Jawad, Khyati Baxi, and Joel A. Strom

Objectives

1. Define the prevalence and age-dependence of valvular heart disease in women.
2. Gender-specific history and physical manifestations of valvular disease.
3. Diagnostic evaluation.
4. Treatment including medical and surgical treatment.
5. Special problems: Pregnancy.

Introduction

Valvular heart disease is an important clinical problem in women as a number of congenital and acquired diseases affecting the cardiac valves occur with greater frequency in women. Women also have differences in physiognomy and physiology that influence the clinical presentation, diagnostic approach, therapeutic options, and results of therapy. Women, on average, tend to be smaller than men. This not only applies to their external dimensions, but also to the dimensions of the cardiovascular system. For example, the heart of a normal woman weighs on average approximately 100 g less than men [1]. They experience differences in cardiovascular remodeling in response to the hemodynamic alterations that result from valvular dysfunction, physiologic changes that accompany a normal pregnancy and the pathologic effects of pregnancy-related complications can deleteriously accelerate valve-related hemodynamic alterations and symptoms of valve dysfunction.

A. Aguila, MD • W. Jawad, MD • K. Baxi, MD • J.A. Strom, MD, MEng (✉)
Division of Cardiology, University of Florida College of Medicine-Jacksonville,
655 West 8th Street, Jacksonville, FL 32209, USA
e-mail: joel.strom@jax.ufl.edu

H.Z. Mieszczanska, G.P. Velarde (eds.),   175
Management of Cardiovascular Disease in Women,
DOI 10.1007/978-1-4471-5517-1_9, © Springer-Verlag London 2014

In this chapter, we will define those areas of valvular heart disease than directly applies to women, and identify those gender-related issues in the diagnosis, evaluation, and treatment of valve disease.

Epidemiology

Certain valvular abnormalities occur with greater frequency in women. For example, rheumatic heart disease manifests as mitral stenosis more often in women than men. Female predominance is also noted in mitral valve prolapse and primary pulmonary hypertension. Congenital valvular abnormalities affect younger women, while acquired disease becomes more prevalent with age. Coronary artery disease-induced mitral regurgitation, calcification of the cardiac skeleton that results in mitral annulus, papillary muscle, aortic valve and aortic calcification, and myxomatous degeneration of the mitral valve and chordae tendineae all increase in frequency with advancing age.

Mitral Valve Disease

The mitral apparatus consists of the mitral valve leaflets, the mitral annulus, the chordae tendineae, the papillary muscles, the left atrium and ventricle. Normal orientation and coordinated performance of all of these structures is required for physiologic valve performance. The normal mitral valve consists of anterior and posterior leaflets attached to the mitral annulus composed of fibromuscular tissue [2]. The anterior mitral leaflet is generally larger than the posterior leaflet, has a triangular shape, and has three segments. It subtends approximately two-thirds of the mitral orifice while attached to 1/3 of the annulus [2]. The posterior leaflet is smaller and has three distinguishable segments or scallops [2]. It is attached to approximately two-thirds of the annulus but occludes only 1/3 of the orifice area. The leaflets are attached to two papillary muscles by chordae tendineae that branch and insert into the free edge and body of the leaflets in order to prevent prolapse during cardiac systole and facilitate diastolic opening [2].

The leaflets themselves are lined with endothelial cells and are composed of three layers: the atrialis located on the atrial side and composed of collagen and elastic fibers, the spongiosa located in the middle of the leaflet and composed of proteoglycans and glycosaminoglycans (GAGs) in which are embedded myofibroblasts, and the ventricularis which lines the ventricular side of the valve and is composed mainly of collagen. In addition, the mitral valve contains cardiac myocytes and stem cells. The fibromuscular annulus is saddle-shaped and undergoes dynamic changes in area during the cardiac cycles to reduce resistance to left ventricular diastolic filling while augmenting systolic leaflet coaptation and thus valve competence. Systolic competence also requires normal chordal geometry, and papillary muscle and adjacent left atrial and ventricular myocardial geometry and performance.

Mitral Regurgitation

Mitral regurgitation (MR), the second most common indication for valve surgery in the United States, may be secondary to structural or functional dysfunction of any or more of the components of the mitral valve apparatus. In women, as in the general population, common causes of (MR) include congenital and acquired mitral apparatus degeneration and remodeling, rheumatic heart disease, endocarditis.

Ischemic Mitral Regurgitation

Coronary artery disease is the most common cause of death and disability in women. Atherosclerosis-induced ischemia can cause MR by a number of mechanisms. Focal left ventricular remodeling typically resulting from a basal inferior-posterior wall infarct involving the region of the posterior medial papillary can cause mitral regurgitation (MR) due to loss of chordal alignment from papillary muscle tethering. The leaflets, particularly the medial side, are apically displaced into the LV preventing normal coaptation. Partial papillary muscle ischemia or infarction can result in incomplete to complete rupture that can result in MR even if LV remodeling does not occur. Complete rupture results in severe acute regurgitation often presenting as acute pulmonary edema and cardiogenic shock often without a typical MR murmur. The ischemic etiology of papillary muscle rupture can be unrecognized in women due to absence of typical symptoms and the fact that it can occur in the setting of a very small infarct.

Both ischemic and non-ischemic cardiomyopathies can induce mitral regurgitation due to loss of normal chordal geometry caused by the spherical LV dilatation and annular enlargement, the latter associated with reduced systolic contraction, all of which decrease the area of leaflet coaptation. The severity of regurgitation is related to levels of pre- and after-load and can be altered by changes in loading conditions [3]. Mitral annular calcification leading to abnormal closure of the mitral leaflets due to restricted mobility is an important cause of mitral regurgitation which is observed with increased frequency in female as compared to males. Annular calcium can also cause chordal abrasion leading to rupture. Finally, a calcified annulus, by in itself can result in effective mitral stenosis due to loss of its ability to dilated in diastole and reduction of the orifice area by exuberant calcification.

Patients with chronic mitral regurgitation experience increased LV wall stress that induces cardiomyocyte apoptosis and hypertrophy and extracellular matrix remodeling, the latter results in increased fibrosis, often perivascular in location. The net result is a spherical LV accompanied by declines in stroke volume, cardiac output and left ventricular ejection fraction [4].

Mitral Valve Prolapse

Mitral valve prolapse (MVP) is twice as prevalent in women as compared to men. In the United States alone, MVP accounts for the majority of cases of severe mitral regurgitation needing surgical mitral valve replacement and also accounts for the most common valvular condition predisposing patients to chordal rupture and infective endocarditis [4]. Myxomatous disease of the mitral valve may affect one or both leaflets and chordae tendinaea. Mitral valve prolapse was first described by Barlow and colleagues and is considered a congenital deficiency of the mitral tissue [2, 5]. Patients with mitral valve prolapse demonstrate focal thickening and lengthening of both the anterior and posterior mitral leaflets from their site of attachment [2]. In addition, there is elongation and thinning of the chordae tendineae predisposing them to rupture in a subset of patients. Dilation of the mitral annulus is the most common cause of associated mitral valve regurgitation in patients with MVP. Myxomatous degeneration, the hallmark of this syndrome, can solely involve the mitral apparatus, but it can involve the tricuspid and aortic valves, especially when associated with identifiable connective tissue disorders. MVP is found in approximately 90 % of patients with Marfan syndrome and 6 % of patients with Ehlers-Danlos syndrome [4]. In those cases, there is involvement of the aorta that can increase the risk for aortic dilatation and dissection.

Histologically, the leaflets show increased deposition of elastic tissue with superimposed fibrous tissue on both the atrial and ventricular aspects of the leaflets and increased production of mucopolyaccharides and GAGs in the spongiosa, produced by transformed myofibroblasts resulting in leaflet thickening [2]. Leaflet remodeling results in an increase in the size of the mitral leaflets and the mitral apparatus. The mitral annulus loses its normal saddle-shape in patients with severe mitral regurgitation. Its area is increased with a decreased ratio of annular height to commissural width, and cyclical changes in the orifice are reduced. Annular flattening leads to increase tension on the annulus itself, leaflets and chords which results in weakening and elongation of the leaflets, prolapse and increased tendency to chordal rupture, all contributing to increased severity of associated mitral regurgitation [6]. The severity of mitral regurgitation depends on the extent and severity of these anatomic and functional derangements and loading conditions and has potential implications at the time of mitral valve repair [6].

Physical Examination

MVP is suggested by the presence of a MR murmur in an otherwise asymptomatic person. The murmur is often mid-late systolic and is frequently proceeded by a click, which occurs coincidental with the maximum systolic excursion of the prolapsing leaflet. The duration and intensity of the murmur is dynamic, varying with position and activity, reflecting a complex interaction of the extent of derangement of the mitral apparatus with changes in LV dimensions and loading conditions. It can become softer and earlier with the straining phase of the Valsalva maneuver, while positional changes, e.g. standing, causes the murmur of MVP to lengthen and to become more intense. Post-ventricular premature contractions and atrial fibrillation cause shortening of the murmur of MVP [7]. The extent of radiation of the murmur depends on the direction of the jet. In particular, posterior leaflet prolapse can result in an anteriorly directed jet that can mimic the murmur of LVOT or semilunar valve stenosis. Posterior directed regurgitation can radiate to the axilla and back. Very early prolapse can result in a holosystolic murmur. The click will merge with the first heart sound. Other findings on cardiac examination include a LV heave and S3 gallop in patients with LV enlargement and/or severe regurgitation. Other physical findings include brisk carotid upstrokes, diminished intensity of the first heart sound (S1) and wide splitting of the second heart sound (S2). Associated pulmonary hypertension is suggested by the presence of a right ventricular heave and increased intensity of the pulmonary component of S2.

Diagnostic Evaluation

Doppler Echocardiography

Transthoracic Doppler-echocardiography (TTE) is the primary test for diagnosis and quantification of mitral valve regurgitation and to determine its effects on left ventricular and atrial size and performance, pulmonary artery pressures, and to diagnose concomitant cardiovascular abnormalities. The complete mitral apparatus should be imaged in multiple planes to define the mechanisms for regurgitation, e.g. prolapse of the mitral valve leaflets, torn chordae chordae tendineae leading to flail leaflets, vegetations, the presence of left ventricular remodeling due to ischemia or cardiomyopathy, etc. MVP is diagnosed by demonstrating ≥2 mm of systolic excursion of one or more mitral into the left atrium in either the parasternal or apical long axis views (Fig. 9.1). Thickening of the involved leaflets greater than 5 mm as well as increased mitral annular diameter supports the diagnosis [8]. Quantification of left ventricular dimensions, wall thicknesses and ejection fraction (LVEF) combined with quantification of left atrial size is important as LV and LA enlargement and decease in LVEF all have prognostic significance and impact the timing of operative repair. Doppler echocardiography is highly sensitive and specific to identify MR and is essential to quantify the severity of MR as well as diagnosing and quantifying the presence and severity of pulmonary arterial hypertension [2]. The severity of MR can be estimated by a number of measurements, e.g. the regurgitant jet area, the diameter of the vena contracta, etc. It can also be quantified in suitable cases by measuring the regurgitant orifice area and volume by proximal isovelocity surface area (PISA) method [9, 10], (Table 9.1). While less accurate than other

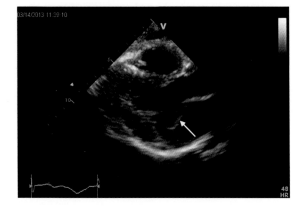

Fig. 9.1 2-D Echocardiogram parasternal long axis view of the left ventricle revealing prolapse of both the anterior and posterior mitral leaflets (*white arrow*)

Table 9.1 Classification of the severity of valve disease in adults

A. Left-sided valve disease

Indicator	Mild	Moderate	Severe
Aortic stenosis			
Jet velocity (m/s)	Less than 3.0	3.0–4.0	Greater than 4.0
Mean gradient (mmHg)[a]	Less than 25	25–40	Greater than 40
Valve area (cm²)	Greater than 1.5	1.0–1.5	Less than 1.0
Valve area index (cm²/m²)			Less than 0.6
Mitral stenosis			
Mean gradient (mmHg)[a]	Less than 5	5–10	Greater than 10
Pulmonary artery systolic pressure (mmHg)	Less than 30	30–50	Greater than 50
Valve area (cm²)	Greater than 1.5	1.0–1.5	Less than 1.0
Aortic regurgitation			
Qualitative			
Angiographic grade	1+	2+	3–4+
Color Doppler jet width	Central jet, width less than 25 % of LVOT	Greater than mild but no signs of severe AR	Central jet. width greater than 65 % LVOT
Doppler vena contracts width (cm)	Less than 0.3	0.3–0.6	Greater than 0.6
Quantitative (cath or echo)			
Regurgitated volume (ml per beat)	Less than 30	30–59	Greater than or equal to 60
Regurgitated fraction (%)	Less than 30	30–49	Greater than or equal to 50
Regurgitated orifice area (cm²)	Less than 0.10	0.10–0.29	Greater than or equal to 0.30

Additional essential criteria

Characteristic	Mitral regulation		
	Mild	Moderate	Severe
Left ventricular size			Increased
Qualitative			
Angiographic grade	1+	2+	3–4+
Color Doppler jet area	Small, central jet (less than 4 cm² or less than 20 % LA area)	Signs of MR greater than mild present but no criteria for severe MR	Vena contracts width greater than 0.7 cm with large central MR jet (area greater than 40 % of LA area) or with a wall-impinging jet of any size, swirling in LA
Doppler vena contracts width (cm)	Less than 0.3	0.3–0.69	Greater than or equal to 0.70
Quantitative (cath or echo)			
Regurgitant volume (ml/beat)	Less than 30	30–59	Greater than or equal to 60
Regurgitant fraction (%)	Less than 30	30–49	Greater than or equal to 50
Regurgitant orifice area (cm²)	Less than 0.20	0.20–0.39	Greater than or equal to 0.40
Additional essential criteria			
Left atrial size			Enlarged
Left ventricular size			Enlarged

B. Right-sided valve disease

Characteristic
Severe tricuspid stenosis: Valve area less than 1.0 cm²
Severe tricuspid regurgitation: Vena contracts width greater than 0.7 cm and systolic flow reversal in hepatic veins
Severe pulmonic stenosis: Jet velocity greater than 4 m/s or maximum gradient greater than 60 mmHg
severe pulmonic regurgitation: Color jet fills outflow tract; dense continuous wave Doppler signal with a steep deceleration slope

Reprinted with permission from Bonow et al. [8] and original modified source Zoghbi et al. [11]

Modified from Zoghbi et al. [11], Copyright 2003, with permission from American Society of echocardiography [12]

AR indicates aortic regurgitation, *cath* catheterization, *echo* echocardiography, *LA* left atrial/atrium, *LVOT* left ventricular outflow tract, and *MR* mitral regurgitation

[a]Valve gradients are flow dependent and when used as estimates or severity or valve stenosis should be assessed with knowledge of cardiac output or forward flow across the valve

methods, a jet/LA area ratio of ≥40 % suggests severe MR. Severe MR is also suggested by a vena contracta diameter of >7 mm, an effective regurgitant orifice area of ≥40 mm^2 area, and/or a regurgitant volume of ≥60 ml. Conversely, mild MR is suggested by values of <3 mm, <20 mm^2, and <30 ml, respectively. Intermediate values suggest moderate MR. MR volume can also be calculated as the difference between the total LV stroke volume and the forward aortic stroke volume by two-D echocardiography and also by magnetic resonance imaging (MRI) [2, 13]. Exercise echocardiography may be helpful to define the response of the mitral apparatus, severity of MR, and LV systolic performance to stress. An exercise induced decrease in LVEF is an indication of early LV dysfunction.

Trans-esophageal Doppler echocardiography (TEE) is helpful in patients with poor imaging windows. In addition to better delineation of the anatomy of the mitral apparatus, left atrial appendage size and function and pulmonary vein flow can be measured. Flow-reversal in the pulmonary veins suggests severe MR. Exclusion of a left atrial thrombus is important for those with embolic symptoms or who are to undergo cardioversion for an atrial tachyarrhythmia. TEE is essential for the preoperative assessment of patients being considered for mitral valve repair. A complete assessment of the three segments of both leaflets is required. Also the chordae tendineae must be imaged and the dimensions the annulus quantified. While most laboratories still employ two dimensional imaging, the use of three dimensional imaging provides superior spatial assessment and can be very useful to define the optimum surgical approach. Other imaging modalities, i.e. CT scanning and MRI may be useful in particular circumstances [14].

Electrocardiography

The electrocardiogram (ECG) is usually normal in the majority of patients, but a small minority of patients demonstrates nonspecific ST-T wave abnormalities. More severe MR is suggested by the presence of electrocardiographic criteria for both left atrial and ventricular enlargement. Paroxysmal supraventricular tachycardia is the most common tachyarrhythmia encountered in patients with MVP syndrome. However, some patients develop ventricular premature contractions and ventricular tachyarrhythmias due to stretch-induced depolarizations of resident cardiomyocytes and QT-segment prolongation. Finally, left atrio-ventricular bypass tracts, including the Wolf-Parkinson-White syndrome, are associated with MVP [4].

Chest Radiography

Chest radiography is often normal in mild MR, but can demonstrate a constellation of findings as the heart responds to worsening disease. Left ventricular and atrial enlargement can occur, the latter manifest by straightening of the left heart border and splaying and posterior deviation of the left main bronchus. With hemodynamic decompensation, pulmonary venous congestion progressing to pulmonary edema, pulmonary artery enlargement, and right atrial and ventricular enlargement may be seen.

Cardiac Catheterization

Invasive hemodynamic assessment of mitral regurgitation can be further evaluated by a left and right heart cardiac catheterization, especially if the non-invasive assessment is ambiguous or for pre-operative evaluation. Measurement of intracardiac pressures and evaluation of pressure waveforms is essential [2]. Increasing MR severity may be manifest by an increase in average left atrial/pulmonary capillary wedge (PCW) pressures accompanied by a late systolic peak ("v" wave) whose height correlates with MR severity [2]. In addition, a right heart catheterization to exclude pulmonary hypertension and tricuspid valve disease, cardiac output measurements, and calculation of pulmonary total and vascular and systemic vascular resistances. A difference between the PCW and LV diastolic pressures should excluded by simultaneous recording of the pressure waveforms. Left ventriculography is used to quantify the degree of mitral regurgitation. Finally, coronary angiography is required in those with suspected or known coronary artery disease, especially if an ischemic etiology to their MR is suspected, those with multiple CAD risk factors, an underlying cardiomyopathy, and those over 40 years of age.

Clinical Course

The majority of patients with mild MR of any etiology remain asymptomatic. However, MVP patients may report atypical chest pain, syncope, presyncope, and palpitations. Worsening MR is characterized by a relatively long asymptomatic period. During this time mitral apparatus, LV and LA remodeling may occur. LV dilatation and remodeling accompanies worsening MR and can in itself increase the degree of valve dysfunction. The increased wall stress can induce apoptosis and fibrosis leading to a decline in systolic performance associated with pulmonary congestion, dyspnea and other manifestations of CHF. Left atrial enlargement also occurs during this asymptomatic period. The first clinical manifestation may be atrial fibrillation or a systemic embolus. Disease progression can result in the development of pulmonary hypertension due to pulmonary venous hypertension or an elevated pulmonary vascular resistance. Development of systemic congestion due to right sided heart failure and tricuspid regurgitation can manifest as, congestive hepatomegaly, edema and ascites.

Progressive mitral regurgitation results in the development of CHF occur in about 15 % of patients with MVP over a course of 10–15 years [10, 14]. Patients are also at increased risk of developing mitral valve infective endocarditis which can accelerate the progression MR, LA and LV remodeling, decline in LVEF. Those factors but especially a decrease in LVEF to below 60% are associated with reduced symptom free survival [2].

Mitral Stenosis

Rheumatic heart disease has a low prevalence in the United States, primarily due to effective prophylaxis against rheumatic fever. However, it remains an important cause of valve disease in developing countries, and because of this reservoir, rheumatic valve disease is often found in immigrant communities in the United States. Acute rheumatic fever results from an autoimmune-mediated inflammatory response to an inadequately treated infection with a Group A β-hemolytic *Streptococcus*. A pancarditis results, involving the mural endocardium, myocardium and epicardium, whose major sequellae involves an inflammatory valvulitis and endocarditis involving the mitral, aortic, and tricuspid valves in decreasing relative frequency [2]. Rheumatic heart disease may be viewed as a disease of the mitral valve as there is always involvement of the mitral valve apparatus. In addition, rheumatic mitral disease is two times more common in women than men [2, 5]. Aschoff bodies, pathognomonic for rheumatic disease, are always found when there is involvement of the mitral valve [2]. Acute rheumatic valve disease is characterized by small vegetations and acute valvulitis and is characterized by mitral regurgitation. Mitral stenosis, with or without mitral regurgitation, is a late finding and is characterized by commissural fusion associated with varying degrees of leaflet thickening due to deposition of fibrous tissue and calcium. Calcium deposition in the mitral leaflets and involvement of the aortic valve are more pronounced in men than women, older patients and those with higher arterial blood pressure.

Other causes of mitral stenosis include congenital leaflet and apparatus deformities, e.g. parachute mitral valve, narrowing of the mitral orifice due to exuberant calcification of the mitral annulus, obstruction due to large vegetations or a left atrial myxoma or rarely a cor triatriatum.

Physical Examination

Patients with mitral stenosis may have a characteristic reddening of the cheeks (malar flush). The cardiovascular finding depend on the severity of the stenosis and whether CHF, pulmonary hypertension and/or primary or secondary tricuspid valve disease is present. The left ventricular apical impulse is usually normal to reduced and may be displaced laterally if RV enlargement is present. The first heart sound is often increased in intensity. An increased pulmonic component of S2 can indicate pulmonary hypertension, as can a RV heave or pulmonary diastolic murmur.

An apical holosystolic mumur suggests the presence of MR. In patients with a pliable valve, an opening snap (OS) can be heard 60–120 ms after S2. The shorter the S2-OS interval is, the higher the left atrial pressure. An apical diastolic rumble following OS and with pre-systolic accentuation is characteristic of MS. It is best heard with the patient in the left lateral decubitus position. The presence of a left or right parasternal systolic or diastolic murmur that increases with inspiration suggests tricuspid regurgitation or stenosis, respective. CHF is manifested by jugular venous distention. An absent "a" wave suggests atrial fibrillation while a "c-v" wave is consistent with tricuspid regurgitation. Systemic venous hypertension is often manifest by hepatomegaly, ascites, and edema. Wheezing may be an early finding of pulmonary venous hypertension, while rales are often present in pulmonary edema.

Diagnostic Evaluation

Doppler-Echocardiography

Transthoracic Doppler-echocardiography (TTE) is the primary imaging modality to diagnose MS, quantify its severity and assess the mitral valve and apparatus morphology, determine its effect on the other cardiac valves, the morphology and performance of the cardiac chambers, determine prognosis, and plan for surgical or catheter-based intervention. Commissural fusion is characteristic of rheumatic mitral valve disease. The leaflets, especially the anterior one may remain pliable resulting in the characteristic diastolic hockey stick appearance in the 2-D parasternal long axis view. As the disease progresses fibrosis and calcification results in decreased mobility Thickening and calcification extends proximally, in contrast to degenerative disease where the process extend from the annulus to the tips. The orifice is reduced and has a characteristic fish mouth appearance in the parasternal short axis view [2]. Thickening and retraction of the chordae tendineae also affect the mobility and the overall degree of stenosis.

Stenosis severity is quantified by determination of the mean gradient (ΔP) across the valve and apparatus calculated by the modified Bernoulli equation ($\Delta P = 4v^2$) and the orifice area (Table 9.1) [15]. The latter can be determined by planimetry performed at the tips of the leaflets in the parasternal short axis view imaged by both 2-D and 3-D echocardiography [2]. Other techniques for quantification of the effective orifice area include the pressure half time PHT (MVA = 220/PHT) and the continuity equation. It is important to recognize that in patients with aortic regurgitation, atrial fibrillation, abnormal left atrial compliance due to left atrial dilatation, abnormal left ventricular compliance, and immediately after balloon valvuloplasty, mitral valve area assessment by PHT has inherent limitations [2]. As mitral regurgitation frequently accompanies stenosis, determination of its severity is an essential part of the Doppler-echocardiographic examination. In addition to assessment of the valve itself, the rest of the mitral apparatus, the atria and ventricles, the other valves, especially the aortic and tricuspid valves, need evaluation.

Table 9.2 Determinants of the echocardiographic mitral valve score

Grade	Mobility	Subvalvular thickening	Thickening	Calcification
1	Highly mobile valve with only leaflet tips restricted	Minimal thickening just below the mitral leaflets	Leaflets near normal in thickness (4–5 mm)	A single area of increased echo brightness
2	Leaflet mid and base portions have normal mobility	Thickening of chordal structures extending up to one third of the chordal length	Midleaflets normal, considerable thickening of margins (5–8 mm)	Scattered areas of brightness confined to leaflet margins
3	Valve continues to move forward in diastole, mainly from the base	Thickening extending to the distal third of the chords	Thickening extending through the entire leaflet (5–8 mm)	Brightness extending into the midportion of the leaflets
4	No or minimal forward movement of the leaflets in diastole	Extensive thickening and shortening of all chorda structures extending down to the papillary muscles	Considerable thickening of all leaflet tissue (greater than 8–10 mm)	Extensive brightness throughout much of the leaflet tissue

Reprinted with permission from Bonow et al. [8]

Trans-esophageal echocardiography (TEE) is employed when TTE imaging is inadequate for diagnosis, to better visualize the mitral apparatus, to diagnose infectious complications, determine the if an intracardiac source of systemic embolus is present e.g. a left atrium or left atrial appendage thrombus. It is also used prior to cardioversion for atrial arrhythmias and as part of the pre-operative and intra-operative assessment of mitral repair surgery or catheter-based intervention. In particular, the Wilkins score derived from a TEE examination of the mitral valve apparatus can be used to predict suitability for mitral balloon valvuloplasty (Table 9.2) [8, 16].

Cardiac magnetic resonance imaging (MRI) is an additional imaging modality which demonstrates thickening of the leaflets and reduced opening of the mitral valve in diastole in patients with mitral stenosis; and the maximal extent of leaflet opening correlates well with the severity of stenosis [2].

Electrocardiography

The electrocardiogram in patients with MS, although often nonspecific in patients with mild disease, shows characteristic changes in patients with moderate to severe stenosis. The most common findings include left atrial enlargement, atrial fibrillation often with coarse fibrillatory waves. Criteria for right ventricular hypertrophy, e.g. right axis deviation, increased R-wave voltage in the V1-3 and associated ST-T wave abnormalities, may be observed in patients with pulmonary hypertension. The presence of left ventricular hypertrophy/enlargement suggests associated MR or aortic valve disease.

Chest Radiography

Early in the course of disease, the cardiac silhouette may be relatively normal, however, straightening of the left heart border due to left atrial appendage enlargement and splaying and posterior displacement of the left main bronchus may be observed. Mitral valve calcification can sometimes be observed on a plain chest X-ray, and is an indicator of advanced disease and occurs most often in older people. Calcification of the mitral annulus may be visible in older patients with either rheumatic or non-rheumatic degenerative valve disease. Elevation of the pulmonary venous pressure can be manifest by prominence of the upper lobe pulmonary veins progressing to interstitial and alveolar infiltrates. Pulmonary hypertension is manifest by enlargement of the main pulmonary artery and right ventricle, while right atrial enlargement suggests the presence of tricuspid regurgitation and right heart failure. LV enlargement suggests associated mitral regurgitation.

Cardiac Catheterization

Cardiac catheterization is required in mitral stenosis patients in order to accurately measure hemodynamics, to assess the presence of concomitant aortic and tricuspid valve and aortic disease, to quantify associated MR and LV size and systolic performance, and to exclude co-existent coronary artery disease. The latter is especially important in patients with ischemic symptoms, pre-existent disease, multiple CAD risk factors, and those generally ≥40 years of age.

Characteristic hemodynamic abnormalities include an elevated left atrial pressure or pulmonary capillary wedge pressure (PCWP) with a diastolic pressure difference between the left atrium and ventricle. A prominent "a"-wave is often observed in patients in sinus rhythm. Cardiac output should be measured simultaneously with the recording of the pressure difference. The Gorlin formula is used to calculate the mitral valve effective orifice area (EOA) [17]. Both the gradient across the mitral valve orifice as well as the mitral valve orifice area are calculated at the time of catheterization. A mean gradient >10 mmHg and a mitral valve area of <1.0 cm^2 defines severe MS, while moderate MS is defined as a gradient of 5–10 mmHg or an EOA of 1.0–1.5 cm^2 and mild stenosis patients generally have a gradient of <5 mmHg and EOA >1.5 cm^2 (Table 9.1) [8, 10].

It is important to recognize some common pitfalls during invasive hemodynamic assessment of mitral valve stenosis. It is important to record an accurate PCWP tracing when it is used as a surrogate for left atrial pressure. The diastolic filling time affects the transvalvular gradient. Irregularity in the diastolic filling time occurs in atrial fibrillation; ten consecutives beats should be averaged to avoid errors when using the Gorlin formula [17]. Finally it is important to recognize coexistent mitral regurgitation as it will lead to overestimation of the true severity of mitral valve stenosis.

Right ventricular, pulmonary artery pressures, and total pulmonary artery and pulmonary vascular resistance may be normal in mild mitral stenosis, but pulmonary arterial pressures and resistances increase with progression of the disease.

There is often a discrepancy between hemodynamic measurements and reported symptoms. Noninvasive exercise stress can help resolve this problem. A significant increase in the gradient across the mitral valve (>15 mmHg) associated with an increase in the pulmonary artery systolic pressure to >60 mmHg during exercise supports the presence of significant disease and are both indications to consider mitral balloon valvuloplasty [8, 10]. In patients with severe mitral stenosis, pulmonary artery pressures are elevated even at rest. However, this is often a reversible process with eventual decrease in the pulmonary artery pressures after valve replacement or balloon valvotomy.

Clinical Course

Patients with rheumatic mitral valve disease may be asymptomatic for many years. However, progressive dyspnea on exertion resulting in reduced exercise capacity is the usual presenting report. A careful history must be obtained with respect to performance of activities of daily living to uncover symptomatic progression. Frequent episodes of bronchitis or pneumonia may suggest mitral valve disease before symptoms and signs of overt CHF occur. Acute pulmonary edema may be the first manifestation of mitral stenosis. It may be precipitated by the onset of an atrial tachyarrhythmia, often atrial fibrillation, acute infection, or the hemodynamic stress of pregnancy and delivery [18]. Acute pulmonary edema occurring during labor and delivery can be the first clinical manifestation mitral stenosis. Rarely, mitral stenosis may present with a systemic embolus resulting in a CVA or TIA. Acute hemoptysis can be observed in pneumonia, a pulmonary embolus or due to rupture of bronchial-pulmonary artery collaterals.

Treatment of Mitral Valve Disease

Valvular heart disease management is similar in women and men, however specific gender related differences related to disease prevalence, body size, age at presentation, differences in left ventricular response to overload states need additional consideration in the management of women with valvular heart disease [18].

Medical treatment of patient with moderate-severe mitral regurgitation relies on improving the hemodynamic milieu to reduce the severity of MR. Patients with left ventricular enlargement and coaptation failure often respond to reduction in pre- and after-load by the use of vasodilators, e.g. ACE-Is or ARBs, and judicious use of diuretics. Systolic blood pressure should be reduced to therapeutically recommended levels. Patients with severely reduced LV systolic performance should be treated as a dilated cardiomyopathy. MVP patient with preserved LV systolic performance may benefit from beta-blocker therapy. Patients with atrial fibrillation, who are not candidates for cardioversion or pulmonary vein isolation, require rate control and anticoagulation with warfarin. Currently, prothrombin and Factor Xa inhibitors are not approved for use in valve disease patients. Mitral stenosis patients should be anticoagulated with warfarin even if they are in sinus rhythm, as they often experience short burst of atrial fibrillation.

The current guidelines for operative intervention for severe MR are presented in Fig. 9.2. Surgical intervention should be considered in patients with severe mitral regurgitation who become symptomatic with functional decline and an enlarging LV associated with a drop in LVEF. However, because even a modest decline in LVEF

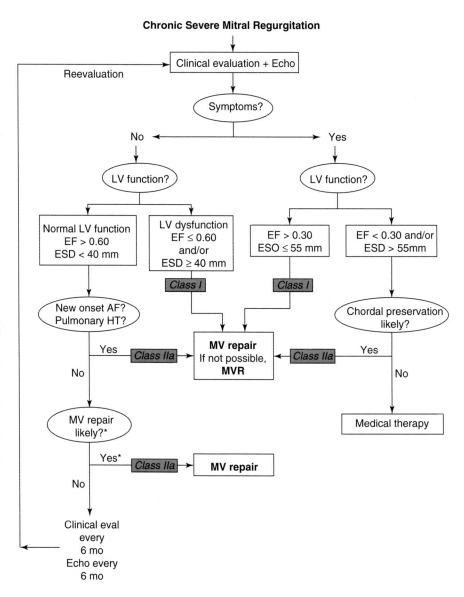

Fig. 9.2 Management strategy for patients with chronic severe mitral regurgitation. *Mitral valve (*MV*) repair may be performed in asymptomatic patients with normal left ventricular (*LV*) function if performed by an experienced surgical team and if the likelihood of successful MV repair is greater than 90 %. *AF* atrial fibrillation, *echo* echocardiography, *EF* ejection fraction, *ESD* end-systolic dimension, *eval* evaluation, *HT* hypertension, and *MVR* mitral valve replacement (Reprinted with permission from Bonow et al. [8])

below 60 % results in increased long-term morbidity and mortality early surgery is now recommended even before significant symptoms have developed [19]. Also, operative repair should be considered in those with progressive atrial enlargement before atrial fibrillation develops. Mitral valve repair is the procedure of choice for suitable candidates when the operation can be performed by an experienced expert surgical team. The high rate of procedural success combined with very low perioperative complications related to primary mitral valve repair has encouraged earlier operation. A bioprosthetic valve is recommended for those patients who are not candidates for valve repair and are not at high risk for prosthetic valve structural deterioration. Mechanical prostheses are generally reserved for patient at high risk for early bioprosthetic valve structural deterioration and those who would require anticoagulation for atrial fibrillation or other reasons. Patients with ischemic MR should undergo coronary revascularization if myocardial viability is demonstrated.

In patients with organic mitral regurgitation mitral valve replacement is usually the procedure of choice. In contrast, there is significant controversy in regards to the procedure of choice in patients with mitral regurgitation secondary to ischemia. In a recent published study there was no significant difference in operative or overall mortality between mitral valve repair as compared to valve replacement in patients with ischemic mitral regurgitation [20]. In patients with coexistent coronary artery disease, mitral valve repair has been reported by a separate group to be superior to valve replacement with significantly decreased peri-operative morbidity and in-hospital mortality [21].

Percutaneous mitral valve repair with placement of a mitral clip device to approximate the edges of the mitral valve at the site of the regurgitant jet has been recently reported to be safe and efficacious in a randomized trial [22]. Percutaneous

————————————————————————————————▶

Fig. 9.3 (**a**): Management strategy for patients with mitral stenosis. †There is controversy as to whether patients with severe mitral stenosis (MVA less than 1.0 cm^2) and severe pulmonary hypertension (pulmonary artery pressure greater than 60 mmHg) should undergo percutaneous mitral balloon valvotomy (*PMBV*) or mitral valve replacement to prevent right ventricular failure. ‡Assuming no other cause for pulmonary hypertension is present. *AF* atrial fibrillation, *CXR* chest X-ray, *ECG* electrocardiogram, *echo* echocardiography, *LA* left atrial, *MR* mitral regurgitation, and *2D* 2-dimensional8. (**b**): Management strategy for patients with mitral stenosis and mild symptoms. *The committee recognizes that there may be variability in the measurement of mitral valve area (*MVA*) and that the mean transmitral gradient, pulmonary artery wedge pressure (*PAWP*), and pulmonary artery systolic pressure (*PP*) should also be taken into consideration. †There is controversy as to whether patients with severe mitral stenosis (MVA less than 1.0 cm^2) and severe pulmonary hypertension (*PH* PP greater than 60–80 mmHg) should undergo percutaneous mitral balloon valvotomy (*PMBV*) or mitral valve replacement to prevent right ventricular failure. *CXR* chest X-ray, *ECG* electrocardiogram, *echo* echocardiography, *LA* left atrial, *MR* mitral regurgitation, *MVG* mean mitral valve pressure gradient, *NYHA* New York Heart Association, *PAP* pulmonary artery pressure, and *2D* 2-dimensional8. (**c**): Management strategy for patients with mitral stenosis and moderate to severe symptoms *The writing committee recognizes that there may be variability in the measurement of mitral valve area (*MVA*) and that the mean transmitral gradient, pulmonary artery wedge pressure (*PAWP*), and pulmonary artery systolic pressure (*PP*) should also be taken into consideration. †It is controversial as to which patients with less favorable valve morphology should undergo percutaneous mitral balloon valvotomy (*PMBV*) rather than mitral valve surgery (see text). *CXR* chest X-ray, *ECG* electrocardiography, *echo* echocardiography, *LA* left atrial, *MR* mitral regurgitation, *MVG* mean mitral valve pressure gradient, *MVR* mitral valve replacement, *NYHA* New York Heart Association, and *2D* 2-dimensional (Reprinted with permission from Bonow et al. [8])

repair was however found to be less effective at reducing the degree of mitral regurgitation compared to conventional mitral valve repair or replacement.

Patients with rheumatic mitral stenosis can be treated with percutaneous balloon valvuloplasty, surgical mitral commisurotomy or mitral valve replacement based on the anatomy and functional status of the valve. Women with symptomatic mitral stenosis of at least moderate severity or new onset atrial fibrillation, as well as those patients which are asymptomatic with moderate mitral stenosis and associated pulmonary hypertension or increased transmitral valvular gradient during exercise and suitable valve anatomy, are recommended to undergo percutaneous mitral balloon valvuloplasty mitral valvulopastly is recommended (Fig. 9.3a–c) [5, 8, 10].

Percutaneous valvulopasty of the mitral valve is accomplished with a single balloon technique which leads to similar results to a double balloon technique with fewer complications [23]. Echocardiography plays a major rule in evaluation of the mitral valve morphology and suitability for mitral balloon valvuloplasty. The

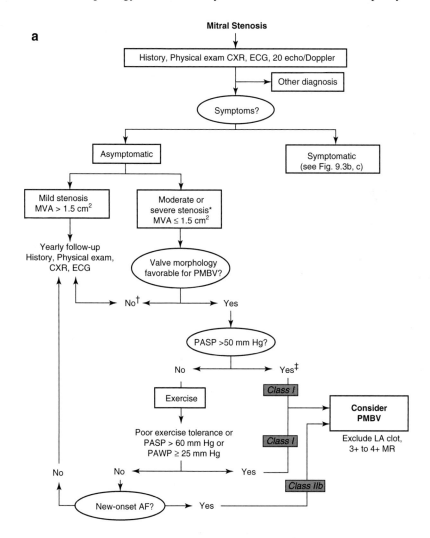

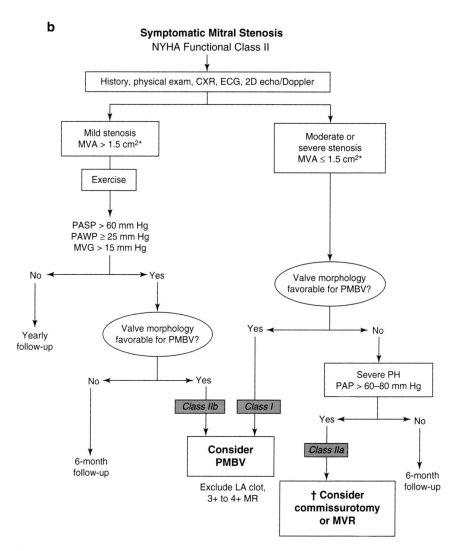

Fig. 9.3 (continued)

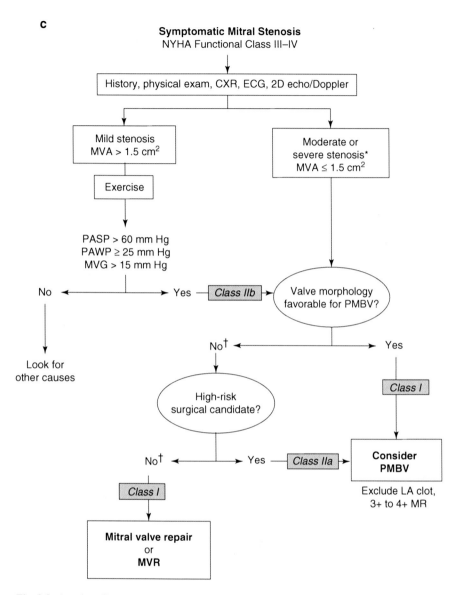

c

Symptomatic Mitral Stenosis
NYHA Functional Class III–IV

History, physical exam, CXR, ECG, 2D echo/Doppler

Mild stenosis
MVA > 1.5 cm^2

Moderate or
severe stenosis*
MVA ≤ 1.5 cm^2

Exercise

PASP > 60 mm Hg
PAWP ≥ 25 mm Hg
MVG > 15 mm Hg

No ← → Yes — *Class IIb* → Valve morphology
favorable for PMBV?

Look for
other causes

No† ← → Yes

Class I

High-risk
surgical candidate?

No† ← → Yes — *Class IIa* → **Consider
PMBV**

Class I

Exclude LA clot,
3+ to 4+ MR

Mitral valve repair
or
MVR

Fig. 9.3 (continued)

Wilkins score (Table 9.2) is a scoring system in which different parts of the mitral valve apparatus are scored depending on mobility, calcification, valve thickening and leaflet thickening with a score less than 9 and less than moderate mitral regurgitation representing a valve favorable for balloon valvotomy [5, 8]. Those patients with mitral valve morphology not favorable for balloon valvotomy can often undergo an open mitral valve comissurotomy or alternatively mitral valve replacement may be needed [5]. If mechanical valve replacement is needed, the choice of valve prosthesis usually depends on the patient's age, contraindications to chronic anticoagulation as well as patient and surgeon's preference. Patients with coexisting rheumatic aortic valve disease and severe valve stenosis or regurgitation can be treated with aortic valve replacement.

Aortic Valve Disease

The normal aortic valve consists of three relatively equal semilunar leaflets attached to a fibrous annulus. The right and left coronary arteries arise from the sinuses of Valsalva above the right and left coronary cusps, respectively. The base of the non-coronary cusp is contiguous with the anterior mitral leaflet. Histologically, the leaflets are covered with endothelium and are composed of three distinct layers: the fibrosa composed of circumferentially oriented collagen, the spongiosa that is rich in extracellular matrix (ECM) and valve interstitial cells (myofibroblasts), and the ventricularis comprised of elastic fibers in addition to collagen. The ECM contains proteoglycans and glycosaminoglycans (GAGs).

Aortic Stenosis

Aortic stenosis (AS) is the most common valvular pathology leading to obstruction of left ventricular outflow in women. The etiologies of AS are depicted in the Table 9.3.

The etiology depends on patient age. A congenital unicuspid or bicuspid valve is most frequent in the pediatric and young adult age groups. A bicuspid valve is the most common congenital malformation in the adult population and accounts for 27 % of AS cases in >70 year old patients. It is encountered in 0.5–2.0 % of people, and while more common in males, it is the most common congenital valve pathology in women [4]. The majority of patients have fusion of the right and left coronary

Table 9.3 Etiologies of aortic stenosis [24]

Congenital	Acquired
Unicuspid valve	Calcific
Bicuspid valve	Trileaflet valve degeneration
Quadricuspid valve	Post-inflammatory
	Rheumatic
	Rheumatoid nodular
	Ochronosis
	Systemic lupus erythematosus

cusps. Increased leaflet stress due to abnormal blood flow induces calcification generally after the age of 40. Bicuspid aortic disease is associated with dilation of the ascending thoracic aorta, coarctation of the aorta, increased risk of aortic dissection, and presence of mitral valve prolapse.

Rheumatic heart disease occurs most frequently in patients between 30 and 60 years of age, but is much less prevalent in the United States and the developing world. As with mitral valve disease with which it is always associated, rheumatic involvement of the aortic valve leads to commissural fusion. A central orifice results with variable degrees of stenosis and regurgitation.

Senile calcific degeneration of a trileaflet aortic is the most frequent cause of AS in the elderly, accounting for 48 % of cases in patients >70 years of age and is also the most common cause of AS in older women [24]. Degeneration results in leaflet thickening, stiffening and calcification, but without commissural fusion. The pathogenesis of calcific aortic valve disease involves proliferative and inflammatory changes, lipid accumulation, increased angiotensin converting enzyme activity, increased oxidative stress, infiltration of inflammatory cells and formation of bone [4, 25]. Calcific aortic valve disease shares a number of similarities with the pathogenesis of atherosclerosis. The two processes also share similar risk factors. Both the aortic valve and annulus can be calcified, and calcific aortic valve disease can be one component of calcification of the mitral annulus, papillary muscles, and the aortic root, especially the sino-tubular junction. The commissures are not generally fused, differentiating from rheumatic and other inflammatory etiologies of aortic valve disease. The severity of leaflet thickening and calcification ranges progresses from mild (termed aortic sclerosis) to severe with increasing age of the orifice [14, 25].

Age-related changes in the aorta can amplify the LV-aortic impedance mismatch that characterizes aortic valve stenosis. Loss of aortic compliance induced systolic hypertension that acts as a secondary obstruction to LV emptying, and can affect measurements of valve stenosis [26]. Aortic calcification that can occur with advanced age can impact therapeutic options.

Physical Examination

A crescendo-decrescendo systolic ejection murmur systolic ejection murmur heard on routine physical examination is often the first sign of AS. In many patients, the murmur is loudest in the right second intercostal space. However, calcific degenerative disease may present with an atypically located murmur, e.g. along the left sternal border. The murmur typically radiates to the carotid arteries, left sternal border, and apex where it may be perceived as more holosystolic. An associated thrill and/or late peaking of the murmur indicate severe obstruction. Patients may also have a diastolic murmur indicating aortic valve insufficiency. Other findings include a left ventricular heave, a palpable or audible fourth heart sound, and diminution of the aortic component of the second heart sound [14]. An ejection click can be perceived in patients with pliable cusps. The presence of a third heart sound suggests predominant aortic regurgitation or LV enlargement with reduced LVEF. The carotid arterial pulse is characteristically slowly rising and sustained (pulsus tardus et parvus); an anacrotic notch may be felt. The association of a typical AS murmur with a rapidly rising carotid pulse suggests with aortic regurgitation or subaortic obstruction, etc.

Fig. 9.4 (**a**) 2-D Echocardiogram parasternal long axis view of the left ventricle revealing calcification of aortic valve leaflets with decreased leaflet opening and impingement of IVS into the LVOT (*white arrow*). (**b**) 2-D Echocardiogram parasternal short axis view at the level of the aortic valve revealing calcification of aortic valve leaflets with decreased leaflet opening (*black arrow*)

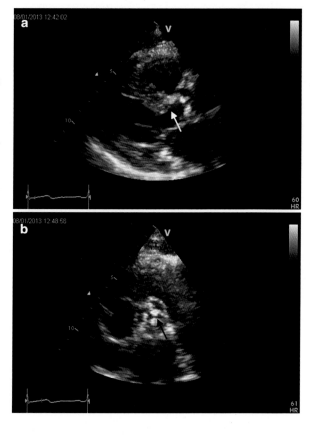

Diagnostic Evaluation

Doppler Echocardiography

Doppler-echocardiography (2-D and 3-D) is the standard non-invasive technique for diagnosis, to assess disease progression, and to help tailor therapy. Calcification of the aortic valve associated with reduced cusp motion is the hallmark of the disease. Stenosis severity can be can be assessed by measurement of the transvalvular peak velocity, peak and mean gradients, hemodynamic effective orifice area, and anatomic area by TEE. The criteria for AS severity are delineated in Table 9.1 [8, 10, 15]. In addition, the effect of aortic stenosis on LA and LV remodeling, hypertrophy, and systolic and diastolic performance can be assessed. Figure 9.4a depicts calcification aortic valve and proximal aortic root with extension of calcium into proximal interventricular septum (IVS). Note the impingement of the hypertrophied IVS into the LVOT (arrow). Figure 9.4b is a short-axis view on the aortic valve from the same patient. The leaflets are heavily calcified and the narrowed orifice is identified by the arrow.

Gender, age, and concomitant diseases all play a role in LV remodeling in AS. Women tend to have higher LV mass/volume ratios, increased relative wall thickness and LVEF [12, 27]. Extreme hypertrophy is more common in elderly women [28]. A sigmoid shape interventricular septum impinging into the LVOT could induce a LVOT gradient and also cause the LVOT to be more ovoid and thus cause overestimation of the severity of obstruction (Fig. 9.4a). These patients at risk to develop low-flow low-gradient (LFLG) severe AS which carries a very poor prognosis [29, 30]. In addition, associated diabetes mellitus, hypertension, coronary artery disease, and primary myocardial disease can impact LV remodeling and performance.

Determination of the aortic area is important as the ratio of the AV orifice area to aortic area can define the need to correct the gradients for pressure recovery, as many women have small aortic roots. Also, assessment of the severity of sino-tubular junction calcification can affect clinical decision making regarding the feasibility and/or approach to valve replacement/ transcatheter aortic valve replacement (TAVR).

TEE is particularly useful to diagnose congenital AV abnormalities. Because of its superior resolution, accurate planimetry of the aortic valve orifice is frequently possible. Also, assessment of the LVOT and aortic annulus geometries are essential to accurately determine prosthesis size. While TEE can visualize the aortic root, often MRI is required to exclude egg-shell calcification that can complicate valve interventions.

Dobutamine stress echocardiography (DSE) is efficacious to separate patients with low-flow low-gradient (LFLG) but truly severe AS from those with either moderate obstruction or very severe LV dysfunction. A dobutamine-induced increase in the AV-gradient without an increase in valve orifice area to 1.0 cm^2 suggests true AS. In contrast, an increase in valve area to >1.0 cm^2 with slight to no increase in gradient suggests moderate obstruction. Failure of both the gradient and valve area to change with dobutamine suggests severely depressed LV systolic performance. Recently, Clavel et al. reported that ESE in asymptomatic patients or DSE in symptomatic ones could distinguish severe AS from moderate disease in patients with LFLG AS with normal EF [31]. Exercise stress testing can be judiciously used in selected patients to define exercise capacity or clarify symptomatic status with a low risk of complications.

High-resolution CAT scans and MRI have significant roles in the assessment of aortic valve disease. Measurement of the LVOT and aortic annulus geometry, quantifying the AV calcium burden, precise visualization of the valve leaflets and aorta, and quantification LV volumes, performance and mass are a few areas where these technologies may have an important role. Imaging of the aorta is should be performed in elderly people as part of the pre-operative evaluation for those being considered for surgical or percutaneous valve replacement.

Electrocardiography

The characteristic findings include left atrial enlargement and voltage criteria for LA hypertrophy with repolarization abnormalities. Extension of calcium into the interventricular septum can result in a LBBB or complete heart block. Atrial fibrillation can be seen, and its acute onset often is manifest by acute clinical deterioration. Ventricular tachyarrhythmias can presage sudden death.

Chest Radiography

Calcification of the aortic valve and aortic root may be seen in chest radiography. Other findings include post-stenotic dilation of the ascending aorta, and the LVH. However, the chest X-ray may be unrevealing.

Cardiac Catheterization

Cardiac catheterization is often required before surgical or catheter-based intervention. Measurement of the effective orifice area requires careful recording of both the LV and aortic pressures. Ideally, the latter should be recorded approximately 5 cm above the valve to account for pressure recovery. Cardiac output must be obtained and the Gorlin equation can be used to calculate the effective orifice area. Discrepancies often occur between catheter and Doppler-echocardiographic calculation of the orifice area. These discrepancies can be due to a number of factors, however, failure to account for pressure recovery and the LVOT pressure are most frequent. Spevack et al. was able to reconcile much of the discrepancy by correcting the Doppler area for the aortic root area [32]. A complete right heart catheterization should be performed, while performance of LV, aortic, and coronary angiography will depend on the clinical presentation of the patient.

Clinical Course

Valvular aortic stenosis patients generally experience a long asymptomatic period. During this time the disease progresses at a variable rate. Serial Doppler-echocardiograms can be used to quantify the progression of valve dysfunction [8, 25]. While the average rate of decrease in valve area, increase in mean gradient, and maximum velocity (V_{max}) is 0.1–0.2 cm²/year, 7–8 mmHg/year, and 0.2–0.3 m/s/year; there is a wide range in progression [33]. Patients at risk for rapid progression include those with a V_{max} >3 m/s, more than mild valve calcification, or multiple CAD risk factors. Asymptomatic patients with severe AS have an excellent survival with low risk of sudden death [34].

Eventually, with increasing stenosis severity patients develop symptoms of angina (35 %), dizziness or syncope (15 %), or dyspnea and heart failure (50 %) [25]. In addition, onset of atrial and ventricular tachyarrhythmias and sudden death increase in frequency in symptomatic patients with severe AS. It is also important to recognize that none of these symptoms are specific for AS, but once one or more develop, patient survival is reduced, ranging from an average of 5 years for angina, 3 years for syncope to less than 2 years for CHF. The V_{max} can predict the time to onset of symptoms. It ranges from 8 %/year if V_{max} <3.0 m/s,

17 %/year if V_{max} of 3.0–4.0 m/s, and 40 %/year once V_{max} >4.0 m/s [35]. The presence of moderate-severe AV calcification, advanced age, CAD and significant associated aortic or mitral regurgitation can accelerate symptom onset in those with mild-moderate AS [34].

Aortic Regurgitation

Aortic regurgitation affects both genders with equal frequency. However, there are important gender-related differences in etiology, pathophysiology and management, including the timing of surgery, between the sexes. We will start with a brief overview of aortic regurgitation, followed by special considerations in women.

Pathophysiology and Etiologies

Aortic valve competence requires normal aortic valve anatomy and that of the surrounding structures, especially the membranous interventricular septum, sinuses of Valsalva, and proximal aortic root. Aortic regurgitation (AR), diastolic backflow of blood into the LV, occurs when there is malcoaptation due to remodeling of surrounding structures, loss of leaflet support, or congenital abnormalities or pathologic distortion, disruption, or destruction of one or more leaflets [8].

The etiologies for AR are numerous [2] as listed in Table 9.4. These include congenital and acquired cardiovascular disease. The latter include degenerative, infectious, inflammatory, heritable and acquired connective tissue disease, the effects of neoplasm, and trauma.

Physical Examination

Patients with mild AR often have no audible murmur; the leak is detected by Doppler-echocardiography. As AR becomes more severe, the patient evinces more of the finding associated with a valve disease and its effects on the cardiovascular system. The murmur of AR is a diastolic high-pitched, decrescendo murmur begins in close proximity to S2 and extends a variable distance into diastole. It is most often loudest in the left third intercostal space and radiates to toward the apex. The duration of the murmur increases with increasing severity in chronic AR, but the reverse is true in acute AR. Patients with AR due to a dilated aortic root may demonstrate a right parasternal murmur. In patient with moderate or severe MR, An aortic systolic ejection murmur may also be present. An apical diastolic rumble (Austin Flint murmur) is sometimes heard in severe AR Other physical findings in those with moderate-severe disease include: An LV heave, an election click in those with pliable leaflets, a resonant S2 in hypertensive patients, an S3 in those with LV dilatation or reduced LVEF. The carotid and peripheral artery pulsations characteristically demonstrate a hyperdynamic circulation with rapid upstrokes (Corrigan's pulse) and descents and a bisferiens systolic wave. The

Table 9.4 Etiologies of aortic regurgitation [2]

Primarily Involves the Valve Leaflets	Primarily Involves the Aortic Root	Involves Both the Valve Leaflets and Aortic Root:	Involves Both Subvavular Structures and Valve Leaflets
1. Physiologic regurgitation	1. Idiopathic aortic root dilation	1. Congenital bicuspid valve	1. Ventricular septal defect
2. Calcific degenerative aortic valve disease	2. Annuloaortic ectasia	2. Marfan's syndrome	2. Discrete membranous subaortic stenosis
3. Congenital leaflet abnormalities.	3. Cystic medial necrosis ± aortic dissection	3. Ankylosing spondylitis	
4. Rheumatic valve disease	4. Systemic arterial hypertension	4. Trauma (either directy from valvotomy or valvuloplasty, or indirect from chest trauma)	
5. Connective tissue diseases (a) heumatoid arthritis (b) ystemic lupus erythematosis	5. Heritable connective tissue diseases (a) Ehler-Danlos syndrome (b) Pseudoxanthoma elasticum (c) Osteogenesis imperfecta		
6. Infective and marantic endocarditis	6. Inflammatory bowel disease		
7. Myxomatous degeneration	7. Giant cell aortitis 8. Syphilitic aortitis 9. Reiter syndrome		

hyperdynamic circulation may also be evidenced by head bobbing (de Musset sign); femoral artery pulses can have "pistol shot" pulses (Traube Sign) and compression-induced bruits (Duroziez sign). Quincke's sign (capillary pulsations in the fingertips via trans illumination, or gentle pressure on the fingernail) may also be elicited in severe AR [4] Patients with progressive disease may also present with heart failure symptoms.

Diagnostic Evaluation

Doppler-Echocardiography

Transthoracic Doppler-echocardiography (TTE) is the primary diagnostic modality to image the AR jet, assess the leaflet anatomy, mobility, and pathology; aortic dimensions; LV dimensions, wall thicknesses, and systolic and diastolic performance; and other associated valvular abnormalities; all are required to grade AR severity and for surgical planning [36, 37]. In particular, an increased LV end-systolic volume has been shown to be a harbinger of worse outcomes [36, 37]. AR severity can be estimated by a number of methods (Table 9.1) All of these methodologies and others that have been proposed have significant sources of errors and limitations. It is best to use a number of them to quantify AR severity. Serial studies are performed to assess for progression of disease [4].

Transesophageal Doppler-echocardiography (TEE), because of its superior resolution, is indicated in order to obtain high-resolution images of the aortic valve, especially when the TTE images are inadequate or ambiguous, especially when a bicuspid valve is suspected. Systolic and diastolic orifice areas can be planimetered. TEE is required to image the aorta. Pre- and intra-operative TEE is required to optimize surgical approach and detect surgical related complications. Three-D echocardiography is also being incorporated in the evaluation of aortic valve disease.

Electrocardiography

Patients with mild isolated AR may have a normal ECG. Typical ECG findings usually manifest in chronic severe AR. These include evidence of LV enlargement due to volume overload, manifest as an increased QRS amplitude with ST-T wave abnormalities. As AR progresses, an interventricular conduction delay may be seen. Lengthening PR-interval an bundle branch block may be seen in exuberant annular calcification that extends into the conduction system and in AR secondary an inflammatory process [4].

Chest Radiography

The chest x-ray may be unrevealing in cases of acute aortic regurgitation, since the heart will likely be of normal size. Increasing AR severity is suggested by enlargement of the cardiac silhouette, aorta, and to assess the presence of pulmonary vascular congestion in patients reporting dyspnea.

Cardiac Catheterization

Invasive hemodynamic studies are indicated when non-invasive studies cannot be obtained, are ambiguous, or in the setting of complex valvular or congenital heart disease. AR severity quantified by measurements of the regurgitant volume and fraction. In addition, aortic angiography can also be used to quantify the severity of AR and evaluate aortic anatomy.

Other Imaging Modalities

Both CT and MRI can be used to diagnose aortic dilatation and pathology. MRI can perform a number of quantitative measurements to determine the etiology of AR and quantify its severity Good correlations have been reported with Doppler-echocardiography.

Acute Aortic Regurgitation

Acute aortic regurgitation occurs in the setting of valve destruction or loss of normal geometry of support. Aortic dissection, infective endocarditis, and traumatic injury to the valve or proximal aorta are main causes. Acute severe regurgitation causes an acute volume overload that occurs before the LV can compensate by dilatation. As a result, the LV end-diastolic and left atrial pressures abruptly increase. The LV diastolic pressure may exceed the left atrial pressure leading to mitral valve closure. Partial closure results in functional mitral stenosis, the cause of the Austin Flint murmur [38]. Premature closure is diagnosed by closure of the mitral valve before the p-wave on echocardiography. Reduced forward cardiac output may be partially compensated by tachycardia. However, hypotension and signs of decreased perfusion are the presenting features. Despite, severely elevated LV diastolic pressures, acute pulmonary edema may not occur in those with competent mitral valves. Development of MR often results in cardiogenic shock. It is also not uncommon for patients to also present with symptoms of ischemia. This occurs when LV end-diastolic pressures approach aortic and coronary artery pressures, thus dropping the myocardial perfusion pressure in the subendocardium. Furthermore, an increased afterload from LV dilation and wall thinning will increase myocardial oxygen demand. Altogether, this combination of events can lead to significant ischemia and all of its sequelae (including infarction, arrhythmia and sudden death).

Management of acute AR is aimed at the correction of its cause [39]. Urgent/emergency surgery is required. Medical therapy to reduce support the blood pressure, reduce LV end-diastolic pressure, and increase forward flow by infusion of nitroprusside, dopamine or dobutamine is only a temporizing measure. Beta-blockers should be used with caution, as they will blunt any compensatory tachycardia. Intra-aortic balloon counterpulsation is contraindicated, as this will worsen the aortic regurgitation [8, 40].

Chronic Aortic Regurgitation

Patients with chronic aortic regurgitation may remain asymptomatic for years before presenting with clinical disease. Initially, exercise capacity is preserved, as the regurgitant volume is dependent on the length of diastole, which inversely correlates with heart rate. Other compensatory processes aimed at accommodating the increased LV volume load on the heart include an increase in LV end-diastolic dimensions and compliance to compensate for the volume load and maintain near normal end-diastolic pressures. These changes also permit a larger stroke volume, which also leads to a preserved ejection fraction. These changes, however, are not without their consequences. The chronically increased regurgitant volume leads to increased LV afterload, which results in LV hypertrophy, dilation and spherical remodeling until the LV can no longer maintain cardiac output and begins to fail. At this point, patients begin to develop exertional dyspnea, and even angina (using the same principles of ischemia described in the previous section). These two symptoms are harbingers of poor outcomes, and are indicators that surgery should be strongly considered. For this reason, taking a thorough history and physical examination is of utmost importance in defining risk of progression and optimal timing of surgery. As left ventricular geometry worsens, the potential benefits of surgery become lessened. Serial echocardiography is an important adjunct to clinical surveillance in managing these patients [8, 40].

Considerations in Women

Unlike coronary artery disease, aortic valvular heart disease can affect patients of all ages. In younger women, the most common etiologies are Marfan syndrome, endocarditis, congenital leaflet anormalities, or associated connective tissue diseases. In older women, the same risk factors as men apply: degenerative calcific disease, hypertension, etc. Furthermore, women tend to develop symptoms before any structural derangements may be detected by echocardiography, and LV enlargement is essentially a late finding in severe AR [41]. It is therefore suggested that any LV chamber enlargement, increase in end-diastolic pressures or impaired function be given strong consideration for surgical evaluation. Over reliance on echocardiographic parameters prior to surgical evaluation may unnecessarily delay AVR, which can result in worse outcomes [18]. Although the guidelines do not differentiate approach to severe aortic regurgitation in men and women, a thorough, symptom-guided evaluation needs to be undertaken in determining timing of surgery. Although this holds true in men as well, it is especially important in women, as delays in surgical referral may lead to poorer outcomes.

Treatment of Aortic Valve Disease

Women require special considerations in the surgical management of aortic valvular heart disease. They tend to have smaller LVOT dimensions, especially if basal IVS hypertrophy develops, aortic annuli and aortic roots compared to their male counterparts. They also may experience incomplete LV remodeling after correction of the hemodynamic derangement. These findings can impact the operative approach and the selection of valve prosthesis in order to avoid patient-prosthesis mismatch.

The echocardiographer plays an important role at the time of valve replacement providing guidance to the surgeon in order to avoid patient-prosthesis mismatch. As

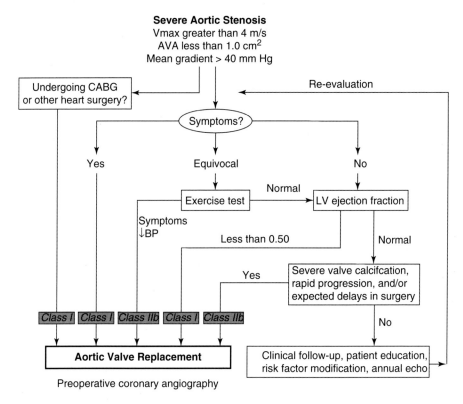

Fig. 9.5 Management Strategy for patients with severe aortic stenosis (Reprinted with permission from Bonow et al. [8])

such, it becomes important to ensure that the predicted functional orifice area of the prosthetic valve will be adequate, as a small effective orifice area when indexed to the patient's body size, can lead to post-operative patient-prosthesis mismatch [18].

The current treatment guidelines for the management of patients with severe aortic stenosis are listed in Fig. 9.5 [8, 10]. Aortic valve surgery is currently the only effective treatment to relieve severe AS. Most patients undergo surgical implantation of a prosthesis. The choice of valve prosthesis largely depends on age, contraindications to anticoagulation, effective orifice area, presence of associated aortic root pathology, e.g. calcification if the sinuses of Valsalva or sino-tubular junction, and subaortic pathology, as well as patient and surgeon preference. Aortic valve replacement is in general a safe surgical procedure with a reported surgical mortality of <3 % [42]. Mortality data shows that at 10 years of follow up, up to 90 %patients with mechanical aortic valve prosthesis are alive compared to 93 % of patients with porcine or pericardial xenografts [42].

There currently is no effective medical therapy for calcific aortic valve disease. While retrospective studies has been reported that statin therapy can slow disease progression in patients with chronic calcific AS, prospective clinical trials have failed to demonstrate this benefit [43, 44]. However, asymptomatic patients with severe AS with preserved left ventricular systolic function (LVEF >50 %), and in whom rapid clinical progression is not expected (based on morphologic assessment of the aortic valve, the absence of risk factors for rapid progression), a conservative approach with routine echocardiograms is appropriate and recommended in the most recent treatment guidelines [8]. Asymptomatic patients with preserved LVEF and in whom rapid clinical progression is expected or in patients with depressed LVEF, aortic valve replacement is recommended [8]. Aortic valve replacement is essential in patients with severe AS once symptoms develop (class I indication and recommended as per the most recent ACC/AHA guidelines [8]). The most common symptoms are angina, dizziness or syncope or those suggestive of CHF, e.g. dyspnea. The last can be due to left ventricular overload and elevated left ventricular pressures whether or not coexistent left ventricular dysfunction is present.

A proportion of patients will experience equivocal symptoms. Exercise or pharmacologic stress testing aids in the objective assessment of symptoms and exercise performance. Patients with severe AS who experience exertional dyspnea, decreased exercise capacity, or a blunted or decreased systolic blood pressure response to exercise (<20 mmHg increase with exercise) should be referred for surgery [45]. Patients with moderate to severe AS in whom non-valve cardiac surgery, e.g. coronary revascularization, is planned, aortic valve replacement at the time of surgery is recommended regardless of presence of symptoms [8]. Coronary angiography before the planned aortic valve replacement is indicated to determine whether the patient has undiagnosed obstructive coronary artery disease which needs to be corrected at the time or the surgical procedure. Special consideration should be given to patients with mixed AS and AR in whom symptoms may be present even with moderate degree of aortic stenosis and therefore aortic valve replacement is recommend with onset of symptoms or evidence of new left ventricular dysfunction even when the severity of mixed AS and AR is only moderate [45]. Patient with bicuspid aortic valve disease may be referred to surgery when there is evidence of severe AS and coexistent aortic dilatation when the diameter of the ascending aorta exceeds 5.0 cm, irrespective of symptoms [8, 10] Patients with dilated aortic roots >5.5 cm may require root replacement or reconstruction.

Recently, a trans-catheter aortic valve replacement (TAVR) procedure has been FDA approved for the treatment of patients with severe AS who are not candidates for surgical valve replacement due to a high surgical risk [46–48]. TAVR has been demonstrated to reduce mortality, symptoms, and re-hospitalization in this patient population [46].

Women with a small annulus size, are at risk for post-operative complications, including patient-prothesis mismatch after a standard aortic valve replacement. Patient-prosthesis mismatch which can result in progressive left ventricular dysfunction, increased incidence of congestive heart failure and increased risk of mortality. TAVR has been proposed as an alternative to surgical AVR in these patients [49]. Women make up to half of patients currently eligible for TAVR, thus the relative importance of these considerations in women. In a small cohort of 35 women with severe aortic stenosis and small aortic annulus size (defined as less than 20 mm), TAVR implantation was successful in the majority of patients.

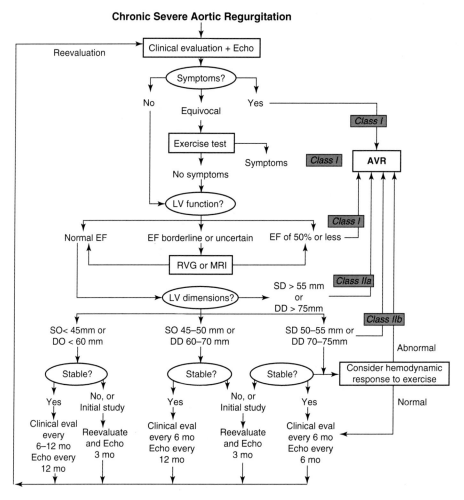

Fig. 9.6 Management strategy for patients with chronic severe aortic regurgitation (Reprinted with permission from Bonow et al. [8])

Post-operative prosthesis mismatch occurred only in a minority of patients, and good post-procedure aortic valve gradient and effective orifice areas were maintained at 14 months of follow up [49]. A recently published study aimed to describe gender-related differences in patients with severe aortic stenosis undergoing TAVR [50]. In this study, of which women accounted for half of the patient cohort, women had smaller aortic annulus size, underwent TAVR more frequently than men and had smaller femoral artery diameter and femoral artery calcification scores [50]. Despite a higher incidence of iliac artery complications in women there was no significant differences in procedural success and 30 day mortality, furthermore female gender was a predictor of survival [50].

The current ACC/AHA guidelines for the management of patients with chronic severe aortic regurgitation are presented in Fig. 9.6 [8, 10]. In contrast to AS, the management of patients with chronic aortic regurgitation requires a complex integration of clinical, imaging, and laboratory data.

Infective Endocarditis and Inflammatory Carditis

Infective endocarditis (IE) has an estimated incidence in the general population of 0.01 % and half the incidence in women as compared to men [51]. Patients at increased risk for IE include valvular abnormalities associated with regurgitation, a previous history of IE, and implantation of a prosthetic heart valve or intra-cardiac device. Diabetes mellitus, end stage renal disease on hemodialysis, human immuno-deficiency virus infection and intravenous drug use are common co-morbidities that increase the risk for IE [51].

Staphylococcus and *Streptococcus* are the most commonly isolated pathogens in native valve disease, while Staphylococcal species are increasingly common pathogens isolated from infected indwelling devices and in nosocomial infections. In patients with streptococcus infection and native valve endocarditis in-hospital mortality is estimated at 10 % however mortality increases in patients with more virulent staphylococcus and prosthetic valve endocarditis [51].

The diagnosis of IE is based on clinical presentation, microbiological data, and echocardiographic findings. Common symptoms include fever, night sweats, loss of appetite, malaise, and fatigue. A new or more prominent regurgitation murmur, anemia, and evidence of micro- or macro-emboli may be observed. An intravascular infection is suspected the same organism is isolated from multiple blood cultures. Clinical suspicion is important as blood cultures should be obtained prior to ini-tiation of antimicrobial therapy, in order to isolate the responsible pathogen, since identification of the responsible organism is important for appropriate management.

Echocardiography plays an important role in early diagnosis and treatment. TTE is indicated in all patients suspected of having IE. The diagnosis is based on the observation of a vegetation characterized by mobile inhomogeneous echogenic mass attached to an intracardiac structure, most often on the low pressure side of a valve, in the appropriate clinic setting. TEE is not routinely indicated in all IE patients. It should be performed in those with suspected prosthetic valve or device infections, especially on indwelling catheters or mechanical prosthetic valves, suspected para-valvular infections (development of conduction system disease), patients at high risk but with negative or inadequate TTEs, and those being evaluated for surgery.

Patients with IE should be cared for by a team consisting of an infectious disease specialist, a cardiologist, and a cardiac surgeon. IE due to antibiotic sensitive organ-ism, should intially be treated with a recommended regimen. However, those with large vegetations (>1 cm on the aortic and mitral valves, and >2 cm on the tricuspid valve), infections with non-penicillin sensitive organisms, and those with infected prostheses should be evaluated for early surgical intervention. Valve surgery is rec-ommended for new onset heart failure, uncontrolled infection, or for prevention of embolic cerebral events which is the most feared complication of valve endocarditis [51, 52]. Early surgery is indicated for IE due to non-penicillin sensitive organisms, especially if left side native valves or prostheses are involved. Surgery should be performed immediately once an indication arises. Temporizing only increases the morbidity and mortality associated with the disease.

New guidelines restrict the use of antibiotics for prophylaxis prior to dental procedures to those patients with the following cardiac conditions associated with the highest risk of adverse outcomes from infective endocarditis: unrepaired cyanotic congenital heart disease, previous infective endocarditis, and prosthetic heart valves [53].

Another cohort subset of women at increased risk for valvular heart disease, include those with systemic autoimmune diseases. Systemic lupus erythematosus (SLE) and rheumatoid arthritis are systemic autoimmune diseases which have higher prevalence in women as compared to men and are associated with significant morbidity and mortality. Valvular heart disease is by far the most common cardiac abnormality and a leading of cause of death in SLE patients [54]. Libman-Sacks endocarditis is suspected by the findings of vegetations on both surfaces along the valve closure lines associated leaflet thickening. Patients with Libman-Sacks endocarditis can develop moderate to severe valvular regurgitation secondary to leaf left or chordal rupture. The vegetations can embolize fibrin and platelet micro-emboli to the brain [54]. Anticoagulation is recommended in patients with valve vegetations and symptoms of stroke or transient ischemic attach (TIA). In those patients with severe disease valve, replacement is recommended [54].

Patients with rheumatoid arthritis can develop a valvulitis due to inflammatory cell deposition leading to leaflet fibrosis and valve nodules which are usually located at the base of the leaflets and valve rings [54]. Patients usually develop symptoms due to cardioembolism, superimposed valve endocarditis as well as valve insufficiency and rarely due to valve stenosis. Echocardiography is an important diagnostic tool. Nodules are visualized accompanied by valve thickening in one third of patients, that can result in valvular regurgitation or stenosis [54]. Finally, noninfected vegetations can occur in patients with debilitating disease (marantic endocarditis).

Pregnancy and Valvular Heart Disease

Pregnancy poses unique challenges to women with valvular hear disease. An extensive discussion of this topic is covered elsewhere in this text. The discussion below covers salient points of valvular disease in the pregnant female.

In order to meet metabolic demands of mother and fetus and to optimize uteroplacental perfusion, blood volume normally increases by 50 %, heart rate increases by 10–20 beats/min, both accompanied by a decline in systemic vascular resistance [8]. Cardiac output begins to increase during the first trimester, probably around the 5th to 10th week of pregnancy, and progressively does so until the end of the second trimester. It remains constant or decreases slightly during the third trimester. The increase in heart rate and stroke volume, due to increased preload and reduced afterload, contribute to the rise in cardiac output. The change in fluid state and hemodynamics is accompanied by mild left atrial and ventricular dilatation. LV systolic performance increases early in pregnancy, progressing until the 20th week of gestation, and then remains constant until end of pregnancy. Blood pressure decreases at the start in the first trimester, but then increases, reaching a peak in mid pregnancy.

Valvular heart disease may be either discovered or worsen during pregnancy depending on the nature of the lesion. Common symptoms of pregnancy, e.g. shortness of breath, fatigue, palpitations, and decreased exercise capacity, edema, mimic those of valvular disease. A systolic flow murmur loudest along the left sternal border can mimic valve aortic or pulmonary stenosis. Splitting of S1, an S3 gallop, mild tachypnea, tachycardia, and lower extremity edema can be found in the normal pregnant women. Additionally, peripartum evaluation is paramount in order to assess for peripartum cardiomyopathy. The management of valvular disease in a pregnant women poses a unique challenge, often requiring pre-conceptual counseling, management, and potential surgical treatment.

Diagnostic Evaluation and Management

The goal of diagnosis and management of valvular disease in pregnancy is not just to diagnose and treat the disease and its complications, but also to minimize the risk of diagnostic and therapeutic modalities to the fetus. Avoidance of radiation exposure and toxic pharmaceuticals (Class D), e.g. ACE-Is and ARBs, is of paramount importance.

Echocardiography is the diagnostic modality of choice in pregnancy. Normal findings during pregnancy include mild ventricular chamber enlargement and minimal valvular regurgitation [8]. The ACC/AHA Class I recommendation for echocardiographic evaluation includes all symptoms or signs of heart failure or structural heart disease, grade 3/6 or louder systolic murmurs, pan-systolic and late-systolic murmurs, murmurs associated with ejection clicks, diastolic murmurs, and murmurs which radiate to the neck and back [8]. Management of mild to moderate valvular disease isolated during pregnancy is by regular interval sonographic evaluation. In the majority of cases, the initial method of treatment irrespective of the affected valve is medical, in order to provide symptomatic control and optimization of cardiac function. Severe disease poses more of a challenge; in the majority of cases, medical therapy is attempted prior to resorting to surgical correction during pregnancy. Failure of medical management and/or further decompensation from severe valvular disease with possible hemodynamic instability may require emergent surgical intervention during pregnancy.

Established valvular disease is also monitored with regards to symptoms, examination findings, and serial echocardiography. Poor functional status is an important consideration for valve surgery prior to conception [2]. Again, as with valvular disease discovered during pregnancy, established disease that is mild-moderate is monitored and medically managed during pregnancy; severe valvular lesions are preferably treated with preservation of the native valve via valvuloplasty or valve repair, as this strategy limits the challenges of anticoagulation in pregnancy.

Mitral Valve Disease

Pregnancy increases the hemodynamic stress in MS. Common complications include congestive heart failure (CHF, 43 %) and atrial arrythmias (20 %), secondary to increased left atrial filling pressures and resultant left atrial expansion, pulmonary congestion, edema, hypertension [2]. Thus, it is recommended to avoid pregnancy in patients with significant MS until underlying valvular disease has been adequately treated [55]. Medical management during pregenancy includes the use of beta-blocker therapy to increase ventricular diastolic filling and coronary perfusion times and judicious use of diuretics. Mitral valvuloplasty is an alternative for severe disease with favorable anatomy. However, given the radiation exposure, it is recommended to delay surgery until weak 14, after organogenesis [55]. Mitral regurgitation (MR) may worsen during pregnancy due to annular dilatation. Symptomatic mitral valve prolapse in pregnancy is secondary to associated MR. Afterload reduction and judicious diuretic use is indicated, with mitral valve repair usually deferred until postpartum state [2].

Aortic Valve Disease

Aortic sclerosis with stenosis (AS) found in women of child-bearing age is most often due to a congenital unicuspid or a bicuspid valve. CHF, the result of increased intravascular volume and limited ventricular compliance, accounts for 40 % of symptomatic AS in pregnancy [2]. Angina can occur due reduced coronary perfusion and increased myocardial oxygen demand, a result to pregnancy-induced tachycardia and decreased afterload. Medical management of symptomatic AS is bed rest and beta- blocker administration. Afterload reduction is contraindicated, and diuresis in the setting of CHF can reduce adequate maternal organ and fetal perfusion. Preterm labor and delivery, intrauterine growth retardation, and increased risk of fetal loss are well described risk of pregnancy in women with severe AS [56].

Aortic Regurgitation (AR) is uncommon with respect to other valvular diseases and can be the result of bicuspid valve, valve damage secondary to endocarditis or rheumatic heart disease, and congenital or acquired aortic root dilatation. Severe AR is predominantly treated with judicious diuretic use and bed rest. Aortic dilatation from decreased collagen synthesis and hormone mediated decreased collagen deposition increases the likelihood of aortic dissection, especially in the setting of weakened structure of aorta from collagen vascular disease [2].

Pulmonic Valve Disease

Pulmonic stenosis (PS) occurs most often as an isolated congenital defect, or more rarely, a a component of Tetralogy of Fallot. PS results in elevated right atrial filling pressures, decreased volume of forward flow to the pulmonary, left heart and systemic circuit, and venous congestion and right sided heart failure. Pulmonic regurgitation (PR) is most often associated with isolated congenital defect or as a result of correction of PS of Tetralogy of Fallot. Additionally, PR can be the result of infective endocarditis and rarely in sarcoidosis. Elevated right ventricular diastolic volume results in eventual dilatation and ventricular failure with predisposition to arrhythmias. PR responds well to medical therapy [55]. Occasionally, PS may require valvuloplasty; yet is markedly responsive to medical therapy as well.

Tricuspid Valve Disease

Tricuspid Stenosis (TS) is rare and may be secondary to rheumatic heart disease in conjunction with mitral and aortic valve disease. Tricuspid atresia is a congenital cause of TS which requires surgery during childhood. Often mild-moderate TS is well tolerated in the setting of pregnancy. Tricuspid regurgitation may be a postoperative consequence of surgical correction of primary or secondary tricuspid disease, e.g. the result IE from intravenous drug abuse. Tricuspid disease is generally well tolerated during pregnancy with medical management used as necessary for symptomatic improvement [57].

Valve Surgery During Pregnancy

Severe valvular disease prior to pregnancy poses a dilemma. Ideally, severe valves disease that could compromise mother and fetus should be addressed prior to pregnancy. However, this is often not the case, especially in the medically underserved community. Most pregnant women with symptomatic valve disease can be treated medically, and catheter-bases or surgical correction can be deferred until after delivery. However, those with life-threatening complications will require intervention. Balloon valvuloplasty could be considered for women with severe symptomatic MS with favorable anatomy, who either are planning to become pregnant or as a therapeutic measure during pregnancy. Balloon mitral valvuloplasty can achieve excellent symptomatic and hemodynamic results with low risk to the mother and fetus [8]. Balloon aortic valvuloplasty is indicated only as a temporizing measure in severely symptomatic AS. The improvement in hemodynamics is often only fair, and there is limited data on the efficacy and rate of restenosis during pregnancy. Careful shielding of the fetus to minimize radiation exposed is essential.

In select instances, progression of valvular disease beyond medical management may occur, as in the case of cardiac decompensation and hemodynamic instability, which may require emergency valve repair. Emergent valve replacement during pregnancy has not been shown to increase maternal mortality. However, there is a significant threat to the fetus secondary to intraoperative decrease in perfusion; 12–20 % fetal loss rate has been reported [55]. Most valvular conditions during pregnancy can be medically managed, with consideration for postpartum replacement surgery if indicated [2].

The choice of tissue versus mechanical valve replacement prior to or during pregnancy hinges on a variety of factors, including patient profile, medication compliance, and risks emboli, hemorrhage, adverse anticoagulation-related events, and risk of structural valve degeneration. Accelerated pregnancy-related structural degeneration is reported [2]. An additional consideration is the likelihood of multiple gestations in the future.

The main benefit of a tissue valve is the lack of need for anticoagulation. Anticoagulation can be difficult to administer and regulate, requires patient cooperation, can induce teratogenicity, and increases risk of peripartum maternal and neonatal hemorrhage. Tissue valves have limited durability, and may require replacement in 5–10 years, exposing the mother to the risk addition surgery.

Mechanical valve prostheses, although more durable than tissue prostheses, require optimized anticoagulation in order to prevent valve thrombosis, thromboemboli, or hemorrhage. Warfarin is associated with embryopathy (6th to 12th week gestation), fetal loss, and increased risk of fetal cerebral hemorrhage; it is therefore avoided [8], especially in the first trimester. Unfractionated heparin, although it does not cross the placental barrier, has been shown to increase the rate of maternal thrombosis and bleeding. Pregnant women should imperatively receive informed counseling concerning anticoagulation treatment options, including increased risk associated with heparin use

(ACC/AHA Class I recommendation) [8]. Additionally, women who are considered high-risk (history of thromboembolic phenomena or older-generation mechanical mitral prosthesis) who opt not to take warfarin first trimester should receive unfractionated heparin continuously with mid-interval prolongation of the aPTT to two to three times control, with subsequent transition to warfarin after first trimester (AHA/ACC Class I recommendation) [8]. Should warfarin be chosen, maintaining INR 2–3 with low dose warfarin and low dose aspirin (Class IIa) [8] is recommended. Women at low risk (no history of thromboembolic disease and newer-generation prosthesis) can be managed with adjusted-dose heparin to prolong the mid-interval aPTT to two to three times control (Class IIb) [8]. Prior to week 36, in anticipation of deliver, warfarin should be discontinued with transition to heparin. Should labor occur while on warfarin, Cesarean section is the preferred delivery method. In the absence of significant bleeding postpartum, the patient can be transitioned to warfarin (Class IIa)

[8]. While data on the safety and efficacy of low molecular weight heparin (LMWH) is limited, current guidelines recommend that pregnant patients with mechanical prosthetic valves who receive dose-adjusted LMWH, the LMWH should be administered twice daily subcutaneously to maintain the anti-Xa level between 0.7 and 1.2 U per ml 4 h after administration (Class IIa) [8]. Anti-Xa levels should be measured weekly throughout gestation. Aspirin at 75 mg daily can be added to this regimen to reduce risk of thrombosis, but with the potential for increased risk of bleeding.

Peripartum Management

Most women with valve disease can be delivered vaginally. Induction of labor and use of forceps are recommended and employed in some centers. Peripartum complications are equivalent to those who undergo a C-section. Careful hemodynamic monitoring may be required, and monitoring should continued for approximately 48 h post partum, because of fluid shifts that occur during this period. Routine IE prophylaxis is not longer recommended [2].

Conclusions

Valve disease in women differs from that in men in a number of important aspects. While the overall prevalence is equal, differences in etiology, structural alterations resulting from valve disease-induced alterations hemodynamic loading condition, and physiognomy affect the diagnosis, severity assessment, and therapy. Pregnancy complicated by valve disease is a challenge that requires specific diagnostic and therapeutic approaches.

References

1. Robbins SL. Pathology. 3rd ed. Philadelphia: W.B. Saunders Company; 1967. p. 512.
2. Otto CM, Bonow R. Valvular heart disease: a companion to Braunwald's heart disease. 3rd ed. Philadelphia: Elsevier; 2009.
3. Yoran C, Yellin EL, Becker RM, Gabbay S, Frater RW, Sonnenblick EH. Dynamic aspects of acute mitral regurgitation: effects of ventricular volume, pressure and contractility on the effective regurgitant orifice area. Circulation. 1979;60:170–6.
4. Bonow R, Mann D, Zipes D, Libby P. Braunwald's heart disease: a textbook of cardiovascular medicine. 9th ed. 2011.
5. Carabello BA. Modern management of mitral stenosis. Circulation. 2005;112:432–7.
6. Jensen MO, Hagege AA, Otsuji Y, Levine RA, Leducq Transatlantic MITRAL Network. The unsaddled annulus: biomechanical culprit in mitral valve prolapse? Circulation. 2013;127:766–8.
7. Devereux RB. Mitral valve prolapse. J Am Med Womens Assoc. 1994;49:192–7.

8. Bonow RO, Carabello BA, Chatterjee K, de Leon AC, Jr FDP, Freed MD, Gaasch WH, Lytle BW, Nishimura RA, O'Gara PT, O'Rourke RA, Otto CM, Shah PM, Shanewise JS, 2006 Writing Committee Members, American College of Cardiology/American Heart Association Task Force. 2008 Focused update incorporated into the ACC/AHA 2006 guidelines for the management of patients with valvular heart disease: a report of the American College of Cardiology/American Heart Association Task Force on Practice Guidelines (Writing Committee to revise the 1998 guidelines for the management of patients with valvular heart disease): endorsed by the Society of Cardiovascular Anesthesiologists, Society for Cardiovascular Angiography and Interventions, and Society of Thoracic Surgeons. Circulation. 2008;118:e523–661.

9. Lambert AS. Proximal isovelocity surface area should be routinely measured in evaluating mitral regurgitation: a core review. Anesth Analg. 2007;105:940–3.

10. American College of Cardiology/American Heart Association Task Force on Practice Guidelines, Society of Cardiovascular Anesthesiologists, Society for Cardiovascular Angiography and Interventions, Society of Thoracic Surgeons, Bonow RO, Carabello BA, Kanu C, de Leon Jr AC, Faxon DP, Freed MD, Gaasch WH, Lytle BW, Nishimura RA, O'Gara PT, O'Rourke RA, Otto CM, Shah PM, Shanewise JS, Smith Jr SC, Jacobs AK, Adams CD, Anderson JL, Antman EM, Faxon DP, Fuster V, Halperin JL, Hiratzka LF, Hunt SA, Lytle BW, Nishimura R, Page RL, Riegel B. ACC/AHA 2006 guidelines for the management of patients with valvular heart disease: a report of the American College of Cardiology/American Heart Association Task Force on Practice Guidelines (writing committee to revise the 1998 guidelines for the management of patients with valvular heart disease): developed in collaboration with the Society of Cardiovascular Anesthesiologists: endorsed by the Society for Cardiovascular Angiography and Interventions and the Society of Thoracic Surgeons. Circulation. 2006;114:e84–231.

11. Zoghbi WA, Enriquez-Sarano M, Foster E, Grayburn PA, Kraft CD, Levine RA, Nihoyannopoulos P, Otto CM, Quinones MA, Rakowski H, Stewart WJ, Waggoner A, Weissman NJ. Recommendations for evaluation of the severity of native valvular regurgitation with two-dimensional and doppler echocardiography. J Am Soc Echocardiogr. 2003;16:777–802.

12. Rohde LE, Zhi G, Aranki SF, Beckel NE, Lee RT, Reimold SC. Gender-associated differences in left ventricular geometry in patients with aortic valve disease and effect of distinct overload subsets. Am J Cardiol. 1997;80:475–80.

13. Keren G, Katz S, Strom J, Sonnenblick EH, LeJemtel TH. Noninvasive quantification of mitral regurgitation in dilated cardiomyopathy: correlation of two Doppler echocardiographic methods. Am Heart J. 1988;116:758–64.

14. Maganti K, Rigolin VH, Sarano ME, Bonow RO. Valvular heart disease: diagnosis and management. Mayo Clin Proc. 2010;85:483–500.

15. Baumgartner H, Hung J, Bermejo J, Chambers JB, Evangelista A, Griffin BP, Iung B, Otto CM, Pellikka PA, Quinones M, American Society of Echocardiography, European Association of Echocardiography. Echocardiographic assessment of valve stenosis: EAE/ASE recommendations for clinical practice. J Am Soc Echocardiogr. 2009;22:1–23; quiz 101–2.

16. Abascal VM, Wilkins GT, O'Shea JP, Choong CY, Palacios IF, Thomas JD, Rosas E, Newell JB, Block PC, Weyman AE. Prediction of successful outcome in 130 patients undergoing percutaneous balloon mitral valvotomy. Circulation. 1990;82:448–56.

17. Gorlin R, Gorlin SG. Hydraulic formula for calculation of the area of the stenotic mitral valve, other cardiac valves, and central circulatory shunts. I. Am Heart J. 1951;41:1–29.

18. Otto CM. Valvular heart disease: focus on women. Cardiol Rev. 2007;15:291–7.

19. Carabello BA. The current therapy for mitral regurgitation. J Am Coll Cardiol. 2008;52: 319–26.

20. Magne J, Girerd N, Senechal M, Mathieu P, Dagenais F, Dumesnil JG, Charbonneau E, Voisine P, Pibarot P. Mitral repair versus replacement for ischemic mitral regurgitation: comparison of short-term and long-term survival. Circulation. 2009;120:S104–11.

21. Reece TB, Tribble CG, Ellman PI, Maxey TS, Woodford RL, Dimeling GM, Wellons HA, Crosby IK, Kern JA, Kron IL. Mitral repair is superior to replacement when associated with coronary artery disease. Ann Surg. 2004;239:671–5; discussion 675–7.

22. Feldman T, Foster E, Glower DD, Kar S, Rinaldi MJ, Fail PS, Smalling RW, Siegel R, Rose GA, Engeron E, Loghin C, Trento A, Skipper ER, Fudge T, Letsou GV, Massaro JM, Mauri L,

EVEREST II Investigators. Percutaneous repair or surgery for mitral regurgitation. N Engl J Med. 2011;364:1395–406.

23. Nobuyoshi M, Arita T, Shirai S, Hamasaki N, Yokoi H, Iwabuchi M, Yasumoto H, Nosaka H. Percutaneous balloon mitral valvuloplasty: a review. Circulation. 2009;119:e211–9.

24. Aortic Stenosis. Available at: http://emedicine.medscape.com/article/150638-overview#aw2aab6b2b4aa.

25. Freeman RV, Otto CM. Spectrum of calcific aortic valve disease: pathogenesis, disease progression, and treatment strategies. Circulation. 2005;111:3316–26.

26. Strom JA, VanAuker MD, Carabello BA. Effects of aging on the diagnostic assessment of valvular heart disease. Am J Geriatr Cardiol. 2006;15:286–90.

27. Kostkiewicz M, Tracz W, Olszowska M, Podolec P, Drop D. Left ventricular geometry and function in patients with aortic stenosis: gender differences. Int J Cardiol. 1999;71:57–61.

28. Aurigemma GP, Gaasch WH. Gender differences in older patients with pressure-overload hypertrophy of the left ventricle. Cardiology. 1995;86:310–7.

29. Clavel MA, Dumesnil JG, Capoulade R, Mathieu P, Senechal M, Pibarot P. Outcome of patients with aortic stenosis, small valve area, and low-flow, low-gradient despite preserved left ventricular ejection fraction. J Am Coll Cardiol. 2012;60:1259–67.

30. Jander N, Minners J, Holme I, Gerdts E, Boman K, Brudi P, Chambers JB, Egstrup K, Kesaniemi YA, Malbecq W, Nienaber CA, Ray S, Rossebo A, Pedersen TR, Skjaerpe T, Willenheimer R, Wachtell K, Neumann FJ, Gohlke-Barwolf C. Outcome of patients with low-gradient "severe" aortic stenosis and preserved ejection fraction. Circulation. 2011; 123:887–95.

31. Clavel MA, Ennezat PV, Marechaux S, Dumesnil JG, Capoulade R, Hachicha Z, Mathieu P, Bellouin A, Bergeron S, Meimoun P, Arsenault M, Le Tourneau T, Pasquet A, Couture C, Pibarot P. Stress echocardiography to assess stenosis severity and predict outcome in patients with paradoxical low-flow, low-gradient aortic stenosis and preserved LVEF. JACC Cardiovasc Imaging. 2013;6:175–83.

32. Spevack DM, Almuti K, Ostfeld R, Bello R, Gordon GM. Routine adjustment of Doppler echocardiographically derived aortic valve area using a previously derived equation to account for the effect of pressure recovery. J Am Soc Echocardiogr. 2008;21:34–7.

33. Joint Task Force on the Management of Valvular Heart Disease of the European Society of Cardiology (ESC), European Association for Cardio-Thoracic Surgery (EACTS), Vahanian A, Alfieri O, Andreotti F, Antunes MJ, Baron-Esquivias G, Baumgartner H, Borger MA, Carrel TP, De Bonis M, Evangelista A, Falk V, Iung B, Lancellotti P, Pierard L, Price S, Schafers HJ, Schuler G, Stepinska J, Swedberg K, Takkenberg J, Von Oppell UO, Windecker S, Zamorano JL, Zembala M. Guidelines on the management of valvular heart disease (version 2012). Eur Heart J. 2012;33:2451–96.

34. Rosenhek R, Binder T, Porenta G, Lang I, Christ G, Schemper M, Maurer G, Baumgartner H. Predictors of outcome in severe, asymptomatic aortic stenosis. N Engl J Med. 2000;343:611–7.

35. Otto CM, Burwash IG, Legget ME, Munt BI, Fujioka M, Healy NL, Kraft CD, Miyake-Hull CY, Schwaegler RG. Prospective study of asymptomatic valvular aortic stenosis. Clinical, echocardiographic, and exercise predictors of outcome. Circulation. 1997;95:2262–70.

36. Sambola A, Tornos P, Ferreira-Gonzalez I, Evangelista A. Prognostic value of preoperative indexed end-systolic left ventricle diameter in the outcome after surgery in patients with chronic aortic regurgitation. Am Heart J. 2008;155:1114–20.

37. Tornos P, Sambola A, Permanyer-Miralda G, Evangelista A, Gomez Z, Soler-Soler J. Long-term outcome of surgically treated aortic regurgitation: influence of guideline adherence toward early surgery. J Am Coll Cardiol. 2006;47:1012–7.

38. Laniado S, Yellin EL, Yoran C, Strom J, Hori M, Gabbay S, Terdiman R, Frater RWM. Physiologic mechanisms in aortic insufficiency. I. The effect of changing heart rate on flow dynamics. II. Determinants of Austin Flint murmur. Circulation. 1982;66:226–35.

39. Strom J, Becker R, Davis R, Matsumoto M, Frishman W, Sonnenblick EH, Frater RW. Echocardiographic and surgical correlations in bacterial endocarditis. Circulation. 1980;62:I164–7.

40. Taylor J. ESC/EACTS guidelines on the management of valvular heart disease. Eur Heart J. 2012;33:2371–2.

41. Morris JJ, Schaff HV, Mullany CJ, Morris PB, Frye RL, Orszulak TA. Gender differences in left ventricular functional response to aortic valve replacement. Circulation. 1994;90:II183–9.
42. Walther T, Blumenstein J, van Linden A, Kempfert J. Contemporary management of aortic stenosis: surgical aortic valve replacement remains the gold standard. Heart. 2012;98 Suppl 4:iv23–9.
43. Cowell SJ, Newby DE, Prescott RJ, Bloomfield P, Reid J, Northridge DB, Boon NA, Scottish Aortic Stenosis and Lipid Lowering Trial, Impact on Regression (SALTIRE) Investigators. A randomized trial of intensive lipid-lowering therapy in calcific aortic stenosis. N Engl J Med. 2005;352:2389–97.
44. Carabello BA, Paulus WJ. Aortic stenosis. Lancet. 2009;373:956–66.
45. Otto CM. Valvular aortic stenosis: disease severity and timing of intervention. J Am Coll Cardiol. 2006;47:2141–51.
46. Makkar RR, Fontana GP, Jilaihawi H, Kapadia S, Pichard AD, Douglas PS, Thourani VH, Babaliaros VC, Webb JG, Herrmann HC, Bavaria JE, Kodali S, Brown DL, Bowers B, Dewey TM, Svensson LG, Tuzcu M, Moses JW, Williams MR, Siegel RJ, Akin JJ, Anderson WN, Pocock S, Smith CR, Leon MB, PARTNER Trial Investigators. Transcatheter aortic-valve replacement for inoperable severe aortic stenosis. N Engl J Med. 2012;366:1696–704.
47. Kodali SK, Williams MR, Smith CR, Svensson LG, Webb JG, Makkar RR, Fontana GP, Dewey TM, Thourani VH, Pichard AD, Fischbein M, Szeto WY, Lim S, Greason KL, Teirstein PS, Malaisrie SC, Douglas PS, Hahn RT, Whisenant B, Zajarias A, Wang D, Akin JJ, Anderson WN, Leon MB, PARTNER Trial Investigators. Two-year outcomes after transcatheter or surgical aortic-valve replacement. N Engl J Med. 2012;366:1686–95.
48. Reynolds MR, Magnuson EA, Wang K, Lei Y, Vilain K, Walczak J, Kodali SK, Lasala JM, O'Neill WW, Davidson CJ, Smith CR, Leon MB, Cohen DJ, PARTNER Investigators. Cost-effectiveness of transcatheter aortic valve replacement compared with standard care among inoperable patients with severe aortic stenosis: results from the placement of aortic transcatheter valves (PARTNER) trial (Cohort B). Circulation. 2012;125:1102–9.
49. Kalavrouziotis D, Rodes-Cabau J, Bagur R, Doyle D, De Larochelliere R, Pibarot P, Dumont E. Transcatheter aortic valve implantation in patients with severe aortic stenosis and small aortic annulus. J Am Coll Cardiol. 2011;58:1016–24.
50. Hayashida K, Morice MC, Chevalier B, Hovasse T, Romano M, Garot P, Farge A, Donzeau-Gouge P, Bouvier E, Cormier B, Lefevre T. Sex-related differences in clinical presentation and outcome of transcatheter aortic valve implantation for severe aortic stenosis. J Am Coll Cardiol. 2012;59:566–71.
51. Hoen B, Duval X. Clinical practice. Infective endocarditis. N Engl J Med. 2013;368:1425–33.
52. Prendergast BD, Tornos P. Surgery for infective endocarditis: who and when? Circulation. 2010;121:1141–52.
53. Nishimura RA, Carabello BA, Faxon DP, Freed MD, Lytle BW, O'Gara PT, O'Rourke RA, Shah PM, Bonow RO, Carabello BA, Chatterjee K, de Leon AC, Jr FDP, Freed MD, Gaasch WH, Lytle BW, Nishimura RA, O'Gara PT, O'Rourke RA, Otto CM, Shah PM, Shanewise JS, Smith Jr SC, Jacobs AK, Buller CE, Creager MA, Ettinger SM, Krumholz HM, Kushner FG, Lytle BW, Nishimura RA, Page RL, Tarkington LG, Yancy Jr CW, American College of Cardiology/American Heart Association Task Force. ACC/AHA 2008 guideline update on valvular heart disease: focused update on infective endocarditis: a report of the American College of Cardiology/American Heart Association Task Force on Practice Guidelines: endorsed by the Society of Cardiovascular Anesthesiologists, Society for Cardiovascular Angiography and Interventions, and Society of Thoracic Surgeons. Circulation. 2008;118:887–96.
54. Roldan CA. Valvular and coronary heart disease in systemic inflammatory diseases: systemic disorders in heart disease. Heart. 2008;94:1089–101.
55. Wang A, Bashore TM. Valvular heart disease. 1st ed. New York: Humana Press; 2009.
56. Loue S, Sajatovic M. Encyclopedia of women's health. 1st ed. New York: Kluwer Academic/ Plenum Publishers; 2004.
57. Wenger NK, Collins P. Women heart disease. 2nd ed. London: Taylor and Francis; 2000.

Chapter 10
Arrhythmias in Women: A Practical Approach

Rachel Lee and Christine Tompkins

Introduction

Gender differences exist in cardiac electrophysiology, which significantly impact the presentation, diagnosis and management of arrhythmias in women. This chapter provides a general understanding of these differences to help guide general practitioners in the daily management of female patients. We start with a basic overview of the proposed mechanisms behind these gender differences, then review specific arrhythmias, highlighting features unique to women.

Cyclical variations in sex hormones influence the clinical presentation of arrhythmias during the menstrual cycle, pregnancy, post-partum period and menopause. Although these mechanisms are not fully understood, they help to explain gender differences in heart rate, heart rate variability, and the surface electrocardiogram (ECG). These concepts provide the foundation for our gender relevant discussion regarding the diagnosis and management of specific cardiac arrhythmias in women.

R. Lee, MD
Division of Cardiology, University of Florida Health Science Center, Jacksonville, FL, USA

Division of Cardiology, University of Florida College of Medicine-Jacksonville, Jacksonville, FL, USA

C. Tompkins, MD (✉)
Division of Cardiology, University of Rochester Medical Center,
601 Elmwood Ave, 679-Y, Rochester, NY 14642, USA
e-mail: christine_tompkins@urmc.rochester.edu

H.Z. Mieszczanska, G.P. Velarde (eds.),
Management of Cardiovascular Disease in Women,
DOI 10.1007/978-1-4471-5517-1_10, © Springer-Verlag London 2014

Gender Differences in Heart Rate, Heart Rate Variability, and the Electrocardiogram

Differences in the heart rate and QT interval on the surface ECG are among the most commonly reported findings between men and women. Women have higher resting heart rates by an average of 3–5 beats/min [1–4] and longer QT intervals than men [5, 6]. Women also exhibit greater heart rate variability (HRV) that gradually diminishes as women age [7–11]. Heart rate variability, a measure of the beat-to-beat variation in heart rate, is largely dependent on a balance between parasympathetic and sympathetic activity and is often used as a surrogate measure of autonomic function. Reduced heart rate variability has been shown to be a predictor of cardiac events [12–16]. Higher HRV is observed in premenopausal women, suggesting that sex hormones (i.e. estrogen and/or progesterone) favorably influence HRV and may play a cardio-protective role in younger woman [17, 18].

Gender differences in the QT interval are also due to differences in sex hormones [19]. Women have a longer corrected QT interval and are more prone to developing acquired long QT syndrome and Torsades de Pointes (TdP) [20, 21]. In fact, up to 65–75 % of drug-induced long QT syndrome occurs in women [22]. Therefore, when caring for the female patient it is important to take into account that women are more susceptible to the effects of QT prolonging medications [23]. In an editorial by Okin, the author points out that gender differences impact the prognostic and diagnostic accuracy of the ECG in women [24]. However there are currently no sex-specific diagnostic ECG criteria to guide management of female patients.

Mechanisms of Gender Differences and Effects of Sex Hormones

In a comprehensive review by Villareal et al. and Yang et al., [25, 26] the mechanisms for gender differences in cardiac electrical properties can be summarized into two postulated mechanisms: (1) direct effects of sex hormones on the distribution, expression and function of cardiac ion channels and (2) influence of sex hormones on autonomic tone. Estrogen (in the form of 17-beta estradiol), progesterone and testosterone mainly influence L-type calcium channels and delayed rectifier potassium channels. In a complex, dose-dependent fashion, these hormones can either prolong or shorten the action potential thereby altering repolarization characteristics [27–34]. In addition, there is evidence that sex hormones influence autonomic tone [35–39].

Understanding the effects of sex hormones on ventricular repolarization provides the basis for understanding gender differences in arrhythmias; why women are at risk for prolonged QTc and TdP, why there is increased risk of syncope and sudden death in congenital long QT syndrome, and why certain arrhythmias are more common during different periods of a woman's reproductive cycle.

Influence on Menstrual Cycle, Pregnancy, Post-partum, and Menopause

Cyclical variations in sex hormones during the menstrual cycle affect the QT interval. During the luteal phase, progesterone levels are high relative to estrogen, while estrogen dominates the follicular phase and ovulation. The QT interval tends to be prolonged during the follicular phase and women with inherited long QT syndrome are found to be at increased risk for TdP [40, 41]. Interestingly, the post-menopausal phase is characterized by an increased risk for recurrent syncope in women with LQT2, but a risk reduction in women with LQT1 [42]. The mechanism underlying this paradox is unknown, but is likely influenced by sex hormone modulation of the delayed rectifier channel based on the specific gene mutations associated with inherited long QT syndrome types 1 (gene mutation in slow component of the delayed rectifier channel, I_{Ks}) and 2 (gene mutation in rapid component of delayed rectifier channel, I_{Kr}). Studies investigating the effect of hormone replacement therapy on the QT interval have provided conflicting results [43–45]. Thus, despite an intriguing association, there is no data to support the use of hormone replacement therapy to reduce the risk of cardiac arrhythmias [46].

During the menstrual cycle, variations in hormone levels also affect the clinical presentation of supraventricular tachycardias (SVT) and should be considered when scheduling ambulatory monitoring or diagnostic electrophysiologic (EP) studies. In a study by Rosano et al., SVT was shown to occur most frequently during the luteal phase of the menstrual cycle when progesterone levels are at their highest [47]. Myerburg et al., applied this information to the timing EP studies and found that women are more easily inducible during the premenstrual (i.e. the luteal phase, within 72 h of the onset of menses) phase [48].

During pregnancy, when estrogen and progesterone levels are at their highest, women without hereditary arrhythmias, congenital or structural heart disease do not appear to be at increased risk for cardiac arrhythmias and sudden cardiac death [49]. Similarly, women with inherited LQTS do not appear to be at increased risk for cardiac events during pregnancy, however, demonstrate a remarkable 40-fold increase of cardiac events during the post-partum period [50]. It is postulated that sinus tachycardia present during pregnancy may have a cardioprotective effect against sudden cardiac death due to a decrease in the QT interval [51]. Beta blocker prophylaxis has been shown to be effective in reducing abnormally elevated heart rates during pregnancy and at reducing the risk of cardiac events during the post-partum phase in women with congenital LQTS.

Syncope and Palpitations

Syncope and palpitations are very common symptoms among women. In a large cohort of patients presenting to the Emergency Room with palpitations and syncope, 60 % were woman. These women were found to have higher proportion of postural tachycardia syndrome (POTS) and orthostatic hypotension [52].

Palpitations can be broadly defined as an unpleasant sensation of a racing or pounding heart. Patients frequently describe skipped beats, irregular heart beats, bursts of fast heart rates or robust cardiac contractions. An understanding of the patient's experience when using the term "palpitations" is an important initial step in the evaluation. Someone describing the occasional "flip-flop" in the chest is likely experiencing either atrial or ventricular premature beats, whereas a patient is likely to have a reentrant arrhythmia such as AV Node Reentrant Tachycardia (AVNRT) or accessory pathway-mediated reentrant tachycardias (AVRT) when describing the abrupt onset of a rapid, regular heart beat that terminates with vagal maneuvers. The history in patients presenting with palpitations should include: onset (abrupt or gradual), duration, termination (abrupt or gradual), frequency (daily, weekly monthly, etc.), triggers, alleviating factors and associated symptoms. Fast heart rhythms with gradual onset and termination suggest sinus tachycardia as can be seen in inappropriate sinus tachycardia (IST) or postural tachycardia syndrome (POTS), whereas the abrupt onset and termination of fast heart beats suggests an arrhythmia (such as AVNRT, AVRT, AT, atrial flutter or fibrillation). Termination with vagal maneuvers, such as bearing down or deep cough can be quite helpful in identifying reentrant arrhythmias dependent on the AV node (such as AVNRT or AVRT).

It is important to inquire specifically about syncope or near-syncope in relation to or independent of palpitations. Syncope is present in approximately 15 % of patients with SVT and is most commonly caused by a prolonged pause following the abrupt termination of an SVT, but can also be observed as a consequence of rapid heart rates during SVT, particularly in the dehydrated state or the presence of structural heart disease. Neck fullness during SVT is a helpful symptom that is often associated with AVNRT and is due to atrial contraction against closed AV (i.e. mitral and tricuspid) valves. It can also occurs in arrhythmias that present with AV dissociation, such as ventricular tachycardia or complete heart block. Polyuria is also an uncommon but helpful symptom associated with supraventricular tachycardias that is caused by release of atrial natriuretic peptide from abrupt increases in atrial pressures when the atria contract against closed AV valves.

Distinguishing between concerning causes of syncope such as arrhythmic syncope versus more benign causes such as neurocardiogenic syncope is paramount. Patients found to have true cardiac syncope (i.e. due to malignant, life-threatening arrhythmias) were found to have a 6-month mortality of 10 % whereas patients with vasovagal syncope had a benign prognosis, similar to those without syncope [53]. The main goal of the initial evaluation of syncope and palpitations is to identify patients who are at high risk for sudden cardiac death and significant life-threatening arrhythmias.

Evaluation of Syncope

The European Society of Cardiology (ESC) Guidelines and the American Heart Association/American College of Cardiology Foundation (AHA/ACCF) Scientific

Statement provides the basis for the initial evaluation of syncope [54]. The initial evaluation of syncope and palpitations in women should start with a thorough history and physical exam. The history should focus on any symptoms present prior to syncope or reversible causes of syncope (i.e. hypoglycemia, simple mechanical falls, etc.) and any history or risk factors for structural cardiac disease. Syncope associated with prolonged standing or changes in body position suggest neurocardiogenic syncope or orthostatic hypotension, while a history lacking orthostatic components may suggest more concerning causes, such as a tachy- or bradyarrhythmias.

The physical exam should include a cardiac exam, orthostatic blood pressure, and in the older patient carotid sinus massage. An ECG will provide valuable information about the heart rate, rhythm, abnormal Q-waves suggestive of prior myocardial infarctions, delta waves suggestive of pre-excitation, large R-wave amplitudes suggestive of hypertensive heart disease or hypertrophic cardiomyopathy (in patients without a history of hypertension); or repolarization abnormalities such as prolonged QT interval due to inherited or acquired LQTS or precordial T-wave inversions seen in ARVC. The ACC/AHA defines an abnormally prolonged QTc in women as ≥460 ms in women and ≥450 ms in men and anything >480 ms is certainly concerning [55, 56].

If after this initial evaluation, a primary cardiac cause for syncope remains possible, then echocardiography, Holter monitoring for 24–48 h, or Event monitoring for 3–4 weeks may be useful. Further testing with tilt table testing can help to identify the presence of neurocardiogenic cause of syncope and define the type of response (i.e. cardioinhibitory or vasodepressor). However, this should be a diagnosis of exclusion in women with a history of syncope or near-syncope. The initial approach to diagnostic testing in a patient with unexplained syncope is shown in Fig. 10.1.

Evaluation of Palpitations

A 12-lead electrocardiogram is the initial evaluation for all patients with palpitations. This should be evaluated for evidence of structural changes (such as left atrial enlargement, left ventricular hypertrophy, pre-excitation, prior myocardial infarction, etc.), and atrial or ventricular ectopy. Efforts to obtain a 12-lead ECG during symptoms are extraordinarily helpful and should be pursued as long as it does not hinder acute management of an unstable patient.

Ambulatory monitoring can be extremely helpful associating symptoms with cardiac rhythms. A 24- or 48-Holter monitor should be pursued in patients with frequent (i.e. daily) symptoms, whereas a 30-day event monitor should be pursued in those with less frequent (i.e. weekly) symptoms. The benefit of these monitors is that they can provide information regarding how the arrhythmias start and end. An implantable loop monitor may be appropriate in patients with very infrequent (episodes occurring less than monthly), but severe symptoms such as syncope with traumatic injuries. An exercise treadmill test is useful in patients with exertion-related symptoms.

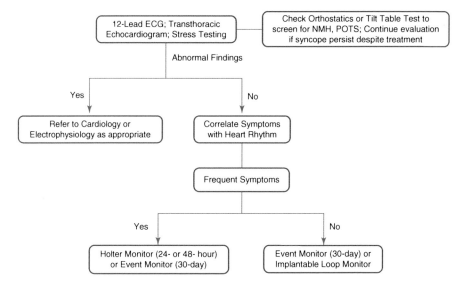

Fig. 10.1 The initial approach to the patient with unexplained syncope

Echocardiography is not necessarily part of the initial assessment in patients with palpitations, but should be considered in those with evidence of structural heart disease on the surface ECG (i.e. hypertrophy, atrial enlargement, Q-waves, etc.). Finally, an invasive electrophysiology study (EPS) with catheter ablation can be considered in patients with a clear history of paroxysmal SVT terminated by vagal maneuvers or evidence of pre-excitation on surface ECG for definitive treatment. The initial approach to diagnostic testing in a patient with palpitations is shown in Fig. 10.2.

Specific Cardiac Arrhythmias

Inappropriate Sinus Tachycardia (IST)

Inappropriate sinus tachycardia is an uncommon and poorly understood syndrome that is defined by non-paroxysmal elevated resting heart rates greater than 100 bpm and/or an exaggerated heart rate response to exercise or stress [57, 58]. The majority of patients with IST are women with the literature citing as many as 90 % of patients [59, 60]. Symptoms include palpitations, weakness, fatigue, lightheadedness, and near syncope. The diagnosis is made when ambulatory monitoring shows elevated resting heart rates (i.e. average heart rate >90 bpm) on a 24-h Holter monitor. It is important to exclude secondary causes of sinus tachycardia, such as drugs, hyperthyroidism, fever, anemia, and infection. There is overlap between the diagnosis of postural orthostatic tachycardia syndrome (POTS) and IST. POTS is defined as the

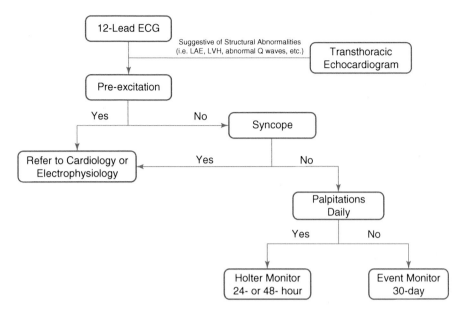

Fig. 10.2 The initial approach to the patient with palpitations

presence of symptoms due to orthostatic intolerance with a heart rate increase of ≥30 bpm (or heart rate that exceeds 120 bpm) within the first 10 min of standing or upright tilt that is not associated with a decline in blood pressure or any debilitating conditions or medications that would diminish vascular tone [61]. POTS can be distinguished from IST by noting an abnormal increase in heart rate that is associated with changes in body position [62] and can be diagnosed using Tilt Table Testing [63]. No proven effective treatment exists for IST. Symptomatic patients can be treated with beta blockers as first line therapy along with lifestyle changes to eliminate any known triggers such as stimulants (caffeine, alcohol, medications). As anxiety can often be superimposed on IST management of anxiety with counseling and benzodiazepines may sometimes be required.

Ivabradine, a specific funny current (I_f) blocker, is currently under investigation as a promising new treatment option for IST. In the first randomized, double-blind placebo controlled crossover trial in patients with IST, Ivabradine significantly reduced heart rates and eliminated >70 % of symptoms reported at baseline; with 50 % of patients reporting complete symptom resolution [64]. In another study of 20 patients, comparing metoprolol succinate and Ivabradine, both drugs were shown to have similar effects on heart rate, however, Ivabradine was more effective than metoprolol in treating symptoms of IST with 70 % of patients reporting elimination of symptoms [65]. Ivabradine is currently not available in the United States and should be avoided in hypotensive, pregnant, and breastfeeding patients [62]. Radiofrequency ablation is rarely effective for IST and should only be considered in extreme symptomatic cases when medical treatment has failed and symptoms have clearly been shown to be associated with fast heart rates [66, 67]. IST is not usually associated with any structural heart disease or secondary causes of sinus tachycardia and tends to have a benign natural history [68].

Atrioventricular Nodal Reentrant Tachycardia (AVNRT)

Atrioventricular Node Reentrant Tachycardia (AVNRT) is the most prevalent paroxysmal supraventricular tachycardia (SVT) in females with a 2:1 predominance over males [69–73]. The diagnosis and management of AVNRT should not be any different from men.

Common signs and symptoms include the abrupt onset of rapid regular palpitations that can be associated with chest tightness, dizziness, and neck pulsations. Heart rates range from 140 to 250 in this rhythm and AVNRT is not typically associated with structural heart disease. Medications have only a modest effect in reducing the frequency of both AVNRT and AVRT. The 2003 ACC/AHA guidelines recommend catheter ablation as first line treatment (Class I) for patients with recurrent symptomatic episodes, patients with infrequent or single episodes who desire definitive treatment, and for patients with infrequent, well-tolerated AVNRT [74].

In those patients who prefer medical management over ablation, standard medical therapy includes non-dihydropyridine calcium channel blockers, beta blockers, or digoxin as first line therapy. Patients should be taught to perform vagal maneuvers (deep cough, bearing down, squatting) immediately at the onset of symptoms as this has greater efficacy than medical therapy. The 30-day recurrence rate following treatment with diltiazem [75] was 60 and 20–40 % with flecainide [76]. The decision to medically manage or ablate should be patient specific and should take into account frequency and duration of symptoms, the effectiveness and tolerance to drugs, and presence of structural heart disease. Radiofrequency ablation is recommended in women who plan to become pregnant in the future to eliminate the possibility of AVNRT complicating the pregnancy. Ablation has a 96 % success rate with recurrence occurring approximately 3–7 %. Patients considering ablation must consider the risk of AV block and need for pacemaker implantation, which can occur in 2–5 % of cases. There is no gender difference in success rates, complications, or recurrence of AVNRT after ablation. However, it has been shown that physicians tend to take a more conservative approach with women; referring women later for ablation after trying more anti-arrhythmic therapy [77, 78].

Atrioventricular Reciprocating Tachycardia (AVRT) (Extra Nodal Accessory Pathways)

AVRT is the second most common paroxysmal SVT in women and is twice as frequent in men. AVRT involves an extranodal accessory pathway that provides a second electrical connection (e.g. in addition to the AV node) between the atria to the ventricles. There are two types of pathways: (a) manifest pathways which conduct electrical signals back and forth between the atrium and ventricle and (b) concealed pathways which can only conduct electrical signals backward from the ventricle to the atrium. Only patients with manifest accessory pathways will have pre-excitation (i.e. delta waves) visible on the surface ECG and represent those patients who are potentially at risk for sudden death.

Delta waves are present on the ECG in 0.15–0.25 % of the general population. Wolf Parkinson White syndrome (WPW) is used to define patients with delta waves on the ECG and symptoms of tachycardia. WPW syndrome is more common in men, and men are more likely to experience atrial fibrillation [70]. The most important consideration in patients with pre-excitation on the ECG is risk stratification for sudden death. Sudden death can occur in the presence of atrial fibrillation/flutter when atrial signals are conducted 1:1 (i.e. at rates ≥200 bpm) to the ventricles over the accessory pathway. Therefore, all patients with delta waves present on the surface ECG must be referred for risk stratification. The clinical features of AVRT are similar to AVNRT and can be distinguished by a thorough electrophysiological study. Like AVNRT, medical therapy tends to be less effective at treating arrhythmias associated with accessory pathways. Drugs used to treat AVRT include, Class I agents such as procainamide, disopyramide, propafenone, and flecainide and Class III agents such as ibutilide, sotalol, and amiodarone. Catheter ablation should be performed for high risk patients, and considered in patients who are symptomatic or fail medical therapy. Outcomes are similar regardless of sex. Because of the increased incidence of SVT in women with accessory pathways during pregnancy, radiofrequency ablation should be considered before these patients attempt pregnancy [77].

Atrial Fibrillation (AFib)/Atrial Flutter (AFl)

Atrial fibrillation is the most common arrhythmia in the United States, affecting over three million people, and the incidence increases with age. It is a supraventricular rhythm with uncoordinated atrial activity demonstrated by fibrillatory (f) waves, with irregular, rapid ventricular response on ECG. Atrial fibrillation is more common in men, however, women tend to have more symptoms that last longer, occur more frequently, and have higher ventricular rates [79, 80]. In addition, women tend to have more impaired quality of life measures than men [81, 82].

Common symptoms include palpitations, fatigue, dyspnea, and dizziness. Physical exam may reveal an irregular pulse, irregular jugular venous pulsations, and variable loudness of first heart sound. Examination should entail seeking for evidence of valvular heart disease, heart failure, sleep apnea or thyroid disorders. Diagnosis is made by documentation on ECG, 24-h Holter or event monitoring.

Management of patients with atrial fibrillation involves the decision to restore and maintain sinus rhythm (i.e. rhythm-control algorithm) versus heart rate control (i.e. rate-control algorithm). Rate control of atrial fibrillation can be achieved with a combination of beta blockers, calcium channel blockers, or digoxin. Restoration of sinus rhythm can be achieved either through electrical cardioversion or pharmacologic cardioversion and sinus rhythm can be maintained with antiarrhythmic medications.

Women tend to fare worse than men with medications for management of atrial fibrillation. Rate-control algorithms are associated with an increased risk of bradycardia, while subgroup analysis of the RACE study (Rate Control versus electrical Cardioversion study) [83] found that women randomized to rhythm-control algorithms did far worse than women managed according to rate-control. Women randomized to rhythm-control were three-times more likely to die from cardiovascular causes, and five-times more likely to develop heart failure or thromboembolic complications than women in the rate-control arm. Similar trends were not observed in men when comparing randomization strategies. Women also experience markedly elevated rates of medication-induced prolonged QT syndrome and torsades de pointes when taking any class of antiarrhythmic medication compared to men. Thus, these factors should be taken into consideration when deciding upon a rhythm-control algorithm with women.

Perhaps as a consequence of the adverse outcomes associated with antiarrhythmic therapy, women are less often treated according to a rhythm-control algorithm and are referred less frequently for cardioversion despite having worse symptoms and longer duration of symptoms than men. Women are also referred less often or later than men for radiofrequency ablation of atrial fibrillation despite similar success rates [84, 85]. Radiofrequency catheter ablation of atrial fibrillation is considered in highly symptomatic patients when symptoms are refractory to medical therapy.

Women have higher rates of thromboembolic complications compared to men, especially those over the age of 75. Elderly women are at especially high risk for disabling strokes, however, despite this finding, are less likely to be started on warfarin [86, 87]. Importantly, anticoagulation should be considered in all women with a CHA2DS2-Vasc score ≥ 2 who do not have any contraindication to anticoagulation.

Associated with atrial fibrillation is atrial flutter, a more organized rhythm with saw-tooth pattern of regular activation called flutter waves (f waves), visible in lead II, III, AVF. In atrial flutter, atrial rates range from 240 to 320 bpm, with inverted flutter waves in the inferior leads (II, III, AVF) and upright flutter waves in V1. Two-to-one AV block is common and can lead to atrial rate of 120–160. Medical therapy of atrial flutter is similar to atrial fibrillation. Because medications tend to be ineffective in atrial flutter, the ACC/AHA guidelines consider catheter ablation to be first line therapy for recurrent atrial flutter regardless of symptoms and cardioversion as first line treatment for the first episode of atrial flutter [74]. Radiofrequency ablation of typical atrial flutter has a 95 % efficacy rate with low procedure-related complication rates.

Atrial fibrillation and atrial flutter are frequently observed together. Following flutter ablation, the incidence of atrial fibrillation is dependent on whether atrial fibrillation was present prior to flutter ablation. For those patients with mostly atrial fibrillation prior to flutter ablation 86 % will develop persistent atrial fibrillation; while 8 % develop atrial fibrillation following flutter ablation when it had not been documented previously.

Atrial Tachycardia

Gender differences in atrial tachycardia have not been as well studied [88]. Rates appear to be similar between men and women with similar outcomes following radiofrequency ablation [88, 89]. Focal atrial tachycardia occurs when an electrical impulse eminate from a site outside of the sinus node. It tends to occur in older patients with structural heart disease or underlying medical and pulmonary conditions. The ECG reveals a non-sinus P wave morphology and axis, and a narrow QRS complex. Although there are no large studies assessing the efficacy of different pharmacological strategies, medications such as beta-blockers or calcium channel blockers are typically the first line of medical therapy. Antiarrhythmic medications (typically class Ia or Ic) can be tried if beta-blockers or calcium channel blockers fail. An EP study should be pursued in cases of incessant atrial tachycardia or if symptoms continue despite medical therapy in paroxysmal atrial tachycardia. However, these procedures can be challenging since atrial tachycardia needs to be observed during the EP study to hone in on the focal site. The sedative medications used to make patients comfortable for the procedure tends to suppress atrial tachycardia.

VT/SCD/Devices in Women

Ventricular Tachycardia (VT)

Sex hormones also influence predisposition to ventricular arrhythmias. One study, demonstrated that postmenopausal women with idiopathic outflow ventricular tachycardia had decreased levels of estradiol compared to control postmenopausal women [90]. Postmenopausal women with idiopathic outflow ventricular tachycardia had a higher arrhythmia burden than controls, which was significantly reduced after 3 months of estrogen replacement therapy. Right ventricular outflow tachycardia, which typically occurs in younger patients and in the absence of structural heart disease, also has gender specific triggers commonly occurring in women during the premenstrual state (i.e. luteal phase) and in men during states of stress and increased exercise [91].

The clinical presentation of ventricular tachycardia (VT) is variable based on underlying structural heart disease, comorbidities, and rate of the tachycardia. Patients can be asymptomatic or present with syncope or sudden cardiac death (SCD). Diagnosis is made by reviewing the ECG. VT needs to be distinguished from SVT with aberrant conduction, bundle branch block, or changes in QRS morphology due to metabolic abnormalities. Management of patients depends primarily on the clinical scenario. Unstable patients should undergo rapid direct current (DC) cardioversion; whereas hemodynamically stable patients can initially be managed with intravenous antiarrhythmics including amiodarone, lidocaine, procainamide and beta blockers. It is important to treat any medical conditions or electrolyte abnormalities, or remove any offending drugs or substances that may be contributing to VT. Antiarrhythmics in general have an uncertain role in the prevention of VT.

Sudden Cardiac Death (SCD)

In the Framingham Study, significant sex-related differences in ventricular tachycardia and sudden cardiac death were found. Women tended to have SCD at an older age than men, usually lagging behind by 10 years, and less coronary heart disease [92, 93]. In addition, women had a lower incidence of SCD, one third of that in men [94]. While women are more likely to present with SCD at an older age they are also more likely than men to have return to spontaneous circulation [95].

Sex differences also exist in the risk factors and etiology of SCD in women. Causes beyond coronary artery disease need to be considered particularly in younger women, such as nonischemic cardiomyopathy, valvular heart disease, hereditary arrhythmias such as Long QT syndrome or congenital heart disease [96]. Thus, classic risk factors for coronary artery disease and ventricular tachycardia that are predictive of events in men may not apply as well to women, making the risk stratification of SCD in women more difficult. Bertoia et al., identified gender specific independent risk factors for SCD in 161,808 women enrolled in the Women's Health Initiative Trial, which included African-American race, increased heart rate, higher hip to waist ratio, elevated white blood cell count, and heart failure [97].

Implantable-Cardioverter Defibrillators (ICD)

Implantable cardioverter defibrillators (ICD) have been shown to decrease mortality when used for both primary and secondary prevention of sudden cardiac death in both men and women. There are some contradictions regarding the mortality outcomes between genders. The Antiarrhythmics Versus Implantable Debfibrillators Trial (AVID) investigators showed no gender difference between men and women with ICD for the secondary prevention of SCD [98]. However, the Sudden Cardiac Death in Heart Failure trial (SCD-HeFT) study found statistically significant decrease in mortality in men who received ICDs but not in women, likely because it was underpowered to detect a difference due to low enrollment of women [99].

A review of the Medicare registry from 1991 to 2005 of a large cohort of subjects diagnosed with ischemic heart disease revealed a two- to threefold increased risk of appropriate ICD therapies for VT/VF at 1 year in men versus women who underwent ICD implantation for either primary or secondary prevention [100]. Importantly, however, subgroup analysis of MADIT II [101] and DEFINITE trial [102] found no difference in ICD effectiveness in patients with either ischemic or nonischemic cardiomyopathy based on gender.

Women are less likely than men to be referred for ICD implantation for both primary and secondary prevention of SCD, with women being 61 % less likely than men to receive an ICD [103, 104]. Reasons for this disparity are unknown [105, 106]. However, it is important to recognize that based on the currently available data ICDs appear to be equally effective at reducing mortality in women and men.

Hereditary Arrhythmias (LQTS-Inherited/Acquired; ARVD; Brugada)

As mentioned earlier, gender differences do exist regarding acquired and inherited long QT syndrome (LQTS), as well as the risk for TdP leading to SCD. Women have increased prevalence of both drug induced and inherited LQTS that appear to correlate with variations in sex hormone levels. Women with prolonged QT intervals are more likely to have increased cardiac events during the post- partum period while men are more likely to suffer syncope and sudden death at a younger age prior to the onset of puberty [91, 107].

Congenital LQTS is characterized by prolonged QT intervals caused by gene mutations that encode sodium or potassium ion channels. Over 300 different LQTS-related mutations have been identified that affect five main genes (KVLQT1, HERG, SCN5A, KCNE1, and KCNE2) [108]. Three major subtypes (LQT1, LQT2, LQT3) comprise the majority of cases. The LQTS subtype can sometimes be inferred from the surface ECG: LQT1 is characterized by broad-based T waves and exercise induced arrhythmic events, LQT2 has low amplitude, notched T waves and auditory induced arrhythmias, and LQT3 has long isoelectric ST segment and SCD events during sleep. Patients are treated with beta blockers and those with high risk markers or with significant symptoms refractory to medications should be considered for ICD implantation. The risk for cardiac events have distinct age and gender predilections in congenital LQTS. Prior to adolescents, boys are at elevated risk for cardiac events. At adolescence, this risk reverses and girls maintain an increased risk of cardiac events into menopause [109].

Women are also more likely to develop drug-induced prolonged QT especially from antiarrhythmics that prolong ventricular repolarization and from electrolyte and metabolic abnormalities. Women are more likely to develop TdP from all classes of antiarrhythmic medications, including Vaughn William Class IA drugs such as quinidine and from Class III drugs such as sotalol [91]. Class IC drugs like flecainide do not increase QT interval. Primary practitioners need to be aware of different gender responses to drugs especially cardiovascular medications. Drug metabolism is affected by changes in hormone levels brought on by menopause, pregnancy and menstruation. Also, women have higher CYP3A4 activity than men which is known to metabolize more than 50 % of medications [110].

Arrhythmogenic Right Ventricular Dysplasia (ARVD) is an important cause of sudden cardiac death and has an autosomal mode of inheritance. This disorder is characterized by fibrofatty infiltration of the ventricles. Diagnosis is made by characteristic epsilon waves seen on ECG and evidence of fatty infiltration on gadolinium-enhanced MRI. Most case series reports ARVD as being more prevalent in men than women, however, there is no difference in the clinical presentation of ARVD between men and women [111].

Brugada is an autosomal dominant arryhythmogenic disorder of cardiac sodium channels caused by mutation in SCNA5 gene that predisposes patients to polymorphic ventricular tachycardia or ventricular fibrillation. It affects men more commonly than women, and men tend to have more syncope, aborted SCD, increased ventricular fibrillation inducibility, greater ST segment elevation, and greater rates of spontaneous type 1 ECG pattern [112]. Finding a type 1 ECG Brugada pattern is recognized as a risk factor for SCD. Women with Brugada syndrome who presented with resuscitated SCD or an appropriate ICD shock were less likely to have spontaneous type 1 ECG pattern when compared to men [113]. Although women appear to be at lower risk it is not clear whether our current risk factors are able to clearly identify women at high risk. High risk patients include patients with syncope, spontaneous type 1 ECG pattern, and those with a family history of SCD. These patients should be considered for cardiac defibrillator implantation.

Pregnancy and Arrhythmias

Pregnancy is a period during which there are numerous physiological, hemodynamic, and hormonal changes. A single-center retrospective study of 136,422 pregnancy-related admissions, reported that SVTs were extraordinarily uncommon during pregnancy and when present were often benign [49]. Only 0.2 % of these admissions were related to arrhythmias. The most common arhythmias during pregnancy are sinus tachycardia, ventricular and atrial ectopy that commonly do not require any treatment [114].

The management of pregnant women should not differ from a non-pregnant woman, with the exception that special considerations need to be taken to minimize risk to the fetus and mother. Documenting the heart rhythm is important as is treating any underlying cause of sinus tachycardia such as infection, metabolic, or endocrine conditions. SVT, specifically AVNRT is the most common arrhythmia during pregnancy and can be treated with vagal maneuvers, adenosine, or IV nodal blocking agents [115]. Early treatment of arrhythmias that have the potential for disrupting hemodynamics is important to avoid compromise to uterine blood flow

[116]. Electrical cardioversion should be performed in hemodynamically unstable pregnant patients.

Medication administration should be limited as much as possible during pregnancy to avoid unnecessary fetal exposure. However, when required, choosing drugs with the longest record of safety in pregnant women should be the first line therapy. Beta blockers have the potential to negatively influence fetal and newborn size, resulting in intrauterine growth retardation. Digoxin, diltiazem, and adenosine can be used safely in the pregnant woman. Amiodarone should be avoided due to the potential for fetal hypothyroidism and increased fetal mortality. Ventricular arrhythmias are rare in pregnancy and its occurrence should prompt an evaluation for underlying cardiomyopathy or post-partum cardiomyopathy with an echocardiogram. Lidocaine and sotalol have been used safely in pregnant women with ventricular tachycardia but have the potential to cause fetal bradycardia. It is preferable to defer any invasive EP procedures until pregnancy is completed to minimize radiation and anesthesia exposure.

Conclusion

Gender differences in arrhythmias exist as a consequence of sex hormone modulation of autonomic tone and cardiac ion channel function. This has important implications for the clinical manifestation of arrhythmias in women especially during menstruation, pregnancy, and menopause. Women tend to have greater symptoms of palpitations and syncope, which are the first symptoms of an arrhythmia. Women have a higher prevalence of AVNRT, but are less likely to have AVRT or atrial fibrillation than men. The QT interval is longer in women than men, increasing the susceptibility to torsades de pointes in women during periods of slow heart rates or upon exposure to QT prolonging medications. Conversely, women have lower rates of SCD due to structural heart disease when compared to men. Particular attention needs to be given to understanding these gender differences and factors unique to women in the management of cardiac arrhythmias.

References

1. Bjerregaard P. Mean 24 hour heart rate, minimal heart rate and pauses in healthy subjects 40–79 years of age. Eur Heart J. 1983;4(1):44–51.
2. Burke JH, Goldberger JJ, Ehlert FA, Kruse JT, Parker MA, Kadish AH. Gender differences in heart rate before and after autonomic blockade: evidence against an intrinsic gender effect. Am J Med. 1996;100(5):537–43.
3. Liu K, Ballew C, Jacobs Jr DR, et al. Ethnic differences in blood pressure, pulse rate, and related characteristics in young adults. The CARDIA study. Hypertension. 1989;14(2):218–26.
4. Molgaard H, Sorensen KE, Bjerregaard P. Minimal heart rates and longest pauses in healthy adult subjects on two occasions eight years apart. Eur Heart J. 1989;10(8):758–64.

5. Rautaharju PM, Zhou SH, Wong S, Calhoun HP, Berenson GS, Prineas R, Davignon A. Sex differences in the evolution of the electrocardiographic QT interval with age. Can J Cardiol. 1992;8:690–5.

6. Borys Surawicz B, Parikh SR. Differences between ventricular repolarization in men and women: description, mechanism and implications. Ann Noninvasive Electrocardiol. 2003;8(4):333–40.

7. Huikuri HV, Pikkujamsa SM, Airaksinen KE, et al. Sex-related differences in autonomic modulation of heart rate in middle-aged subjects. Circulation. 1996;94(2):122–5.

8. Liao D, Barnes RW, Chambless LE, Simpson Jr RJ, Sorlie P, Heiss G. Age, race, and sex differences in autonomic cardiac function measured by spectral analysis of heart rate variability–the ARIC study. Atherosclerosis risk in communities. Am J Cardiol. 1995;76(12):906–12.

9. Stein PK, Kleiger RE, Rottman JN. Differing effects of age on heart rate variability in men and women. Am J Cardiol. 1997;80(3):302–5.

10. Barantke M, Krauss T, Ortak J, et al. Effects of gender and aging on differential autonomic responses to orthostatic maneuvers. J Cardiovasc Electrophysiol. 2008;19(12):1296–303.

11. Sloan RP, Huang MH, McCreath H, et al. Cardiac autonomic control and the effects of age, race, and sex: the CARDIA study. Auton Neurosci. 2008;139(1–2):78–85.

12. Tsuji H, Larson MG, Jr Venditti FJ, et al. Impact of reduced heart rate variability on risk for cardiac events. The Framingham heart study. Circulation. 1996;94(11):2850–5.

13. Bigger Jr JT, Fleiss JL, Steinman RC, Rolnitzky LM, Kleiger RE, Rottman JN. Frequency domain measures of heart period variability and mortality after myocardial infarction. Circulation. 1992;85(1):164–71.

14. Kleiger RE, Miller JP, Bigger Jr JT, Moss AJ. Decreased heart rate variability and its association with increased mortality after acute myocardial infarction. Am J Cardiol. 1987;59(4):256–62.

15. Lown B, Verrier RL. Neural activity and ventricular fibrillation. N Engl J Med. 1976;294(21):1165–70.

16. Fei L, Anderson MH, Katritsis D, et al. Decreased heart rate variability in survivors of sudden cardiac death not associated with coronary artery disease. Br Heart J. 1994;71(1):16–21.

17. Ramaekers D, Ector H, Aubert AE, Rubens A, Van de Werf F. Heart rate variability and heart rate in healthy volunteers. Is the female autonomic nervous system cardioprotective? Eur Heart J. 1998;19(9):1334–41.

18. Umetani K, Singer DH, McCraty R, Atkinson M. Twenty-four hour time domain heart rate variability and heart rate: relations to age and gender over nine decades. J Am Coll Cardiol. 1998;31(3):593–601.

19. Hreiche R, Morissette P, Turgeon J. Drug-induced long QT syndrome in women: review of current evidence and remaining gaps. Gend Med. 2008;5(2):124–35.

20. Merri M, Benhorin J, Alberti M, Locati E, Moss AJ. Electrocardiographic quantitation of ventricular repolarization. Circulation. 1989;80(5):1301–8.

21. Stramba-Badiale M, Locati EH, Martinelli A, Courville J, Schwartz PJ. Gender and the relationship between ventricular repolarization and cardiac cycle length during 24-h Holter recordings. Eur Heart J. 1997;18(6):1000–6.

22. Abi-Gerges N, Philp K, Pollard C, Wakefield I, Hammond TG, Valentin JP. Sex differences in ventricular repolarization: from cardiac electrophysiology to torsades de pointes. Fundam Clin Pharmacol. 2004;18(2):139–51.

23. Stramba-Badiale M, Priori SG. Gender-specific prescription for cardiovascular diseases? Eur Heart J. 2005;26(16):1571–2.

24. Okin PM. Electrocardiography in women: taking the initiative. Circulation. 2006;113(4):464–6. doi:10.1161/CIRCULATIONAHA.105.581942.

25. Villareal RP, Woodruff AL, Massumi A. Gender and cardiac arrhythmias. Tex Heart Inst J. 2001;28(4):265–75.

26. Yang PC, Clancy CE. Effects of sex hormones on cardiac repolarization. J Cardiovasc Pharmacol. 2010;56(2):123–9.

27. Johnson BD, Zheng W, Korach KS, Scheuer T, Catterall WA, Rubanyi GM. Increased expression of the cardiac L-type calcium channel in estrogen receptor-deficient mice. J Gen Physiol. 1997;110(2):135–40.

28. Kurokawa J, Tamagawa M, Harada N, et al. Acute effects of oestrogen on the guinea pig and human IKr channels and drug-induced prolongation of cardiac repolarization. J Physiol. 2008;586(Pt 12):2961–73.
29. Ranki HJ, Budas GR, Crawford RM, Jovanovic A. Gender-specific difference in cardiac ATP-sensitive K(+) channels. J Am Coll Cardiol. 2001;38(3):906–15.
30. Wu ZY, Yu DJ, Soong TW, Dawe GS, Bian JS. Progesterone impairs human ether-a-go-go-related gene (HERG) trafficking by disruption of intracellular cholesterol hemostasis. J Biol Chem. 2011;285(25):22186–94.
31. Nakamura H, Kurokawa J, Bai CX, Asada K, Xu J, Oren RV, Zhu ZI, Clancy CE, Isobe M, Furukawa T. Progesterone regulates cardiac repolarization through a nongenomic pathway: an in vitro patch-clamp and computational modeling study. Circulation. 2007;116:2913–22.
32. Bai CX, Kurokawa J, Tamagawa M, Nakaya H, Furukawa T. Nontranscriptional regulation of cardiac repolarization currents by testosterone. Circulation. 2005;112:1701–10.
33. Drici MD, Burklow TR, Haridasse V, Glazer RI, Woosley RL. Sex hormones prolong the QT interval and downregulate potassium channel expression in the rabbit heart. Circulation. 1996;94(6):1471–4.
34. Xiao L, Zhang L, Han W, Wang Z, Nattel S. Sex-based transmural differences in cardiac repolarization and ionic-current properties in canine left ventricles. Am J Physiol Heart Circ Physiol. 2006;291(2):H570–80.
35. Liu CC, Kuo TB, Yang CC. Effects of estrogen on gender-related autonomic differences in humans. Am J Physiol Heart Circ Physiol. 2003;285(5):H2188–93.
36. Ng AV, Callister R, Johnson DG, Seals DR. Age and gender influence muscle sympathetic nerve activity at rest in healthy humans. Hypertension. 1993;21(4):498–503.
37. Shimizu W, Antzelevitch C. Cellular basis for the ECG features of the LQT1 form of the long-QT syndrome: effects of beta-adrenergic agonists and antagonists and sodium channel blockers on transmural dispersion of repolarization and torsade de pointes. Circulation. 1998;98(21):2314–22.
38. Nakagawa M, Ooie T, Ou B, et al. Gender differences in autonomic modulation of ventricular repolarization in humans. J Cardiovasc Electrophysiol. 2005;16(3):278–84.
39. Conrath CE, Wilde AA, Jongbloed RJ, et al. Gender differences in the long QT syndrome: effects of beta-adrenoceptor blockade. Cardiovasc Res. 2002;53(3):770–6.
40. Nakagawa M, Ooie T, Takahashi N, et al. Influence of menstrual cycle on QT interval dynamics. Pacing Clin Electrophysiol. 2006;29(6):607–13.
41. Ciaccio EJ. Torsades, sex hormones, and ventricular repolarization. J Cardiovasc Electrophysiol. 2011;22(3):332–3.
42. Buber J, Mathew J, Moss AJ, et al. Risk of recurrent cardiac events after onset of menopause in women with congenital long-QT syndrome types 1 and 2. Circulation. 2011;123(24):2784–91.
43. Haseroth K, Seyffart K, Wehling M, Christ M. Effects of progestin-estrogen replacement therapy on QT-dispersion in postmenopausal women. Int J Cardiol. 2000;75(2–3):161–5; discussion 165–6.
44. Kadish AH, Greenland P, Limacher MC, Frishman WH, Daugherty SA, Schwartz JB. Estrogen and progestin use and the QT interval in postmenopausal women. Ann Noninvasive Electrocardiol. 2004;9(4):366–74.
45. Saba S, Link MS, Homoud MK, Wang PJ, Estes 3rd NA. Effect of low estrogen states in healthy women on dispersion of ventricular repolarization. Am J Cardiol. 2001;87(3):354–6. A9–10.
46. Grady D, Herrington D, Bittner V, et al. Cardiovascular disease outcomes during 6.8 years of hormone therapy: Heart and Estrogen/progestin replacement study follow-up (HERS II). JAMA. 2002;288(1):49–57.
47. Rosano GM, Leonardo F, Sarrel PM, Beale CM, De Luca F, Collins P. Cyclical variation in paroxysmal supraventricular tachycardia in women. Lancet. 1996;347(9004):786–8.
48. Myerburg RJ, Cox MM, Interian Jr A, et al. Cycling of inducibility of paroxysmal supraventricular tachycardia in women and its implications for timing of electrophysiologic procedures. Am J Cardiol. 1999;83(7):1049–54.

49. Li JM, Nguyen C, Joglar JA, Hamdan MH, Page RL. Frequency and outcome of arrhythmias complicating admission during pregnancy: experience from a high-volume and ethnically-diverse obstetric service. Clin Cardiol. 2008;31(11):538–41.
50. Rashba EJ, Zareba W, Moss AJ, et al. Influence of pregnancy on the risk for cardiac events in patients with hereditary long QT syndrome. LQTS investigators. Circulation. 1998;97(5):451–6.
51. Seth R, Moss AJ, McNitt S, et al. Long QT syndrome and pregnancy. J Am Coll Cardiol. 2007;49(10):1092–8.
52. Ulas UH, Chelimsky TC, Chelimsky G, Mandawat A, McNeeley K, Alshekhlee A. Comorbid health conditions in women with syncope. Clin Auton Res. 2010;20(4):223–7.
53. Soteriades ES, Evans JC, Larson MG, et al. Incidence and prognosis of syncope. N Engl J Med. 2002;347(12):878–85.
54. Strickberger SA, Benson DW, Biaggioni I, et al. AHA/ACCF scientific statement on the evaluation of syncope. J Am Coll Cardiol. 2006;47(2):473–84. doi:10.1016/j.jacc.2005.12.019.
55. Rautaharju PM, Surawicz B, Gettes LS, et al. AHA/ACCF/HRS recommendations for the standardization and interpretation of the electrocardiogram: part IV. J Am Coll Cardiol. 2009;53(11):982–91.
56. Misiri J, Candler S, Kusumoto FM. Evaluation of syncope and palpitations in women. J Womens Health (Larchmt). 2011;20(10):1505–15.
57. Morillo CA, Klein GJ, Thakur RK, Li H, Zardini M, Yee R. Mechanism of 'inappropriate' sinus tachycardia. role of sympathovagal balance. Circulation. 1994;90(2):873–7.
58. Morillo CA, Guzman JC. Inappropriate sinus tachycardia: an update. Rev Esp Cardiol. 2007;60 Suppl 3:10–4.
59. Lee RJ, Shinbane JS. Inappropriate sinus tachycardia. diagnosis and treatment. Cardiol Clin. 1997;15(4):599–605.
60. Krahn AD, Yee R, Klein GJ, Morillo C. Inappropriate sinus tachycardia: evaluation and therapy. J Cardiovasc Electrophysiol. 1995;6(12):1124–8.
61. Grubb BP. Postural tachycardia syndrome. Circulation. 2008;117(21):2814–7.
62. Olshansky B, Sullivan RM. Inappropriate sinus tachycardia. J Am Coll Cardiol. 2013;61(8):793–801.
63. Pandian JD, Dalton K, Henderson RD, McCombe PA. Postural orthostatic tachycardia syndrome: an underrecognized disorder. Intern Med J. 2007;37(8):529–35.
64. Cappato R, Castelvecchio S, Ricci C, et al. Clinical efficacy of ivabradine in patients with inappropriate sinus tachycardia: a prospective, randomized, placebo-controlled, double-blind, crossover evaluation. J Am Coll Cardiol. 2012;60(15):1323–9.
65. Ptaszynski P, Kaczmarek K, Ruta J, Klingenheben T, Wranicz JK. Metoprolol succinate vs. ivabradine in the treatment of inappropriate sinus tachycardia in patients unresponsive to previous pharmacological therapy. Europace. 2013;15(1):116–21.
66. Lee RJ, Kalman JM, Fitzpatrick AP, et al. Radiofrequency catheter modification of the sinus node for "inappropriate" sinus tachycardia. Circulation. 1995;92(10):2919–28.
67. Man KC, Knight B, Tse HF, et al. Radiofrequency catheter ablation of inappropriate sinus tachycardia guided by activation mapping. J Am Coll Cardiol. 2000;35(2):451–7.
68. Still AM, Raatikainen P, Ylitalo A, et al. Prevalence, characteristics and natural course of inappropriate sinus tachycardia. Europace. 2005;7(2):104–12.
69. Deneke T, Muller P, Lawo T, et al. Gender differences in onset of symptoms in AV nodal re-entrant and accessory pathway-mediated re-entrant tachycardia. Herzschrittmacherther Elektrophysiol. 2009;20(1):33–8.
70. Rodriguez LM, de Chillou C, Schlapfer J, et al. Age at onset and gender of patients with different types of supraventricular tachycardias. Am J Cardiol. 1992;70(13):1213–5.
71. Gowd BM, Thompson PD. Effect of female sex on cardiac arrhythmias. Cardiol Rev. 2012;20(6):297–303.
72. Liuba I, Jonsson A, Safstrom K, Walfridsson H. Gender-related differences in patients with atrioventricular nodal reentry tachycardia. Am J Cardiol. 2006;97(3):384–8.

73. Liu S, Yuan S, Hertervig E, Kongstad O, Olsson SB. Gender and atrioventricular conduction properties of patients with symptomatic atrioventricular nodal reentrant tachycardia and wolff-parkinson-white syndrome. J Electrocardiol. 2001;34(4):295–301.

74. Blomstrom-Lundqvist C, Scheinman MM, Aliot EM, et al. ACC/AHA/ESC guidelines for the management of patients with supraventricular arrhythmias–executive summary. J Am Coll Cardiol. 2003;42(8):1493–531.

75. Clair WK, Wilkinson WE, McCarthy EA, Pritchett EL. Treatment of paroxysmal supraventricular tachycardia with oral diltiazem. Clin Pharmacol Ther. 1992;51(5):562–5.

76. Pritchett EL, DaTorre SD, Platt ML, McCarville SE, Hougham AJ. Flecainide acetate treatment of paroxysmal supraventricular tachycardia and paroxysmal atrial fibrillation: dose–response studies. The flecainide supraventricular tachycardia study group. J Am Coll Cardiol. 1991;17(2):297–303.

77. Dagres N, Clague JR, Breithardt G, Borggrefe M. Significant gender-related differences in radiofrequency catheter ablation therapy. J Am Coll Cardiol. 2003;42(6):1103–7.

78. Santangeli P, di Biase L, Pelargonio G, Natale A. Outcome of invasive electrophysiological procedures and gender: are males and females the same? J Cardiovasc Electrophysiol. 2011;22(5):605–12.

79. Volgman AS, Manankil MF, Mookherjee D, Trohman RG. Women with atrial fibrillation: greater risk, less attention. Gend Med. 2009;6(3):419–32.

80. Potpara TS, Marinkovic JM, Polovina MM, et al. Gender-related differences in presentation, treatment and long-term outcome in patients with first-diagnosed atrial fibrillation and structurally normal heart: the Belgrade atrial fibrillation study. Int J Cardiol. 2012;161(1):39–44.

81. Paquette M, Roy D, Talajic M, et al. Role of gender and personality on quality-of-life impairment in intermittent atrial fibrillation. Am J Cardiol. 2000;86(7):764–8.

82. Dagres N, Nieuwlaat R, Vardas PE, et al. Gender-related differences in presentation, treatment, and outcome of patients with atrial fibrillation in Europe: a report from the euro heart survey on atrial fibrillation. J Am Coll Cardiol. 2007;49(5):572–7.

83. Rienstra M, Van Veldhuisen DJ, Hagens VE, et al. Gender-related differences in rhythm control treatment in persistent atrial fibrillation: data of the rate control versus electrical cardioversion (RACE) study. J Am Coll Cardiol. 2005;46(7):1298–306.

84. Michelena HI, Powell BD, Brady PA, Friedman PA, Ezekowitz MD. Gender in atrial fibrillation: ten years later. Gend Med. 2010;7(3):206–17.

85. Forleo GB, Tondo C, De Luca L, et al. Gender-related differences in catheter ablation of atrial fibrillation. Europace. 2007;9(8):613–20.

86. Friberg L, Benson L, Rosenqvist M, Lip GY. Assessment of female sex as a risk factor in atrial fibrillation in Sweden: nationwide retrospective cohort study. BMJ. 2012;344:e3522.

87. Humphries KH, Kerr CR, Connolly SJ, et al. New-onset atrial fibrillation: sex differences in presentation, treatment, and outcome. Circulation. 2001;103(19):2365–70.

88. Hu YF, Huang JL, Wu TJ, et al. Gender differences of electrophysiological characteristics in focal atrial tachycardia. Am J Cardiol. 2009;104(1):97–100.

89. Anguera I, Brugada J, Roba M, et al. Outcomes after radiofrequency catheter ablation of atrial tachycardia. Am J Cardiol. 2001;87(7):886–90.

90. Hu X, Wang J, Xu C, He B, Lu Z, Jiang H. Effect of oestrogen replacement therapy on idiopathic outflow tract ventricular arrhythmias in postmenopausal women. Arch Cardiovasc Dis. 2011;104(2):84–8.

91. Ghani A, Maas AH, Delnoy PP, Ramdat Misier AR, Ottervanger JP, Elvan A. Sex-based differences in cardiac arrhythmias, ICD utilisation and cardiac resynchronisation therapy. Neth Heart J. 2011;19(1):35–40.

92. Kannel WB, Wilson PW, D'Agostino RB, Cobb J. Sudden coronary death in women. Am Heart J. 1998;136(2):205–12.

93. Kannel WB, McGee DL, Schatzkin A. An epidemiological perspective of sudden death. 26-year follow-up in the framingham study. Drugs. 1984;28 Suppl 1:1–16.

94. Kannel WB, Schatzkin A. Sudden death: lessons from subsets in population studies. J Am Coll Cardiol. 1985;5(6 Suppl):141B–9.

95. Teodorescu C, Reinier K, Uy-Evanado A, et al. Survival advantage from ventricular fibrillation and pulseless electrical activity in women compared to men: the Oregon sudden unexpected death study. J Interv Card Electrophysiol. 2012;34(3):219–25.
96. Rizzo S, Corrado D, Thiene G, Basso C. Sudden cardiac death in women. G Ital Cardiol (Rome). 2012;13(6):432–9.
97. Bertoia ML, Allison MA, Manson JE, et al. Risk factors for sudden cardiac death in post-menopausal women. J Am Coll Cardiol. 2012;60(25):2674–82.
98. A comparison of antiarrhythmic-drug therapy with implantable defibrillators in patients resuscitated from near-fatal ventricular arrhythmias. The antiarrhythmics versus implantable defibrillators (AVID) investigators. N Engl J Med. 1997;337(22):1576–83.
99. Bardy GH, Lee KL, Mark DB, et al. Amiodarone or an implantable cardioverter-defibrillator for congestive heart failure. N Engl J Med. 2005;352(3):225–37.
100. Curtis LH, Al-Khatib SM, Shea AM, Hammill BG, Hernandez AF, Schulman KA. Sex differences in the use of implantable cardioverter-defibrillators for primary and secondary prevention of sudden cardiac death. JAMA. 2007;298(13):1517–24.
101. Zareba W, Moss AJ, Jackson Hall W, et al. Clinical course and implantable cardioverter defibrillator therapy in postinfarction women with severe left ventricular dysfunction. J Cardiovasc Electrophysiol. 2005;16(12):1265–70.
102. Albert CM, Quigg R, Saba S, et al. Sex differences in outcome after implantable cardioverter defibrillator implantation in nonischemic cardiomyopathy. Am Heart J. 2008;156(2):367–72.
103. Havmoeller R, Reinier K, Teodorescu C, et al. Low rate of secondary prevention ICDs in the general population: multiple-year multiple-source surveillance of sudden cardiac death in the Oregon sudden unexpected death study. J Cardiovasc Electrophysiol. 2013;24(1):60–5.
104. Mezu U, Ch I, Halder I, London B, Saba S. Women and minorities are less likely to receive an implantable cardioverter defibrillator for primary prevention of sudden cardiac death. Europace. 2012;14(3):341–4.
105. LaPointe NM, Al-Khatib SM, Piccini JP, et al. Extent of and reasons for nonuse of implantable cardioverter defibrillator devices in clinical practice among eligible patients with left ventricular systolic dysfunction. Circ Cardiovasc Qual Outcomes. 2011;4(2):146–51.
106. Cook NL, Orav EJ, Liang CL, Guadagnoli E, Hicks LS. Racial and gender disparities in implantable cardioverter-defibrillator placement: are they due to overuse or underuse? Med Care Res Rev. 2011;68(2):226–46.
107. Engelstein ED. Long QT, syndrome: a preventable cause of sudden death in women. Curr Womens Health Rep. 2003;3(2):126–34.
108. Splawski I, Shen J, Timothy KW, et al. Spectrum of mutations in long-QT syndrome genes. KVLQT1, HERG, SCN5A, KCNE1, and KCNE2. Circulation. 2000;102(10):1178–85.
109. Goldenberg I, Moss AJ. Long QT syndrome. J Am Coll Cardiol. 2008;51(24):2291–300.
110. Kurokawa J, Kodama M, Furukawa T, Clancy CE. Sex and gender aspects in antiarrhythmic therapy. Handb Exp Pharmacol. 2012;214:237–63.
111. Bauce B, Frigo G, Marcus FI, et al. Comparison of clinical features of arrhythmogenic right ventricular cardiomyopathy in men versus women. Am J Cardiol. 2008;102(9):1252–7.
112. Benito B, Sarkozy A, Mont L, et al. Gender differences in clinical manifestations of brugada syndrome. J Am Coll Cardiol. 2008;52(19):1567–73.
113. Sacher F, Meregalli P, Veltmann C, et al. Are women with severely symptomatic brugada syndrome different from men? J Cardiovasc Electrophysiol. 2008;19(11):1181–5.
114. Joglar JA, Page RL. Antiarrhythmic drugs in pregnancy. Curr Opin Cardiol. 2001;16(1):40–5.
115. Ruys TP, Cornette J, Roos-Hesselink JW. Pregnancy and delivery in cardiac disease. J Cardiol. 2013;61(2):107–12.
116. McAnulty JH. Arrhythmias in pregnancy. Cardiol Clin. 2012;30(3):425–34.

Chapter 11
Women with Adult Congenital Heart Disease

Rebecca E. Pratt and James Eichelberger

Complex congenital heart disease (CHD) is no longer just a pediatric problem. Advancements in pediatric cardiothoracic surgery and pediatric cardiology management are leading patients with complex CHD to significantly longer lives well into adulthood and often beyond an age where pediatric caregivers have been traditionally trained. In 2002, the incidence of total CHD cases was 12–14 per 1,000 live births of which 6 per 1,000 live births were severe or moderately severe forms [1]. A large percentage of children with CHD, 80–85 % up to as much as 95 % in some reports, are now reaching adulthood [2, 3] and require lifelong medical surveillance. Although prevalence of adult patients with congenital heart disease (ACHD) has variability in reporting, the overall prevalence has been estimated to be approximately 3,000 per million adults [4]. This is further classified by severity with 177 per million severe ACHD cases, 1,172 per million moderate, and 1,880 per million mild. The increasing prevalence of congenital heart disease in adults has led to recent establishment of specialty board certification in ACHD beginning in 2013. As seen in childhood, there remains a gender predominance within certain diagnoses in adults [3].

Diagnosis Specific Gender Differences

Certain CHD diagnoses are known to have gender predominance. For instance, patent ductus arteriosus (PDA), secundum atrial septal defect (ASD), Ebstein's malformation [displacement of the tricuspid valve], atrioventricular septal defects (AVSD),

R.E. Pratt, MD (✉)
Division of Pediatric Cardiology,
University of Rochester Medical Center, Rochester, NY, USA
e-mail: rprattmd@gmail.com

J. Eichelberger, MD
Division of Cardiology, University of Rochester Medical Center, Rochester, NY, USA

H.Z. Mieszczanska, G.P. Velarde (eds.),
Management of Cardiovascular Disease in Women,
DOI 10.1007/978-1-4471-5517-1_11, © Springer-Verlag London 2014

Table 11.1 Diagnosis-specific gender predominance

Females	Males
Patent ductus arteriosus	Transposition of the great arteries
Secundum atrial septal defect	Aortic valve stenosis
Ebstein's malformation	Bicuspid aortic valve disease
Atrioventricular septal defect	Coarctation of the aorta
Mitral valve prolapse	Tetralogy of Fallot
Pulmonary atresia	Single ventricle lesions
	Tricuspid atresia
(Inflow tract defects)	(Outflow tract defects)

and mitral valve prolapse are seen more commonly in girls whereas transposition of the great arteries (TGA), aortic valve stenosis (AS), bicuspid aortic valve disease (BAV), coarctation of the aorta [discrete narrowing of the descending thoracic aorta], tetralogy of Fallot (TOF) [ventricular septal defect, overriding aorta, pulmonary stenosis, right ventricular hypertrophy], and single ventricle lesions [hypoplastic left or right ventricle] are seen more commonly in boys [5, 6]. Similar gender differences are seen in ACHD. PDA and secundum ASD remain more common in women, in addition to pulmonary atresia (PA). Adult males still are more likely to have TGA, AS, coarctation of the aorta, TOF and single ventricle anatomy as well as tricuspid atresia (TA) in comparison to women [3, 5]. In general, defects that involve the inflow tract are predominant in women and defects involving the outflow tract are predominant in men [3] (Table 11.1).

Reasons behind these observed gender variations for a specific congenital heart disease diagnosis are largely unknown since most of these conditions do not demonstrate linkage to either X or Y chromosomes, with few exceptions. In Turner syndrome, for example, the absence of a second X chromosome in women is associated with an increased risk of congenital heart disease, mostly aortic coarctation.

Mortality Differences Between Genders

In childhood, there is no evidence to suggest that gender influences survival [3]. In adulthood, there may be gender-related factors contributing to mortality differences. The Dutch CONgenital CORvitia (CONCOR) registry and the national mortality registry, as reviewed by Verheugt et al. [7], demonstrates 2.8 % of patients with ACHD died at a median age of 48.8 years, 42 % of whom were female, which is significantly greater than the general Dutch population. The majority of patients died from cardiovascular causes, primarily chronic heart failure and sudden death. Defects with the highest mortality were single ventricle lesions, tricuspid atresia, and double outlet right ventricle. Complications, including endocarditis, supraventricular and ventricular arrhythmias, conduction disturbances, myocardial infarction and pulmonary hypertension, were all associated with increased risk of mortality. All-cause and cardiovascular mortality was slightly higher in men, although this was not significant. Patients with Eisenmenger were found to have a small, although not significant, predominance in women [3]. Verheugt et al. [3] also report a lower female mortality in patients with coarctation of the aorta or aortic valve-related problems, which is primarily explained by the male predominance in these diseases.

The European Heart Survey database, as reviewed by Engelfriet and Mulder [8], demonstrates higher 5-year mortality in men over women, which appears particularly so in certain diagnoses: TGA, single ventricle anatomy status-post Fontan procedure (original procedure named after Francis Fontan), and cyanotic patients. Conversely, there was a greater mortality in women with Eisenmenger compared to men with Eisenmenger. Neither of these findings though were found to be statistically significant, perhaps due to the relatively low number of deaths.

Before the age of 40, women with Eisenmenger are more likely to die compared to men with Eisenmenger [5]. There is speculation regarding factors associated with mortality as reported by Jane Somerville [5]. Somerville lists that these factors may include effects of pregnancy, gynecologic surgeries with associated complications, cerebral abscesses, hormone-related fluid retention and a female predisposition to thrombosis, particularly in patients where oral contraception is being prescribed.

Morbidty Differences Between Genders

Although research is limited, women have been shown to be at a higher risk for certain outcomes and sequelae compared to their male counterparts. Verheugt et al. [3] and Somerville [5] report women with ACHD are at higher risk than men with ACHD of developing pulmonary hypertension. Pulmonary arterial hypertension, defined as mean pulmonary pressure greater than 25 mmHg at rest or 30 mmHg during exercise [9], is seen in 33–35 % more women [3, 10]. Eisenmenger physiology is characterized by severe, irreversible pulmonary arterial hypertension with resultant cyanosis [9]. There is speculation that puberty effects play a role in development of pulmonary arterial hypertension in women, as do hormonal differences between genders and pregnancy effects [3, 10]. There is potential that specific diagnoses, those more often seen in women, may contribute to the higher risk of pulmonary hypertension; however, ventricular septal defects (VSD), which do not have gender predominance, are more common in patients with Eisenmenger physiology compared to ASD for which there is a higher female predominance. The female predominance in pulmonary hypertensive patients decreases after the age of 40 [5]. This may be explained by the increased mortality in female Eisenmenger patients seen between the ages of 20–39 [5].

Among patients with congenital aortic pathology, women are at approximately 30 % lower risk of aortic complications or long-term sequelae, including dissection, surgery, and aneurysm formation, compared to their male counterparts [3, 8]. This is primarily explained by the greater male predominance in congenital aortic valve and outflow disease [3, 5, 6, 8, 10]. Surgical intervention is more likely in men based on the overall smaller size of the aorta in women and lack of gender-specific criteria for aortic surgery [3]. However, women have worse surgical outcome and a higher mortality following acute aortic dissection, which may represent inadequate diagnosis and treatment in women [3]. Women with bicuspid or mildly abnormal aortic valves demonstrate calcification later compared to males [5]. This is supported by the later mean age in women at the time of surgical intervention.

The risk of endocarditis has been observed to be less in women, perhaps due to better oral hygiene as well as lower rates of intravenous drug abuse [3, 10].

Indications for implantable cardioverter defibrillator (ICD) in patients with CHD were primarily derived from adult randomized trials and have evolved from secondary prevention of sudden cardiac death to treatment of sustained ventricular arrhythmias to primary prevention in patients with increased risk of sudden cardiac death [11]. Current recommendations for ICD placement in patients with CHD are for secondary prevention following sudden cardiac arrest or for symptomatic sustained ventricular tachycardia; for recurrent syncope of undetermined origin when either ventricular dysfunction is present or ventricular arrhythmias are inducible during electrophysiological study; or for recurrent syncope and significant systemic ventricular dysfunction [11]. Tracy et al. [12] report observational studies have shown systemic ventricular dysfunction in patients with CHD to be the most predictive risk factor for sudden cardiac death or appropriate ICD use, however, current guidelines have not been changed.

Women with ACHD are at a 55 % lower risk of implantation of an ICD compared to their male counterparts with only a slightly lower risk of developing arrhythmias [3]. There is a slight predominance of supraventricular arrhythmias in men, but no difference between genders in ventricular arrhythmias, which is a major indication for ICD placement in ACHD [3]. The ICD survival benefit demonstrates no significant gender difference which does not explain the significant gender difference between ICD placement [3, 10].

Reproductive Health Counseling

Only 34–51 % of women with ACHD recall discussing contraception or pregnancy issues regarding potential risks with their physicians [12, 13]. The importance of discussing and managing contraception is crucial when caring for women in general and particularly important in women with ACHD as pregnancy risks to both mother and child can be increased [13–15]. Most female patients with ACHD can and should be managed as normal with respect to contraceptive discussions and treatment. Exceptions are women with certain forms of complex congenital heart disease, significant aortic pathology, pulmonary hypertension, cyanotic congenital heart disease, valve replacements and congestive heart failure [5, 14]. These groups of female ACHD patients are at higher risk for development of side effects and complications with estrogen based contraceptives, and counseling must address both maternal risks as well as fetal [15].

Natural methods of contraception (withdrawal and safe period) as well as barrier methods (condom and diaphragm) have high failure rates and are not recommended [15]. Low-estrogen contraceptive pills, or combined contraceptive pills, come with significant side effects such as fluid retention, elevated blood pressure, additional risk of thromboembolic events in patients with an already increased risk, alteration in warfarin control which is particularly concerning in patients with prosthetic valves, and worsening pulmonary vascular disease [5, 15, 16]. Within the first 6 months of starting a low-estrogen contraceptive, approximately 15 % of cyanotic patients experience a thromboembolic event; if this risk is acceptable to both patient and provider, aspirin therapy should also be initiated [5]. Progesterone contraceptive pills do not carry the increased thromboembolism risk [15] although there may be a slight increased risk in polycythemic patients [5]. There are few serious side effects such as irregular menstrual bleeding, although women often experience a general unwell feeling [5, 15]. There is a high failure rate on the progesterone contraceptive pills in comparison to the combination contraceptive pills [15, 16].

Intrauterine devices (IUD) are highly effective in preventing pregnancy as in the general population, but come with a small risk of endocarditis at the time of insertion along with bleeding and sepsis [5, 15]. Mirena, a slow-release progestogen IUD, carries a slightly lower risk of endocarditis due to the suppression of endometrium, in addition to a very low pregnancy rate and a substantially reduced amount of menstrual bleeding [17]. Tubal ligation should be considered in women with ACHD who carry a significantly high risk of morbidity and mortality or when a woman with ACHD decides she does not want to have children [16–18].

Pregnancy

Although heart disease in pregnancy accounts for only 1 % of all pregnancies, the majority of heart disease in pregnancy (70–80 %) is now due to ACHD [5] (Fig. 11.1).

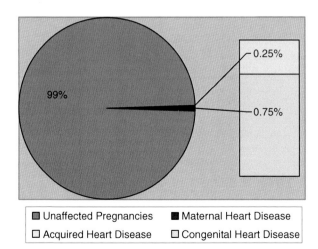

Fig. 11.1 Pregnancy and heart disease

Pregnancy in women with ACHD poses several potential problems in this generally higher-risk population. Pregnancy is a circulatory burden to women in general healthy states with subsequent increased cardiac output, heart rate and blood volume and decreased systemic vascular resistance, and in women with certain ACHD diagnoses, their ability to adapt to these physiological changes is compromised [14, 15, 19, 20]. While many ACHD diagnoses are associated with a normal pregnancy and normal outcomes, there is a higher incidence of miscarriages, premature deliveries, worsening heart failure and overall clinical deterioration [5, 14, 15, 18]. A systematic review by Drenthen et al. [14] reported 11 % of completed pregnancies in patients with ACHD experienced arrhythmias, heart failure and cardiovascular events that are generally rare in a healthy population.

Specific conditions that place women with ACHD at a higher risk include cyanotic lesions, presence of pulmonary hypertension, severe aortic stenosis, significant aortic pathology, congestive heart failure, and prosthetic, particularly mechanical, valves [5, 14, 17–19, 21]. Other conditions are less worrisome during pregnancy and include mild pulmonary valve stenosis, mild AS, bicuspid aortic valve without aortic stenosis, ASD without pulmonary hypertension, small VSD, mitral valve prolapse, TOF without sequelae, and small PDA [5, 18]. Obstetric complications do not appear to be more predominant in ACHD compared to the general population although infant mortality is higher, 4 % compared with <1 % in the general population and as high as 30 % in women with Eisenmenger physiology (Tables 11.2 and 11.3).

Table 11.2 High-risk adult congenital heart disease during pregnancy

Eisenmenger physiology – contraindication for pregnancy
Severe pulmonary hypertension, without cyanosis
Cyanotic lesions – right to left shunt creates risk of thromboembolism
Severe aortic stenosis
Significant aortic pathology
Congestive heart failure
Prosthetic valve replacements – anticoagulation risk, both maternal and fetal

Table 11.3 Diagnoses in which pregnancy is reasonably well tolerated

Atrial septal defect, with no evidence of pulmonary hypertension
Ventricular septal defect
Patent ductus arteriosus, with no evidence of pulmonary hypertension
Coarctation of the aorta
Mild aortic valve stenosis
Bicuspid aortic valve, without valve stenosis
Mild pulmonary stenosis
Mitral valve prolapse
Tetralogy of Fallot, without significant sequelae

Maternal Risks

The most frequent complication in women with ACHD during pregnancy is onset of or worsening heart failure in nearly 5 % [5, 14]. Women at particular risk are those with cyanotic congenital heart disease, Eisenmenger syndrome, stenotic valvar lesions, and pulmonary atresia. Symptoms that are able to be adequately treated with medical therapy often resolve without long-term sequelae.

Arrhythmias, most often supraventricular, occurred in 4.5 %, greater than in the general population [5, 14]. Women at greatest risk of developing an arrhythmia are those with AVSDs, TGA (particularly following atrial switch operation, where systemic venous return is routed to the left ventricle and pulmonary venous return to the right ventricle, rather than the current arterial switch operation where the great arteries are switched to the corresponding ventricles), Fontan circulation, and Ebstein's malformation [5, 14, 17]. The presence of scar tissue following repair or palliation of these defects appears to play a causative role of arrhythmia in the setting of increased volume load and enhanced adrenergic receptors [14]. Antiarrhythmics should be avoided as a general rule; adenosine is safe in pregnancy for atrial arrhythmias and lidocaine for ventricular tachycardia [17]. Beta-blockers, digoxin and calcium channel blockers are also considered relatively safe during pregnancy and cardioversion is usually safely performed [17, 22]. Amiodarone, at its lowest effective dose, should be used only when all other therapies have failed [22].

Cardiovascular events during pregnancy, including myocardial infarction, cerebrovascular accidents, and mortality, occurred in 1 out of every 50 pregnancies [14]. Eisenmenger syndrome carries a particularly high mortality risk [14]; these patients should be generally counseled against becoming pregnant and to consider early termination if pregnancy occurs. Women with ACHD are at greater risk for thromboembolic events anywhere from six times that of a healthy woman to 20 times, particularly in ACHD diagnoses with arrhythmias, sluggish blood flow, and prosthetic heart valves [14, 15]. Anticoagulation is needed, however warfarin crosses the placenta and poses significant risks to the fetus [15]. Heparin does not cross the placenta but is reported to be less effective for prophylaxis prompting individualized assessment on anticoagulant therapy [15].

Premature deliveries in mothers with ACHD occur at a higher rate than the general population, 16 % compared to 10 %, and even greater in more complex ACHD [14]. At time of membrane rupture, there is a low risk of bacterial endocarditis necessitating consideration of the use of antibiotic prophylaxis [5, 17]. This is seen particularly in patients with secundum ASD [14]. The prevalence of hypertension related to pregnancy was not significantly increased compared to the general population with the exception of those patients with aortic stenosis, coarctation of the aorta and TGA [14]. Preeclampsia occurs more commonly in the same subgroup of women [14].

Lesion-Specific Risks

Cyanotic Lesions Without Pulmonary Hypertension

Cyanotic patients without pulmonary hypertension have a high incidence of spontaneous abortion [5]. This is directly related to degree of maternal systemic oxygen desaturation; pulse oximetry less than 85 % is associated with early miscarriage [5]. At an oxygen saturation between 85 and 90 %, babies are frequently born prematurely and small for gestational age. Cyanotic mothers should be instructed to rest often as the pregnancy progresses since cyanosis often worsens [5]. Anticoagulation should be considered if there is high thromboembolic risk especially in association with decreased mobilization. Maternal complications occur in one-third of cyanotic women, but these are usually treatable [5]. The risk of having children with cardiac defects is the same as that of women who are acyanotic [5].

Pulmonary Hypertension

Women with significant pulmonary hypertension, regardless of whether they are cyanotic (Eisenmenger physiology) or acyanotic, are at a significantly higher risk of both maternal and fetal complications and mortality [5]. Many women experience miscarriages and all women experience a clinical deterioration compared to their pre-pregnancy state. Mortality in women with Eisenmenger syndrome appears to be related more to effects on the pulmonary vascular bed rather than thromboembolic events. Babies are very often small for gestational age as well as born prematurely [5].

In Eisenmenger patients, the fall in systemic vascular resistance leads to greater shunting and increased cyanosis due to the lack of change in pulmonary vascular resistance with resultant worsening heart failure [17]. In some cases, maternal mortality may be as high as 50 %. Most maternal deaths occur in the first 7 days following delivery, despite aggressive therapy [17]. In general, pregnancy is contraindicated in women with severe pulmonary hypertension due to both maternal and fetal mortality risks [16].

Tetralogy of Fallot

The majority of women with TOF have undergone complete repair prior to reaching adulthood and, if acyanotic, typically have a good prognosis [17, 22]. There is limited data on pregnancy in the setting of TOF, however, pregnancy is felt to be well tolerated for both mother and fetus following a successful repair. Complications have been reported in up to as many as 12 % of women with TOF during pregnancy, including arrhythmias and heart failure [22]. In women with unrepaired TOF, surgical repair is indicated prior to pregnancy [22].

Aortic Stenosis

Women with significant aortic stenosis are also at increased risk during pregnancy. Women with a peak systolic gradient across the aortic valve below 60 mmHg tend to have no or few problems during pregnancy while women with severe stenosis often experience pulmonary edema requiring intervention with diuretics and rest [5]. It is recommended that these patients deliver via caesarian section. Should intervention be required prior to completion of pregnancy, surgery is possible with acceptable risks as well as potential for interventional percutaneous cardiac procedures [5]. The risk of aortic dissection, particularly in the setting of a bicuspid aortic valve, is increased during pregnancy; aortic dimensions should be measured prior to pregnancy as well as during [22]. Aortic insufficiency carries less risk than does aortic stenosis due to the fixed obstruction in stenosis [17].

Coarctation of the Aorta

In women with coarctation of the aorta, close observation of blood pressures is needed to ensure that pressures are not excessively reduced in the setting of hypertension otherwise the risk of miscarriage is significant [5]. However, in general, pregnancy is often well tolerated if repaired prior to pregnancy [22]. With coarctation of the aorta and other conditions associated with aortic pathology there is a small risk of developing an aortic aneurysm, aortic dissection or aortic rupture during pregnancy [5].

Valve Replacement

Women who are status-post mechanical valve replacement require special considerations of management and risk related to anticoagulation during pregnancy. Concern of potential teratogenicity during the first trimester as well as bleeding complications at the end of pregnancy make warfarin use less favorable during these time periods [5]. Moreover, pregnancy confers a prothrombotic state where increases in coagulation factors I, VII, VIII, X, a decrease in protein S and an inhibition of fibrinolysis have all been demonstrated. Usual dosing strategies of heparinoids therefore may not provide adequate anticoagulation during pregnancy [5]. Indeed, there are case series of prosthetic valve thromboses in pregnant patients treated with low molecular weight heparins particularly when anti-Xa levels are not closely monitored. There are also case reports of accelerated disintegration of porcine or bovine bioprosthetic valves during pregnancy. Homografts and autografts, on the other hand, may be less likely to be affected by pregnancy [5].

Transposition of the Great Arteries

In transposition of the great arteries (D-TGA), with a systemic left ventricle following arterial switch operation, limited research is available on pregnancy outcomes as this operation has been performed relatively more recent. However, there are no major difficulties anticipated [17]. Women with a systemic right ventricle, as in congenitally corrected (L-) TGA, repaired TGA status post atrial switch operations or single right ventricle anatomy, can experience worsening right ventricular function as a result of pregnancy and an increased risk of arrhythmias [17, 22]. Pulmonary edema ensues but is often treatable with careful management. In certain conditions, cardiac function does not recover following pregnancy and may in fact continue to worsen.

Single Ventricle Anatomy

Women with single ventricular anatomy status post Fontan circulation are reported to have good outcomes, although there is increased risk of a thromboembolic event as Fontan circulation itself is prothrombotic with its low-flow state in addition to the state of pregnancy [5]. However, women with a low resting oxygen saturation, decreased ventricular function, significant atrioventricular valve regurgitation or with protein-losing enteropathy have a high risk of complication and should be counseled against pregnancy [22].

Fetal Risk

There is a higher incidence of fetal and neonatal adverse events in pregnant women with congenital heart disease compared to the general population, including intrauterine growth restriction, prematurity, and mortality [15]. Poor fetal growth often requires early delivery further increasing the issues of prematurity. Mothers with ACHD at particular risk of these fetal events are cyanotic CHD and left heart obstruction, such as severe aortic stenosis [15, 17]. In the general population, fetal mortality is less than 1 %; in women with ACHD, fetal mortality is increased to 4 % and as high as 28 % in complex CHD or Eisenmenger physiology [14].

Also a concern is the inheritable risk. Detailed genetic counseling should be provided to all women with ACHD who are considering pregnancy. Mothers with ACHD have an overall significantly greater risk of having affected offspring compared to fathers with ACHD [5, 15, 17]. Women with ACHD have as much as four to six times the risk of having a fetus with congenital anomalies compared to mothers without ACHD. Certain maternal syndromes have as high as a 90 % chance of recurrence, such as in Noonan's syndrome. Other conditions have up to a 50 % chance of transmission to offspring in cases where chromosomal abnormalities are identified, such as in patients with ACHD and 22Q11 gene deletion, for example. All pregnancies in women with ACHD should be considered for evaluation by fetal echocardiography.

Hormone Therapy

A recurring theme is women with ACHD at particularly greater risk during hormone therapy include those who are cyanotic, have pulmonary hypertension, are in borderline heart failure, and those with arrhythmias or are prone to developing an arrhythmia [5]. Clomiphene, used in fertility issues, in-vitro fertilization and egg harvesting, has been reported to precipitate atrial fibrillation, heart failure and worsen cyanosis. Danazol, used in endometriosis, may elicit vomiting and a general unwell feeling. Effects of post-menopausal hormonal therapy in patients with ACHD remains unknown as women with ACHD are only recently reaching this age. However, it does present potential risks of thrombosis and fluid retention. Thyroid disease is an important finding in women particularly since amiodarone-induced thyrotoxicosis affects women more often than men and should be monitored for in such patients [5].

Lifestyle Differences Between Genders

Specific lifestyles can have long-term effects on cardiac conditions, both acquired and congenital. Women have lifestyle differences compared to men and this is also true of women with CHD [5, 8]. Smoking is less common in women with ACHD compared to men, as is drug and alcohol abuse. More women with ACHD remain single compared with men with ACHD and adults without CHD. There is a higher incidence of divorce in women with ACHD compared with men with ACHD. Women with ACHD have greater overall health concerns. With respect to appearance, women with ACHD have unique concerns regarding physical immaturity in those who have experienced growth delay and abnormal breast development. Cyanosis and badly placed or poorly healed scars are often of significant concern to women compared to men with ACHD. The development of kyphoscoliosis has both appearance concerns and potential adverse effects on cardiorespiratory function. In general, scoliosis is more in common in females and is much more so in females with ACHD. Obesity, although less commonly seen in ACHD, is more of a concern in women than men [5, 8].

As patients with ACHD are aging, concern regarding coronary artery disease (CAD) is increasing. In cyanotic patients, coronary arteries are larger than average and lead to less acquired CAD than is seen in the general population, although a difference between women and men with cyanotic disease has yet to be reported. Women in general have an overall lower risk of developing significant obstructive coronary disease compared to age-matched men and this is also probably true for women with ACHD [5, 8].

Cardiac Surgery Differences Between Genders

Unique problems arise in adults with congenital heart disease requiring cardiac surgery. For example, conduit replacements may require special modifications in the presence of associated defects, bypass techniques may need to be modified and risk is increased in patient subsets with cyanosis [2]. In the pediatric population, females have a higher in-hospital mortality compared to males undergoing cardiac surgery [23]. Despite adjusting for a larger number of low-risk procedures and a lower number of high-risk procedures, females had 50 % higher odds of mortality than males. It is unclear as to why this gender difference exists despite no difference in surgical approach.

The case series by Izquierdo et al. [24] on heart transplantation in ACHD demonstrates 1-year survival to be 75 % compared to patients with dilated cardiomyopathy and ischemic heart disease, 78 %. The majority of patients undergoing transplant were single ventricle anatomy without a Fontan procedure. Half of the cases with ACHD were female but no gender-related differences were reported based on the small number of patients [24].

Conclusion

Adults with CHD have become a new entity in adult medicine and women have their own set of mortality and morbidity risks independent of those for men. These patients need specialized care by providers who are not only familiar with adult medicine, but also with congenital heart disease. Overall, women with ACHD are at a lower mortality risk than men possibly related, in part, to a lower prevalence of more complex outflow defects relative to women. However, in the setting of Eisenmenger physiology, younger women have a higher mortality than younger men. Morbidity also differs between genders; puberty and hormonal differences are thought to play a role in these dissimilarities.

Of significant concern in women with ACHD is that of reproductive health and pregnancy risks. In the majority of ACHD diagnoses, contraception and pregnancy should be approached as normal. In a small subgroup of ACHD, women should be counseled and forewarned regarding certain risks and complications. Diagnoses of most concern, particularly during pregnancy, are cyanotic lesions, the presence of pulmonary hypertension, and/or congestive heart failure, significant aortic pathology and prosthetic valves.

Women with ACHD require special consideration as they differ from their male counterparts. Provider awareness of these differences will benefit these women and most will be able to lead a full life with only a few limitations.

References

1. Hoffman JI, Kaplan S. The incidence of congenital heart disease. J Am Coll Cardiol. 2002;39:1890–900.
2. Party BCSW. Grown-up congenital heart (GUCH) disease: current needs and provision of service for adolescents and adults with congenital heart disease in the UK. Heart (British Cardiac Society). 2002;88 Suppl 1:i1–14.
3. Verheugt CL, Uiterwaal CS, van der Velde ET, Meijboom FJ, Pieper PG, et al. Gender and outcome in adult congenital heart disease. Circulation. 2008;118:26–32.
4. van der Bom T, Bouma BJ, Meijboom FJ, Zwinderman AH, Mulder BJ. The prevalence of adult congenital heart disease, results from a systematic review and evidence based calculation. Am Heart J. 2012;164:568–75.
5. Somerville J. The Denolin Lecture: the woman with congenital heart disease. Eur Heart J. 1998;19:1766–75.
6. Samanek M. Boy:girl ratio in children born with different forms of cardiac malformation: a population-based study. Pediatr Cardiol. 1994;15:53–7.
7. Verheugt CL, Uiterwaal CS, van der Velde ET, Meijboom FJ, Pieper PG, et al. Mortality in adult congenital heart disease. Eur Heart J. 2010;31:1220–9.
8. Engelfriet P, Mulder BJ. Gender differences in adult congenital heart disease. Neth Heart J. 2009;17:414–7.
9. Duffels MG, Boersma E, Mulder B. Pulmonary arterial hypertension in adults with congenital heart disease. Eur Cardiol. 2008;4:86–8.
10. Warnes CA. Sex differences in congenital heart disease: should a woman be more like a man? Circulation. 2008;118:3–5.
11. Epstein AE, DiMarco JP, Ellenbogen KA, Estes 3rd NA, Freedman RA, et al. ACC/AHA/HRS 2008 Guidelines for Device-Based Therapy of Cardiac Rhythm Abnormalities: a report of the American College of Cardiology/American Heart Association Task Force on Practice Guidelines (Writing Committee to Revise the ACC/AHA/NASPE 2002 Guideline Update for Implantation of Cardiac Pacemakers and Antiarrhythmia Devices) developed in collaboration with the American Association for Thoracic Surgery and Society of Thoracic Surgeons. J Am Coll Cardiol. 2008;51:e1–62.
12. Tracy CM, Epstein AE, DiMarco JP, Estes 3rd NA, Hammil SC, et al. ACCF/AHA/HRS Focused Update of the 2008 Guidelines for Device-Based Therapy of Cardiac Rhythm Abnormalities: a report of the American College of Cardiology Foundation/American Heart Association Task Force on Practice Guidelines developed in collaboration with the American Association for Thoracic Surgery, Heart Failure Society of America, and Society of Thoracic Surgeons. J Am Coll Cardiol. 2012;60:1297–1313.
13. Kaemmerer M, Vigl M, Seifert-Klauss V, Nagdyman N, Bauer U, et al. Counseling reproductive health issues in women with congenital heart disease. Clin Res Cardiol. 2012;101:901–7.
14. Drenthen W, Pieper PG, Roos-Hesselink JW, van Lottum WA, Voors AA, et al. Outcome of pregnancy in women with congenital heart disease: a literature review. J Am Coll Cardiol. 2007;49:2303–11.
15. Uebing A, Steer PJ, Yentis SM, Gatzoulis MA. Pregnancy and congenital heart disease. BMJ. 2006;332:401–6.
16. Warnes CA, Williams RG, Bashore TM, Child JS, Connolly HM, et al. ACC/AHA 2008 Guidelines for the Management of Adults with Congenital Heart Disease: Executive Summary: a report of the American College of Cardiology/American Heart Association Task Force on Practice Guidelines (writing committee to develop guidelines for the management of adults with congenital heart disease). Circulation. 2008;118:2395–451.

17. Broberg CS, Yentis SM, Steer PJ, Gatzoulis MA. Women and congenital heart disease. Wenger N, Collins P, editors. Women and heart disease. London/New York: Taylor & Francis; 2005. p. 455–71.
18. Colman JM, Siu SC. Pregnancy in adult patients with congenital heart disease. Prog Pediatr Cardiol. 2003;17:53–60.
19. Bowater SE, Thorne SA. Management of pregnancy in women with acquired and congenital heart disease. Postgrad Med J. 2010;86:100–5.
20. Stout K. Pregnancy in women with congenital heart disease: the importance of evaluation and counselling. Heart (British Cardiac Society). 2005;91:713–4.
21. Khairy P, Ouyang DW, Fernandes SM, Lee-Parritz A, Economy KE, Landzberg MJ. Pregnancy outcomes in women with congenital heart disease. Circulation. 2006;113:517–24.
22. European Society of Gynecology, Association for European Paediatric Cardiology, German Society for Gender Medicine, Authors/Task Force M, Regitz-Zagrosek V, et al. ESC Guidelines on the management of cardiovascular diseases during pregnancy: the Task Force on the Management of Cardiovascular Diseases during Pregnancy of the European Society of Cardiology (ESC). Eur Heart J. 2011;32:3147–97.
23. Chang RK, Chen AY, Klitzner TS. Female sex as a risk factor for in-hospital mortality among children undergoing cardiac surgery. Circulation. 2002;106:1514–22.
24. Izquierdo MT, Almenar L, Martinez-Dolz L, Moro J, Aguero J, et al. Mortality after heart transplantation in adults with congenital heart disease: a single-center experience. Transplant Proc. 2007;39:2357–9.

Chapter 12
Hypertension in Women

Illena Antonetti and John D. Bisognano

Overview

Hypertension affects nearly a billion people world-wide with more than 67 million of them diagnosed in the United States [1]. Known colloquially as the "silent killer," hypertension, along with obesity, hyperlipidemia, and diabetes, contributes to the development of cardiovascular, cerebrovascular, and renal disease. With nearly one in three Americans diagnosed with hypertension, increased responsibility has been placed upon medical providers to appropriately diagnose and treat the disease. In women, studies have supported they are generally more aware of their diagnosis when compared to men, and similarly treated with similar control [2]. Most concerning, however, is the underdiagnosis of hypertension in the primary care setting, with findings suggesting that less than 33 % of new cases of hypertension in women are appropriately diagnosed [3]. The goal of this chapter is to review the diagnosis, treatment, and special considerations present in women with hypertension.

I. Antonetti, MD (✉)
Department of Cardiovascular Disease,
University of South Florida,
Tampa, FL, USA
e-mail: illena.antonetti@orlandohealth.com

J.D. Bisognano, MD, PhD
Division of Cardiology,
University of Rochester Medical Center,
Rochester, NY, USA
e-mail: john_bisognano@urmc.rochester.edu

H.Z. Mieszczanska, G.P. Velarde (eds.),
Management of Cardiovascular Disease in Women,
DOI 10.1007/978-1-4471-5517-1_12, © Springer-Verlag London 2014

Table 12.1 Classification of blood pressure

BP classification	SBP (mmHg)	DBP (mmHg)
Normal	<120	and <80
Prehypertension	120–139	or 80–89
Stage 1 hypertension	140–159	or 90–99
Stage 2 hypertension	>160	or >100

Source: National Heart, Lung, and Blood Institute; National Institutes of Health; U.S. Department of Health and Human Services [2]

Definitions, Terms, and Classifications (Table 12.1)

Practical Points in Diagnosis and Treatment

Epidemiological Differences Between Women and Men

Differences in blood pressure between the sexes exist bimodally in adulthood and in later age. In early adulthood men generally have higher systolic blood pressures, while in later age women's pressures are higher starting at age 60 [1]. Women typically are less hypertensive than men until age 50, where at that age the incidence of newly diagnosed hypertension in women exceeds that of men. Older African-American women above the age of 75 years are the most prevalent hypertensives, with 75 % of them diagnosed by this age. Again, women are thought to be more aware of their hypertension diagnosis than men, and have it treated and better controlled (according to NHANES III data). This is possibly due to more doctor encounters and primary care opportunities in women [1]. There is also an increased incidence of diastolic dysfunction and diastolic heart failure in women, especially older women greater than 70 years, when compared to men. Diastolic dysfunction occurs when there is impaired relaxation of the left ventricle, and when fully developed can lead to diastolic heart failure, or heart failure with preserved ejection fraction. Older women greatly outnumber men in diastolic heart failure, and they have higher rates of hypertension pre-diagnosis. Older women who develop diastolic heart failure with preserved ejection fraction have also higher rates of hypertension than women without diastolic failure, and less incidence of myocardial infarction than do patients with systolic heart failure [4].

Diagnosis

The diagnosis of hypertension in men and women is the same. Table 12.1 shows the classification of blood pressure according to The Seventh Report of the Joint National Committee on Prevention, Detection, Evaluation and Treatment of High Blood pressure (JNC-7). Hypertension is appropriately diagnosed after two separate blood pressure readings in the seated position after two or more separate office visits. The inclusion of a "prehypertensive" category, defined as a systolic blood pressure of 120–139 mmHg or diastolic blood pressure of 80–89 mmHg was created to support targeted lifestyle interventions in this group to avoid escalation in the blood pressure to hypertensive levels in the future. Unless other indications are present to prompt treatment to lower the blood pressure (other risk factors such as diabetes or evidence of target organ damage such as chronic renal insufficiency), the prehypertensive category is useful to encourage providers to prescribe exercise and additional lifestyle modifications such as weight loss and diet modification that may be warranted at that point. In women, review of additional contributors, such as oral contraceptive therapy in younger women or hormonal therapy in perimenopausal women, should be discussed should evidence of prehypertension be found.

Ideally, measurement of blood pressure should involve both right and left arms to evaluate for any significant discrepancies between the two which may herald a larger problem such as vascular stenosis or aortic coarctation. When using a manual cuff, care should be taken to ensure the right size is used (the cuff bladder itself should encircle 80 % of the arm).

Thorough history and physical examination should follow with careful search for identifiable reversible causes of secondary hypertension. In women in particular these may include Cushingoid features suggestive of glucocorticoid excess, variable extremity blood pressures indicative of possible coarctation of the aorta, obesity with increased neck girth and fatigue or daytime somnolence suggestive of obstructive sleep apnea. Young women less than 35 years of age with resistant hypertension should be screened for renovascular hypertension/fibromuscular dysplasia with ultrasound of the renal arteries. Occult hypertension in the morbidly obese young woman could suggest a diagnosis of polycystic ovarian syndrome. Again, in young women consideration should be given to the use of oral contraceptives and elevated blood pressure readings. Women are more predisposed to developing certain rheumatologic and collagen vascular disorders including systemic sclerosis and systemic lupus which in themselves can promote hypertension. Other etiologies of secondary hypertension include untreated pheochromocytoma and thyroid disease, which should be considered based on clinical presentation.

Basic laboratory tests and procedures that are recommended after a diagnosis of hypertension is made include the 12-lead electrocardiogram to evaluate for presence of left ventricular hypertrophy or atrial enlargement which would suggest long-standing hypertension, urinalysis to evaluate for proteinuria and intrinsic renal dysfunction from hypertension, basic metabolic profile with glomerular filtration rate (GFR) to evaluate electrolytes and renal involvement, and routine lipid screening. Additional studies may be warranted should there be suspicion of the reversible causes described above (sleep study, thyroid secreting hormone (TSH), plasma metanephrines, renal ultrasound, cortisol levels, etc). There is some evidence that elevated C-reactive protein (CRP) in women with no other risk factors is associated with a higher cardiovascular event rate but in isolation its clinical utility remains unclear.

Treatment

Once the diagnosis of hypertension is made, treatment of hypertension for women is essentially the same as that for men with the exception of the consideration of current reproductive goals. Care should be taken with determining where the woman is in terms of family planning and discussion of birth control should always be included if angiotensin converting enzyme (ACE) inhibitors or angiotensin-receptor blockers (ARBs) are being considered. ACE inhibitors and ARBs should be avoided in women actively planning a pregnancy or in women who are not reliably using birth control or similarly effective anti-contraceptive modalities.

Recent data shows that both the diagnosis and treatment of hypertension is suboptimal. In 2010, only 47 % of Americans with hypertension reported theirs as controlled, an actual increase from 29 % 10 years prior (NHANES study data). Women are more likely than men to report their blood pressure as being controlled (approximately 51 % compared to 43 %). Certain sub-populations, including the elderly, diabetic, those with chronic kidney disease, and African-Americans have higher rates of having treated, but uncontrolled, hypertension [5].

Overall trial data shows no difference between different antihypertensive classes in terms of effect on outcomes in women when compared to men. The Seventh Report of the Joint National Committee on Prevention, Detection, Evaluation and Treatment of High Blood pressure (JNC-7) provides a step-wise method of therapy (see Fig. 12.1), beginning with lifestyle modifications including a balanced, low salt (2.4 g of sodium) and low fat diet, weight loss, smoking cessation, reduced alcohol intake, and exercise. Initial treatment goals are that of a systolic blood pressure (SBP) of less than 140 or 130 mmHg if the patient is diabetic or with renal insufficiency. Thiazide diuretics typically are first-line in therapy, with use of 12.5–25 mg of hydrochlorothiazide or even chlorthalidone (see Table 12.2). Should the patient have diabetes or chronic kidney disease, an ACE inhibitor or an ARB should be utilized with close monitoring of electrolytes and renal function to ensure stability in the first few weeks. Those with stage 2 hypertension ($\geq$ 160/100) or above should be treated initially with two antihypertensives. A diagnosis of congestive heart failure or coronary disease warrants using ACE inhibitors and adding beta-blockers should blood pressure allow.

Special Considerations

Pregnancy

The diagnosis of hypertension during pregnancy, whether chronic or gestational, is associated with fetal growth restriction, preterm birth, still birth, and pre-eclampsia. Different definitions of hypertension in pregnancy exist, including that of chronic hypertension, which is defined as hypertension present and observed prior to

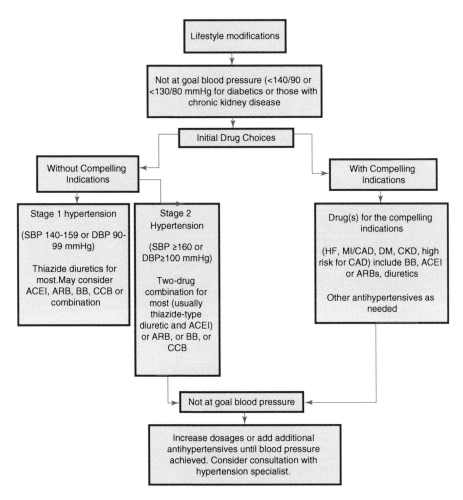

Fig. 12.1 Treatment Algorithm – JNC 7 (*Source*: National Heart, Lung, and Blood Institute; National Institutes of Health; U.S. Department of Health and Human Services [2]). *ACEI* Angiotensin converting enzyme (*ACE*) inhibitor, *ARB* angiotensin receptor blocker, *BB* beta blocker, *CCB* calcium channel blocker, *SBP* systolic blood pressure, *DBP* diastolic blood pressure, *HF* heart failure, *MI* myocardial infarction, *CAD* coronary artery disease, *DM* diabetes mellitus, *CKD* chronic kidney disease

pregnancy or that which is diagnosed before the 20th week. Hypertension that is diagnosed during pregnancy and does not go away after delivery of the baby is also termed chronic hypertension. Chronic hypertension is more common in older women and African-American women. Gestational hypertension is defined as transient hypertension during pregnancy should pre-eclampsia not be present and if blood pressure stabilizes once the baby is delivered or by 12 weeks post-partum. Pre-eclampsia is defined by increased blood pressure of greater than 140/90 mmHg with proteinuria of greater than or equal to 0.3 g of protein in a 24 h collection.

Table 12.2 Oral antihypertensive drugs – JNC –7

Class	Drug (trade name)	Usual dose range (mg/day)	Usual daily frequency
Thiazide diuretics	HCTZ	12.5–25	1
	Chlorthalidone	12.5–25	1
BBs	Atenolol (Tenormin)	25–100	1
	Bisoprolol (Zebeta)	2.5–10	1
	Metoprolol (Lopressor)	50–100	2
	Metoprolol XL (Toprol XL)	50–100	1
Combined α and BBs	Carvedilol (Coreg)	12.52–50	2
	Labetalol (Normodyne)	200–300	2
ACE-I	Benazepril (Lotensin)	10–40	1
	Captopril (Capoten)	25–100	1
	Enalapril (Vasotec)	5–40	1
	Lisinopril (Zestril)	10–40	1
	Quinapril (Accupril)	10–80	1
	Ramipril (Altace)	2.5–20	1
ARBs	Irbesartan (Avapro)	150–300	1
	Losartan (Cozaar)	25–100	1–2
	Olmesartan (Benicar)	20–40	1
	Telmisartan (Micardis)	20–80	1
	Valsartan (Diovan)	80–320	1–2
CCBs	Amlodipine (Norvasc)	2.5–10	1
	Nicardipine SR (Cardene SR)	60–120	2
	Nifedipine (Adalat, Procardia)	30–60	1
α agonists	Clonidine (Catapres)	0.1–0.8	2
	Clonidine patch	0.1–0.3	weekly
	Methyldopa	250–1000	2
Direct vasodilators	Hydralazine (Apresoline)	25–100	2
	Minoxidil	2.5–80	1–2

Source: National Heart, Lung, and Blood Institute; National Institutes of Health; U.S. Department of Health and Human Services [2]

Without proteinuria, pre-eclampsia is still entertained should the woman develop headache, blurry vision, abdominal pain, elevation in liver enzymes, or thrombocytopenia. Pre-eclampsia can progress to development of eclampsia once seizures develop [6].

Women who become pregnant with severely elevated, uncontrolled hypertension are at risk for superimposed pre-eclampsia, increased morbidity including left ventricular dysfunction, pulmonary edema, encephalopathy, cerebral hemorrhage, acute renal failure, placental abruption, and risk of death. Severe elevations should be evaluated and treated as an inpatient. Young women less than 30 years of age presenting with systolic blood pressure greater than 160 mmHg, or hypertensive crisis with anxiety symptoms should be evaluated with 24 h catecholamines which provide greater sensitivity and specificity than plasma metanephrine levels for potentially fatal pheochromocytoma during pregnancy, which carries a risk as high as 58 % to the mother and 56 % to the fetus, making early diagnosis critical.

Table 12.3 Oral antihypertensives during pregnancy

Name	Starting dose	Max dose in 24 h	Onset of action	Mechanism of action	Breastfeeding
Methyldopa	250 mg BID	4 g	2 days	Central alpha 2 adrenergic agonist	Safe[a]
Labetalol	100 mg BID	2400 mg	2–3 days	Alpha and beta blocker	Safe
Nifedipine XL	30 mg daily	120 mg daily	7–14 days	Ca channel blocker	Safe
HCTZ	12.5 mg daily	50 mg, ideally only 25 mg	2–3 week	Diuretic[b]	No adequate studies, may reduce milk supply

Adapted from Ames et al. [6]
[a]Avoid with history of depression, usually changed at delivery due to association with post partum depression
[b]See text for considerations prior to use

The aforementioned screening for renal artery stenosis, thyroid dysfunction, glucocorticoid excess or Cushings syndrome, or mineralcorticoid excess can be done as well. Primary aldosteronism is not recommended to be screened in pregnancy due to elevated levels of the hormone that naturally occur in the gravid state. Aldosterone and renin levels can be checked 6 weeks post-partum. Patients with history of long-standing hypertension without prior evaluation or treatment before pregnancy should have routine electrocardiogram, echocardiogram, and work up for other end-organ dysfunction such as renal injury or retinopathy [6].

Treatment of hypertension during pregnancy should occur when elevated greater than 160/110 mmHg with debate existing at levels less than this. Mild chronic hypertension (less than 160/110 mmHg) treated in pregnancy has been studied without improvement in preterm deliveries, mortality, or reduced incidence in superimposed pre-eclampsia. There was also some association between decreased birth weight and treatment of mild chronic hypertension, with a reduction in weight by 145 g with every 10 mm of mercury drop in mean arterial pressure [7]. Most pregnancies go uncomplicated should blood pressure remain mildly elevated without superimposed pre-eclampsia. When treatment is needed for elevation greater than 160/110 mmHg or by clinical discretion from the obstetrician, first-line therapy usually includes administration of methylodopa, which has the largest literature base and safety data, or labetalol (See Tables 12.3 and 12.4) [8]. Nifedipine is also commonly used. Care must be taken to screen for depression or history of depression prior to starting methyldopa as it can be associated with post-natal depression. For this reason it is commonly changed to another agent (e.g. labetalol, atenolol, nifedipine) after delivery [9]. Up to 5 % of methyldopa users have elevations in liver transaminases and can have Coombs positivity with hemolytic anemia being rare [9]. Earlier reports showed an association between atenolol and babies being born small for gestational age [10]. ACE inhibitors and ARBs are thoroughly avoided given their association with

Table 12.4 Intravenous antihypertensives to use for emergencies during pregnancy

Name	Dose	Activity time (min)	Mechanism of action	Side effects
Labetalol	20–40 mg IV every 30 min as needed	2–4	Alpha and beta blocker	Tremulousness, headache
Hydralazine	10 mg IV every 2 h as needed	20–30	Direct vasodilator	Lupus-like syndrome with chronic use
Diazoxide	30–50 mg IV every 5–15 min	2–4	Direct vasodilator	Hypotension, hypoglycemia
Nitroprusside drip	0.25–5 µg/kg/min	1–2	Direct vasodilator	Hypotension, cyanide toxicity if used >4 h, dose with pharmacist

Modified from Yoder et al. [8]

cardiac and CNS defects in the first trimester and growth restriction, oligohydramnios, fetal renal failure and renal tubular dysplasia, pulmonary hypoplasia, hypocalvaria (incomplete ossification of the skull) and still birth in second and third trimester exposure [6, 9]. Should severely elevated blood pressure fail to be controlled by a single agent, additional ones can be added and slowly titrated for desired goal. Careful avoidance of diuretics is often done, although study data has demonstrated use of thiazides without difference in outcomes. The risk-benefit of decreased intravascular volume should be taken into account and use in known fetal growth restriction or preeclampsia is generally discouraged. Delivery is usually guided by presence of hypertension, clinical circumstances, and the judgment of the obstetrician. With severe hypertension the recommended time of delivery is usually shorter at 36–37 weeks (compared to normal 38–39 weeks) and superimposed pre-eclampsia with it moves delivery often to 34 weeks. Risk of hypertension is increased for subsequent pregnancies, and risk of developing hypertension later in life is also elevated. For instance, a first pregnancy complicated with gestational hypertension has a risk of 70 % to have a recurrent hypertensive disorder in the second pregnancy [6]. Care should be taken for regular blood pressure follow up by the involved primary care physician and referral for management of target organ damage if detected. For breast feeding, several anti-hypertensives are usable although some, such as ACE-inhibitors enalapril and captopril, require the woman to use strict birth control to avoid pregnancy and the aforementioned fetal side effects (see Table 12.5).

Oral Contraceptives

Women on oral contraceptives should be routinely screened for occult hypertension by their primary care providers on routine office visit examinations, particularly when other factors such as obesity and strong family history of hypertension are present. Should they become hypertensive on oral contraceptive therapy consideration to

Table 12.5 Hypertensives compatible with breast feeding

Labetalol
Nifedipine
Enalapril/captopril (avoid if planning another pregnancy or if not using birth control method reliably)
Hydrochlorothiazide
Verapamil
Methyldopa
Hydralazine
Minoxidil
Nadolol
Oxprenolol
Propranolol
Timolol
Diltiazem (weak antihypertensive effect)
Spironolactone (weak antihypertensive effect)

Modified from Yoder et al. [8]

switching the class of oral contraceptive can be made and blood pressure resolution followed accordingly. Should blood pressure remain elevated cessation of the oral contraceptive with institution of alternative form of birth control is recommended.

Renal Fibromuscular Dysplasia

A rare condition, renal fibromuscular dysplasia should be entertained in young women (age <35 years) who present with either isolated hypertension or hypertension that is refractory to medications. This disease disproportionately affects women more so than men, and although rare it is easily treatable with balloon angioplasty (without stenting) in the hypertensive woman. Interestingly, fibromuscular dysplasia can affect any artery, with the most common being the renal arteries followed by the carotids. Those with carotid disease usually present in their mid- fifties with either an asymptomatic carotid bruit or if symptomatic with stroke. If renal fibromuscular dysplasia is suspected in a young woman, diagnosis involves careful examination which may reveal an abdominal bruit with both a systolic and diastolic component (reflecting fibromuscular disease with stenosis). Duplex ultrasound of the renal arteries should be ordered with special attention noted to request evaluation of the middle and distal renal arteries as these are most affected by the disease. Up to a third of patients can have both renal arteries involved. Therapy is usually reserved for those with hypertension, hypertension refractory to medication, those with evidence of renal impairment, and those with medication non-compliance or intolerance. Treatment consists of angioplasty alone without stenting although some cases rarely involve renal macroaneurysms that can be treated surgically. Evaluation post angioplasty with duplex ultrasound is usually recommended to ensure resolution of stenosis with repeat angioplasty recommended should evidence of it remain [11].

Menopause

Women after the age of 60 demonstrate greater risk in developing hypertension than their male counterparts as previously reviewed. Care should be taken for prompt recognition and treatment in the newly hypertensive woman, and often providers will hear that the patient has never had hypertension before and how this elevation is new for them. A new diagnosis of hypertension may ensue due to the patients age and onset of menopause with decline in the cardioprotective effect of estrogen. Vigilant monitoring, which can be done at home by the patient, should ensue and hypertension appropriately treated if it persists.

Obesity

The obesity epidemic, especially in the United States, has grown to overwhelming proportions. Estimates from the CDC show that 35 % of Americans in the year 2009–2010 were obese, affecting an alarming 78 million adults. Obesity is defined as having a body mass index (BMI) of greater than or equal to 30, with calculation of BMI being the patients weight in kilograms divided by their height in meters squared and rounded off to the nearest decimal point. Several studies support direct correlation between increased BMI and increased blood pressure. Of the obese in the United States, there is a current trend of more women being obese than men (40.6 % versus 37.5 % in the year 2009–2010) (see Fig. 12.2). Over the past 10 years, however, the percentage of obese women in the US has changed insignificantly (33.4 % in 1999–2000 versus 35.8 % in 2009–2010), in comparison to men who have increased in their percentage of being obese (27.5–35.5 % respectively) [12]. Although often not included in routine assessment and plans, vigilance in diagnosing and counseling women with an elevated BMI has documented benefit in reduction of blood pressure.

Obstructive Sleep Apnea

Obstructive sleep apnea is characterized by multiple nocturnal episodes of upper airway obstruction or occlusion which results in oxyhemoglobin desaturation, central nervous system hyperarousal, and swings in intrathoracic pressure. These phenomena, along with peripheral vasoconstriction and inflammation result in secondary hypertension, which often goes untreated due to lack of diagnosis [13]. Sleep apnea is diagnosed two to three times more in men than in women, but similarly women may have deleterious effects including uncontrolled hypertension and symptoms of daytime somnolence [13]. Women are thought to have less rates of sleep apnea than men due to carrying their obesity in the lower parts of their bodies rather than their upper airways and chest [14, 15]. Given similar BMIs men will have more severe and more frequent rates of sleep apnea than women [15]. Women

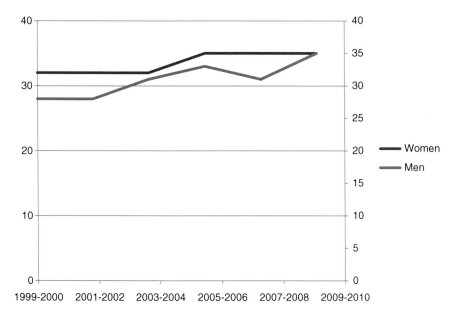

Fig. 12.2 Percentage trends in the prevalence of obesity in the United States in adults >20 years from 1999 to 2010 (Adapted from CDC/NCHS, National Health and Nutrition Examination Survey, 2009–2010)

with polycystic ovarian syndrome (PCOS) also have higher rates of obstructive sleep apnea even when BMI is adequately controlled [16].

Women are thought to present with less classic symptoms of sleep apnea. Rather than the typical somnolence and nighttime snoring, women can present with insomnia, morning headaches, chronic fatigue, and variations in mood [17]. Treatment of obstructive sleep apnea consists of continuous positive airway pressure (CPAP) therapy overnight to reduce the incidence of apnea and is superior to placebo or supplemental oxygen alone. On average, treatment with CPAP therapy has been shown in several small trials and meta-analyses to reduce mean blood pressure a mere 1.5–2 mmHg from baseline in both normotensive and hypertensive individuals. There was a correlation between the severity of sleep disordered breathing, increase in the mean systolic and diastolic blood pressure, and prevalence of hypertension, but this correlation weakened when obesity was used in a multi-variate analysis [18, 19].

Summary

- Hypertension is a highly prevalent disease in women, which can be successfully treated to prevent cardiovascular morbidity and mortality.
- Diastolic heart failure is more common in older women over the age of 70. Many of them have a prior diagnosis of hypertension.

- Work up includes determining if there is essential hypertension, hypertension due to secondary causes, and end organ damage. Therapy depends on which of these is diagnosed.
- Most individuals require 2 plus antihypertensives for adequate control.
- Pregnant women with hypertension prior to pregnancy have increased morbidity, mortality, and risk of fetal complications. A team approach between obstetrics, primary care, and cardiology is optimal in treating hypertension in pregnancy.
- First-line agents for treatment during pregnancy are methyldopa, labetalol, and nifedipine. After delivery methyldopa is usually exchanged due to risk of peripartum depression and another agent (atenolol, HCTZ, labetalol, nifedipine, captopril/enalapril if not planning another pregnancy) is started.
- Renal fibromuscular dysplasia should be considered in hypertensive young women under the age of 35 with isolated hypertension or hypertension refractory to medications. Work up consists of renal duplex ultrasound with special attention to the mid and distal renal arteries. Treatment consists of renal artery angioplasty, not stenting.
- Increasing rates of obesity and sedentary lifestyles contribute to the rising hypertension prevalence in women. Care should be taken to provide counseling for obesity, diet, and appropriate exercise as integral parts of hypertension treatment.
- Obstructive sleep apnea, although less common in women, is a secondary cause of hypertension that often presents in women with non-classic symptoms such as insomnia, irritability, and fatigue. Treatment involves use of CPAP therapy.

References

1. Ong KL, Cheung BM, Man YB, et al. Prevalence, awareness, treatment, and control of hypertension among United States adults 1999–2004. Hypertension. 2007;49:69–75.
2. National Heart, Lung, and Blood Institute; National Institutes of Health; U.S. Department of Health and Human Services. National High Blood Pressure Education Program. The seventh report of the Joint National Committee on prevention, detection, evaluation, and treatment of high blood pressure. Aug 2004. Report No.: 04–5230.
3. Schmittdiel J, Selby JV, Swain B, et al. Missed opportunities in cardiovascular disease prevention? Low rates of hypertension recognition for women at medicine and obstetrics-gynecology clinics. Hypertension. 2011;57:717–22.
4. Owan TE, Redfield MM. Epidemiology of diastolic heart failure. Prog Cardiovasc Dis. 2005;47:320–32.
5. Gu Q, Burt VL, Dillon CF, et al. Trends in antihypertensive medication use and blood pressure control among United States adults with hypertension: the National Health and Nutrition Examination survey, 2001 to 2010. Circulation. 2012;126:2105–14.
6. Ames M, Rueda J, Caughey AB, et al. Ambulatory management of chronic hypertension in pregnancy. Clin Obstet Gynecol. 2012;55:744–55.
7. Von Dadelszen P, Ornstein MP, Bull SB, et al. Fall in mean arterial pressure and fetal growth restriction in pregnancy hypertension: a meta-analysis. Lancet. 2000;355:87–92.
8. Yoder S, Thornburg LL, Bisognano JD. Hypertension in pregnancy and women of childbearing age. Am J Med. 2009;122:890–5.

9. James PR, Nelson-Piercy C, et al. Management of hypertension before, during, and after pregnancy. Heart. 2004;90:1499–504.
10. Magee LA, Elran E, Bull SB, et al. Risks and benefits of beta-receptor blockers for pregnancy hypertension: overview of the randomized trials. Eur J Obstet Gynecol Reprod Biol. 2000;88:15–26.
11. Olin JW. Recognizing and managing fibromuscular dysplasia. Cleve Clin J Med. 2007;74:273–82.
12. Ogden CL, Carroll MD, Kit BK, et al. Prevalence of obesity in the United States, 2009–2010. NCHS Data Brief. 2012;82:1–8.
13. Bradley TD, Floras JS. Obstructive sleep apnea and its cardiovascular consequences. Lancet. 2009;373:82–93.
14. Millman RP, Carlisle CC, Eveloff SE, et al. Body fat distribution and sleep apnea severity in women. Chest. 1995;107:362–6.
15. Kapsimalis F, Kryger MH. Gender and obstructive sleep apnea syndrome, part 2: mechanisms. Sleep. 2002;25:497–504.
16. Tasali E, Van Cauter E, Ehrmann DA. Polycystic ovary syndrome and obstructive sleep apnea. Sleep Med Clin. 2008;3:37–46.
17. Kapsimalis F, Kryger MH. Gender and obstructive sleep apnea syndrome, part 1: clinical features. Sleep. 2002;25:409–13.
18. Okcay A, Somers VK, Caples SM. Obstructive sleep apnea and hypertension. J Clin Hypertens. 2008;10:549–55.
19. Nieto FJ, Young TB, Lind BK, et al. Association of sleep-disordered breathing, sleep apnea, and hypertension in a large community-based study. JAMA. 2000;283:1829–36.

Chapter 13
Impact of Diabetes Mellitus and the Metabolic Syndrome on the Female Heart

Illena Antonetti and Gladys P. Velarde

Introduction

Over 12.6 million of women over the age of 20 in the United States have either diagnosed or undiagnosed diabetes mellitus. The overwhelming majority (>90 %) of these cases are type 2 diabetes mellitus, related to overall insulin resistance and eventual abnormal insulin secretion. In comparison, type 1 diabetes mellitus affects only 5 % of diabetics [1]. Surprisingly, women with the diagnosis of diabetes bear higher mortality when afflicted with coronary artery disease than their male counterparts, negating the premise that female gender offers cardio-protection [2–4]. The metabolic syndrome also confers worse outcomes for women with increased morbidity and cardiovascular mortality in those affected, even after controlling for other risk factors. This chapter will review the epidemiological impact of both the metabolic syndrome and diabetes in women's heart disease and review important aspects of early diagnosis, medical and life-style modifying, goal-directed therapy to avoid increased morbidity.

I. Antonetti, MD
Department of Cardiovascular Medicine, University of South Florida,
Tampa, FL, USA

G.P. Velarde, MD, FACC (✉)
Division of Cardiology, University of Florida Health Cardiology Center – Jacksonville,
University of Florida College of Medicine-Jacksonville,
ACC Building 5th floor, 655 West 8th Street, Jacksonville, FL, USA
e-mail: gladys.velarde@jax.ufl.edu

H.Z. Mieszczanska, G.P. Velarde (eds.),
Management of Cardiovascular Disease in Women,
DOI 10.1007/978-1-4471-5517-1_13, © Springer-Verlag London 2014

Table 13.1 ATP III clinical identification of the metabolic syndrome

Risk factor	Defining level
Abdominal obesity, given as waist circumference	
Men	>102 cm (>40 in.)
Women	>88 cm (>35 in.)
Triglycerides	≥150 mg/dL
HDL cholesterol	
Men	<40 mg/dL
Women	<50 mg/dL
Blood pressure	≥130/≥85 mmHg
Fasting glucose	≥110 mg/dL

Adapted from Grundy et al. [6]

Epidemiology

The Ominous Epilogue: Metabolic Syndrome in Women

The increasing rates of obesity and sedentary lifestyle are the leading causes for the development of the metabolic syndrome, the ominous predecessor to type 2 diabetes mellitus. Currently more than 47 million Americans are estimated to have the metabolic syndrome in the United States.

More than 80 % of individuals considered obese (BMI >30 Kg/m^2) develop the metabolic syndrome prior to developing diabetes mellitus. More than 80 % of those newly diagnosed with type 2 diabetes mellitus had the metabolic syndrome prior to their diagnosis, and of them a significant majority are women more so than men (89.9 % versus 78.2 %; $p < 0.001$) [5]. The metabolic syndrome, even when adjusted for traditional risk factors, independently confers at least a 1.5 fold increase in cardiovascular disease and all-cause mortality, a twofold increase in cardiovascular events, and a fivefold increase in developing overt diabetes mellitus. Despite having similar age-adjusted prevalence (women 23 % vs. men 24 %), women with metabolic syndrome have a higher cardiovascular disease risk than men. In the San Antonio Heart Study, when using the Third Report of the National Cholesterol Education Program Adult Treatment Panel (ATP III) definition of metabolic syndrome (Table 13.1) to predict cardiac mortality, the hazard ratios for women were 4.65 (95 % CI 2.35–9.21) and in men 1.82 (95 % CI 1.14–2.91) [7, 8]. This increased gender risk was also found in the Atherosclerosis Risk in Communities (ARIC) study, which showed hazard ratios of 2.05 (95 % CI 1.59–2.64) in women compared to 1.46 (95 % CI 1.23–1.74) in men (shown in Fig. 13.1) [7, 9].

There have been a number of definitions of the metabolic syndrome since first described by Reaven in 1988 [10]. The metabolic syndrome was termed then "Syndrome X" after dyslipidemia, hypertension, and hyperglycemia were found to be strongly associated with development of overt diabetes and future cardiovascular disease. Due to the high prevalence of relative insulin resistance observed in these

Fig. 13.1 Hazard ratios for cardiovascular disease according to gender and number of components of the MBS in the Atherosclesosis Risk in Communities (ARIC) study.

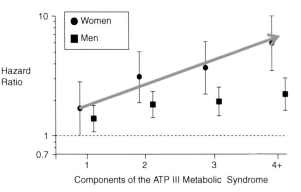

individuals, the term 'Insulin Resistance Syndrome' emerged, which was then followed by the term 'metabolic syndrome' now commonly adopted. The definition most widely used in studies and clinical practice is one recommended by the ATP III [6] where the syndrome is defined by having at least three of the following (Table 13.1):

- Abdominal obesity (>40 in. (102 cm) in men or >35 in. (88 cm) in women)
- High triglycerides (≥150 mg/dl)
- Low HDL cholesterol (<40 mg/dl in men or <50 mg/dl in women)
- Elevated blood pressure (≥130/85 mmHg)
- Impaired fasting plasma glucose (≥110 mg/dl)

In addition to the development of cardiovascular disease and diabetes, the metabolic syndrome is associated with polycystic ovarian syndrome, hepatosteatosis, asthma, cholesterol gallstones, and some cancers [11].

It is well-documented that the metabolic syndrome affects women of ethnic minority groups disproportionately. Caucasian men and women seemingly have nearly the same rates, whereas within African Americans, women have a 57 % higher prevalence than African American men and within Mexican Americans women have a 26 % higher prevalence than Mexican-American men (Fig. 13.2) [12]. Independent of ethnicity, it appears that the prevalence of metabolic syndrome is increasing more in women than in men [6]. According to the National Health and Nutrition Examination Survey data from 1988 to 1994 compared to data from 1999 to 2000, the age-adjusted prevalence in metabolic syndrome in women increased by nearly 24 % compared to 2 % in men [7, 12]. The increased prevalence of metabolic syndrome in women is thought to be due to their increasing rates of hypertension, central obesity and elevated triglycerides. These individual risk factors and components of metabolic syndrome appear to be increasing in higher rates in women compared to men [7, 12–14]. Increased waist circumference, independent of BMI, increases the risk of developing metabolic syndrome in women more than men. In the San Antonio Heart Study participants with a BMI ≥30 kg/m² versus those with a BMI < 25 kg/m², men had an odds ratio of developing metabolic syndrome of 3.7 compared to 8.3 in women [8]. With higher waist circumference the findings are similar. For waist circumferences greater than 102 cm in men or greater than 88 cm

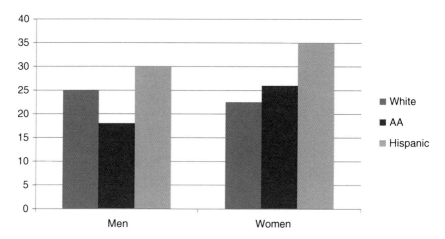

Fig. 13.2 Age-adjusted prevalence of metabolic syndrome among US adults by gender and race or ethnicity [12]

in women the odds ratio for developing metabolic syndrome in men was 2.8 and much higher at 5.9 in women [7, 8]. Several meta-analysis have shown increased rates of cardiovascular events and death in both sexes with metabolic syndrome, with worsened hazard ratios in those studies done solely in women (see Figs. 13.3 and 13.4) [14].

The Silent Foe: Diabetes Mellitus in Women

Women in general are more likely to have diabetes than men [12]. It affects a higher total percentage of ethnic minority women in the United States with African-American women (12.6 %) and Mexican-American women (11.3 %) surpassing white women (4.7 %) in those over the age of 20.

According to the Third National Health and Nutrition Examination Survey (NHANES III, 1988–1994), the prevalence of diabetes in women, increases with age, doubling the amount of diabetes in women of middle age as compared to younger women [12, 13]. In fact, it was estimated at the time that nearly 2.7 million American women aged 40–59 had diabetes. Moreover, ethnic disparities that exist in the metabolic syndrome again ring true in diabetes. For women of middle age, diabetes is at least twice as common in ethnic minorities compared to Caucasian women. For example, according to the NHANES III data set for women ages 50–59, the prevalence of diabetes was 9.7 % for Caucasian women, 23 % for African American women, and 24 % for Mexican American women [12, 13]. No other national survey data exists for other ethnic groups regarding comparative trends unfortunately. Similarly, the death rate differences between these groups are more formidable. Between the ages of 45–64 the death rate in diabetic women was nearly

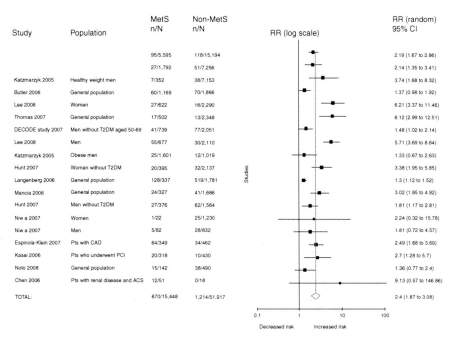

Fig. 13.3 Metabolic syndrome increases risk of cardiovascular disease in a meta-analysis 2.4 fold, with many of the studies above show worse hazard ratios for women (Reproduced with permission from Mottillo et al. [14])

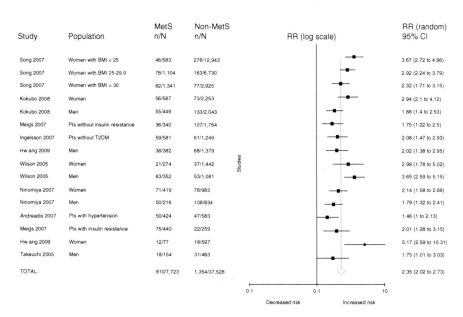

Fig. 13.4 Metabolic syndrome increases risk of cardiovascular death 2.4 fold, with several studies showing higher hazard ratios in women (Reproduced with permission from Mottillo et al. [14])

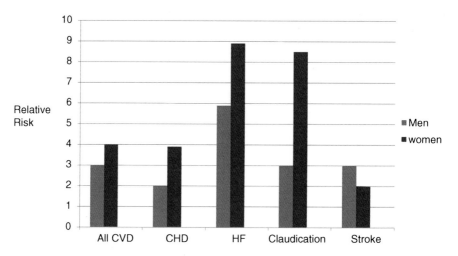

Fig. 13.5 Relative risk of cardiovascular events in patients with diabetes. (Ages 35–64) (Framingham Heart Study 30 year follow-up). $P<0.001$ for all values except $*P<0.05$ (Adapted by Velarde from Wilson and Kannel [17])

three times more than that of non-diabetic women. But when death rates are examined by race, again ethnic differences among women become evident, with all-cause mortality rate in this age group being nearly doubled in African-American women 44.8 % compared to 26.9 % in Caucasian women despite control for cardiovascular risk factors [12, 13].

The original 1979 Framingham data provided interesting data regarding diabetic women. Initial data from this cohort showed diabetic women had similar cardiovascular disease risk as diabetic men. They were five times more likely than non-diabetic women and two times more likely than non-diabetic men to develop cardiovascular disease [2, 3]. Subsequent analyses have demonstrated that diabetic women also have significantly higher mortality than diabetic men, especially after a coronary event. Data shows that both, early and late, mortality after a myocardial infarction is significantly higher in diabetic women compared to diabetic men, with rates of 22 % versus 14 % and 28.9 % versus 19.6 %, respectively [2, 15, 16], (Fig. 13.5). The recent decreasing trend in cardiovascular mortality observed in men and in women without diabetes has not been seen in women with diabetes, who in fact have trended towards increased cardiovascular mortality, regardless of whether they were known diabetics or developed it after myocardial infarction [18]. Twenty year follow up data from the Nurses' Health Study on approximately 1,700 female registered nurses, found impressive trends towards higher mortality in those women with diabetes. In that study women with diabetes were three times more likely to die of any cause than their non-diabetic colleagues. Furthermore, among women with known CAD at baseline, diabetic women were almost seven times more likely to die than nondiabetic women with CAD (Hazards Ratio 6.84). A very important observation in this study was the impact of length of exposure to diabetes. Duration

Table 13.2 Criteria for the diagnosis of diabetes

1. A1C $\geq$6.5 %. The test should be performed in a laboratory using a method that is NGSP certified and standardized to the DCCT assay[a]
OR
2. FPG $\geq$126 mg/dl (7.0 mmol/l). Fasting is defined as no caloric intake for at least 8 h[a]
OR
3. 2-h plasma glucose $\geq$200 mg/dl (11.1 mmol/l) during an OGTT. The test should be performed as described by the World Health Organization, using a glucose load containing the equivalent of 75 g anhydrous glucose dissolved in water[a]
OR
4. In a patient with classic symptoms of hyperglycemia or hyperglycemic crisis, a random plasma glucose $\geq$200 mg/dl (11.1 mmol/l)

Adapted from American Diabetes Association [20]

[a]In the absence of unequivocal hyperglycemia, criteria 1–3 should be confirmed by repeat testing

of diabetes correlated with increased mortality risk, and demonstrated a 30-fold increased risk of fatal coronary heart disease in women with CAD and with diabetes of greater than 25 years [19].

Practical Points in Diagnosis and Treatment

Diagnosis of Diabetes

The diagnosis of diabetes mellitus is rendered in the same way for both genders. Type 2 diabetes has a more insidious onset than type 1. Patients can typically escape formal diagnosis due to lack of overt symptoms early on and which usually occur years later. Type 2 diabetes has a complex genetic linkage which is stronger than for type 1 diabetes mellitus. It is often diagnosed more in women with hypertension and hyperlipidemia, thus causing additive or multiplicative effects in increasing CV risk.

Table 13.2 reviews the diagnostic criteria and evaluation for diabetes as recommended by the American Diabetes Association [21]

Gestational diabetes, a slightly separate entity, is defined as any degree of glucose intolerance during pregnancy, with most cases resolving after delivery. Currently mothers with the standard criteria for diabetes, as seen in Tables 13.2 and 13.3, are diagnosed with formal diabetes mellitus and not just gestational diabetes. To diagnose gestational diabetes an oral glucose tolerance test is administered between weeks 24 and 28 of gestation. Defined cut-offs exist for fasting, 1 and 2 h plasma glucose levels as stated on Table 13.3. Gestational diabetes in itself confers up to a 30 % increased risk of future development of adult onset diabetes, thus recommendations of post-delivery screening in the mother at least once every 3 years. Of importance is the addition of considering gestational diabetes (along with other pregnancy related complications) as a

Table 13.3 Definitions, terms, classifications

Disorder/syndrome	Definition/criteria for diagnosis
Metabolic syndrome	A group of risk factors when associated together predict future risk for cardiovascular disease and diabetes. Consist of 3 of 5 of the following:
	1. Abdominal obesity >102 cm (>40 in) in men, >88 cm (>35 in) in women
	2. Triglycerides ≥150 mg/dL
	3. HDL cholesterol <40 mg/dL in men, <50 mg/dL in women
	4. Blood pressure ≥130/85 mmHg
	5. Fasting glucose ≥110 mg/dL
Prediabetes	Glucose intolerance as defined by the presence of:
	1. Fasting plasma glucose 100
	2. Oral glucose tolerance test 140
	3. HgA1C 5.7
Diabetes mellitus type 1	Diabetes with hyperglycemia that results from a lack of insulin from the autoimmune destruction of beta-islet pancreatic cells
Diabetes mellitus type 2	Diabetes where there is primary insulin resistance and secondary progressive insulin secretory deficiency. Diagnosed with either:
	1. Fasting plasma glucose ≥126 mg/dL on more than one occasion
	2. 75-g oral glucose tolerance test with 2 h value of ≥200 mg/dL
	3. Random plasma glucose of ≥200 mg/dL with typical diabetes symptoms[a]
	4. HgA1C ≥6.5 %
Gestational diabetes	Diabetes diagnosed during pregnancy that is not clearly overt new onset diabetes currently or known diabetes. Diagnosed by:
	1. 75-g oral glucose tolerance test at 24–28 gestation with
	(a) Fasting glucose ≥92 mg/dL
	(b) 1 h glucose ≥180 mg/dL
	(c) 2 h glucose ≥153 mg/dL
Polycystic ovarian syndrome (PCOS)	Oligo or anovulation with signs of androgen excess activity (either clinically or by bioassay), polycystic ovaries, and exclusion of other causes

[a]Includes excessive thirst, urination, fatigue/weakness, weight loss, or overt clinical presentation of hyperglycemic crisis

contributing risk factor for CVD in the revised American Heart Association guidelines of 2011 [22] stressing the importance of early assessment and diagnosis of life-time risk.

Treatment of Diabetes and the Metabolic Syndrome

The American Diabetic Association endorses aggressive treatment of those with A1C levels within the abnormal range of 6–6.4 % with lifestyle modifications. These include, weight loss, diet and exercise as they are more than ten times at risk for developing diabetes than their normal A1C counterparts.

After the diagnoses of the metabolic syndrome, prediabetes or diabetes mellitus are made; care must be taken to meet therapeutic goals of glycosylated hemoglobin levels (HgA1C levels), blood pressure, cholesterol, and most importantly weight. Treatment of the metabolic syndrome consists primarily on emphasizing therapeutic lifestyle changes and in some instances may include medical treatment of prehypertension and or prediabetes, although guidelines are not clear on that. Women diagnosed with prediabetes or diabetes should be counseled on weight loss to a normal BMI if obesity is present, on a lean, low-fat diet, and recommended at least 30 min of cardiovascular exercise daily.

Glycosylated hemoglobin A1C (HgA1C) levels of less than or equal to 7 % should be attained through a combination of, diet, exercise, weight loss and medication.

Evidence supports aggressive lifestyle modification that promotes healthy diet and exercise as key parts of the treatment. Initial observational studies and small clinical trials suggested diet and exercise could curtail the development of diabetes. These studies were helpful and provided initial insight. The Diabetes Prevention Program (DPP) study was however the first sentinel trial to establish that weight loss and exercise can significantly reduce the development of diabetes.

Diabetes Prevention Program Study

The Diabetes Prevention Program Research Group was the first large cohort, with over 3,000 Americans, 68 % of which were women and 45 % of ethnic minority groups, that provided impressive evidence of decreased incidence of diabetes with weight loss and exercise in patients with impaired glucose levels (an elevated fasting plasma glucose or elevated post-load plasma glucose) that were not yet diabetic. When randomized to at least a 7 % weight loss and at least 150 min of physical activity a week, patients reduced their incidence of diabetes mellitus 58 % (95 % CI, 48–66 %) in a mean follow up of 2.8 years. Treatment with metformin reduced the incidence of diabetes as well, but only by 31 % (95 % CI, 17–43 %). There was no treatment difference between either sex nor were there differences between ethnic groups [23]. The results of the Diabetes Prevention Program empower health care providers to clearly and strongly advocate for weight loss, exercise, and healthy eating habits as a way to significantly reduce the risk of developing diabetes even more effectively than medications. Figuratively, to prevent a single case of diabetes during 3 years, 6.9 patients would have to commit to the above lifestyle intervention, while 13.9 would have to be placed on metformin.

Treatment of Hypertension in Diabetes

The most recent blood pressure goals have been established by The Seventh Report of the Joint National Committee on Prevention, Evaluation, and treatment of High

Blood Pressure (JNC-7) and currently include a blood pressure of ≤130/80 and treatment with an angiotensin converting enzyme (ACE) inhibitor or angiotensin receptor blocker (ARB) as first line in those with diabetes due to their cardiac and renal protective effects. In women of child-bearing age, care must be taken to ensure that they are on oral contraceptives or similar birth control while on ACE inhibitors or ARBs to avoid adverse fetal effects. Nonetheless, they are both considered first line therapy for hypertension in diabetics of both sexes, with benefits shown both in cardiovascular outcomes and associated microvascular outcomes, including retinopathy, nephropathy, and neuropathy. There have been several important landmark clinical trials that have delineated the treatment algorithm for hypertension (Table 13.4). Although none of them directly studied hypertension solely in diabetic women, there were significant numbers of women enrolled in of these trials [24].

UKPDS

Spanning from 1977 to 1997 and involving 23 centers, the United Kingdom Prospective Diabetes Study (UKPDS) had over 5,000 patients with a new diagnosis of diabetes and was the first hallmark study to show definitively that complications can be reduced by blood glucose and blood pressure control. The treatment arms consistent of a tight blood pressure group with goal of blood pressure 150/85 versus a less tight blood pressure control group with goal of blood pressure 180/105. Forty-six percent of the tight blood pressure group were women, 42 % of the less tight blood pressure group were women. Patients in the tight blood pressure group treated with captopril and atenolol had decreased risk of in the combined endpoint of myocardial infarction, sudden death, stroke, and peripheral vascular disease, with a relative risk of 0.66. Risk in primary retinopathy was also seen, but significant reduction in myocardial infarctions alone was not seen [24, 25]. Interestingly, the risk reductions were not significant 10 years after the trial as during the post-trial period patients were no longer on their intensive hypertensive regimen [26].

HOT Trial

The Hypertension Optimal Treatment study was important to establish the benefit in reduction in diastolic blood pressure. Approximately 47 % of those enrolled were women. A large randomized trial with over 18,000 patients between the ages of 50–80 years old, it used first-line treatment of felodipine with additional antihypertensives as needed. Results showed benefit in decreasing blood pressure to less than 140/85. Additionally, there was a remarkable 51 % reduction in cardiovascular events in diabetic patients with diastolic blood pressures ≤80 mmHg in comparison to diabetic patients with diastolic blood pressures ≤90 mmHg (p = 0.005) [24, 27].

Table 13.4 Clinical trials of BP medications in patients with diabetes

Study	n	Follow up period (years)	Blood pressure (mmHg)	Drugs tested	Impact on outcomes
UKPDS	5,102	20	Tight goal 150/85 versus less stringent goal <180/105	Tight: captopril or atenolol	Favors tight control: decreased death from diabetes, stroke, and microvascular disease (retinopathy)
HOT	18,790	3.8	Diastolic goal <80 versus ≤90	Calcium channel blocker plus others	≤80 group: decreased major cardiovascular events
HOPE, MICRO-HOPE	9,297 (3,577 with diabetes)	3.5 (4.5)	Mean BP for both groups 139/79 at baseline	Ramipril versus placebo	Ramipril group: decreased MI, stroke, cardiovascular death, all-cause mortality, nephropathy
ALLHAT	42,418 (13,101 with diabetes)	4.9	Mean BP 146/83 at baseline	Amlodipine versus lisinopril versus chlorthalidone	Chlorthalidone group: lower systolic BP than amlodipine or lisinopril; no difference for fatal/nonfatal MI: increased heart failure for amlodipine and lisinopril versus chlorthalidone
ABCD	470	5	Diastolic goal: Intensive ≤75 versus moderate ≤80–89	Nisoldipine versus enalapril	Intensive: decreased death; no difference for retinopathy or neuropathy; increased MI for nisoldipine versus enalapril; renal function stabilized with both drugs
ACCORD BP	4,733	4.7	Systolic goal <120 versus <140	Stepped care to reach goals	No difference in nonfatal MI, nonfatal stroke, or cardiovascular death

[a]Adapted by Velarde and Antonetti from Salanitro and Roumie [24]

HOPE Trial

The Heart Outcomes Prevention Evaluation study was a sentinel trial to establish the benefits of ACE inhibitors to reduce future cardiovascular events in patients with cardiovascular disease or risk factors for it. It studied over 9,000 patients with over 4,000 randomized to receive either ramipril or placebo. Approximately 40 % of those enrolled had diabetes. Thirty-eight percent of those assigned to the ramipril arm were women compared to 35 % in the placebo group. The study was stopped 6 months early (after 4.5 years) due to the consistent benefit of ramipril compared to placebo. Significant findings included a 22 % risk reduction for myocardial infarction, 33 % risk reduction for stroke, and 24 % risk reduction for total mortality in the ramipril group when compared to the placebo group [24, 28]. Additionally, the Microalbuminuria, Cardiovascular, and Renal Outcomes in the Heart Outcomes Prevention Evaluation trial (MICRO-HOPE) demonstrated a 22 % risk reduction in the development of nephropathy in those treated with ramipril [24, 29].

ALLHAT Trial

The Antihypertensive and Lipid Lowering Treatment to Prevent Heart Attack trial was conducted to compare treatment with calcium channel blockers, ACE inhibitors, and or thiazide diuretics as blood pressure treatment in patients with elevated blood pressure and another cardiovascular disease risk factor. Of those enrolled, 36 % had diabetes. The combined primary outcome consisted of fatal or non-fatal myocardial infarction and there were no significant differences between the three drug classes, despite a slight increase in blood sugar and increased risk of diabetes with chlorthalidone after a year therapy (thiazide diuretic used in the trial) that an increased risk in heart failure was seem for those patients on amlodipine (40 % more) and lisinopril (15 % more) compared to chlorthalidone. With this disparity, the authors alluded to diuretics as preferable treatment for hypertension [24, 30].

ABCD Trial

The Appropriate Blood Pressure Control in Diabetes study aimed to study microvascular disease progression with moderate versus intensive control of blood pressure as well as to compare nisoldipine, a calcium channel blocker, with enalapril, an angiotensive converting enzyme, as a first-line anti-hypertensive. The two study arms consisted of intensive blood pressure control with diastolic goal of ≤75 mmHg compared to moderate blood pressure control with diastolic goal of ≤80–89 mmHg. Thirty-two percent of those enrolled were women. Mean blood pressure at study end was 132/78 mmHg in the intensive blood pressure control group and 138/86 mmHg in the moderate blood pressure control group. When compared to the moderate blood pressure control group, the incidence in death was reduced 51 % in the intensive blood pressure control group. Regarding microvascular outcomes, there was no difference between the rate of progression in retinopathy and neuropathy. It was also found that in those treated with nisoldipine compared to enalapril there were significantly higher rates (a total of 25 versus 5) of fatal and non-fatal myocardial infarctions (9.5 RR, 95 % CI 2.3–21.4) [24, 31, 32].

ACCORD Trial

The Action to Control Cardiovascular Risk in Diabetes blood pressure trial was conducted to determine the outcome on cardiovascular disease in diabetics with aggressive systolic blood pressure lowering to <120 mmHg. 47.7 % of those enrolled were women. Over 4,500 patients were randomized to the intensive blood pressure control group (goal systolic blood pressure of <120 mmHg) or the standard blood pressure control group (systolic <140 mmHg). Follow up was approximately 5 years and showed no significant difference between the composite primary outcome of non-fatal myocardial infarction, stroke or cardiovascular death. There were, however, fewer cardiovascular events (208 versus 237) and fewer strokes (36 versus 62) in the intensive treatment arm despite this not reaching statistical significance. Notably there were significantly more adverse events (p<0.001), such as syncope and dizziness, in the intensive group compared to the standard group (3.3 % versus 1.3 %) [24, 33].

In summary, there is much data to support controlling hypertension in diabetics, with the first-line therapy being ACE inhibitors or ARBs, bearing in mind that women of child-bearing age should be counseled on the teratogenicity of both and the need to be on reliable birth control. Gender specific differences in outcomes with any specific therapy have not been seen, although women have not been uniquely studied in these aforementioned landmark trials. However, as opposed to other areas of cardiovascular research, women often composed a sizable number of the study participants in hypertension clinical trials and meaningful therapeutic applications, can still be inferred.

Goal blood pressure should be ≤ 130/80 (as long as this is well tolerated without symptoms) to best avoid future cardiovascular events and microvascular diabetic disease.

Treatment of Hyperlipidemia in Diabetes and Metabolic Syndrome

In ATP III, diabetes mellitus is regarded as a coronary disease equivalent. Thus the LDL goal of less than or equal to 100 mg/dL with option to go as low as 70 mg/dl has been made. Aggressive lifestyle modifications with option of statin drug therapy for levels 100–129 mg/dL and/or initiation of statin therapy for LDL greater than 130 mg/dL is recommended [34]. Aggressive treatment to these goals is recommended for women with either diabetes or the metabolic syndrome given their increased risk for developing cardiovascular disease.

Recent concerns have been raised regarding the use of statins and increased risk of future diabetes.

At least six, large, randomized studies have reported conflicting results of increased rates of diabetes in the statin treatment arm despite decreased risk for cardiovascular events. The JUPITER trial, one of the largest studies, was designed to assess cardiovascular endpoints in patients without overt hyperlipidemia, but with an elevated CRP. JUPITER enrolled over 17,000 patients and assigned them to either placebo or rosuvastatin for on average 1–9 years. On follow up, a significant higher number of individuals in the rosuvastatin group developed physician-reported diabetes (270 in the rosuvastatin group versus 216 in the placebo group, p=0.01) despite having the same fasting blood glucose levels during follow up [35]. Other studies, including one from the West of Scotland Coronary Prevention Study (WOSCOPS) study which used pravastatin, provided evidence to the contrary. It showed that pravastatin may reduce the incidence of diabetes [36]. Two large meta-analyses that have followed, including one in 2010 which included a total of 13 statin trials (over 91,000 participants), including both the JUPITER trial and WOSCOPS study, found statins were associated with a 9 % increased risk for incidence of diabetes (OR 1.09; 95 % CI 1.02–1.17) with little heterogeneity between trials [37]. Risk for developing diabetes with statins was highest in trials with older patients, but neither change in LDL concentration nor BMI explained the increased risk in diabetes. One extra case of diabetes resulted for every 255 patients treated for 4 years in this study. The subsequent meta-analysis, comprised of five trials (over 32,000 participants), studied whether intensive-dose statin therapy was associated with increased risk of diabetes compared to moderate-dose statin therapy [38]. Intensive-dose statin therapy consisted of atorvastatin 80 mg daily, or simvastatin 40–80 mg daily while moderate-dose statin therapy consisted of pravastatin 40 mg daily, simvastatin 20–40 mg daily, atorvastatin 10 mg daily, or placebo. There were two additional cases of diabetes in the intensive-treatment group per 1,000 patient-years but 6.5 fewer cardiovascular events per 1,000 patient years, with odds ratios of 1.12 (95 % CI 1.04–1.22) for development of diabetes and 0.84 (95 % CI 0.75–0.94) for sustaining a cardiovascular events. Compared to moderate-dose statin therapy, the NNH (number needed to harm) per year for intensive-dose statin therapy was 498 for one newly diagnosed diabetic, while the NNT (number needed to treat) per year for intensive-dose statin therapy was 155 to avoid a cardiovascular event. These findings support that there seems to be a small increased risk for developing diabetes while on statin therapy, independent of BMI and LDL reduction intensity, that is outweighed by a higher reduction in cardiovascular events with their use.

The Women's Health Initiative also investigated the correlation between statin use and incidental development of diabetes, but in a unique cohort of only post-menopausal women [39]. In this group of nearly 150,000 post-menopausal women average age of 63 years, treated with trial medication in addition to treatment of other medical conditions such as hyperlipidemia, those who were taking a statin at baseline showed an increased risk of diabetes, notably much larger than the above mentioned meta-analyses. This increased risk was present even when adjusting for possible confounders of age, race, BMI, physical activity, smoking status, family history of diabetes, clinical study arm, and personal history of cardiovascular disease, with a hazard ratio of 1.48 (95 % CI, 1.38–1.59).

Surmising from all the data available to date, it does appears to be an associated small risk with statins in developing incident diabetes, but this has been found to be overpowered by the cardio-protective benefits they offer. This risk, albeit small, needs to be discussed with patients.

As discussed earlier, women generally have increased morbidity and mortality after their sentinel myocardial infarction compared to men [15]. The pathophysiology behind this remains poorly understood and whether there are specific risk factors to which to attribute this increased risk is unclear.

Limited gender specific data on the use of statins however shows a clear benefit of statins with decrease in cardiovascular mortality in the subset of women with coronary artery disease.

In a large meta-analysis of 13 trials and over 17,000 women (two thirds of whom came from two studies), there were differences in outcomes with statins depending on whether women had known cardiovascular disease or not [40]. Lipid lowering with statins in women without known cardiovascular disease did not reduce overall mortality (RR 0.95, 95 % CI 0.62–1.46), cardiovascular mortality (RR 1.07, 95 % CI 0.47–2.40), non-fatal myocardial infarction (RR 0.61, 95 % CI 0.22–1.68), revascularization (RR 0.87, 95 % CI 0.33–2.31), or cardiovascular events (RR 0.87, 95 % CI 0.69–1.09). However, some analyses were limited because of low cardiovascular event rates in those trials. In 8 of the trials that included over 8,000 women with known coronary artery disease, statins significantly reduced cardiovascular mortality (RR 0.74, 95 % CI 0.55–1.00), non-fatal myocardial infarction (RR 0.71, 95 % CI 0.58–0.87), revascularization (RR 0.70, 95 % CI 0.55–0.89), and total cardiovascular events (RR 0.80, CI 0.71–0.91) [40]. However, statins did not reduce total mortality (RR 1.00, 95 % CI 0.77–1.29). In summary, data suggests that for women without coronary artery disease, lipid lowering with statins does not affect all-cause or cardiovascular mortality. Lipid lowering with statins may or may not reduce cardiovascular events in this cohort of women, i.e. no primary prevention, but more data is needed. For women with known cardiovascular disease, lipid lowering with statins is effective in reducing cardiovascular mortality, cardiovascular events including revascularization, and non-fatal myocardial infarctions but no demonstrated effect on total mortality.

Low HDL, high amounts of small particle serum LDL, and hypertriglyceridemia appears to be a least favorable lipid profile for women when compared to men. There is some suggestion in recent trial data that omega-3 fatty acids in women without known heart disease, but deemed at risk, benefit with significantly lowered rates of cardiovascular death and hospitalization for cardiovascular cause when compared to their male cohorts who did not experience any benefit (HR 0.82, 95 % CI 0.67–0.99, p=0.04) [41]. Findings from the JELIS (Japan Eicosapentaenoic Acid Lipid Intervention) study, the first large-scale, prospective, randomized trial of combined treatment with a statin and an omega-3 fatty acid originally derived from fish, eicosapentaenoic acid (EPA), has shown that the addition of EPA to statin therapy provides additional benefit in preventing major coronary events, apparently through lipid-independent mechanisms in patients with CVD [42]. The majority of the participants in this study were women. The results add support to previous evidence of the beneficial effect of omega-3 fatty acids in patients with known coronary heart disease [42].

Diagnosis of Coronary Artery Disease in the Diabetic Woman

Diagnosis of asymptomatic coronary artery disease in the diabetic population is often recommended in diabetic patients with risk factors, regardless of gender [43].

However, most recent consensus from different organizations including American Diabetic Association (ADA) shy away from this practice [44, 45] and specific testing and modality of testing in asymptomatic diabetic individuals (irrespective of sex) remains controversial. It has been shown that adenosine stress nuclear testing is equally prognostic in diabetic men and women undergoing stress testing [41]. Furthermore, Berman et al. prospectively followed adenosine myocardial perfusion single photon emission tomographic studies in women versus men and demonstrated that amongst diabetic patients, women had worse outcome than men for any degree of perfusion defects [46]. Nuclear stress testing has been the modality that has been most researched in diabetic populations for both diagnosis and prognosis, but data is lacking to support an actual improvement in their outcome with directed cardiovascular treatment [47]. Normal stress testing even in higher-risk diabetics is useful in short term risk stratification only. Conflicting guidelines from the American Heart Association and the ADA exist; with the former emphasizing that there are no outcome data to support stress testing in asymptomatic diabetic patients. On the contrary the American Diabetic Association has advocated for stress testing in diabetics with any of the following (1) typical or atypical cardiac symptoms (2) resting electrocardiogram (ECG) suggestive of ischemia or infarction (3) peripheral or carotid arterial occlusive disease (4) sedentary lifestyle, with age greater than or equal to 35 with plans to begin a vigorous exercise program and (5) two or more of the following risk factors in addition to diabetes: total cholesterol greater than 240 mg/dL, $LDL > 160$, $HDL < 35$, blood pressure $> 140/90$, smoking, family history of premature coronary artery disease, and micro or macroalbuminuria [43]. Of note, the ADA committee in 1998 acknowledged these recommendations were based on expert consensus clinical judgment as there were no published data supporting these recommendations. As mentioned earlier the most recent standard of medical care guidelines from the ADA do not advocate for routine screening of asymptomatic diabetic patients with high cardiovascular disease risk [44, 45].

However, both the American College of Cardiology, American Heart Association and the ADA recommend that an exercise ECG test be done among patients with diabetes with known or suspected CAD, type 1 diabetes for more than 15 years, type 2 diabetes for more than 10 years or age greater than 35, microvascular disease, peripheral arterial disease or autonomic neuropathy prior to engaging in an aggressive exercise program. The United States Preventative Services Task Force (USPSTF) however, concluded that there is insufficient evidence to recommend for or against this type of screening for coronary disease in asymptomatic patients, including before an exercise program [48]. Hence, presently there is inadequate evidence to recommend routine stress testing in asymptomatic diabetic patients.

Special Considerations

Polycystic Ovarian Syndrome

Estimated to occur in about 6–7 % of premenopausal women, polycystic ovarian syndrome (PCOS) is a syndrome that consists of hyperandrogenism and oligo-ovulation when other medical disorders have been excluded. Key components of the metabolic syndrome are present in PCOS, of these central adiposity and low HDL levels are the most common. The lipoprotein profile in women with polycystic ovaries is significantly distorted. They usually have high concentrations of serum triglycerides and total and low-density lipoprotein cholesterol. Furthermore, the levels of high density lipoprotein (HDL) and particularly HDL2 subfraction are suppressed [20, 49]. Insulin resistance, increased glucose levels, and hypertension are also more frequently present in PCOS than weight-matched controls. Women with PCOS have a higher rate of developing overt diabetes mellitus when compared to women of the same BMI who do not have PCOS [7]. Of all women with PCOS, up to 30 % have impaired glucose tolerance and another 7.5 % have the diagnosis of diabetes. In those that have PCOS without obesity, 10.3 % of them have impaired glucose tolerance. The exact cause of the insulin resistance is unclear and suppression of androgen excess does not appear to change insulin resistance. Despite observations that women with PCOS appear to have more extensive coronary artery disease on angiography, higher coronary artery calcification scores, more endothelial dysfunction and pro-inflammatory and pro-thrombogenic markers [50, 51] and an indisputable presence of multiple cardiovascular risk factors at a young age, prospective limited study data surprisingly does not support an increased risk of cardiovascular disease in women with PCOS [7, 21]. However, no prospective longitudinal study has assessed CVD outcomes specifically in women with PCOS. Uncertainty thus remains in women with PCOS regarding increased incidence of cardiovascular disease and mortality later in life. Even in the absence of definitive outcome studies, the evidence supports a strong recommendation that women with PCOS should undergo comprehensive evaluation for recognized cardiovascular risk factors and receive appropriate treatment based on findings.

Gestational Diabetes

Not all women are recommended by the American Diabetic Association to be tested for gestational diabetes. Women who meet all the low-risk criteria are exempt from such testing as it has been found not to be useful and cost-ineffective. These criteria, which all must be met, include age less than 25, normal body weight, no first-degree relatives with diabetes, no history of abnormal glucose metabolism, no history of prior poor obstetric outcome, and women who are not members of ethnic groups with high prevalence of diabetes mellitus such as Hispanics, Native Americans, Asian Americans, African Americans and Pacific Islanders [52]. Timing of the risk assessment for gestational diabetes is important. It is recommended that women with increased risk factors such as obesity, strong family history, history themselves of gestational diabetes in the past, should undergo glucose testing as soon pregnancy is confirmed. They are then again tested at the routine 24–28 weeks of gestation. Average risk women without these risk factors are usually tested within 24–28 weeks. There are typically two approaches, the one step approach consisting of a diagnostic oral glucose tolerance test without prior serum glucose screening, and the two step approach, consisting of initial serum glucose screening 1 h after a 50 g oral glucose load followed by a diagnostic oral glucose tolerance test in women with abnormal glucose level after the 50 g challenge.

Immediately after pregnancy, up to 5–10 % of women with gestational diabetes are diagnosed with diabetes [53]. Women diagnosed with gestational diabetes have a 35–60 % chance of developing diabetes in the following 10–20 years. Non-Caucasian and Hispanic women with a history of gestational diabetes and those who fail to lose their pregnancy weight or are obese are at the highest risk for developing overt diabetes. It is recommended then that women with gestational diabetes get tested for diabetes 6–12 weeks after the baby is delivered and then at least every 3 years thereafter [52, 53].

Women with Diabetes and Known Cardiovascular Disease

Women with diabetes and established coronary have worse outcomes than men with higher cardiac morbidity and mortality as previously outlined [2, 15, 16]. Given their risk, aggressive attempts should be made to reach goals for lipids, blood pressure, and fasting blood sugar levels as per guidelines. Modification of other risk factors such as obesity, nicotine and alcohol dependence should be aggressively pursued. In women with established coronary artery disease and diabetes, a lower LDL target level (70 mg/dl or less) appears to be associated with the greatest outcome benefits [6, 22]. This is usually achieved through statin therapy which has the strongest evidence as reviewed previously.

The increased mortality seen in diabetic women, particularly in those with established coronary disease compared to diabetic men, remains poorly understood and highlights the importance to include more women (diabetic in particular) in cardiovascular trials with pre-defined gender specific analysis. Increasing rates of obesity affecting women more than men, as well as psychological variables such as depression, isolation, poor stress coping mechanisms, have been cited as additional factors for increased cardiovascular disease in women particularly. However, more research is needed in the field to determine if gender specific pathophysiological differences exist in the diabetic female heart that could explain some of the disparities in outcomes. The impact of risk factors in the micro and macrovascular circulation in the diabetic heart within the context of hormonal status, aging and psychosocial influences need to be better explored.

Summary

- The metabolic syndrome is an important predictor of cardiovascular morbidity and mortality, especially in women of ethnic minority groups with increased cardiovascular disease risk when compared to men.
- The metabolic syndrome is a well-recognized antecessor to diabetes mellitus type 2 and as such offers an opportunity for aggressive therapeutic lifestyle changes.

- Aggressive treatment of risk factors for diabetes, including obesity, prediabetes, and the metabolic syndrome, are essential for primary prevention
- Subgroups of women are more likely to develop diabetes. Ethnic minorities and women with gestational diabetes, are particularly at risk, and should be counseled on risk factor modification early on.
- Women with diabetes have worse cardiovascular outcomes, with increased morbidity and mortality, particularly after first myocardial infarction and in those with established coronary artery disease.
- Therapeutic goals for women with diabetes include blood pressure of less than 140/90 with option of tighter control in certain younger diabetics to goal of <130/80 if it can be achieved without undue treatment burden.
- Therapeutic goals for women with diabetes and hyperlipidemia include the use of moderate intensity statins for those with diabetes alone and high intensity statins for those with diabetes and high risk of atherosclerotic of cardiovascular disease.
- A normal BMI, appropriate diet and exercise are paramount for treatment for women with diabetes.
- Treatment of hypertension should include ACE inhibitors or ARBs if tolerated (and if of child bearing age on oral contraceptives or similar birth control)
- The role of diagnostic stress testing for asymptomatic diabetic women remains controversial. This is mostly due to lack of data in diabetic women and stress testing specifically and lack of mortality benefit of stress testing in asymptomatic individuals in general.

Addendum

Since the completion of this book, two new guidelines have come out that slightly modify some of the text above. The new JNC 8 hypertension guidelines [54] have loosened the blood pressure target for older patients >60 years old to <150/90 and also loosen recommendation for treatment of diabetics >18 years old to <140/90 not differentiating them from the general adult population. These guidelines represent a consensus of a committee of experts that are not all in agreement with the final document and it has not yet been endorsed by the AHA/ACC and deviates from recent updated recommendations by other expert committees. The American Society of Hypertension (ASH) jointly with the International Society of Hypertension (ISH) recently released their new guidelines [55] upholding the prior recommendations for a goal and treatment initiation level of blood pressure in those <80 years of age of 140/90 mmHg, consistent with the most recent guidelines of the European Society of Hypertension (ESH) [56]. As it relates to diabetic patients >18 years old, they concur that should be treated to <140 mmHg systolic, <85 mmHg diastolic (ESH) and to lower target of <130 mmHg systolic for certain younger diabetics if it can be achieved without undue treatment burden [55, 57].

The AHA and the ACC have issued a 'HYPERLINK "http://content.onlinejacc.org/article.aspx?articleid=1778408" scientific advisory' [58] on the treatment of hypertension, and likely will produce their own hypertension guideline in the future.

Regarding the new cholesterol guidelines published recently by the ACC/AHA [59], the focus has shifted from goal directed or specific target levels of LDL or non-HDL to degree of strength of statin needed to treat patients with different risk profiles. Statins continue to form the basis for treatment of patients with moderate or high risk for atherosclerotic cardiovascular disease (ASCVD). Statins continue to be recommended for adult diabetic patients regardless of gender from moderate reduction statins (pravastatin and simvastatin) for adults 40–75 years old age with diabetes alone to high intensity statins (atorvastatin and rosuvastatin) for adults 40–75 years old age with diabetes and a $\geq$7.5 % 10 year of ASCVD risk unless contraindicated.

References

1. National Diabetes Fact Sheet, Centers for Disease Control; 2011. www.cdc.gov.
2. Koerbel G, Korytkowski M. Coronary heart disease in women with diabetes. Diab Spectr. 2003;16:148–53.
3. Kannel WB, McGee DL. Diabetes and cardiovascular disease. The Framingham Study. JAMA. 1979;241:2035–8.
4. Howard BV, Cowan LD, Go O, et al. Adverse effects of diabetes on multiple cardiovascular disease risk factors in women: the Strong Heart Study. Diabetes Care. 1998;21:1258–65.
5. Guzder RN, Gatling W, Mullee MA, et al. Impact of metabolic syndrome criteria on cardiovascular disease risk in people with newly diagnosed type 2 diabetes. Diabetologia. 2006;49:49–55.
6. Grundy SM, Brewer Jr BB, Cleeman J, et al. Definition of the metabolic syndrome: report of the National Heart, Lung, and Blood Institute/American Heart Association Conference on scientific issues related to definition. Circulation. 2004;109:433–8.
7. Bentley-Lewis R, Koruda K, Seely EW. The metabolic syndrome in women. Nat Clin Pract Endocrinol Metab. 2007;3:696–704.
8. Hunt KJ, Resendez RG, Williams K, et al. National Cholesterol Education Program versus World Health Organization metabolic syndrome in relation to all-cause and cardiovascular mortality in the San Antonio Heart Study. Circulation. 2004;110:1251–7.
9. McNeill AM, Rosamond WD, Girman CJ, et al. The metabolic syndrome and 11-year risk of incident cardiovascular disease in the atherosclerosis risk in communities study. Diabetes Care. 2005;28:385–90.
10. Reaven GM, et al. Abnormal lipoprotein metabolism in non-insulin- dependent diabetes mellitus: pathogenesis and treatment. Am J Med. 1987;83:31–40.
11. Margolin E, Zhornitzki T, Kopernik G, et al. Polycystic ovary syndrome in post-menopausal women–marker of the metabolic syndrome. Maturitas. 2005;50:331–6.
12. Ford ES, Giles WH, Dietz WH. Prevalence of the metabolic syndrome among US adults. Findings from the third National Health and Nutrition Examination Survey. JAMA. 2002;287:356–9.
13. Ford ES, Giles WH, Mokdad AH. Increasing prevalence of the metabolic syndrome among US adults. Diabetes Care. 2004;27:2444–9.
14. Mottillo S, Filion KB, Genest J, et al. The metabolic syndrome and cardiovascular risk. A systematic review and meta-analysis. J Am Coll Cardiol. 2010;56:1113–32.
15. Miettinen H, Lehto S, Salomaa V, et al. Impact of diabetes on mortality after the first myocardial infarction. Diabetes Care. 1998;21:69–75.
16. Vaccarino V, Krumholz HM, Yarzebski J, et al. Sex differences in 2-year mortality after hospital discharge for myocardial infarction. Ann Intern Med. 2001;134:173–81.

17. Wilson PWF, Kannel WB. In: Hyperglycemia, diabetes and vascular disease. Ruderman N et al., eds. Oxford; 1992.
18. Gu K, Cowie CC, Harris MI. Diabetes and decline in heart disease mortality in US adults. JAMA. 1999;281:1291–7.
19. Hu FB, Stampfer MJ, Solomon CG, et al. The impact of diabetes mellitus on mortality from all causes and coronary heart disease in women. 20 years of follow up. Arch Intern Med. 2001;161:1717–23.
20. Giallauria F, Orio F, Palomba S, et al. Cardiovascular risk in women with polycystic ovary syndrome. J Cardiovasc Med. 2008;9:987–92.
21. Sharpless JL. Polycystic ovary syndrome and the metabolic syndrome. Clinl Diabetes. 2003;21:154–61.
22. Mosca L, Benjamin EJ, Berra K, et al. A guideline from the American Heart Association. Effectiveness-based guidelines for the prevention of cardiovascular disease in women—2011 update: guidelines for the prevention of cardiovascular disease in women. Circulation. 2011;123(11):1243–62.
23. Diabetes Prevention Program Research Group. Reduction in the incidence of type 2 diabetes with lifestyle intervention or metformin. N Engl J Med. 2002;346:393–403.
24. Salanitro AH, Roumie CL. Blood pressure management in patients with diabetes. Clin Diabetes. 2010;28:107–14.
25. U.K. Prospective Diabetes Study Group. Tight blood pressure control and risk of macrovascular and microvascular complications in type 2 diabetes: UKPDS 38. BMJ. 1998;317:703–13.
26. Holman RR, Paul SK, Bethel MA, et al. Long-term follow-up after tight control of blood pressure in type 2 diabetes. N Engl J Med. 2008;359:1565–76.
27. Hansson L, Zanchetti A, Carruthers SG, et al. Effects of intensive blood pressure lowering and low-dose aspirin in patients with hypertension: principal results of the Hypertension Optimal Treatment (HOT) randomized trial. Lancet. 1998;351:1755–62.
28. Yusuf S, Sleight P, Pogue J, et al. Effects of an angiotensin-converting enzyme inhibitor, ramipril, on cardiovascular events in high-risk patients. N Engl J Med. 2000;342:145–53.
29. Heart Outcomes Prevention Evaluation Study Investigators. Effects of ramipril on cardiovascular and microvascular outcomes in people with diabetes mellitus: results of the HOPE study and MICRO-HOPE substudy. Lancet. 2000;355:253–9.
30. Whelton PK, Barzilay J, Cushman WC, et al. Clinical outcomes in antihypertensive treatment of type 2 diabetes, impaired fasting glucose concentration, and normoglycemia: Antihypertensive and Lipid-Lowering Treatment to Prevent Heart Attack Trial (ALLHAT). Arch Intern Med. 2005;165:1401–9.
31. Estacio RO, Jeffers BW, Hiatt WR, et al. The effect of nisoldipine as compared with enalapril on cardiovascular outcomes in patients with non-insulin dependent diabetes and hypertension. N Engl J Med. 1998;338:645–52.
32. Estacio RO, Jeffers BW, Gifford N, et al. Effect of blood pressure control on diabetic microvascular complications in patients with hypertension and type 2 diabetes. Diabetes Care. 2000;23 Suppl 2:B54–64.
33. The ACCORD study group. Effects of intensive blood-pressure control in type 2 diabetes mellitus. N Engl J Med. 2010;362:1575–85.
34. Grundy SM, Cleeman JI, Bairey Merz N, et al. Implications of recent clinical trials for the National Cholesterol Education Program adult treatment panel III guidelines. Circulation. 2004;110:227–39.
35. Ridker PM, Danielson E, Fonseca FA, et al. Rosuvastatin to prevent vascular events in men and women with elevated C-reactive protein. N Engl J Med. 2008;359:2195–207.
36. Freeman DJ, Norrie J, Sattar N. Pravastatin and the development of diabetes mellitus: evidence for a protective treatment effect in the West of Scotland Coronary Prevention Study. Circulation. 2001;103:357–62.
37. Sattar N, Preiss D, Murray HM, et al. Statins and risk of incident diabetes: a collaborative meta-analysis of randomised statin trials. Lancet. 2010;375:735–42.
38. Preiss D, Seshasai SRK, Welsh P, et al. Risk of incident diabetes with intensive-dose compared with moderate-dose statin therapy. JAMA. 2011;305:2556–64.

39. Culver AL, Ockene IS, Balasubramanian R, et al. Statin use and risk of diabetes mellitus in postmenopausal women in the Women's Health Initiative. Arch Intern Med. 2012;172: 144–52.
40. Walsh JME, Pignone M. Drug treatment of hyperlipidemia in women. JAMA. 2004; 291:2243–52.
41. The Risk and Prevention Study Collaborative Group. n-3 fatty acids in patients with multiple cardiovascular risk factors. N Engl J Med. 2013;368:1800–8.
42. Yokoyama M, Origasa H, Matsuzaki M, et al. Effects of eicosapentaenoic acid on major coronary events in hypercholesterolaemic patients (JELIS): a randomised open-label, blinded endpoint analysis. Lancet. 2007;369:1090–8.
43. American Diabetes Association. Standards of medical care for patients with diabetes mellitus (Position Statement). Diabetes Care. 2003;26(Suppl 1):S33–50.
44. Bax JJ, Young LH, Frye RL, Bonow RO, Steinberg HO, Barrett EJ. ADA Screening for coronary artery disease in patients with diabetes. Diabetes Care. 2007;30:2729–36
45. American Diabetes Association. Standard of Medical Care in Diabetes Diabetes Care 2014;37(Suppl 1):S14–S80.
46. Berman DS, Kang X, Hayes SW, et al. Adenosine myocardial perfusion single-photon emission computed tomography in women compared with men. J Am Coll Cardiol. 2003;41:1125–33.
47. Albers AR, Krichavsky MZ, Balady GJ. Stress testing in patients with diabetes mellitus. Diagnostic and prognostic value. Circulation. 2006;113:583–92.
48. U.S. Preventive Services Task Force – USPSTF (2012) Agency for healthcare research and quality. Rockville, MD. http://www.ahrq.gov/professionals/clinicians-providers/guidelines-recommendations/uspstf/index.html.
49. Raikowha M, Glass MR, Rutherford AJ, Michelmore K, Balen AH. Polycystic ovary syndrome: a risk factor for cardiovascular disease? Br J Obstet Gynecol. 2000;107:11–8.
50. Cho LW, Jayagopal V, Kilpatrick ES, et al. The biological variation of C-reactive protein in polycystic ovarian syndrome. Clin Chem. 2005;51:1905–7.
51. American Association of Clinical Endocrinologists Position Statement on metabolic and cardiovascular consequences of Polycistic Ovary Syndrome. Polycystic Ovary Syndrome Writing Committee. Endocr Pract. 2005;11(2):125–34.
52. American Diabetes Association. Diagnosis and classification of diabetes mellitus. Position statement. Diabetes Care. 2010;33:562–9.
53. Centers for Disease Control and Prevention. National diabetes fact sheet: general information and national estimates on diabetes in the United States. Atlanta: U.S Department of Health and Human Services, Centers for Disease Control and Prevention; 2011. www.cdc.gov.
54. James PA, Oparil S, Carter BL, et al. 2014 evidence-based guideline for the management of high blood pressure in adults: report from the Panel Members Appointed to the Eighth Joint National Committee (JNC 8). JAMA. 2014;311(5):507–20. doi:10.1001/jama.2013.284427.
55. Weber MA, Schiffrin EL, White WB, et al. Clinical practice guidelines for the management of hypertension in the community: a statement by the American Society of Hypertension and the International Society of Hypertension. J Clin Hypertens (Greenwich). 2014;16:14–26.
56. Mancia G, Fagard R, Narkiewicz K, et al. 2013 ESH/ESC guidelines for the management of arterial hypertension: the Task Force for the Management of Arterial Hypertension of the European Society of Hypertension (ESH) and of the European Society of Cardiology (ESC). Eur Heart J. 2013;34:2159–219.
57. American Diabetes Association. Standard of medical care in diabetes diabetes care. 2014; 37(Suppl 1).
58. Go AS, Bauman M, Coleman King SM, Fonarow GC, Lawrence W, Williams KA, Sanchez E. AHA/ACC/CDC Science Advisory: An Effective Approach to High Blood Pressure Control A Science Advisory From the American Heart Association, the American College of Cardiology, and the Centers for Disease Control and Prevention. J Am Coll Cardiol. 2013.
59. Stone NJ, Robinson J, Lichtenstein AH, et al. 2013 ACC/AHA guideline on the treatment of blood cholesterol to reduce atherosclerotic cardiovascular risk in adults: a report of the American College of Cardiology/American Heart Association Task Force on Practice Guidelines. J Am Coll Cardiol. 2013. doi:10.1016/j.jacc.2013.11.002.

Part III
Pregnancy and Heart Disease

Chapter 14
Heart Disease in Pregnancy

Erica O. Miller, Stephanie J. Carter, and Sabu Thomas

Introduction

Cardiovascular disease affects only 1–4 % of pregnancies, yet still accounts for nearly 12 % of pregnancy related deaths in the United States, making this the leading cause of non-obstetric mortality [1, 2]. It is also the most important cause of non-obstetric morbidity during pregnancy. Unfortunately, cardiovascular disease in pregnancy is often under recognized as a result of its rather low prevalence, even when pregnant women exhibit concerning signs or symptoms. Contributing to the diagnostic challenges, normal physiologic changes that occur during pregnancy can often mimic cardiac disease. The morbidity and mortality from cardiovascular disease in this population can be attributed to a combination of normal physiological changes, previously unrecognized heart disease, and higher risk pre-existing cardiac conditions. The epidemiology of pregnant women is also changing, with more pregnancies complicated by advanced maternal age, assistive reproductive technologies and congenital heart disease [2]. Cardiovascular disease does not necessarily preclude successful pregnancy, but can increase maternal and neonatal risk. Patients with pre-existing cardiac lesions and those at significant risk for acquired heart disease during pregnancy should be counseled in advance about their risk. To assist clinicians in counseling and management of cardiovascular disease in pregnancy, we have reviewed the pertinent literature. In this chapter, we will summarize changes in cardiovascular physiology that occur during pregnancy and then outline approaches to pre-existing and acquired heart disease in pregnancy.

E.O. Miller, MD (✉)
Department of Medicine, University of Rochester Medical Center, Rochester, NY, USA
e-mail: erica_miller@urmc.rochester.edu

S.J. Carter, MD • S. Thomas, MD
Division of Cardiology, University of Rochester Medical Center, Rochester, NY, USA
e-mail: stephanie_carter@urmc.rochester.edu

H.Z. Mieszczanska, G.P. Velarde (eds.),
Management of Cardiovascular Disease in Women,
DOI 10.1007/978-1-4471-5517-1_14, © Springer-Verlag London 2014

Normal Cardiovascular Physiology of Pregnancy

Physiologic Changes in Pregnancy

Significant physiologic changes occur during pregnancy. These include an increase in blood volume and cardiac output, an increase in red blood cell mass, a reduction in systemic vascular resistance and shifts in blood flow between organ systems [3]. These changes can even persist for up to 3 months post-partum [4].

It is vital that clinicians understand these changes to assess and interpret symptoms, physical findings, and electrocardiographic and echocardiographic findings, which can either mimic or truly represent cardiac disease in pregnancy. Understanding these physiologic changes and their consequences in the setting of abnormal cardiac anatomy and physiology will also assist in risk stratification of women with known cardiac disease. In general, those at highest risk include women with the Eisenmenger syndrome, pulmonary hypertension or Marfan Syndrome with aortopathy [5]. In these settings, pregnancy poses significant risk and should be avoided (Table 14.1).

During pregnancy, plasma volume increases by approximately 30–50 % [4]. This is accomplished through an increase in sodium retention and total body water. Women accumulate sodium during pregnancy from increased estrogen plus increased hepatic production of angiotensinogen and renin production in the liver, uterus, and kidney. Total body water is also increased through a variety of endocrine pathways including deoxycorticosterone, prostaglandins, prolactin, placental lactogen, growth hormone, and ACTH. Red cell mass is also increased by approximately 20–30 % and is mediated by progesterone, placental chorionic somatomammotropin and prolactin [3]. The disproportionate increase in plasma volume relative to red cell volume results in the well-recognized anemia of pregnancy. The normal range for hematocrit in pregnancy is 33–38 % [3, 4].

Cardiac output, a product of stroke volume and heart rate, is increased in pregnancy by as much as 50 %. This results from increases in both stroke volume and heart rate. Early in pregnancy, stroke volume is the predominant contributor, increasing by around 30 % [4]. Later in gestation, increases in heart rate have a larger role in maintaining cardiac output. Both atrial natriuretic peptide and brain natriuretic

Table 14.1 Conditions in which pregnancy is contraindicated

Eisenmenger syndrome
Cyanosis from any cause
Marfan syndrome with aortopathy
Severe/symptomatic mitral or aortic stenosis
Pulmonary arterial hypertension from any cause
Symptomatic heart failure from any cause

Adapted from Thorne et al. [20] with permission of BMJ Publishing Group Ltd and Regitz-Zagrosek et al. [17] with permission of Oxford University Press (UK) © European Society of Cardiology. www.escardio.org/guidelines

Table 14.2 Physiologic changes during pregnancy, labor and delivery, and the post-partum period

	Pregnancy	Labor and delivery	Postpartum
Plasma volume	↑ by 30–50 %	↓ due to blood loss	↓
Heart rate	↑ by 15–20 beats per minute	↑	↓
Cardiac output	↑ by up to 50 %	↑ again by up to 50 %	↓
Stroke volume	↑ by 30 % during first and second trimesters	↑	↓
Blood pressure	↓ systolic and diastolic	↑	↓
Systemic vascular resistance	↓	↑	↓

peptide are increased in pregnancy, which causes peripheral vasodilation and afterload reduction with resulting increase in cardiac output [3].

Systemic vascular resistance decreases during pregnancy by up to 30 % at 8 weeks [4]. This decrease is due to increased estrogens, progesterone, prostaglandins, prolactin. Increased prostacyclin decreases the vasoconstrictive effect of angiotensin II during pregnancy. Nitric oxide is also increased, resulting in vasodilation. Relaxin is also thought to contribute to decreased systemic vascular resistance [3].

In addition to changes in blood volume, there are also shifts in blood flow between organ systems. Blood flow is increased to the uterus and kidneys [3]. Changes in coronary blood flow are not well understood, though it is likely increased to meet myocardial demand from increased ventricular wall muscle mass and end diastolic volume [6, 7]. Normal physiologic changes during pregnancy, labor and delivery, and the post-partum period are summarized in Table 14.2.

Symptoms During Pregnancy

Many symptoms that occur commonly during normal pregnancy would be concerning for cardiac disease in other settings. Pregnancy is typically associated with fatigue, dyspnea on exertion, and decreased exercise capacity due to a combination of normal physiologic changes [8]. Many women also feel lightheaded and may even experience syncope from aortocaval compression from the gravid uterus. Lower extremity edema likely results from sodium retention, and may be worsened by decreased venous return from the lower extremities due to caval compression [3].

Physical Exam of Pregnant Patient

Pertinent vital sign changes during pregnancy include tachycardia, with heart rate increasing by 15–20 beats per minute and peaking at 32 weeks gestation. Blood pressure is decreased, particularly the diastolic pressure, resulting in a widened pulse pressure [3]. Physical exam demonstrates displaced apical impulse due to increased left ventricular mass and the more horizontal position of heart due to diaphragmatic elevation from the uterus. Pregnant women have more pronounced jugular venous pulsations, which is likely related to increased volume and decreased systemic vascular resistance. Auscultation reveals a split S1, probably due to early closure of the mitral valve. The second heart sound is widely split, likely because of increased pulmonary blood flow. A systolic murmur is often audible due to increased flow and relative valvular stenosis. A physiologic third heart sound (S₃), reflecting the increased blood volume, can sometimes be auscultated.

Electrocardiographic changes during pregnancy include an increase in heart rate and leftward shift of the QRS and T-wave axis because of upward and horizontal displacement of the heart by the gravid uterus [9]. Interestingly, estrogen may have a digoxin-like effect on the ECG, causing ST segment depressions [9]. Echocardiography during pregnancy may reveal an increase in left atrial size and left ventricular wall mass [10, 11]. It is important to consider the patient's position when interpreting symptoms, vital signs, and physical exam findings due to increased inferior vena cava compression while supine. This may be relieved by having the patient move to the left lateral decubitus position, where inferior vena cava compression is minimized [3]. Up to 11 % of women are diagnosed formally with the supine hypotensive syndrome of pregnancy, which is due to the same phenomenon of inferior vena cava compression [12]. These women have tachycardia and symptomatic hypotension with weakness, lightheadedness, nausea, dizziness, and syncope [3].

Labor and Delivery

Labor and delivery are associated with dramatic hemodynamic changes, which vary with duration of labor and associated pain as well as type of anesthesia. During labor, cardiac output may increase by as much as 50 % [3]. Oxygen consumption also increases, by as much as 30 % [13]. Uterine contractions are associated with dramatic shifts in blood distribution, with autotransfusion of 300–500 ml of blood from the uterus to the systemic circulation [14]. Transient hypotension occurs in 60 % of cesarean deliveries with either epidural or spinal anesthesia [15]. Vaginal deliveries are typically result in 300–400 ml estimated blood loss, while cesarean deliveries are associated with 500–800 ml of blood loss.

Postpartum Changes

Some changes in pregnancy persist following delivery, in subsequent pregnancies, and beyond. In particular, cardiac output and left ventricular volumes increase during pregnancy and remain elevated in the year following pregnancy, with greater increase in women who have had multiple pregnancies [11]. While many of the cardiovascular changes during pregnancy appear to be adaptive, women with higher parity appear to be at increased cardiovascular risk later in life, at least based on prospective data [16]. The long-term consequences of pathologic changes to cardiovascular function such as peripartum cardiomyopathy will be addressed in a later section.

Medication Adjustment

Whether medically managing cardiac disease or an unrelated chronic or acute medical condition, the impact of the cardiovascular changes during pregnancy on medication pharmacokinetics must be considered. Plasma volume is increased and plasma proteins are decreased, which results in variable binding, delivery, and elimination of drugs. Glomerular filtration is increased, which leads to more rapid elimination of renally cleared medications. Similarly, there is increased hepatic blood flow with faster hepatic clearance [4]. Medical management of specific cardiac conditions will be addressed later in the chapter.

Summary of Cardiovascular Changes in Pregnancy

Cardiovascular disease, while rare in pregnancy, is an important cause of morbidity and mortality. Profound hemodynamic changes include increased blood volume and cardiac output, decreased systemic vascular resistance, and shifts in blood flow between different organ systems. Pregnant women have faster heart rates and lower blood pressure than their non-pregnant counterparts. Their cardiac exam also differs, with changes in point of maximum impulse and new murmurs. They may demonstrate electrocardiographic changes including T wave inversions and ST segment depression. Echocardiograms performed on pregnant women may reveal increased left ventricular mass. These changes can vary dramatically from minute to minute based on body position and from week to week based on gestational age. It is important for obstetricians, anesthesiologists, and cardiologists to be familiar with the normal changes in pregnancy and their effects on women with and without cardiac disease during their pregnancies and beyond.

Risk Stratification of Women with Pre-existing Heart Disease Considering Pregnancy

Overview

Cardiac disease is the leading cause of non-obstetric mortality in pregnancy. Given that certain pregnant women are at higher risk than others, risk assessment should be tailored to the individual patient and potential pathology. However, this is complicated by limited data on disease-specific predictors of outcome as well as changing demographics of pregnant women and advances in diagnostic testing and therapeutic interventions [17]. As there are a growing number of adults surviving with congenital heart disease, it comes as no surprise that this is the most common form of heart disease presenting to high-risk obstetrical referral centers in North America [18]. In general, the risk of pregnancy complications increases with the complexity of congenital heart disease [19]. Women of childbearing age with cardiac disease should be counseled on issues of contraception, maternal and fetal risks of pregnancy, and potential long-term maternal morbidity and mortality. Pregnancy-related risk is cumulative, therefore risk increases with each additional cardiac or non-cardiac condition (i.e. diabetes) [18, 20]. Furthermore, there is an increasing number of pregnancies complicated by advanced maternal age [21]. Capabilities exist now to detect and monitor cardiac disease in both the mother and the fetus, for instance with troponin assays and fetal echocardiography [22]. Diagnosis, management, and counseling regarding risks for the mother and fetus during pregnancy is limited by the lack of prospective or randomized studies so the onus remains on clinicians to apply available data and guidelines to individual patients [17]. First, a more generalized approach to risk stratification of women with heart disease that pre-exists pregnancy will be presented. Following this, risks of specific congenital, valvular, and rhythm abnormalities will be addressed.

Assessment of Risk in Patients with Preexisting Cardiac Disease

Siu and colleagues [18] have developed a risk stratification tool to further quantify cardiac risk during pregnancy in women with both congenital and acquired heart disease. Cardiac events in these women are most commonly pulmonary edema or arrhythmia. Four risk factors should be assessed:

1. Prior cardiac event, including heart failure, transient ischemic attack, stroke or arrhythmia preceding pregnancy
2. New York Heart Association Class III or IV, or cyanosis
3. Left atrial outlet obstruction with mitral valve area <2 cm² or left ventricular outflow tract obstruction with aortic valve area <1.5 cm² or peak left ventricular outflow gradient >30 mmHg on echocardiogram
4. Left ventricular systolic dysfunction with ejection fraction <40 % [18].

This validated risk score may be used to predict the risk for cardiac complications (Table 14.3). In patients with pre-existing cardiac disease and no risk factors, the risk for a maternal cardiac event during pregnancy or peripartum is 5 %. The presence of one risk factor increases this to 25 %. Women with known cardiac disease and more than one risk factor are at a significantly higher risk for a cardiac event (75 %) [18].

Maternal functional class is an important predictor of outcome with NYHA functional class III (marked limitation of physical activity) and IV (symptomatic at rest) predicting higher maternal cardiac events.

Table 14.3 Quantifying cardiac risk during pregnancy

Number of risk factors	Risk for cardiac event during pregnancy (%)
0	5
1	25
2	75

Adapted from Regitz-Zagrosek et al. [17]. With permission of Oxford University Press (UK) © European Society of Cardiology. www.escardio.org/guidelines

Table 14.4 WHO classification of maternal cardiovascular risk

WHO class	Pregnancy risk	Frequency of cardiac follow-up
I	Low: risk of maternal morbidity or mortality no higher than in general population	Once or twice during pregnancy
II	Moderate: small increase in risk of maternal morbidity or mortality	At least every trimester
III	High: significant increase in risk of severe maternal morbidity or mortality	Monthly during pregnancy
IV	Very high: pregnancy contraindicated due to very high risk of severe maternal morbidity or mortality	Every 2–4 weeks during pregnancy

Adapted from Thorne et al. [20] with permission of BMJ Publishing Group Ltd.

The World Health Organization (WHO) has also developed a tool for risk stratification (Table 14.4), which has been adopted by the European Society of Cardiology [17]. In this schema, pregnancies are classified into one of four risk classifications:

WHO class I is considered low risk, II corresponds to moderate risk, III is high risk, and IV is very high risk. Distinction between class II and III must be especially individualized, with increased risk with more risk factors or a combination of conditions.

It may be appropriate for women in class I to be seen by a cardiologist only one or two times during pregnancy. Cardiology follow-up for women in class II should occur at least every trimester. Due to the high risk for morbidity and mortality in class III, these women benefit from preconception counseling from an expert cardiologist and a high risk obstetrician, should be evaluated by a cardiologist approximately monthly during pregnancy, and require close monitoring postnatally [17]. Higher risk pregnancies should be managed by maternal and fetal medicine obstetricians in conjunction with cardiologists. Preferred mode of delivery for women with significant cardiac risk is usually vaginal given the smaller volume blood loss and less dramatic changes in hemodynamics. However, this should be tailored to the individual patient and in some instances early cesarean delivery is required [17]. Conditions in which pregnancy is contraindicated (WHO Class IV) are listed in Table 14.1 above. When women with these lesions reach child bearing age, they should be counseled that pregnancy is contraindicated.

Congenital, valvular, and acquired cardiac conditions are categorized into WHO classes I through IV in Table 14.5.

Table 14.5 WHO risk categories for specific cardiac conditions

WHO class	Congenital	Valvular	Acquired prior to pregnancy
I	Uncomplicated, small, or mild:	Uncomplicated, small, or mild:	Isolated ventricular extrasystoles
	Pulmonary stenosis	Mitral valve prolapse with no more than trivial mitral regurgitation	Atrial ectopic beats
	Ventricular septal defect		
	Patent ductus arteriosus		
	Successfully repaired simple lesions		
	Ostium secundum atrial septal defect		
	Ventricular septal defect		
	Patent ductus arteriosus		
	Total anomalous pulmonary venous return		
II	Unoperated atrial septal defect		Most arrhythmias
	Repaired tetralogy of Fallot		
II or III	Hypertrophic cardiomyopathy	Native or tissue valvular heart disease not considered WHO class IV	Heart transplantation
	Marfan syndrome without aortic root dilatation		Mild left ventricular impairment
	Aorta <45 mm in aortic disease associated with bicuspid aortic valve		
III	Systemic right ventricle	Mechanical valve	
	Congenitally corrected transposition of the great arteries		
	Simple transposition status post Mustard or Senning repair		
	Complex congenital heart disease status post Fontan		
	Unrepaired cyanotic heart disease		
	Other complex congenital heart disease		
	Marfan syndrome with aortic dilatation of 40–45 mm		
	Aortic dilatation of 45–50 mm in aortic disease associated with bicuspid aortic valve		

IV	Eisenmenger syndrome	Severe mitral stenosis	Pulmonary arterial hypertension from any cause
	Uncorrected cyanotic congenital heart disease with resting oxygen saturation <85 %	Severe symptomatic aortic stenosis	Severe systemic ventricular dysfunction with LVEF <30 % or NYHA class III or IV
	Native severe coarctation of the aorta		Previous peripartum cardiomyopathy with residual impairment of left ventricular function
	Marfan syndrome with aortic dilatation of >45 mm		
	Aortic dilatation of >50 mm in aortic disease associated with bicuspid aortic valve		

Adapted from Thorne et al. [20] with permission of BMJ Publishing Group Ltd and Regitz-Zagrosek et al. [17] with permission of Oxford University Press (UK) © European Society of Cardiology. www.escardio.org/guidelines

LVEF left ventricular rejection fraction, NYHA New York Heart Association

Very High Risk Lesions

Congenital

As outlined above, one of the highest risk conditions is the Eisenmenger syndrome whereby a left to right shunt caused by a congenital heart defect causes increased flow through the pulmonary vasculature, causing pulmonary hypertension, which in turn causes increased pressures in the right side of the heart and reversal of the shunt into a right-to-left shunt. This is high risk from the combination of pulmonary hypertension and systemic cyanosis from the resultant right to left shunting. Pulmonary hypertension is generally considered to be elevated pulmonary arterial pressures (with varying cut-offs for mean pulmonary artery pressures) with impairment of right ventricular function. Potential consequences of pulmonary hypertension in pregnant and postpartum women include pulmonary hypertensive crises, pulmonary thrombosis, and refractory right heart failure [17]. Additional risks of the Eisenmenger syndrome that can be attributed to cyanosis include heart failure, supraventricular tachycardia, infective endocarditis, and thromboembolism. The risk for thromboembolism must be balanced with concurrent risk for hemoptysis and thrombocytopenia [17]. Maternal mortality in the Eisenmenger syndrome varies from 28 to 36 %, with the time period of highest risk being the month following delivery [23, 24]. Risk is increased with late presentation to the hospital, more severe pulmonary hypertension, and requirement of delivery under general anesthesia [24]. Given the significant maternal risk, women with the Eisenmenger syndrome or pulmonary hypertension should be counseled to avoid pregnancy. It is important to note that some pulmonary hypertension medications like bosentan decrease the efficacy of hormonal contraception [25]. The fetus is at risk for premature delivery or demise in the presence of maternal cyanosis, with <12 % chance of live birth with maternal oxygen saturation <85 % or polycythemia to hemoglobin of >20 g/dL preceding pregnancy [17, 26]. Management includes continuation of pulmonary hypertensive medications, possible bedrest, consideration of prophylaxis of thromboembolism, judicious use of diuretics to avoid volume depletion, treatment of iron deficiency, and frequent monitoring of oxygen saturation and complete blood counts. During delivery, regional anesthesia is preferable to general, and early cesarean delivery may become necessary if maternal or fetal deterioration is evident [17].

Severe coarctation of the aorta is also a high risk lesion. It poses a significant risk for hypertensive disease to the mother, which can result in rupture to aortic or cerebral aneurysms [17]. In one series, risk for maternal mortality during pregnancy was 2 % [27]. Good control of blood pressure is critical, though this must be balanced by avoiding placental hypoperfusion with overly aggressive blood pressure control. Percutaneous intervention for coarctation is possible during pregnancy, though the risk dissection with the procedure is higher during pregnancy. Thus, this is typically only attempted in the peripartum period when medical management has failed and there is clear evidence of fetal or maternal compromise [17].

The major risk for Marfan syndrome with aortopathy is aortic dissection during pregnancy, and patients with higher degree of aortic dilatation are considered WHO pregnancy class IV. As in non-pregnant patients, risk for dissection correlates directly with aortic root diameter, with the largest risk occurring in patients with aortic diameter >40 mm. It is thought that historically, the risk for dissection was over-estimated due to case reports with potential biases. Now, studies have demonstrated that pregnancy apparently has little effect on aortic dilatation in Marfan syndrome [28]. Complications of dissection include worsening mitral regurgitation, supraventricular arrhythmias, heart failure, and acute blood loss. Since pregnant women and the fetus have decreased ability to tolerate these complications, Marfan patients at greatest risk for dissection with aortic root diameter >45 mm should be counseled that pregnancy is contraindicated. Monitoring includes echocardiography every 1–3 months during pregnancy and again 6 months postnatally [17]. Medical management typically includes beta blockade due to potential for protection from more rapid aortic dilatation, though there is limited data confirming this effect [29]. Fetal growth must be monitored with mothers on beta blockers, with greater risk for fetal growth impairment with atenolol [17]. Both vaginal and cesarean delivery may be considered, with the primary goal of minimizing the cardiovascular stress of delivery as much as possible through continuation of beta blockade and expedition of some stages of labor and delivery [17] (Table 14.6).

Valvular

Mitral stenosis (MS) due to rheumatic heart disease is the most common valvular anomaly that becomes clinically significant in pregnancy, and if severe (with valve area <1.0 cm^2), is a contraindication to pregnancy [17, 30]. Women should be counseled that their symptoms will worsen during pregnancy. The increase in heart rate and stroke volume during pregnancy increases the pressure gradient across the narrowed mitral valve. This leads to further increase in left atrial volume and pressure with subsequent pulmonary congestion, worsening dyspnea, orthopnea, reduced exercise tolerance, and potentially atrial fibrillation [17, 31]. Maternal mortality is reported between 1 and 3 % [17]. Requirement for hospitalization was uniform in one series of women with severe mitral stenosis, and 15 % required surgical repair during pregnancy [32]. Fetal risks include prematurity, intrauterine growth retardation, and fetal or neonatal demise (up to 3 %) [31]. Both severity of mitral stenosis and resulting heart failure symptoms are directly correlated with maternal and fetal complications. Maternal complications include worsening heart failure, need for surgery or balloon valvuloplasty, thromboebmolism, and death. Fetal complications include premature birth, small for gestational age, respiratory distress, and death [33, 34]. Ideally, severe mitral stenosis would be repaired prior to pregnancy, which can decrease pregnancy risk from WHO class IV to class II or III [20]. During pregnancy, echocardiograms should be performed monthly, or sooner if symptoms warrant. The goal of medical management of mitral stenosis during pregnancy is to decrease heart rate and minimize left atrial enlargement [35]. If symptomatic

Table 14.6 Maternal risk associated with pre-existing cardiac disease

Low risk
Mild pulmonic stenosis
Small ventricular septal defect
Small patent ductus arteriosus
Repaired atrial septal defect
Repaired ventricular septal defect
Repaired total anomalous pulmonary venous return
Mitral valve prolapse without significant mitral regurgitation
Isolated premature ventricular contractions
Isolated premature atrial contractions
Moderate risk
Unrepaired atrial septal defect
Repaired tetralogy of Fallot
Most arrhythmias
Moderate to high risk
Hypertrophic cardiomyopathy
Marfan syndrome without aortic root dilatation
Native or bioprosthetic valvular heart disease not considered very high risk
Heart transplantation
Mild left ventricular impairment
High risk
Repaired transposition of the great arteries
Previous Fontan repair
Mechanical valve
Very high risk
Eisenmenger syndrome
Uncorrected congenital cyanotic heart disease with hypoxia at rest
Severe coarctation of the aorta
Marfan syndrome with aortopathy
Severe mitral stenosis
Severe aortic stenosis with symptoms
Pulmonary hypertension
Heart failure with LVEF <30 % or NYHA Class III or IV

Adapted from Thorne et al. [20] with permission of BMJ Publishing Group Ltd and from Regitz-Zagrosek et al. [17] with permission of Oxford University Press (UK) © European Society of Cardiology. www.escardio.org/guidelines

pulmonary hypertension develops, women should have their activity restricted and they should be started on a selective beta 1 antagonists. Selective beta 1 antagonists are preferred due to the role of beta 2 receptors in uterine relaxation. Metoprolol is preferred over atenolol due to the potential for greater fetal growth restriction with atenolol [17]. Fluid status should be monitored closely and managed with fluid restriction or gently diuresis, avoiding hypotension and potentially catastrophic placental hypoperfusion [35]. Women with mitral stenosis during pregnancy are at increased risk for atrial arrhythmias, and management of these will be addressed in the following section on acquired heart disease during pregnancy. Percutaneous mitral valve balloon valvotomy may be considered after 20 weeks gestation in women with significant heart failure symptoms (NYHA Class III or IV) who have failed medical management [35]. Delivery should be vaginal in women without pulmonary hypertension and NYHA class I or II heart failure symptoms, while cesarean delivery is favored in women with NYHA class III or IV heart failure symptoms and pulmonary hypertension [17].

Severe aortic stenosis places women at very high risk for complications during pregnancy. The most common cause of aortic stenosis in women of childbearing age is congenital bicuspid aortic valve [17]. Symptomatic severe aortic stenosis is defined as a valve area ≤ 1 cm^2 or peak gradient ≥ 64 mmHg in the presence of dyspnea on exertion, chest pain, or syncope, or an abnormal exercise stress test. The risk for maternal mortality was previously thought to be as high as 17 % [36]. More recent series show that maternal mortality is rare [37]. Symptoms of aortic stenosis, including angina, dyspnea, and syncope, typically worsen or even appear for the first time during pregnancy. In all grades of aortic stenosis, increased cardiac output during pregnancy leads to increases in transvalvular aortic gradients [32]. 10 % of patients with severe aortic stenosis experience signs and symptoms of heart failure during pregnancy, and anywhere between 3 and 25 % will develop arrhythmias [38]. Such complications are rare in mild or moderate disease [37]. Women with aortic stenosis should be monitored carefully during pregnancy with monthly or bimonthly echocardiograms [17]. If signs or symptoms of heart failure develop, patients should be managed with activity restriction, gentle diuresis, and treatment of arrhythmias. Percutaneous valvuloplasty may be attempted during pregnancy in patients without evidence of calcification or aortic regurgitation [39]. Delivery in severe symptomatic aortic stenosis should be by cesarean section with general anesthesia, and in some cases early cesarean delivery with subsequent surgical aortic valve replacement is required [17].

Acquired

Pulmonary hypertension from an acquired causes such as lung disease, hypoxia, and chronic thrombo-embolic disease is managed the same as pulmonary hypertension from congenital heart disease, which was addressed previously. A mean PAP ≥ 25 mmHg at rest is indicative of pulmonary hypertension. The risk probably increases with more elevated pulmonary pressures.

High Risk

Congenital

Patients with transposition of the great arteries generally fall into WHO class III for pregnancy risk. Whether corrected in utero (known as congenitally corrected transposition of the great arteries or atrioventricular and ventriculo-arterial discordance), or surgically after birth with an arterial switch operation (Senning or Mustard repair), risk is apparently similar [17]. Pregnancy complications include potentially life-threatening arrhythmias, hypertensive disease, worsening heart failure symptoms, and irreversible decline in right ventricular function [17, 40]. Patients with transposition of the great arteries are at increased risk for AV nodal blockade and bradycardia, so beta blockers must be used with caution. Cardiac follow up should occur frequently during pregnancy, with echocardiograms and ECGs every 1–2 months. Vaginal delivery is usually appropriate in the absence of any hemodynamic decompensation [17].

Pregnancy risk for women with who have had the Fontan procedure depends on the hemodynamics of the circuit, with better prognosis and lower risk in women with a more optimal circuit [17]. Maternal complications include atrial arrhythmias and worsening heart failure symptoms, and there is increased risk for fetal loss, premature birth, and small for gestational age size [41]. Patients should be evaluated by a cardiologist monthly during and immediately following pregnancy. ACE inhibitors must be discontinued, and anticoagulation to prevent thrombo-embolism should be considered. Vaginal delivery is preferred, though early cesarean delivery may be necessary if worsening heart failure occurs [17].

Valvular

Mechanical valves are WHO class III. In women of child-bearing age, mechanical valves have the advantage of excellent hemodynamics and higher durability when compared with bioprosthetic valves. The major disadvantage is the risk for valve thrombosis, which can be fatal, and the potential complications of full anticoagulation during pregnancy. The risk for teratogenicity on warfarin is 6.4 %. Warfarin crosses the placenta and typically causes primarily central nervous system abnormalities. The risk for warfarin embryopathy can be effectively eliminated with substitution of heparin beginning by 6 weeks gestation through 12 weeks, and then resumption of oral anticoagulation with warfarin until delivery is planned [42]. Women requiring lower warfarin doses (<5 mg per day) have a 2.6 % risk of teratogenesis while women on higher doses (>5 mg per day) have an 8 % risk [43]. However, the risk for valve thrombosis is directly related to the time spent on heparin in place of warfarin, with 3.9 % thrombosis with only oral anticoagulation, 9.2 % for heparin in the first trimester, and 33 % for heparin throughout pregnancy [42]. These risks must be weighed by the patient and physician, and will inform the decision regarding anticoagulation regimen. Close monitoring of anticoagulation and evidence of possible valve thrombosis should be performed throughout pregnancy. Vaginal delivery is contraindicated for pregnant women on warfarin due to the risk for neonatal intracranial hemorrhage. Given the concurrent risk for maternal hemorrhage with cesarean section on warfarin, planned vaginal delivery with transition back to heparin is preferred [17].

Moderate to High Risk

Congenital

Hypertrophic cardiomyopathy is the most common heritable cardiac disease, and it is frequently diagnosed during pregnancy [17]. Fortunately, women without symptoms or high ventricular outflow gradient preceding pregnancy typically tolerate pregnancy well and are considered WHO class II. Risks include worsening heart failure and pulmonary congestion, and signs and symptoms of left ventricular outflow tract obstruction such as syncope. Management includes beta blockade in patients with septal wall thickness >15 mm or with moderate to severe left ventricular outflow tract obstruction [44]. Delivery should be planned in most cases, and decision for regional versus general anesthesia must be decided based on patient characteristics. Epidural anesthesia can cause worsening of left ventricular outflow tract obstruction due to systemic vasodilation [17].

Valvular

Many valvular lesions and those that have been replaced with a bioprosthetic valve are WHO class II-III. Bioprosthetic valves are generally well tolerated in pregnancy, and pregnancy appears to have no effect on valve durability [45]. Mitral valve prolapse is the most common cause of mitral regurgitation in pregnancy, and is generally well tolerated. In contrast to mitral stenosis, mitral regurgitant lesions benefit from the favorable effects of decreased systemic vascular resistance and increased blood volume [46].

Moderate Risk

Congenital

Uncorrected atrial septal defects place pregnant women in WHO class II. Women of childbearing age with atrial septal defects that are hemodynamically significant should be offered closure prior to pregnancy, as this would significantly decrease pregnancy risk related to the atrial septal defect [17]. Maternal risks include thromboembolism, and arrhythmias, with the risk for arrhythmias especially high in pregnant women over the age of 30 [19, 47]. Fetal risks include pre-eclampsia and small for gestational age birth [17]. A cardiologist typically need only see pregnant women with unrepaired atrial septal defects twice during pregnancy. Transcatheter device closure may be considered during pregnancy if the patient is deteriorating. Given the risk of paradoxical embolism, attempts should be made to minimize venous stasis, including compression stockings, mobilization as able, and potentially medical deep venous thrombosis prophylaxis if bedrest is required for other reasons. Vaginal delivery is usually appropriate [17].

Women with repaired tetralogy of Fallot typically tolerate pregnancy well, and are considered WHO class II. Maternal risks include arrhythmias, heart failure, right ventricular dilatation, thrombo-embolism, aortic root dilatation, and endocarditis, and occur in up to 12 % of women [48]. Fetal risk is likely increased as well. Most women with repaired tetralogy of Fallot can be seen by a cardiologist once per trimester. Those with severe pulmonary regurgitation are at increased risk for cardiac complications, especially irreversible right ventricular dilatation, and should have more frequent follow up with monthly or bimonthly echocardiograms. Vaginal delivery is almost always appropriate [17].

Acquired

Most arrhythmias are considered WHO pregnancy risk class II, with moderate risk to mother and fetus. Most occur in the setting of congenital or valvular heart disease, endocrine abnormalities such as hyperthyroidism, or cardiomyopathy [17]. Management of arrhythmias during pregnancy will be addressed later in the chapter.

Low Risk

Congenital

Uncomplicated, mild pulmonary stenosis, ventricular septal defect, and patent ductus arteriosus are all low risk congenital heart lesions, falling into WHO pregnancy risk class I. However, clinicians should be aware that dramatic increases in cardiac output may lead to right heart failure or atrial arrhythmias despite mild or asymptomatic disease prior to pregnancy [49].

Severe pulmonary stenosis with peak Doppler gradient >64 mmHg should be repaired prior to pregnancy. In women with mild pulmonary stenosis, there is increased risk for hypertensive diseases of pregnancy, and likely some risk of increased fetal complications as well, though this has not been well quantified. Cardiac follow-up once per trimester is appropriate, and vaginal delivery is well tolerated in asymptomatic patients. Small, non-hemodynamically significant ventricular septal defects are similarly well tolerated during pregnancy. Patients should have a pre-pregnancy evaluation of the size of the defect, cardiac dimensions, and estimated pulmonary pressures with an echocardiogram. The main maternal risk is likely hypertensive disease of pregnancy. Cardiac follow-up should occur twice during pregnancy and vaginal delivery is appropriate. Women with repaired ostium secundum atrial septal defects, ventricular septal defects, patent ductus arteriosus, and total anomalous pulmonary venous return are all similarly at low pregnancy risk [17].

Valvular

Mitral valve prolapse without mitral regurgitation is low risk, while mitral valve prolapse with more than trivial mitral regurgitation would be considered WHO pregnancy risk class II-III [17].

Acquired

Isolated premature ventricular contractions and premature atrial contractions are low risk in pregnancy [17].

Risk to the Fetus/Neonate

A general approach to assessing risk for adverse neonatal outcomes has also been developed, with the most common risks to the infant being premature birth or small-for-gestational-age birth weight [18]:

1. New York Heart Association Class III or IV, or cyanosis
2. Left atrial outlet obstruction with mitral valve area <2 cm^2 or left ventricular outflow tract obstruction with aortic valve area <1.5 cm^2 or peak left ventricular outflow gradient >30 mmHg on echocardiogram
3. Heparin or warfarin administration during pregnancy
4. General pregnancy risk factors, including smoking during pregnancy and multiple gestation pregnancies.

Additional Counseling Considerations

For pregnant women with congenital heart disease or a heritable cardiovascular condition, detailed family history and genetic counseling are warranted. Family history should include questions about any cardiac disease and specifically sudden death for unclear causes [17]. Women with congenital heart disease should be counseled that their children would be at an approximately tenfold higher risk of congenital heart disease when compared with the general population. The risk for transmission varies of course, depending on the underlying disease. Interestingly, left sided obstructive lesions have a higher rate of transmission to offspring than other types of congenital heart disease [5]. Some lesions, such as atrioventricular septal defects, follow single gene inheritance. Others, such as tetralogy of Fallot, are polygenic. Marfan syndrome, hypertrophic cardiomyopathy, and long QT syndrome are autosomal dominant, with 50 % risk of transmission to offspring [17]. Transposition of the great arteries appears to be sporadic [26]. Genetic testing should be considered in cardiomyopathies and chanellopathies, when other family members are affected, and if there are other anatomic or developmental abnormalities due to risk for a genetic syndrome. For pregnancies in women affected by congenital heart disease, fetal echocardiography should be offered in the 19th–22nd week of pregnancy. Nuchal fold thickness offers earlier screening for congenital heart disease in the 12th–13th week of pregnancy [17].

Summary of Pre-existing Heart Disease in Pregnancy

Cardiac risk stratification is an important part of counseling and management of pregnant women. Risk is variable, but general principles can be applied help quantify risk to both the mother and fetus in women with congenital heart disease as well as previously acquired valvular disease, arrhythmias, or cardiomyopathies. Risk assessment should be used to guide counseling, management, and monitoring.

Acquired Heart Disease During Pregnancy

Overview

The prevalence of cardiovascular disease during pregnancy is increasing. This is, in part, due to the increasing age (25–44 years) of women at first pregnancy. Older women are more likely to have the traditional risk factors of chronic hypertension, diabetes and preexisting coronary artery disease. Emerging risk factors, such as maternal obesity and gestational hypertension also contribute to the rise in heart disease associated with pregnancy [2]. This section describes the cardiac diseases that are commonly encountered during pregnancy, including hypertensive disorders, cardiomyopathies, coronary artery disease and arrhythmias.

Hypertension

Hypertension is a major cause of maternal, fetal and neonatal morbidity and mortality and occurs in up to 15 % of pregnancies [50]. The hypertensive disorders in pregnancy consist of: (1) chronic, or preexisting, hypertension; (2) gestational hypertension, including preeclampsia; (3) preexisting hypertension with superimposed gestational hypertension plus proteinuria, and; (4) hypertension [51]. These disorders are summarized in Table 14.7.

Pregnant women with untreated hypertension have higher incidences of stroke, abruptio placentae, disseminated intravascular coagulation and end-organ damage. The fetal complications of untreated hypertension include premature birth, intrauterine growth retardation and death.

Table 14.7 Hypertensive disorders of pregnancy

Hypertensive disorder	Definition	Incidence (%)	Proteinuria present
Chronic	BP≥140/90 mmHg that precedes pregnancy, develops before 20 weeks of gestation or persists beyond the 42nd day postpartum	1–5	±
Gestational	Hypertension that develops after 20 weeks of gestation, is not associated with proteinuria and resolves by 12 weeks postpartum	6–7	±
Preeclampsia	De novo hypertension plus new-onset proteinuria, usually occurring during the third trimester	5–7 (25 % in women with preexisting hypertension)	Yes, >0.3 g/24 h

Preeclampsia is a complication of pregnancy that is characterized by hypertension and proteinuria in a previously normotensive woman. It develops in the later stages of pregnancy, usually during the third trimester, but can present as early as 20 weeks of gestation. The etiology of preeclampsia is unclear. Proposed mechanisms include mutations in angiotensinogen [52] and associations with certain human leukocyte antigen (HLA) types [53].

Risk factors for preeclampsia include [54]:

- previous preeclampsia
- first pregnancy
- multiple fetuses
- diabetes
- chronic hypertension
- hydatiform mole

Complications of untreated severe preeclampsia include:

- headache with visual disturbance
- blindness
- right upper quadrant pain
- hyperreflexia
- HELLP syndrome (hemolysis, transaminitis, thrombocytopenia)

Eclampsia is the development of a seizure disorder in the setting of preeclampsia.

Treatment

For all types of hypertensive disorders during pregnancy, management depends on degree of hypertension, gestational age and risk factors; however, close monitoring is always recommended (Table 14.8).

Table 14.8 Antihypertensive medications and their uses during pregnancy

Classification	Medication	FDA category	Common adverse effects
ACE inhibitor	Benazepril, Captopril, Enalapril, Ramipril	D	Renal or tubular dysplasia, oligohydramnios, growth retardation, ossification disorders of skull, lung hypoplasia, contractures, large joints, anemia, intrauterine fetal death
ARB	Candesartan, Irbesartan, Valsartan	D	See above (ACE Inhibitor)
Aldosterone antagonist	Eplerenone	–	Unknown
	Spironolactone	D	Antiandrogenic effects, oral clefts
Alpha-agonist	Methyldopa	B	Mild neonatal hypotension
Alpha-/ beta-blocker	Labetalol	C	Intrauterine growth retardation, neonatal bradycardia and hypotension
Beta-blocker (class II)	Atenolol	D	Hypospadias, birth defects, low birth weight; bradycardia and hypoglycemia in fetus
	Bisoprolol	C	Bradycardia and hypoglycemia in fetus
	Metoprolol	C	Bradycardia and hypoglycemia in fetus
	Propranolol	C	Bradycardia and hypoglycemia in fetus
Calcium channel blocker	Diltiazem (IV)	C	Possible teratogenic effects
	Nifedipine	C	Tocolytic
	Verapamil (PO)	C	Well-tolerated, though limited experience
	Verapamil (IV)	C	May be associated with a greater risk of hypotension and subsequent fetal hypoperfusion
Direct renin inhibitor	Aliskiren	D	Unknown
Diuretic	Furosemide	C	Oligohydramnion
	Hydrochlorothiazide	B	Oligohydramnion
Nitrate	Isosorbide dinitrate	B	Bradycardia
Vasodilator	Hydralazine	C	Fetal tachyarrhythmias, lupus-like symptoms (maternal)

Adapted from Regitz-Zagrosek et al. [17]. With permission of Oxford University Press (UK) © European Society of Cardiology. www.escardio.org/guidelines

Patients with preexisting hypertension may usually continue their medications during pregnancy, with the exception of angiotensin converting enzyme (ACE) inhibitors, angiotensin receptor blockers (ARB) and direct renin inhibitors, all of which are contraindicated during pregnancy. The treatment of mild-to-moderate hypertension (systolic blood pressure (SBP) 140–169 mmHg and diastolic blood pressure (DBP) 90–109 mmHg) without superimposed gestational hypertension or proteinuria is controversial, given the potential effects on perfusion to the fetus [17]. Cases of severe hypertension (SBP 160–180 mmHg and DBP >110 mmHg) may require immediate hospitalization for aggressive blood pressure control. The treatment of preeclampsia is delivery of the fetus.

Women with hypertensive disorders during pregnancy are at increased risk for recurrence in subsequent pregnancies. In addition, these women have increased risks for developing hypertension, stroke and coronary disease later in life [55, 56].

Cardiomyopathies

Cardiomyopathies are rare but potentially fatal complications of pregnancy [57]. The incidence of cardiomyopathies during pregnancy is unknown, as many cases are not diagnosed. The common cardiomyopathies consist of peripartum cardiomyopathy, hypertrophic cardiomyopathy and dilated cardiomyopathy and are discussed in this section. A group of miscellaneous cardiomyopathies, including infiltrative or toxic cardiomyopathies, as well as storage diseases, may also become apparent during pregnancy.

Peripartum Cardiomyopathy

Peripartum cardiomyopathy (PPCM) is defined as de novo left ventricular systolic dysfunction (left ventricular ejection fraction <45 % by echocardiography) of unclear etiology that develops between the last month of pregnancy and 5 months postpartum. As such, it is a diagnosis of exclusion. Reported incidences of PPCM range from approximately 1:100 live births in Zaria, Nigeria to 1:4,000 live births in the United States [58, 59].

Risk factors for PPCM include [17]:

- Family history
- Multiparity or multiple childbirths
- Smoking
- Hypertension
- Diabetes
- Preeclampsia, eclampsia, or postpartum hypertension
- Malnutrition
- Advanced maternal age or teenage pregnancy
- Prolonged use of oral tocolytic beta-agonists, such as terbutaline
- African descent

PPCM may be considered a subset of pregnancy-associated cardiomyopathy (PACM) [60]. PACM, first described in 1937, encompasses women who develop heart failure earlier than the last gestational month. Figure 14.1 illustrates the time of diagnosis among 123 patients with PACM versus PPCM [61].

More than 50 % of women with PPCM recover normal heart function, usually within 6 months of delivery. A left ventricular ejection fraction (LVEF) of greater than 30 % at the time of diagnosis has been associated with better outcomes [61]. Figure 14.2 reflects the findings of a study conducted by Elkayam et al. [61] among 40 patients with PPCM. Timing of recovery in these women is illustrated below.

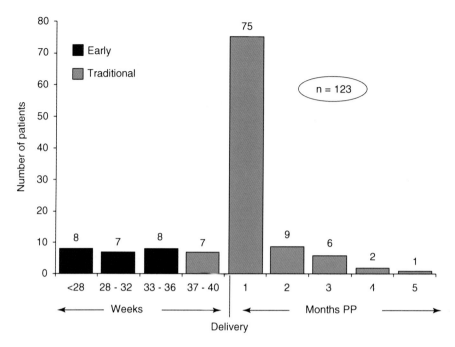

Fig. 14.1 Timing of diagnosis of peripartum cardiomyopathy (Reprinted with permission from Elkayam et al. [61])

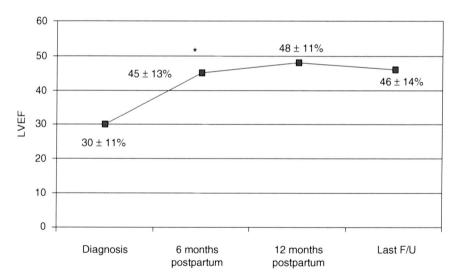

Fig. 14.2 Recovery of left ventricular function in peripartum cardiomyopathy (Reprinted From Elkayam et al. [61])

The risk of recurrence of PPCM in subsequent pregnancies is discussed in a paper by Elkayam et al. [62]: among 28 patients whose LVEFs recovered normal function, 21 % developed heart failure symptoms, 21 % experienced a decrease in LVEF of more than 20, 11 % had premature deliveries and mortality rate was 0 %; among 16 patients whose LVEFs remained less than 50, 44 % developed heart failure symptoms, 25 % experienced a decrease in LVEF of more than 20, 37 % had premature deliveries and mortality rate was 19 %.

Repeat pregnancy is contraindicated in women whose left ventricular function does not normalize. Severe heart failure requiring cardiac transplant occurs in approximately 4 % of women with PPCM, and overall maternal mortality from PPCM is approximately 9 % [62].

The treatment of PPCM is similar to that of other cardiomyopathies (see below). Case reports and experimental studies have also demonstrated the potential benefits of prolactin blockade in mice by the agent bromocriptine [63, 64]; however, current data are not sufficient to recommend the routine use of bromocriptine to treat PPCM.

Hypertrophic Cardiomyopathy (HCM)

Pregnancy is generally well-tolerated in women with clinically-silent HCM. By contrast, women who have symptoms of heart failure before pregnancy are more likely to develop atrial fibrillation and syncope and have higher risks of symptomatic progression and maternal death. Syncope may also develop as a result of potentially severe left ventricular outflow tract obstruction.

Dilated Cardiomyopathy (DCM)

During pregnancy, women with DCM develop left ventricular dilation and systolic dysfunction of unclear etiology. This disease manifests as heart failure symptoms and is differentiated from PPCM by time course. Whereas PPCM is diagnosed later in pregnancy or postpartum, DCM is diagnosed early in pregnancy, often during the first or second trimester.

Treatment

Medical therapy for all cardiomyopathies may be initiated during pregnancy and continue postpartum. In general, standard heart failure medications, including beta blockers, digoxin, diuretics and hydralazine may be used safely. In addition, most ACE inhibitors and angiotensin receptor blockers, which are contraindicated during pregnancy, may be given postpartum.

Coronary Artery Disease

Acute myocardial infarction (AMI) during pregnancy is rare, occurring in approximately 3–6 per 100,000 pregnancies. Coronary artery dissection, spasm and in situ thrombosis occur more frequently than atherosclerosis. The incidence of maternal mortality after acute coronary syndrome (ACS) is approximately 5–10 % and is highest in the peripartum period [22, 65, 66]. This percentage is expected to grow with advancing maternal age and increasing numbers of high-risk pregnancies.

Independent risk factors of AMI during pregnancy include maternal age (usually older than 33 years), chronic hypertension, preeclampsia, diabetes, thrombophilia, postpartum infection and severe postpartum hemorrhage [67, 68]. Diagnostic criteria of ACS during pregnancy are the same as those for non-pregnant patients. Of note, T-wave inversions on the electrocardiogram occur commonly in pregnancy and may not necessarily suggest ischemia.

Spontaneous coronary artery dissection occurs with greater frequency in pregnant women. The cause for this phenomenon is unclear, though the effect of high progesterone levels on the intima and media layers of the arterial wall has been implicated [66].

Treatment

Medical therapy for AMI in pregnant women is similar to that used in non-pregnant patients. Bare metal stents (BMS) require a shorter duration of dual anti-platelet therapy, as compared to drug-eluting stents (DES). For this reason, BMS are recommended over DES to minimize the risk of in-stent thrombosis if clopidogrel is discontinued in the setting of bleeding during delivery [69]. Thrombolytic agents are permitted in cases where cardiac catheterization facilities are not available; however, these agents increase the risk of maternal hemorrhage by approximately 8 % [18]. Standard therapies, including aspirin, short-term heparin, nitrates and beta-blockers are generally safe. ACE inhibitors and statins are contraindicated. Clopidogrel and glycoprotein IIb/IIIa receptor inhibitors should be used with caution, as information regarding the effects of these medications during pregnancy is limited. If cardiac catheterization is performed, abdominal lead shielding is used to protect the fetus. Medications commonly used in the treatment of coronary artery disease (CAD), along with their pregnancy risk categories, are listed in Table 14.9.

Coronary artery bypass grafting has been performed, though rarely, in pregnant women; however, this surgery is associated with a significantly increased risk of fetal loss [66, 69].

Arrhythmias

During pregnancy, arrhythmias can be induced by a hyperdynamic state, altered hormone levels and exacerbation of underlying heart disease [62]. Arrhythmias

Table 14.9 Common CAD medications and their uses during pregnancy

Classification	Medication	FDA category	Common adverse effects
Anticoagulant	Fondaparinux	–	Limited experience
	Heparin (low molecular weight)	B	Rare osteoporosis (long-term use)
	Heparin (unfractionated)	B	Osteoporosis and thrombocytopenia (long-term use)
Antiplatelet	Acetylsalicylic acid	B	No known teratogenic effects
	Clopidogrel	C	No information during pregnancy available
	Ticlopidine	C	Unknown
Lipid-lowering drug	Colestipol, cholestyramine	C	May impair absorption of fat-soluble vitamins
	Fenofibrate	C	No adequate human data
	Gemfibrozil	C	No adequate human data
	Statins	X	Congenital anomalies

Adapted from Regitz-Zagrosek et al. [17]. With permission of Oxford University Press (UK) © European Society of Cardiology. www.escardio.org/guidelines

See also Table 14.8 for ACE inhibitors, ARBs and beta-blockers

requiring treatment occur in up to 15 % of women with congenital heart disease during pregnancy [19]. Women with preexisting arrhythmias are at a higher risk of recurrence during pregnancy [70].

The most common arrhythmias during pregnancy are premature atrial or ventricular complexes, which do not require antiarrhythmic therapy. Episodes of symptomatic paroxysmal supraventricular tachyarrhythmias also commonly occur and can often be treated with vagal maneuvers. Sustained tachyarrhythmias, such as atrial fibrillation and atrial flutter, bradyarrhythmias, atrioventricular blocks and life-threatening ventricular arrhythmias are rare during pregnancy.

Women with preexisting bradyarrhythmias may develop symptoms during pregnancy, due to the need for increased cardiac output. Women with congenital long QT syndrome have a greater risk of sudden cardiac death in the postpartum period than either before or during pregnancy [71].

Treatment

Ventricular rate control in pregnant women can be achieved with similar therapies used in non-pregnant patients. These medications include beta-blockers, digoxin and adenosine. Antiarrhythmic drugs and their pregnancy risk categories are listed in Table 14.10. Direct current cardioversion, if required, is also safe during pregnancy. General treatment guidelines for common arrhythmias encountered during pregnancy are listed in Table 14.11.

Table 14.10 Common antiarrhythmic medications and their uses during pregnancy

Classification	Medication	FDA category	Common adverse effects
Class IA antiarrhythmic	Disopyramide	C	Uterine contractions
Class IB antiarrhythmic	Procainamide	C	Unknown
	Quinidine	C	Thrombocytopenia, premature birth, CNVIII toxicity
	Lidocaine	C	Fetal bradycardia, acidosis, central nervous system toxicity
	Mexiletine	C	Fetal bradycardia
Class IC antiarrhythmic	Propafenone	C	Unknown
Class III antiarrhythmic	Amiodarone	D	Thyroid insufficiency, hyperthyroidism, goiter, bradycardia, growth retardation, premature birth
	Sotalol	B	Bradycardia and hypoglycemia in fetus
Antiarrhythmic	Adenosine	C	Limited human data
Cardiac Glycoside	Digoxin	C	Serum levels are unreliable, safe

Adapted from Regitz-Zagrosek et al. [17]. With permission of Oxford University Press (UK) © European Society of Cardiology. www.escardio.org/guidelines

See also Table 14.8 for beta-blockers and calcium-channel blockers

Summary of Heart Disease in Pregnancy

Despite the fact that heart disease is a significant risk factor for pregnant women in terms of morbidity and mortality, most women are able to have a successful pregnancy. This chapter discussed the normal cardiovascular physiology of pregnancy and the risks associated with preexisting and acquired heart disease during pregnancy. Key points from this chapter include the following:

- Normal physiologic changes in pregnancy include increased blood volume and cardiac output and decreased systemic vascular resistance.
- The pharmacokinetics of drugs can be altered during pregnancy, and some common medications to treat heart disease are contraindicated in pregnancy.
- There is an increasing number of women with congenital heart disease who are now able to survive into adulthood and become pregnant.
- Risk stratification tools have been developed to quantify cardiac risk during pregnancy in women with congenital and acquired heart disease.
- Preconception counseling should be performed for all women with heart disease to assess for maternal and fetal risk.
- Pregnancy is contraindicated in women with the following conditions: Eisenmenger syndrome, uncorrected cyanotic congenital heart disease with resting hypoxia, native severe coarctation of the aorta and Marfan syndrome with significant aortic dilatation with or without bicuspid aortic valve.
- The common acquired heart diseases during pregnancy include hypertensive disorders, cardiomyopathies, coronary artery disease, and arrhythmias.
- The treatment of women who are at high-risk for cardiac complications during pregnancy requires a team-based approach, which includes a maternal-fetal medicine specialist and a cardiologist.

Table 14.11 General treatment guidelines for commonly encountered arrhythmias during pregnancy

Arrhythmia	Examples	Recommended treatment
Supraventricular tachycardia (SVT)		
	Atrial fibrillation	Vagal maneuvers for the acute conversion of paroxysmal SVT
	Atrial flutter	Immediate electrical cardioversion for the acute treatment of any tachycardia with hemodynamic instability
	Atrial tachycardia	Digoxin or metoprolol/propranolol for long-term management of SVT
	AV nodal reentry tachycardia	
	AV reentry tachycardia involving an accessory pathway	
Ventricular tachycardia (VT)		
	RV outflow tract tachycardia	Implantation of ICD, if clinically-indicated, prior to or during pregnancy
	Non-long QT sustained VT	Beta-blocking agents for the long-term management of congenital long QT syndrome
	Monomorphic VT	Metoprolol, Propranolol or Verapamil for the long-term management of idiopathic sustained VT
		Immediate electrical cardioversion of VT for sustained stable or unstable VT
Sinus bradycardia		
	Valsalva maneuver during delivery	Usually transient
	Supine hypotensive syndrome	Temporary pacemaker if symptoms persist
Atrioventricular blocks		
	First degree AV block	No treatment required
	Second degree AV Block, usually associated with underlying structural heart disease	No treatment required if Type I (Wenckebach) and asymptomatic
	Complete heart block, usually associated with congenital heart disease	Supportive pacing if required, but usually not necessary

Adapted from Regitz-Zagrosek et al. [17]. With permission of Oxford University Press (UK) © European Society of Cardiology. www.escardio.org/guidelines

References

1. Berg CJ, Callaghan WM, Syverson C, Henderson Z. Pregnancy-related mortality in the United States, 1998 to 2005. Obstet Gynecol. 2010;116:1302–9.
2. Sahni G, Elkayam U. Cardiovascular disease in pregnancy. Preface. Cardiol Clin. 2012;30:xi–xii.
3. Ouzounian JG, Elkayam U. Physiologic changes during normal pregnancy and delivery. Cardiol Clin. 2012;30:317–29.
4. Abbas AE, Lester SJ, Connolly H. Pregnancy and the cardiovascular system. Int J Cardiol. 2005;98:179–89.
5. Siu S, Colman JM. Cardiovascular problems and pregnancy: an approach to management. Cleve Clin J Med. 2004;71:977–85.
6. Laird-Meeter K, van de Ley G, Bom TH, Wladimiroff JW, Roelandt J. Cardiocirculatory adjustments during pregnancy – an echocardiographic study. Clin Cardiol. 1979;2:328–32.

7. Estensen ME, Beitnes JO, Grindheim G, et al. Altered left ventricular contractility and function during normal pregnancy. Ultrasound Obstet Gynecol. 2013;41(6):659–66.
8. Zeldis SM. Dyspnea during pregnancy. Distinguishing cardiac from pulmonary causes. Clin Chest Med. 1992;13:567–85.
9. Veille JC, Kitzman DW, Bacevice AE. Effects of pregnancy on the electrocardiogram in healthy subjects during strenuous exercise. Am J Obstet Gynecol. 1996;175:1360–4.
10. Vered Z, Poler SM, Gibson P, Wlody D, Perez JE. Noninvasive detection of the morphologic and hemodynamic changes during normal pregnancy. Clin Cardiol. 1991;14:327–34.
11. Clapp 3rd JF, Capeless E. Cardiovascular function before, during, and after the first and subsequent pregnancies. Am J Cardiol. 1997;80:1469–73.
12. Kinsella SM, Lohmann G. Supine hypotensive syndrome. Obstet Gynecol. 1994;83:774–88.
13. Winner W, Romney SL. Cardiovascular responses to labor and delivery. Am J Obstet Gynecol. 1966;95:1104–14.
14. Adams JQ, Alexander Jr AM. Alterations in cardiovascular physiology during labor. Obstet Gynecol. 1958;12:542–9.
15. Ouzounian JG, Masaki DI, Abboud TK, Greenspoon JS. Systemic vascular resistance index determined by thoracic electrical bioimpedance predicts the risk for maternal hypotension during regional anesthesia for cesarean delivery. Am J Obstet Gynecol. 1996;174:1019–25.
16. Ness RB, Harris T, Cobb J, et al. Number of pregnancies and the subsequent risk of cardiovascular disease. N Engl J Med. 1993;328:1528–33.
17. Regitz-Zagrosek V, Blomstrom Lundqvist C, Borghi C, et al. ESC Guidelines on the management of cardiovascular diseases during pregnancy: the Task Force on the Management of Cardiovascular Diseases during Pregnancy of the European Society of Cardiology (ESC). Eur Heart J. 2011;32:3147–97.
18. Siu SC, Sermer M, Colman JM, et al. Prospective multicenter study of pregnancy outcomes in women with heart disease. Circulation. 2001;104:515–21.
19. Drenthen W, Pieper PG, Roos-Hesselink JW, et al. Outcome of pregnancy in women with congenital heart disease: a literature review. J Am Coll Cardiol. 2007;49:2303–11.
20. Thorne S, MacGregor A, Nelson-Piercy C. Risks of contraception and pregnancy in heart disease. Heart. 2006;92:1520–5.
21. Stephanie J, Ventura BEH. QuickStates: birth rates among women aged 15–44 years, by maternal age group – National Vital Statistics System, United States, 1961, 2007, and 2011. Morb Mortal Wkly Rep. 2012;61:978.
22. James AH, Jamison MG, Biswas MS, Brancazio LR, Swamy GK, Myers ER. Acute myocardial infarction in pregnancy: a United States population-based study. Circulation. 2006;113:1564–71.
23. Weiss BM, Zemp L, Seifert B, Hess OM. Outcome of pulmonary vascular disease in pregnancy: a systematic overview from 1978 through 1996. J Am Coll Cardiol. 1998;31:1650–7.
24. Bedard E, Dimopoulos K, Gatzoulis MA. Has there been any progress made on pregnancy outcomes among women with pulmonary arterial hypertension? Eur Heart J. 2009;30:256–65.
25. van Giersbergen PL, Halabi A, Dingemanse J. Pharmacokinetic interaction between bosentan and the oral contraceptives norethisterone and ethinyl estradiol. Int J Clin Pharmacol Ther. 2006;44:113–8.
26. Presbitero P, Somerville J, Stone S, Aruta E, Spiegelhalter D, Rabajoli F. Pregnancy in cyanotic congenital heart disease. Outcome of mother and fetus. Circulation. 1994;89:2673–6.
27. Beauchesne LM, Connolly HM, Ammash NM, Warnes CA. Coarctation of the aorta: outcome of pregnancy. J Am Coll Cardiol. 2001;38:1728–33.
28. Rossiter JP, Repke JT, Morales AJ, Murphy EA, Pyeritz RE. A prospective longitudinal evaluation of pregnancy in the Marfan syndrome. Am J Obstet Gynecol. 1995;173:1599–606.
29. Gersony DR, McClaughlin MA, Jin Z, Gersony WM. The effect of beta-blocker therapy on clinical outcome in patients with Marfan's syndrome: a meta-analysis. Int J Cardiol. 2007;114:303–8.

30. Reimold SC, Rutherford JD. Clinical practice. Valvular heart disease in pregnancy. N Engl J Med. 2003;349:52–9.
31. Silversides CK, Colman JM, Sermer M, Siu SC. Cardiac risk in pregnant women with rheumatic mitral stenosis. Am J Cardiol. 2003;91:1382–5.
32. Lesniak-Sobelga A, Tracz W, KostKiewicz M, Podolec P, Pasowicz M. Clinical and echocardiographic assessment of pregnant women with valvular heart diseases–maternal and fetal outcome. Int J Cardiol. 2004;94:15–23.
33. Bhatla N, Lal S, Behera G, et al. Cardiac disease in pregnancy. Int J Gynaecol Obstet. 2003;82:153–9.
34. Barbosa PJ, Lopes AA, Feitosa GS, et al. Prognostic factors of rheumatic mitral stenosis during pregnancy and puerperium. Arq Bras Cardiol. 2000;75:215–24.
35. Elkayam U, Bitar F. Valvular heart disease and pregnancy part I: native valves. J Am Coll Cardiol. 2005;46:223–30.
36. Arias F, Pineda J. Aortic stenosis and pregnancy. J Reprod Med. 1978;20:229–32.
37. Silversides CK, Colman JM, Sermer M, Farine D, Siu SC. Early and intermediate-term outcomes of pregnancy with congenital aortic stenosis. Am J Cardiol. 2003;91:1386–9.
38. Yap SC, Drenthen W, Pieper PG, et al. Risk of complications during pregnancy in women with congenital aortic stenosis. Int J Cardiol. 2008;126:240–6.
39. Bhargava B, Agarwal R, Yadav R, Bahl VK, Manchanda SC. Percutaneous balloon aortic valvuloplasty during pregnancy: use of the Inoue balloon and the physiologic antegrade approach. Cathet Cardiovasc Diagn. 1998;45:422–5.
40. Therrien J, Barnes I, Somerville J. Outcome of pregnancy in patients with congenitally corrected transposition of the great arteries. Am J Cardiol. 1999;84:820–4.
41. Canobbio MM, Mair DD, van der Velde M, Koos BJ. Pregnancy outcomes after the Fontan repair. J Am Coll Cardiol. 1996;28:763–7.
42. Chan WS, Anand S, Ginsberg JS. Anticoagulation of pregnant women with mechanical heart valves: a systematic review of the literature. Arch Intern Med. 2000;160:191–6.
43. Sillesen M, Hjortdal V, Vejlstrup N, Sorensen K. Pregnancy with prosthetic heart valves – 30 years' nationwide experience in Denmark. Eur J Cardiothorac Surg. 2011;40:448–54.
44. Spirito P, Autore C. Management of hypertrophic cardiomyopathy. BMJ. 2006;332:1251–5.
45. North RA, Sadler L, Stewart AW, McCowan LM, Kerr AR, White HD. Long-term survival and valve-related complications in young women with cardiac valve replacements. Circulation. 1999;99:2669–76.
46. Rayburn WF, LeMire MS, Bird JL, Buda AJ. Mitral valve prolapse. Echocardiographic changes during pregnancy. J Reprod Med. 1987;32:185–7.
47. Yap SC, Drenthen W, Meijboom FJ, et al. Comparison of pregnancy outcomes in women with repaired versus unrepaired atrial septal defect. BJOG. 2009;116:1593–601.
48. Veldtman GR, Connolly HM, Grogan M, Ammash NM, Warnes CA. Outcomes of pregnancy in women with tetralogy of Fallot. J Am Coll Cardiol. 2004;44:174–80.
49. Gelson E, Johnson M. Effect of maternal heart disease on pregnancy outcomes. Expert Rev Obstet Gynecol. 2010;5:605–17.
50. James PR, Nelson-Piercy C. Management of hypertension before, during, and after pregnancy. Heart. 2004;90:1499–504.
51. Helewa ME, Burrows RF, Smith J, et al. Report of the Canadian Hypertension Society Consensus Conference 1. Definitions, evaluation and classification of hypertensive disorders in pregnancy. CMAJ. 1997;157:715–25.
52. Ward K, Hata A, Jeunemaitre X, et al. A molecular variant of angiotensinogen associated with preeclampsia. Nat Genet. 1993;4:59–61.
53. Kilpatrick DC, Liston WA, Jazwinska EC, et al. Histocompatibility studies in pre-eclampsia. Tissue Antigens. 1987;29:232–6.
54. Steegers EA, von Dadelszen P, Duvekot JJ, et al. Pre-eclampsia. Lancet. 2010;376:631–44.
55. Hargood JL, Brown MA. Pregnancy-induced hypertension: recurrence rate in second pregnancies. Med J Aust. 1991;154:376–7.

56. Wilson BJ, Watson MS, Prescott GJ, et al. Hypertensive diseases of pregnancy and risk of hypertension and stroke later in life: results from cohort study. BMJ. 2003;326:845.
57. Pearson GD, Veille JC, Rahimtoola S, et al. Peripartum cardiomyopathy: National Heart, Lung, and Blood Institute and Office of Rare Diseases (National Institutes of Health) workshop recommendations and review. JAMA. 2000;283:1183–8.
58. Sliwa K, Hilfiker-Kleiner D, Petrie MC, et al. Current state of knowledge on aetiology, diagnosis, management, and therapy of peripartum cardiomyopathy: a position statement from the Heart Failure Association of the European Society of Cardiology Working Group on peripartum cardiomyopathy. Eur J Heart Fail. 2010;12:767–78.
59. Sliwa K, Fett J, Elkayam U. Peripartum cardiomyopathy. Lancet. 2006;368:687–93.
60. Elkayam U, Akhter MW, Singh H, et al. Pregnancy-associated cardiomyopathy: clinical characteristics and a comparison between early and late presentation. Circulation. 2005;111:2050–5.
61. Elkayam U. Clinical characteristics of peripartum cardiomyopathy in the United States: diagnosis, prognosis, and management. J Am Coll Cardiol. 2011;58:659–70.
62. Elkayam U, Tummala PP, Rao K, et al. Maternal and fetal outcomes of subsequent pregnancies in women with peripartum cardiomyopathy. N Engl J Med. 2001;344:1567–71.
63. Sliwa K, Blauwet L, Tibazarwa K, et al. Evaluation of bromocriptine in the treatment of acute severe peripartum cardiomyopathy: a proof-of-concept pilot study. Circulation. 2010;121:1465–73.
64. Hilfiker-Kleiner D, Meyer GP, Schieffer E, et al. Recovery from postpartum cardiomyopathy in 2 patients by blocking prolactin release with bromocriptine. J Am Coll Cardiol. 2007;50:2354–5.
65. Ladner HE, Danielsen B, Gilbert WM. Acute myocardial infarction in pregnancy and the puerperium: a population-based study. Obstet Gynecol. 2005;105:480–4.
66. Roth A, Elkayam U. Acute myocardial infarction associated with pregnancy. J Am Coll Cardiol. 2008;52:171–80.
67. Joyal D, Leya F, Koh M, et al. Troponin I levels in patients with preeclampsia. Am J Med. 2007;120:819.
68. George D, Erkan E. Antiphospholipid syndrome. Prog Cardiovasc Dis. 2009;52:115–25.
69. Roos-Hesselink JW, Duvekot JJ, Thorne SA. Pregnancy in high risk cardiac conditions. Heart. 2009;95:680–6.
70. Silversides CKHL, Haberer K, et al. Recurrence rates of arrhythmias during pregnancy in women with previous tachyarrhythmia and impact on fetal and neonatal outcomes. Am J Cardiol. 2006;97:1206.
71. Rashba EJ, Zareba W, Moss AJ. Influence of pregnancy on the risk for cardiac events in patients with hereditary long QT syndrome. LQTS Investigators. Circulation. 1998;97:451–6.

Part IV
Special Considerations

Chapter 15
Antithrombotic Issues in Women

Ana Muñiz-Lozano, Fabiana Rollini, Francesco Franchi,
Jung Rae Cho, and Dominick J. Angiolillo

Overview

Despite the numerous randomized trials that have evaluated the use of anti-thrombotic therapy in the setting of acute coronary syndromes (ACS) and atrial fibrillation (AF), the heterogeneity of the population enrolled in the majority of these studies represents an important limitation and extrapolating data to under-represented populations does not come without concerns. In particular, women are underrepresented in most trials [1–4]. In line with this, in general gender differences in clinical response to antithrombotic therapies, in terms of thrombosis and bleeding risks, remain poorly understood. Accordingly, the association between possible sex differences in platelet biology and pharmacodynamic response to antithrombotic therapies warrants further understanding [5–7]. Table 15.1 provides a detailed description of the existing sex-related features regarding antiplatelet and anticoagulant therapies and the main studies conducted, which will be better outlined in the sections below [8–38]. The present chapter provides an overview on the impact of antithrombotic therapy, from bench to bedside, thus evaluating basic aspects of biology of thrombosis, response to antithrombotic therapies, and their impact in various clinic setting in which these are utilized.

A. Muñiz-Lozano, MD • F. Rollini, MD • F. Franchi, MD
J.R. Cho, MD • D.J. Angiolillo, MD, PhD (✉)
Division of Cardiology,
University of Florida College of Medicine-Jacksonville,
655 West 8th Street, Jacksonville, FL 32209, USA
e-mail: dominick.angiolillo@jax.ufl.edu

H.Z. Mieszczanska, G.P. Velarde (eds.),
Management of Cardiovascular Disease in Women,
DOI 10.1007/978-1-4471-5517-1_15, © Springer-Verlag London 2014

Table 15.1 Gender-related differences of antithrombotic therapies

Agent		Class	Gender-specific variable analysed	Gender-related variances	References
Antiplatelets	Aspirin	COX-1 inhibitor	Platelet reactivity in women treated with aspirin.	Higher agonist-induced platelet reactivity in women	Becker et al. [9]
			Pharmacokinetic properties	Quicker absorption and larger distribution volume in women	Buchanan et al. [10]
			Drug bioavailability	Slower drug clearance in females	Ho et al. [11]
			Clinical outcome for primary and secondary prevention in females versus male patients	No difference observed in meta-analysis of clinical trials	Woodfield et al. [12] Baigent et al. [13]
	P2Y$_{12}$ receptor inhibitors	Clopidogrel	Thienopyridine	Platelet function inhibition by clopidogrel	No gender-related differences	Ferreiro et al. [14]
			Reduction of the combined risk of death, MI or stroke at one year	Greater risk reduction among women	Steinhubl et al. [15]
			Meta-analysis of five large phase III clinical trials focused on sex-related differences in clinical outcome	No statistical significant heterogenicity with regard to gender	Berger et al. [16]
		Prasugrel Thienopyridine	Reduction in ischemic events comparing prasugrel with clopidogrel	No interactions between treatment effect, bleeding and gender	Wiviott et al. [17]
		Ticagrelor Cyclopentyl-triazolopyrimidine	Composite ischemic event rate comparing ticagrelor with clopidogrel	No interactions between treatment effect, bleeding and gender	Wallentin et al. [18]

GPI	Abciximab	GP IIb/IIIa antagonist	*In vitro* platelet response to abciximab	No gender-related differences	Coller et al. [19]
			Meta-analysis of large clinical trials with regard to major adverse events	No differences with regard to adverse outcome, higher major and minor bleeding rates in women	Cho et al. [20]
	Eptifibatide	GP IIb/IIIa antagonist	Composite adverse clinical events and bleeding rate	No differences in death, MI or target vessel revascularization, higher major and minor bleeding rates in women	Fernandes et al. [21]
	Tirofiban	GP IIb/IIIa antagonist	Biomarker in ACS	CRP and brain natriuretic peptide more likely elevated in women than men	Wiviott et al. [22]
Anticoagulants	Heparins	UFH	Indirect factor Xa and Thrombin inhibitor	aPTT values	Higher in women	Granger et al. [23]
		LMWH	Indirect factor Xa and Thrombin inhibitor	Reduction in the composite of death and MI	Larger reduction of the primary endpoint and more minor bleedings in female patients	FRICS study group [24]
				Meta-analysis of phase III clinical trials focused on sex-related differences in clinical outcome	No gender-related interactions with regard to triple endpoint, death or MI significantly reduced in women but not men	Toss et al. [25]
				Clinical adverse outcome in fibrinolysis plus heparins	No gender-related interactions	Cohen et al. [26] Mega et al. [27]
	Warfarin	Vitamin K antagonist	Risk of thromboembolism under treatment with a vitamin K antagonist	Higher benefit in women	Fang et al. [28]
			Major bleeding risk	No gender-related interactions	Hughes et al. [29]

(continued)

Agent	Class	Gender-specific variable analysed	Gender-related variances	References
Bivalirudin	Direct factor IIa inhibitor	Ischemic outcomes and major bleeding rates under treatment with bivalirudin plus provisional use of GPI	Female gender significantly associated with major bleeding risk	Chacko et al. [30]
		Ischemic outcomes and bleeding rates under monotherapy with bivalirudin	No gender-related differences with regard to ischemic outcomes	Manoukian et al. [31]
			No gender-related differences	Mehran et al. [32]
Dabigatran	Oral direct factor IIa inhibitor	Thromboembolic events and bleeding risk in patients with atrial fibrillation	No gender-related interactions, safe and effective in women and men	Connolly et al. [33]
Fondaparinux	Indirect factor Xa inhibitor	Reduction in the composite endpoint of death, MI, refractory ischemia or major bleeding	Higher absolute reduction of major bleeding in women with a trend for statistical interaction	Yusuf et al. [34, 35]
		Reduction in the composite of death or re-infarction	No gender-related interactions	Oldgren et al. [36]
Rivaroxaban	Oral direct factor Xa inhibitor	Thromboembolic events and bleeding risk in patients with atrial fibrillation	No gender-related interactions, safe and effective in women and men	Patel et al. [37]
Apixaban	Oral direct factor Xa inhibitor	Thromboembolic events and bleeding risk in patients with atrial fibrillation	No gender-related interactions, safe and effective in women and men	Granger et al. [38]

Adapted with permission from Rauch [8]

GP glycoprotein, *GPI* glycoprotein IIb/IIIa inhibitors, *aPTT* activated partial thromboplastin time, *COX* cyclooxygenase, *MI* myocardial infarction, *ACS* acute coronary syndromes, *CRP* C-reactive protein

Definitions, Terms and Classifications

Epidemiology of Thrombotic Disorders in Women

Atherothrombotic disorders (ischemic heart disease and stroke) cause approximately a quarter of the total women mortality worldwide [39]. Coronary artery disease (CAD), just in the United States, accounted for 15.6 % of deaths in women in 2007, and cerebrovascular disease (CVD) accounted for another 6.7 % [40]. In 2007, among the 607,000 American women hospitalized for CAD approximately one million underwent cardiac catheterization, percutaneous coronary intervention (PCI), stenting, or coronary artery bypass graft procedures. The average length of hospital stay was 5.3 days for acute myocardial infarction (MI) alone. The same year, 458,000 women were hospitalized for CVD, with an average hospital stay of 5.4 days [41].

Underestimation of cardiac risk and misconception of symptoms of CAD in women usually lead to less referral for cardiac testing, appropriate treatment and coronary catheterization during ACS [42–44]. Moreover, women used to be older than men when they present CAD and thus excluded more frequently from randomized studies [45, 46]. The prevalence of CAD is higher among men until the age of 39 (15.9 % vs. 7.8 %, respectively), although in the range 40–59 years (37.9 % and 38.5 %) and in the range 60–79 years (73.3 % and 72.6 %) the prevalence is very similar [47]. On the contrary, after 80 years of age women have more CAD than men [48]. Therefore, the onset of clinical manifestations of CAD occurs about 10 years later in women versus men [42]. Figure 15.1 shows how as women become older the incidence of CAD, stroke, and peripheral artery disease increases considerably [5]. Essentially, around the time of menopause, the incidence of CAD more than triples [40]. Additionally, there are growing proportions of costs of CAD and CVD, estimated at $505 billion in the United States alone [49], given the longer life expectancy of women relative to men worldwide [38].

Currently, the rate of recurrent MI and cardiovascular death among women has increased compared with men, despite the decrease of CAD mortality among men because of the advances in the diagnosis and treatment of ACS [50, 51]. Even though women present a higher risk profile compared with men, the Can Rapid Risk Stratification of Unstable Angina Patients Suppress Adverse Outcomes with Early Implementation of the ACC/AHA Guidelines? (CRUSADE) National Quality Improvement Initiative showed that ACS women less often receive guideline-recommended antithrombotic therapies [42].

Gender Disparities in Platelet Biology

Platelet Reactivity

There are described differences in platelet reactivity across populations using several methods and in response to variable stimuli [52] (Fig. 15.2). Compared with platelets from men, those from women without CAD are more reactive in response

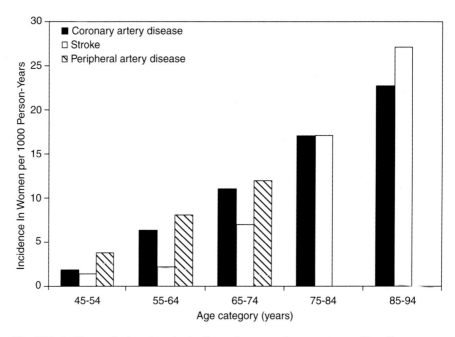

Fig. 15.1 Incidence of atherothrombotic disease in women by age category. Data for coronary artery disease and stroke are from the Framingham original and offspring cohort, and data on peripheral arterial disease are from the ARIC (atherosclerosis risk in communities) cohort (per 1,000 person-years) (Reprinted with permission Wang et al. [5])

to standard concentrations of agonists such as adenosine diphosphate (ADP) and thrombin receptor agonist protein [53, 54]. The total of glycoprotein (GP) IIb/IIIa receptors that can bind PAC-1 antibody in response to ADP or thrombin receptor agonist protein stimulation seems to be 50–80 % greater in women than in men [54]. Compared with men after adjustment for risk factors such as smoking, hypertension, diabetes, hyperlipidemia, and aspirin use, platelets from women, in particular, white women, bound more fibrinogen in response to low and high concentrations of ADP and showed more spontaneous aggregation among asymptomatic patients [55]. High platelet reactivity was related with an increased risk of downstream MI (two- to three-fold increased risk compared with those with normal platelet reactivity) in a population-based study of asymptomatic, premenopausal women [56]. Considerably higher levels of signaling cascade proteins expressed on platelets from male versus female donors were found in a recent study of signaling proteomes in platelets [57]. These initial findings suggest that sex-specific platelet proteomic signaling mechanisms could contribute to variances in platelet reactivity and outcome differences between women and men, even though this concept entails further investigation.

Healthy men and women were also studied in the Genetic Study of Aspirin Responsiveness (GeneSTAR) study, which proved higher platelet reactivity among

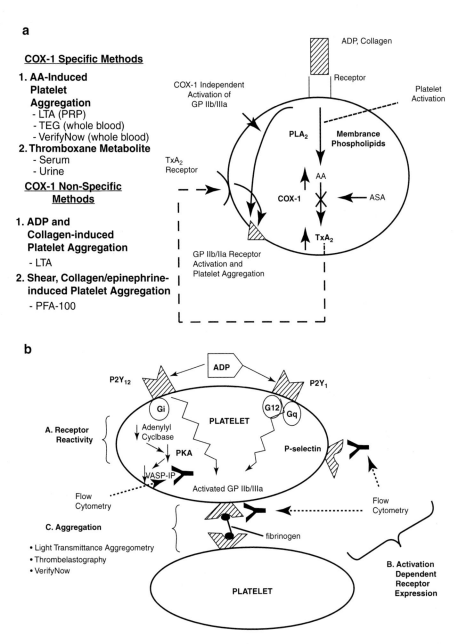

Fig. 15.2 Platelet responsiveness to aspirin and clopidogrel. Laboratory measurement of platelet responsiveness to aspirin (**a**) and clopidogrel (**b**). *AA* arachidonic acid, *ADP* adenosine diphosphate, *ASA* acetylsalicylic acid (aspirin), *COX* cyclooxygenase, *GP* glycoprotein, *LTA* light transmittance aggregometry, *PFA* platelet function analyzer, *PKA* protein kinase A, *PLA2* phospholipase A2, *PRP* platelet-rich plasma, *TEG* thrombelastography, *VASP* vasodilator-stimulated phosphoprotein, *Y* monoclonal antibodies (Reprinted with permission Gurbel et al. [52])

women compared with men in response to varying concentrations of arachidonic acid, ADP, or epinephrine after adjustment for age, risk factors, race, menopausal status, and hormone therapy [9]. Nevertheless, the study found comparable grades of platelet inhibition among men and women, in response to arachidonic acid after receiving a low-dose of aspirin. However, women's platelets were more reactive than those of men in response to collagen or ADP stimulation after aspirin therapy, suggesting upregulation of platelet activation pathways indirectly related to cyclo-oxygenase-1 (COX-1) [9]. Moreover platelet-related gender differences, compared with men a greater prothrombotic tendency (augmented speed and strength of platelet-fibrin clotting) among women was also shown by thromboelastography-based studies [58, 59].

Inflammation

An inflammatory response mediated by activated platelets, releasing cytokines and immunomodulatory ligands, additionally intensifies platelet response and endothelial activation during plaque rupture [60]. Exposure of its core contents on acute plaque rupture, promotes adhesion of platelet receptors and integrins to von Willebrand factor and collagen in the subendothelium [61, 62]. Releasing of proinflammatory cytokines and inflammatory factors and binding to leukocytes to form platelet-leukocyte coaggregates are also facilitated by activated platelets, which may promote an inflammatory response within the vessel wall [62, 63]. In the Women's Health Study, a higher C-reactive protein (CRP) level, the most frequently investigated marker of inflammation, independently predicted among healthy postmenopausal women the risk of cardiovascular death, nonfatal MI, stroke, or need for coronary revascularization (relative risk: 1.5 for the highest quartile versus the lowest; 95 % confidence interval [CI]: 1.1–2.1) [64].

A recent meta-analysis showed a risk ratio for CAD of 1.41 (95 % CI: 1.13–1.75) among women in five studies whose CRP level was 3.0 mg/l versus 1.0 mg/l, even though the Cardiovascular Health Study showed that CRP did not add to risk prediction for women but only for intermediate-risk men [65, 66]. There are other inflammatory markers, such as leukocyte count and P-selectin, which can be higher among healthy women and predictive of imminent cardiovascular events [67, 68]. Beyond their direct platelet-mediated effects, antiplatelet therapies have also been related with pleiotropic anti-inflammatory effects [69]. The synergy of aspirin in addition to statins in lowering CRP levels in a population-based, longitudinal stroke study in which 50 % of the participants were women did not vary by gender [70]. In one nonrandomized study, even after adjustment for gender, clopidogrel therapy was correlated with less level of inflammatory markers [71]. CRP levels increased 1 month after clopidogrel interruption without significant sex variances in another small study in which 50 % of the participants were women [72]. Regarding novel and more potent antithrombotic therapies, if these drugs can lead to selective improvements in clinical outcomes according to gender through a greater reduction in inflammation remains unknown.

Role of Hormones in Platelet Biology and Inflammation

Genomic effects in megakaryocytes, signaling properties in platelets, or both, might contribute to sex differences in platelet function given that megakaryocytes and platelets express the estrogen receptor [73] and androgen receptor [73, 74], and platelet nitric oxide synthase release and thromboxane A2 (TXA2) generation can be modulated by estrogens and/or androgens [74, 75]. Moreover, during mega-karyocyte differentiation transcripts from both estrogen receptor and androgen are upregulated [74].

The evidence on the effect of female menstrual-cycle hormones on platelet biology is controversial. One study suggested that hormones may regulate platelet GP IIb/IIIa activation, showing that platelets bound more fibrinogen during the luteal phase than the follicular phase [55]. During the menstrual cycle, platelet adhesion to vascular collagen also shows biphasic peaks [73]. On the contrary, no significant relationship between platelet aggregability and menstrual cycle phase, oral contraceptive use, or menopausal state was found by other studies [57, 76, 77]. The expression of proteins in the coagulation-fibrinolytic pathways is altered by both oral contraceptive and perimenopausal hormonal agents, and may contribute to increased thrombotic risk promoting fibrinogen binding to platelets, increasing factor VII levels and activity, and levels of fibrinogen and plasminogen activator inhibitor-1 [78]. The relationship between hormones and atherothrombotic risk could be mediated also by the systemic inflammation. Among post-menopausal women treated with estrogen, randomized [79] and cross-sectional [80] studies have shown increased CRP levels. Nevertheless, baseline CRP did not found a significant statistical interaction with hormone therapy in predicting CAD risk in a nested case–control analysis from the two randomized, controlled studies of the Women's Health Initiative [81].

A link between genetic polymorphisms for platelet glycoproteins and the risk of atherothrombotic events has been investigated in several studies [82–84], whether sex-specific differences influence the impact of these polymorphisms on platelet biology, treatment response, and patient outcomes remains still unknown. The HERS (Heart Estrogen–Progestin Study) showed that among women who received placebo women homozygous for the GP Ibα-5 T allele, heterozygotes and homozygotes for the GP Ibα-5C allele had a significantly lower incidence of the composite endpoint (death, MI, or unstable angina) at 5.8 years of follow-up [85]. In women with the -5C allele versus the -5TT genotype postmenopausal hormone treatment was associated with a 46 % lower adjusted cardiovascular risk (p < 0.001 for interaction) [85]. In women who had the GP Ibα-TT and GP VI-TC/CC genotypes (21.2 %) hormone therapy was associated with significant harm, but women with the GP IbαTC/CC and GP VI-TT genotypes (16.6 %) it was associated with significant benefit [85]. Thus, the risk-benefit ratio for proposed antiplatelet treatment may be altered by pharmacogenomic testing which can determine underlying cardiovascular risk in postmenopausal women. However, additional investigations are indeed warranted.

Sex Differences in Bleeding with Antithrombotic Therapy

Patients with ACS who receive antithrombotic drugs have shown to be associated with a fivefold increased risk of death at 30 days and a 1.5-fold increased risk of death between 30 days and 6 months [86–88]. Women randomized to receive aspirin for primary prevention of cardiovascular disease versus placebo in the Associated With Antiplatelet Therapies The Women's Health Study, experienced more frequently serious gastrointestinal (GI) bleeding requiring transfusion (relative risk: 1.40; 95 % CI: 1.07–1.83) [89]. Nevertheless, 2.5 major bleeding events per 1,000 women versus three major bleeding events per 1,000 men after aspirin use over an average 6.4 years occurred according to a meta-analysis by Berger et al. [90]. There was no evidence of difference of effect between women and men for major bleeding (p<0.24) for clopidogrel treatment, but the odds ratio for bleeding was numerically higher among women than men (1.43; 95 % CI: 1.15–1.79 vs. 1.22; 95 % CI: 1.05–1.42) [90]. In a multivariable risk model, Subherwal et al. consistently identified sex as an independent predictor of in-hospital major bleeding (odds ratio: 1.31; 95 % CI: 1.23–1.39) [91]. Additionally, women who underwent invasive treatment with PCI had significantly higher rates of in-hospital major bleeding compared with men (14.1 % vs. 5.9 %, p<0.001) in the CRUSADE registry [92]. Despite GI bleeding after MI is more common in men, access-site complications are more frequent in women undergoing PCI (e.g., access site bleeding, retroperitoneal bleeding) [93, 94].

Other sex-specific differences, such as in vascular reactivity [95], could also contribute to differences in bleeding risk in addition to bleeding-site differences may relate in part to the smaller blood vessels in women [96]. Overall among women with less body mass, the question of weight-based dosing has been raised for antiplatelet agents such as clopidogrel [97], given that it could provide a mechanism for variations in antiplatelet response. Therefore, there was identified a significant interaction between sex, GP IIb/IIIa inhibitors (GPI) use, and bleeding risk (p<0.014) in the CRUSADE registry (Fig. 15.3) [92]. Inappropriate dosing when using antithrombotic therapy is one of the main reasons of the higher bleeding risk in some women. In fact, an excess dosing of unfractionated heparin, low molecular weight heparin, or GPI could explained an estimated 15 % of the major bleeding showed in CRUSADE [98]. In fact, women remained at higher risk of excess dosing and bleeding than did men even after adjustment for age, weight, and renal function. Only 27 % of the risk in men is due to excess dosing of these agents while it reaches 72 % of the increased bleeding risk among women [92]. Compared with men, women receiving appropriately dosed bivalirudin had also higher rates of bleeding complications in the Intracoronary Stenting and Antithrombotic Regimen: Rapid Early Action for Coronary Treatment (ISAR-REACT) [99] and Acute Catheterization and Urgent Intervention Triage strategy (ACUITY) trials [100]. In the setting of ACS there are also important implications of bleeding like a lower probability to be discharge on antiplatelet therapy [101], maybe because its reinitiation is postponed until the patient is considered "safe" from additional bleeding although this treatment "gap" can last up to 6 months after the initial event [101]. A higher probability to have a heightened systemic inflammatory response has also been described [102]. Importantly, the higher incidence of in-hospital bleeding among women has major implications for their risk of future ischemic events.

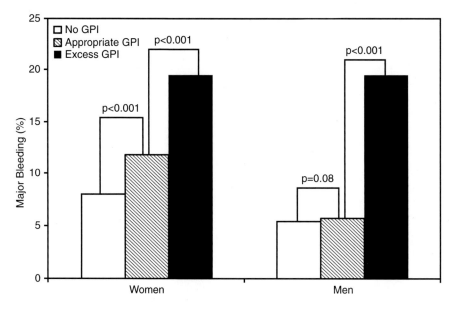

Fig. 15.3 Major bleeding by sex and GPI dosing. Incidence of in-hospital major bleeding among women and men with acute coronary syndromes who did not receive a GP IIb/IIIa inhibitor (*GPI*), those who received appropriate GPI dosing, and those who received excess GPI dosing in the CRUSADE registry. Probability values represent unadjusted comparisons (Adapted with permission from Alexander et al. [92])

AF, stroke, prosthetic heart valve replacement, MI and venous thrombosis are included among the indications of vitamin K antagonists (VKA). The main contributors which determine the bleeding risks in patients on oral anticoagulation have extensively been investigated [103]. In patients treated with VKA, patient characteristics, such as age and comorbidity, intensity of anticoagulant effects, length of therapy, and interaction with drugs that interfere with hemostasis are the determinants which primarily influence the risk of bleeding [14, 104]. However, female sex has not been described to be associated with major bleeding, including life-threatening bleeding events, such as intracranial hemorrhage [29]. However, in patients on oral anticoagulant therapy female sex appears to be an independent risk factor for minor bleeding [105, 106]. The association of sex and heparin-induced bleeding has not been consistently reported [107].

Antiplatelet Therapy

Gender-Related Differences in Response to Antiplatelet Drugs

Aspirin

Numerous studies have proved that aspirin reduces the risk of thrombotic events in patients with CAD [38, 108, 109]. In both sexes, aspirin inhibits similarly the formation of TXA2 synthesis in platelets by blocking selectively and irreversibly acetylating COX-1 [10, 11, 108]. However, in women pathways that are indirectly related to COX-1, such as those stimulated by collagen, ADP and epinephrine, are less inhibited compared with men [9]. Several ex vivo assays have shown that these differences persist after adjustment for several potential confounders, such as race, and results in higher platelet reactivity in aspirin-treated women with CAD [110–112]. A substudy of the Clopidogrel for High Atherothrombotic Risk and Ischemic Stabilization, Management and Avoidance (CHARISMA) and the Heart Outcomes Prevention Evaluation (HOPE) trial showed higher risk of cardiovascular events among women. These trials found greater in vivo platelet activation related with female gender that was demonstrated to be a determinant of 11-dehydro thromboxane B2 concentration, a marker of aspirin resistance [113, 114].

Despite 6 randomized trials (95,456 patients) that were included in the aforementioned meta-analysis from Berger et al. showed that primary prevention with aspirin therapy significantly reduced the risk of cardiovascular events in both sexes [12 and 14 % reductions in women and men, respectively] [97], the benefit was primarily driven by a reduction of MI in men (odds ratio [OR] 0.68, 95 % confidence interval [CI] 0.54–0.86, p=0.001) and ischemic stroke in the 51,342 women included (OR 0.76, 95 % CI 1.35–2.20, p<0.001). Notably, as above mentioned, the risk of bleeding was significantly increased by aspirin to a similar degree in both sexes [97]. Tests for heterogeneity of treatment effect were not reported. Significant reductions in major coronary events and serious vascular events with aspirin therapy were found in men, but not women in both primary and secondary prevention studies from the ATT (Antithrombotic Trialists) Collaboration meta-analysis, that included the same studies but had access to individual participant data, estimating consequently in a more accurate way the magnitude of several risk factors, such as gender, in influencing selected outcomes [13]. Nevertheless, no heterogeneity of treatment effect was distinguished by sex for any of the endpoints evaluated after adjustment for multiple comparisons. These results suggested that the absolute risk reduction essentially depends on the individual's absolute risk without treatment, given that the relative risk reduction among men and women is similar.

Aggregate data from 16 randomized trials of aspirin use in the secondary prevention setting, with stratification by sex were additionally reported (Fig. 15.4) [13]. Equally, the decrease in vascular mortality with aspirin versus placebo therapy after acute MI compared with men (22 %) was just 16 % (p<0.05 for heterogeneity), in the International Study of Infarct Survival-2 (ISIS-2) trial [38]. In line with this, gender mix may be the cause of around a 25 % of the variation in the reported efficacy of aspirin in reducing the rates of cardiovascular events across placebo-controlled trials [115]. Accordingly, greater benefits of aspirin in decreasing non-fatal MI rates have been proved in trials primarily with men compared with those containing mostly women [115].

Compared with lower doses, no clear overall benefit with aspirin doses 100 mg was found in secondary analyses from previous clinical trials [116–118]. Additionally, no particular benefit related with a higher aspirin dose among women in these secondary studies was found, even though the higher platelet reactivity

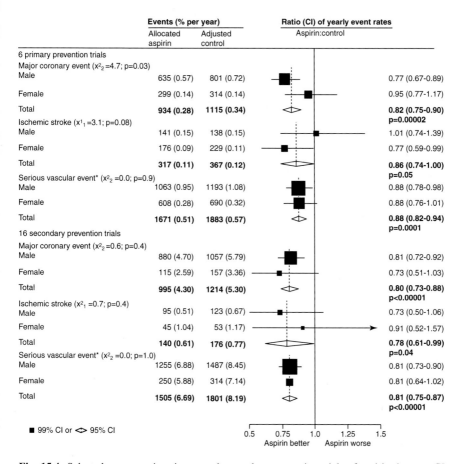

	Events (% per year)		Ratio (CI) of yearly event rates
	Allocated aspirin	Adjusted control	Aspirin:control
6 primary prevention trials			
Major coronary event (x^2_2 =4.7; p=0.03)			
Male	635 (0.57)	801 (0.72)	0.77 (0.67-0.89)
Female	299 (0.14)	314 (0.14)	0.95 (0.77-1.17)
Total	**934 (0.28)**	**1115 (0.34)**	**0.82 (0.75-0.90)** p=0.00002
Ischemic stroke (x^1_1 =3.1; p=0.08)			
Male	141 (0.15)	138 (0.15)	1.01 (0.74-1.39)
Female	176 (0.09)	229 (0.11)	0.77 (0.59-0.99)
Total	**317 (0.11)**	**367 (0.12)**	**0.86 (0.74-1.00)** p=0.05
Serious vascular event* (x^2_2 =0.0; p=0.9)			
Male	1063 (0.95)	1193 (1.08)	0.88 (0.78-0.98)
Female	608 (0.28)	690 (0.32)	0.88 (0.76-1.01)
Total	**1671 (0.51)**	**1883 (0.57)**	**0.88 (0.82-0.94)** p=0.0001
16 secondary prevention trials			
Major coronary event (x^2_2 =0.6; p=0.4)			
Male	880 (4.70)	1057 (5.79)	0.81 (0.72-0.92)
Female	115 (2.59)	157 (3.36)	0.73 (0.51-1.03)
Total	**995 (4.30)**	**1214 (5.30)**	**0.80 (0.73-0.88)** p<0.00001
Ischemic stroke (x^2_1 =0.7; p=0.4)			
Male	95 (0.51)	123 (0.67)	0.73 (0.50-1.06)
Female	45 (1.04)	53 (1.17)	0.91 (0.52-1.57)
Total	**140 (0.61)**	**176 (0.77)**	**0.78 (0.61-0.99)** p=0.04
Serious vascular event* (x^2_2 =0.0; p=1.0)			
Male	1255 (6.88)	1487 (8.45)	0.81 (0.73-0.90)
Female	250 (5.88)	314 (7.14)	0.81 (0.64-1.02)
Total	**1505 (6.69)**	**1801 (8.19)**	**0.81 (0.75-0.87)** p<0.00001

■ 99% CI or ◇ 95% CI

0.5   0.75   1.0   1.25   1.5
Aspirin better   Aspirin worse

Fig. 15.4 Selected outcomes in primary and secondary prevention trials of aspirin, by sex. *CI* confidence interval (Reprinted with permission from the ATT (Antithrombotic Trialists) Collaboration Baigent et al. [13])

demonstrated in women [9, 53–55]. Moreover, in cases where the potential benefit compensates the potential risk of GI bleeding, the U.S. Preventive Services Task Force recommends low-dose aspirin for the prevention of MI among men age 45–79 years and for prevention of stroke among women age 55–79 years, according to sex differences in the epidemiology of cardiovascular disease and available evidence supporting therapy [119]. Likewise, for persons whose 10-year cardiovascular risk is at least 6 % aspirin therapy is recommended by the American Stroke Association and American Heart Association [120]. The 2007 update to the AHA guidelines for CVD prevention in women defined women at high risk as those with "established CHD, CVD, peripheral arterial disease, abdominal aortic aneurysm, end-stage or chronic renal disease, DM, and 10-year Framingham risk >20 %" [121]. The 2011 AHA guidelines for prevention of CVD in women recommended aspirin (75–325 mg/day) as a consideration in those who are at high risk regardless of age or for women >65 years of age who are at risk or healthy, depending on risk of hemorrhage and consideration of risk for ischemic stroke. These guidelines also recommended the use of specific risk prediction instruments that include CVD as part of global risk assessment [122–124].

Adenosine Diphosphate P2Y$_{12}$ Receptor Antagonists

Thienopyridines inhibit irreversibly platelet activation blocking platelet ADP P2Y$_{12}$ receptor. The first generation thienopyridine ticlopidine has been largely replaced in clinical practice by clopidogrel, a second generation thienopyridine because of its more favorable safety profile [125]. There is no difference between men and women in plasmatic levels of clopidogrel's active metabolite [126]. Nevertheless, clopidogrel-induced inhibition of platelet aggregation presents some gender variability [127–129]. In patients presenting with unstable angina (UA)/non-ST elevation myocardial infarction (NSTEMI), the Clopidogrel in Unstable Angina to Prevent Recurrent Ischemic Events (CURE) trial, demonstrated a smaller absolute (1.2 % vs. 2.8 %) and relative (12 % vs. 25 %) risk reduction in the composite endpoint of cardiovascular death, non-fatal MI or stroke at 1 year in women compared with men with clopidogrel plus aspirin compared to aspirin alone at 1 year [130], with similar findings in the subgroup of patients undergoing PCI [131]. On the contrary from the CURE trial, in patients undergoing elective PCI, the Clopidogrel for the Reduction of Events During Observation (CREDO) trial showed a 26.9 % relative risk reduction in favour of clopidogrel for the composite of death, MI and stroke at 1 year in the overall population, but demonstrated a greater risk reduction of the combined risk of death, MI or stroke at 1 year (32 % vs. 25 %) among women [15]. Patients treated with fibrinolytic therapy within 12 h after the beginning of STEMI symptoms in the CLARITY-TIMI 28 (Clopidogrel as Adjunctive Reperfusion Therapy – Thrombolysis in Myocardial Infarction 28), were randomized to dual antiplatelet therapy with aspirin plus clopidogrel versus clopidogrel alone. Despite a higher event rate among women in both treatment arms, a 36 % reduction in the risk of the composite ischemic endpoint with clopidogrel in the overall population, with similar reduction for men and women (35 % vs. 38 %, respectively) was observed [132]. In patients undergoing PCI 3 days after starting the assigned study medication the OR of the composite endpoint of cardiovascular death, recurrent MI or stroke at 30 days was 59 % in women and 41 % in men. The ClOpidogrel and Metoprolol in Myocardial Infarction Trial (COMMIT) trial enrolled Chinese patients with suspected MI and compared the effect of clopidogrel plus aspirin versus aspirin alone. This trial demonstrated similar reductions in the primary ischemic endpoint at 28 days with no heterogeneity in effect related to sex, but with higher event rate in women [133]. Also in the CHARISMA trial, aforementioned, no clinical benefit was associated to the combination of a low-dose aspirin and clopidogrel in asymptomatic patients with at least three atherothrombotic risk factors without statistically significant differences between men and women [134].

These five main randomized trials (CURE, CREDO, CLARITY-TIMI 28, COMMIT, CHARISMA) were included in a meta-analysis of focused on sex-related differences between men and women on dual antiplatelet therapy with aspirin versus clopidogrel versus aspirin alone [16]. Particularly in patients with known risk factors for CAD clopidogrel treatment was associated with a significant reduction in the risk of cardiovascular events (cardiovascular death, MI, or stroke). Nevertheless, merely the risk of MI was significantly reduced with clopidogrel (relative risk: 0.81; 95 % CI: 0.70–0.93) but not the risk for stroke or all-cause mortality, among the 23,533 women evaluated. On the contrary, significant reductions were shown in all 3 endpoints among the 56,091 men evaluated. Overall, the study found a significant 16 % relative reduction among men (7.8 % vs. 9.0 %, OR 0.84; 95 % CI 0.78–0.91) in major cardiovascular events with clopidogrel vs. placebo compared with a nonsignificant 7 % of relative reduction among women (11.0 % vs. 11.8 % OR 0.93; 95 % CI 0.86–1.01). No evidence of statistical heterogeneity between women and men was shown regarding to mortality, MI, stroke and major bleeding. However, much of the difference between men and women could be chance finding, and only a trend towards statistical heterogeneity based on gender was found (p=0.092).

Variable responses to clopidogrel have been independently associated with polymorphisms of the cytochrome P450 (CYP) 2C19, in particular clopidogrel prodrug metabolism to its active metabolite. According with the presence of a gain-of-function and loss-of-function genotype, higher risks of both major bleeding [135] and stent thrombosis [136] have been detected respectively. There are not expected genotype-driven variances in outcome between men and women given that these polymorphisms are similarly distributed among men and women. Further investigations are still needed because it would be important to clarify if other gene-gene or gene-environment interactions could drive possible sex differences.

No significant interaction between sex and treatment assignment was found in the pivotal randomized trials of the novel antiplatelet agents prasugrel [17] and ticagrelor [18], despite the reductions in the primary endpoint relatively smaller in women than in men, these studies were not powered to examine treatment interactions among subgroups. Prasugrel is a third generation oral thienopyridine with more potent platelet $P2Y_{12}$ inhibitory effects, because of the fact that a more favorable metabolic conversion produces higher concentrations of its active metabolite compared to clopidogrel [137]. In moderate to high-risk ACS patients undergoing PCI prasugrel was associated with a significant 19 % reduction in ischemic events compared to clopidogrel, in the Trial to assess improvement in therapeutic outcomes by optimizing platelet inhibition with prasugrel– Thrombolysis In Myocardial Infarction 38 (TRITON-TIMI 38) trial [17]. In the overall population, in spite of an increased risk of bleeding compared with clopidogrel, the net clinical benefit (defined as death from any cause, non-fatal MI, non-fatal stroke, and TIMI major hemorrhages) was favorable to prasugrel. Even with a higher absolute (2.4 % vs. 1.6 %) and relative (21 % vs. 12 %) reduction of the primary ischemic endpoint with prasugrel among men compared to women, no significant interactions between treatment and sex were found. On the other hand, underwriting the existence of less pharmacological variability compared with clopidogrel, a genetic subanalysis of the TRITON-TIMI 38 demonstrated that functional CYP genetic variants did not influence active metabolite levels, platelet inhibition and cardiovascular outcomes of 1,466 patients allocated to treatment with prasugrel [138]. Ticagrelor, the first member of a new class of reversible $P2Y_{12}$ receptor antagonists called CycloPentylTriazoloPyrimidine (CPTP), demonstrated to be associated with a 16 % reduction in the composite ischemic endpoint compared to clopidogrel in patients with ST-elevation ACS who underwent primary PCI or with non-ST-elevation ACS planned for an invasive or medical approach in the phase III results of the Platelet Inhibition and Patient Outcomes (PLATO) trial [18]. Despite ticagrelor was associated with higher rates of major bleeding not related to coronary-artery bypass grafting, including more cases of fatal intracranial bleeding, in the overall population among ticagrelor and clopidogrel groups no differences in bleeding were found conferring to different definitions. Compared to clopidogrel, ticagrelor showed similar absolute (2.0 % vs. 1.9 %) and relative reduction (17.0 vs. 15.0 %) of the primary endpoint in women in comparison with men. Also among different sexes similar effects were also found regarding major bleeding.

Glycoprotein IIb/IIIa Inhibitors

GPI (abciximab, tirofiban and eptifibatide) block the binding of fibrinogen to the GP IIb/IIIa receptor on the surface of activated platelets and in this way inhibit the final common pathway leading to platelet aggregation. *In vitro*, no sex differences in platelet response to GPI were observed [19, 139]. Among the trials of GPI, a significant interaction between treatment and sex was found regarding cardiovascular events. In fact, between women and men, despite women had a higher rate of major and minor bleeding, no gender difference regarding major adverse outcomes was found at 30 days, 6 months and 1 year in a pooled analysis of data from three large randomized trials of patients undergoing PCI with adjunctive use of abciximab [20]. Also for eptifibatide the Enhanced suppression of the platelet GP IIb/IIIa receptor with Integrilin therapy (ESPRIT) trial, observed no statistical interaction between sex and treatment regarding death, MI or urgent target vessel revascularization either at 48 h or 1 year [21].

Six randomized trials on the efficacy and safety of GPI in patients with ACS not routinely scheduled for early coronary revascularization were included in a meta-analysis in which, despite a highly significant interaction between sex and use of GPI regarding cardiac events, GPI diminish the incidence of death or MI, particularly in patients at high risk of thrombotic complications [140]. Possibly because of the higher percentage of men with positive baseline troponins than women (49 % vs. 37 %), the interaction showed (an increased risk of 19 % in men vs. 15 % in women in the odds of 30-day death or MI compared with placebo or control), remained significant even after adjustment for baseline clinical characteristics, including age and co-morbidities (given that women were older, had more comorbid conditions, and more frequently had larger infarctions). Neither after risk stratification by troponin level sex differences were found. Actually, in both men and women with positive baseline troponins a reduction in the 30-day rate of death or MI by GPI was observed, while with negative troponins this effect was not beneficial in both sexes. Posteriorly in patients with UA/NSTEMI a different pattern of presenting biomarkers was observed [22]. Men were more likely to have elevated creatine kinase-MB and troponins, while women were more likely to have elevated CRP and brain natriuretic peptide. These findings suggested that a multimarker approach may be useful in the initial risk assessment of UA/NSTEMI, particularly in women. On the other hand, perhaps because of the concomitant use of clopidogrel, more recent investigations have not shown sex-related differences in outcome in ACS patients [141].

Anticoagulat Therapy

Anticoagulation in Coronary Artery Disease

The mentioned underrepresentation of women in clinical trials could be possibly related with an underestimation of cardiac risk or a misconception of symptoms of CAD and leads to the imperative necessity of gender-specific evidence related with the management and outcomes of ACS, particularly regarding differences in platelet reactivity and response to antithrombotic therapies [9, 54–59]. In fact, some investigations have already demonstrated many variances concerning women, such as different clinical presentation (symptoms and age), management or outcomes, different thrombotic profiles and response to antithrombotic therapies and propensity for increased bleeding [86–88]. In line with this, in addressing anticoagulant therapy in CAD, these need to be specifically addressed.

Indirect Thrombin Inhibitors

Unfractionated (UFH) and low-molecular-weight (LMWH) heparins enhance inactivation of factor Xa and, to a less extent, thrombin by binding to antithrombin III. The lack of necessity of laboratory monitoring of activity and the more predictable dose–response are the main advantages of LMWH. Another kinetic advantage of LMWH over UFH is that they inhibit the early steps of coagulation cascade and thrombin generation, due to a higher anti-factor Xa:IIa ratio and prolonged duration of anti-factor Xa activity. Sex is considered one of the clinical factors that affect the response to UFH, in addition to body weight, age, smoking history and diabetes mellitus [142, 143]. Particularly, in response to the anticoagulant effect of heparin women are expected to achieve higher activated partial thromboplastin time (aPTT) [23]. On the contrary, the pharmacokinetic (PK) and pharmacodynamic (PD) profiles after enoxaparin were found to be consistent between sexes in a post-hoc analysis of the Thrombolysis in Myocardial Infarction 11A (TIMI 11A) study, a multicenter dose-ranging trial to assess the safety of enoxaparin in patients with ACS [144, 145].

The Fragmin and Fast Revascularization during In- Stability in Coronary artery disease (FRISC) trial was the only placebo controlled trial of LMWH use reporting data stratified by sex [146]. This study compared dalteparin and placebo in patients with ACS, and it found that dalteparin was associated with a 63 % risk reduction in the composite of death and MI during the first 6 days, with a larger absolute (4.5 % vs. 2.2 %) and relative reduction (13.1 % vs. 28.9 %) of the primary endpoint in women compared with men. Nevertheless, regarding the frequency of minor bleedings, either with weight adjusted and fixed dose treatment it was higher in women compared with men. A significant interaction between sex and anti-Xa activity determined in samples obtained during the acute and the standard dosing phase of treatment was demonstrated in multiple regression analysis [25]. The FRISC II study reported a larger absolute and relative risk reduction in the composite endpoint of death and MI in women than in men [24].

A direct comparison between LMWH and UFH based on sex has been reported in few trials. In ACS patients the superiority of enoxaparin over UFH in reducing the risk of death and severe cardiac events in patients with ACS, was showed to be applicable to a plethora of subgroups in a pooled data meta-analysis of two large trials [26]. Nevertheless a significant benefit of enoxaparin over UFH regarding the double composite endpoint of death or MI was significantly observed in women, but not in man, despite a significant relative risk reduction was seen independently from sex with regards to the composite triple endpoint of death, MI or recurrent angina prompting urgent revascularisation [26]. Additionally, enoxaparin demonstrated to be not superior but also noninferior to UFH with a modest increase in the risk of major bleeding in the Superior Yield of the New Strategy of Enoxaparin, Revascularization and Glycoprotein IIb/IIIa Inhibitors (SYNERGY) study [147]. Multiple subgroups, including the ones stratified by sex and study site presented this absence of differences [147]. STEMI patients with programmed fibrinolysis where randomized to a regimen of enoxaparin or UFH as adjunctive antithrombin therapy in the Enoxaparin and Thrombolysis Reperfusion for Acute Myocardial Infarction Treatment– Thrombolysis in Myocardial Infarction (ExTRACT-TIMI 25) study. In this study, women were older and more likely to have hypertension and diabetes. Despite increased rates of short term mortality, compared with men, women treated with enoxaparin had a similar relative benefit (16 % vs. 19 %) and a greater absolute benefit (2.9 % vs. 1.9 %) [27].

Direct Thrombin Inhibitors

Direct thrombin inhibitors (hirudin, bivalirudin, melagatran, argatroban, dabigatran, lepirudin and desirudin) block directly the interaction of thrombin with its substrates. Their property to decrease thrombin-mediated activation of platelets, consequently exerting some degree of antiplatelet effects, is one of the characteristics of this class of antithrombotic agents. In the guidelines for the management of non ST elevation ACS and for primary PCI in patients with STEMI, with or without pre-treatment with heparin, bivalirudin is currently recommended as a class Ib [148, 149]. The safety and efficacy of bivalirudin in CAD have been observed in several registries and randomized trials supporting guidelines recommendations. The benefits associated with the administration of bivalirudin appear to be independent from sex. Therefore, it is likely that the higher risk of bleeding observed was related with baseline co-morbidities of women. In patients with stable or unstable angina undergoing PCI the Randomized Evaluation in PCI Linking Angiomax to Reduced Clinical Events-2 (REPLACE-2) trial showed similar ischemic outcomes at 30 days for treatment with bivalirudin plus provisional GPI compared with heparin plus GPI, with similar mortality at 1 year, and a significant decrease of bleeding complications, without differences based on sex [150, 151]. Female gender demonstrated to be significantly associated with a 1.5-fold increased risk of major bleeding in a post-hoc multivariate analysis [30].

In patients with ACS undergoing an early invasive strategy also similar ischemic event rates at 30 days, less bleedings, and superior net clinical outcomes were associated with bivalirudin plus provisional GPI compared with heparin plus GPI in the aforementioned ACUITY trial. No significant interactions regarding net clinical outcomes, composite ischemia and major bleeding between the use of bivalirudin and numerous variables, including gender were observed in the subgroup analysis [152, 153]. Moreover, an almost twofold increased risk of major bleeding was demonstrated to be associated with female gender [31]. Among patients enrolled in the ACUITY, a further study specifically focused on sex-related difference trial corroborated these findings [100]. According the results of this study, women with ACS have higher rates of net clinical adverse event because of their higher risk of bleeding, but they do not experience an increased risk of one- and 12-month ischemic complications or mortality compared with men, even though differences in risk factors. Nevertheless, regardless of the treatment strategy chosen, bivalirudin monotherapy is related to similar short- and long-term protection from ischemic events and significantly less bleeding compared with a regimen of UFH plus GPI in women with ACS.

The Harmonizing Outcomes with Revascularization and Stents in Acute Myocardial Infarction (HORIZONS AMI) trial, showed that in patients with acute MI bivalirudin monotherapy significantly decreased net adverse cardiac events, cardiac death and major bleedings at 30 days and 1 year compared with heparin plus a GPI [32, 154]. Bivalirudin demonstrated to early reduce net adverse cardiac events and major bleeding independently from gender [155]. Additionally, with the use of bivalirudin in-hospital bleeding occurred in 1.7 % of patients and female gender was significantly associated with an increase in bleeding events, in a large European registry of 3,799 patients undergoing PCI [156]. Also a multi-center trial that assessed the feasibility of bivalirudin in renal, iliac and femoral interventions, the Angiomax Peripheral Procedure Registry of Vascular Events Trial (APPROVE) Registry, found that women had a trend towards higher risk of bleeding events at 30 days [157]. Moreover, a significant univariate association between female gender and a composite of early ischemic events and bleeding events with bivalirudin was showed in a further small study on patients undergoing PCI found [158]. On the contrary, a significant interaction between female sex and major bleeding was not demonstrated by the multivariate analysis.

Factor Xa Inhibitors

Fondaparinux blocks selectively the coagulation factor Xa by binding antithrombin III leading to a conformational change which results in intensified affinity for factor Xa and maximizes its inhibitory effect [159]. A predictable and persistent antico-agulation which requires only a single daily subcutaneous administration and a long half-life are some of the advantages of fondaparinux. In patients with ACS fondaparinux and enoxaparin presented similar efficacy in decreasing the risk of ischemic events at 9 days in the Fifth Organization to Assess Strategies in Acute Ischemic Syndromes (OASIS-5) trial, but fondaparinux was related to reduced rates of major bleeding and long-term mortality and morbidity [34]. In both sexes as compared with enoxaparin the composite endpoint of death, MI, refractory isch-emia or major bleeding was reduced with fondaparinux. Conversely, among women a trend for statistical interaction was found compared with men (p for interac-tion=0.07), because of a higher absolute reduction of major bleeding (3.0 % vs. 1.3 %) with the use of fondaparinux [34]. In patients with STEMI, the Sixth Organization to Assess Strategies in Acute Ischemic Syndromes (OASIS-6) trial found that fondaparinux reduced the primary endpoint of a composite of death or reinfarction at 30 days compared to usual care (UFH for up to 48 h followed by placebo for up to 8 days or placebo in those in whom UFH was not indicated) [35]. In the overall population and in a prespecified subgroup of patients not receiving reperfusion treatment similar trends for a reduction by fondaparinux treatment in the primary endpoint for women and men were observed [35, 36].

Anticoagulation in Atrial Fibrillation

Gender differences in cardiac arrhythmias have been poorly investigated [3, 4, 28, 160]. The most frequent clinically relevant arrhythmia is AF, which is a major risk for stroke and other thromboembolic events. Sex differences in AF patients have been reported [28, 50, 160–168] and numerous studies indicate a higher stroke risk in females with AF independently of the other known risk factors. In fact, the female gender was included as clinically important parameter for stroke risk assessment in both the Stroke Prevention in Atrial Fibrillation and Framingham risk scores as well as CHADS2-VASC scoring system [89, 169, 170]. In patients with first diagnosed AF gender differences were also observed. Women were older and more likely to have symptomatic AF, hypertension, diabetes and thyroid disease, compared with males with first-diagnosed AF. Moreover, in patients with heart failure, women have a higher risk to develop AF than men [39].

Female AF patients have a 1.6-fold increase risk of stroke [171], and cohort studies such as the Anticoagulation and risk factors in atrial fibrillation (ATRIA) study [28], the Copenhagen Heart Study [162], surveys (e.g. The Euro Heart survey [167]) and subgroup analyses from clinical trials (e.g. SPORTIF [172]) have clearly revealed a higher incidence of stroke and thromboembolism in females compared to males, even while on oral anticoagulation. The 2010 European Society of Cardiology guidelines include female gender as a 'clinically relevant non-major' stroke risk modifier, which could affect a decision on thromboprophylaxis [173].

The ATRIA study demonstrated that women who are not treated with anticoagulation therapies present higher risk than men for AF-related thromboembolic events [28]. Additionally, in the Framingham study the risk of death in patients with non-valvular AF was associated with an OR of 1.5 (95 % CI, 1.2–1.8) in men and 1.9 (95 % CI, 1.5–2.2) in women in up to 40 years of follow-up [174]. Compared to men's AF, moreover, women's AF was independently associated with a 2.5-fold higher mortality because of cardiovascular diseases in female in the Copenhagen City Heart Study [162]. Therefore, the mortality is greater for women than in men with AF [175]. It has not been well investigated if AF may be the cause for death or only an indirect marker of more co-morbidities that lead to death. In fact, the reason of gender-related differences in thromboembolic risk associated with AF has not been well elucidate. In patients with AF higher levels of prothrombotic factors and increased platelet activation have been observed. Increased concentrations of pro-thrombin fragment F1.2, von Willebrand factor and tissue plasminogen activator antigen within the circulating blood have been observed in female patients with AF [176–178]. It is necessary to better understand the mechanisms that may influence to the increased AF-related thromboembolic risk-associated with female sex. To date, an increased risk of stroke in AF related to these prothrombogenic factors has not been prospectively proved. The rates of thromboembolism in patients not taking warfarin in the ATRIA study were: 3.5 % per year for women vs.1.8 % per year for men (adjusted rate ratio [RR] =1.6; 95 % CI, 1.3–1.9) [28]. In females, a significantly larger reduction in thromboembolic events with oral anticoagulation has been observed compare with male patients (adjusted RR=0.4 versus 0.6, respectively; p=0.01). The stroke risk was significantly more reduced in women than in men in another prospective study of 780 patients with AF who received anticoagulation therapy [161].

In general, there is not so much information on elderly AF patients and it remains uncertain if stroke and bleeding risk could be different between elderly women and elderly men. The prevalence of AF grows with age, and it is up to 8 % in subjects older than 80 years [173]. Although AF is more frequent in men, among elderly patients the proportion of women is higher than men, because of their longer life expectancy. The Euro Heart Survey on AF subgroup analysis has shown that females with AF were older, with more comorbidities and a lower quality of life, but under-went less electrical cardioversion, compared with males [167]. Additionally, in female patients with AF the Rate Control Versus Electrical Cardioversion (RACE) study, showed that a rhythm control approach had led to more cardiovascular morbidity and mortality [166].

In conclusion, the optimal anticoagulant therapy of AF remains unclear because of the lack of representation of women in the large trials. In the sections below, we will review the data available regarding the most relevant anticoagulant agents currently available.

Vitamin K Antagonists (VKA)

The oral anticoagulants reduce anticoagulant activity by inhibiting the effects of vitamin K and consequently impairing γ-carboxylation of the coagulation factors II, VII, IX, and X in the liver. In woman some studies underlined a potential higher benefit of warfarin, which has demonstrated at least not to be inferior in reducing the risk of thromboembolism in both sexes [28, 179]. Major bleeding risk associated with warfarin use shows increasingly to be similar between men and women [28, 169, 172]. Nevertheless, the necessary dose to maintain a therapeutic INR may be affected by gender [180].

For a number of decades VKA have regularly been prescribed for the primary and secondary prevention of thromboembolic events in patients with AF [90, 173]. Compared with older males, older female AF patients were less likely to receive warfarin, and more likely to experience a major bleed on warfarin therapy [165]. In general, no difference in bleeding complications related to the use of VKA was found between genders [28, 161, 181]. In a retrospective analysis of 18,867 patients with AF no significant bleeding differences regarding to gender were found. In this study anticoagulant therapy with warfarin was associated with a 0.47 % annual risk for intracranial hemorrhage compared with 0.15 % without warfarin use [182].

The Elderly Patients followed by Italian Centres of Anticoagulation (EPICA) Study (n = 4,093) was a large, multicenter observational study that included elderly patients who started VKA treatment after the age of 80 years for the thromboprophylaxis of AF or after venous thromboembolism (VTE) (first event or recurrence) [183]. The study population had a higher percentage of women (54 %) compared with other studies [28, 160]. A posterior analysis of the AF patients (n = 3,015), aimed specifically to assess the potential bleeding and stroke risks differences between genders. The study did not find clear gender related differences in the risk of major adverse events in elderly patients, but elderly males showed a non-statistically significant higher rate of bleeding complications (OR 1.5), and females showed a slightly higher rate of stroke, therefore suggesting the possibility of a higher net clinical benefit of anticoagulant treatment in females. History of major bleeds, history of falls and active cancer are risk factors independently associated to bleeding when multivariate analysis was performed.

VKA are expected to be largely replaced from the new oral anticoagulants (NOAC) for primary and secondary prevention of thromboembolic events. However, in the large phase 3 trials no gender-related differences have been documented regarding to the safety and efficiency (as described below). Nonetheless, the superiority of these NOAC over the traditional VKA results a main step forward, allowing efficient and safe anticoagulation for both women and men.

Direct Thrombin Inhibitors

Dabigatran is a new oral direct competitive thrombin inhibitor which is administered twice daily. This agent is characterized by a pharmacologic profile, which is better than that of warfarin, and does not require regular monitoring, such as measuring the INR level under treatment with vitamin K antagonists. The Randomized Evaluation of Long-Term Anticoagulation Therapy (RE-LY) trial randomized 18,113 patients with AF to two fixed doses of dabigatran (110 and 150 mg) compared with warfarin, evaluating the reduction of the risk of stroke or systemic embolism [33]. In this study, both dabigatran dosages compared with warfarin were associated with similar rates of periprocedural bleeding (p=0.28 and p=0.58 respectively). No sex interaction and noninferiority between both dabigatran doses (110 mg twice daily and 150 mg twice daily) were observed [33].

Factor Xa Inhibitors

Rivaroxaban, an oral factor Xa inhibitor, has also demonstrated to have a more consistent and predictable anticoagulant effect compared with VKA. A double-blind trial randomized 14,264 patients with nonvalvular AF who were at increased risk for stroke, to receive either rivaroxaban (at a daily dose of 20 mg) or dose-adjusted warfarin [37]. Rivaroxaban was noninferior to warfarin for the prevention of stroke or systemic embolism (event rates 1.7 % per year for rivaroxaban vs. 2.2 % per year for warfarin, hazard ratio in the rivaroxaban group, 0.79; 95 % confidence interval, 0.66–0.96; p<0.001 for noninferiority) in patients with AF. No significant difference in the risk of major bleeding was found between groups. Notably, with rivaroxaban the incidence of intracranial and fatal bleeding was lower than in warfarin group. No sex differences were observed [37].

Apixaban is another novel oral direct factor Xa inhibitor with better PK and PD properties than warfarin that has been studied for preventing thromboembolic events in AF patients. This agent has demonstrated to reduce the risk of stroke or systemic embolism without significantly increasing the risk of major bleeding or intracranial hemorrhage in patients with AF for whom VKA was unsuitable [184]. Because of the superiority of apixaban compared to warfarin The Apixaban versus Acetylsalicylic Acid to Prevent Stroke in Atrial Fibrillation Patients Who Have Failed or Are Unsuitable for Vitamin k Antagonist Treatment (AVERROES) trial was prematurely terminated. No sex significant interaction was observed [184]. The Apixaban for reduction in stroke and other ThromboemboLic events in atrial fibrillation (ARISTOTLE) trial (n=18,201) randomized AF patients with at least one additional risk factor for stroke to apixaban at a dose of 5 mg twice daily vs. warfarin at an INR of 2.0–3.0. The primary outcome was defined as a composite of ischemic or hemorrhagic stroke or systemic embolism. Compared with warfarin, apixaban showed to be superior in the prevention of the primary endpoint. As compared with 1.60 % in the warfarin group, the annual rate of the primary outcome was 1.27 % in the apixaban group, (hazard ratio with apixaban, 0.79; 95 % confidence interval, 0.66–0.95; p = 0.01 for superiority). Additionally, in patients suffering from nonvalvular AF less bleeding and lower mortality was found with apixaban compared to warfarin [38]. No sex differences were observed.

Fibrinolytic Therapy

The relative benefit of fibrinolytic treatment among patients presenting with STEMI or bundle-branch block is irrespective of sex according to a review of the larger placebo-controlled trials of fibrinolytic therapy [185]. The observed higher rates of mortality in women compared to men in clinical trials of fibrinolytic therapy may partially be explained by the fact that most of women enrolled are older and more commonly have co-morbidities [12, 38, 185–189]. However, regarding the risk of morbidity and mortality compared to men in the setting of thrombolysis after adjustment for worse baseline characteristics, available data present several incongruences [190–192]. Compared to men women presented comparable adjusted risk of morbidity and mortality but showed a higher incidence of hemorrhagic stroke according to the International Tissue Plasminogen Activator/Streptokinase Mortality Study [190]. Moreover, women who receive thrombolytic therapy for treatment of acute MI are at greater risk for both fatal and nonfatal complications than men [12, 191]. Higher rates of bleeding complicating fibrinolysis for acute MI have been independently associated with female gender [193, 194]. A large contemporary cohort of women and men with STEMI undergoing fibrinolytic therapy was enrolled in the Global Utilization of Streptokinase and Tissue Plasminogen Activator for Occluded Coronary Arteries (GUSTO) V trial [195]. Patients were randomized to reteplase alone vs. half-dose of reteplase plus abciximab. Non inferiority was found for half-dose of reteplase plus abciximab which showed a 0.3 % absolute and 5 % relative reduction in the rate of 30-day mortality. Among fibrinolysis-treated patients with MI a post-hoc analysis of the GUSTO V study confirmed that female sex is independently associated with death and bleeding complications [196].

Special Considerations

The fact that trials sponsored by pharmaceutical companies do not have a federal mandate for inclusion of women and minorities, may partially explain the inadequate prevalence of women, which reflects fears related to drug administration in women of childbearing potential. Sex specific analyses were rarely performed in the pivotal safety trials of antithrombotic drugs (even when women are included), which leads to the fact that recommendations of clinical guidelines are typically "gender neutral". A recent regulation changes (Women's Health Study, Women's Health Initiative) enhances that more women would be enrolled in NIH-sponsored phase 3 trials since the NIH Revitalization Act. Growing literature is slowly accumulating regarding gender-based differences in the presentation, treatment and clinical outcomes of CAD and AF.

Clinical Consequences and Shadow Areas of Knowledge

Higher risk of both thrombosis and bleeding among women compared with men has been underlined as an enigma by the cumulative evidence [99]. Despite the effort to carry out measures for improving the quality avoiding the excess antithrombotic drug dosing [197], even with appropriate dosing sex differences in bleeding risk may continue. As aforementioned, intrinsic discrepancies in platelet reactivity and causative effects from inflammatory and hormonal processes may elucidate these differences. The way to reduce cardiovascular risk without increasing bleeding risk remains unknown.

Platelet function testing or pharmacogenomics have been suggested to lead drug selection and dosing [128]. In fact, women presented significantly higher residual platelet reactivity after standard clopidogrel dosing compared with men when a point-of-care ADP specific platelet aggregation assay was used, in the Gauging Responsiveness With A VerifyNow Assay-Impact On Thrombosis And Safety (GRAVITAS) trial [128]. Nevertheless, no improvement of clinical outcomes was found using in response to platelet testing results a higher clopidogrel dosing strategy empirically [198]. In a small study by Cuisset et al., on the contrary, patients with high platelet reactivity on clopidogrel who were randomized to routine (vs. provisional) GPI therapy during PCI presented greater 30-day cardiovascular event rates without a significant increase in bleeding [199]. However, based on small studies gender-specific implications are difficult to define.

Another therapeutic option could be targeting other platelet pathways, such as cilostazol, which has demonstrated to achieve additional platelet inhibition among patients with high on-treatment reactivity to clopidogrel by rising intracellular cyclic adenosine monophosphate via selective phosphodiesterase inhibition. In ACS patients undergoing PCI and in addition to aspirin and clopidogrel therapy, cilostazol has demonstrated to reduce long-term cardiovascular risk without an increase in bleeding [200] showing a significant benefit for women but not for men [201]. The use of tailored therapy in routine practice is limited by the absence of an established standardized test and dubiety about alternative therapeutic options to improve outcomes, despite it would be a very advantageous method [202].

As mentioned above women remain underrepresented in both early and later phase studies [2] and consequently there is systematic knowledge gap regarding sex differences in platelet biology, genomics, and response to therapeutics. The fact that the prevalence of ACS and AF in women is predominant in older ages, could be a reason for that underrepresentation, given that also elderly people is usually excluded from the research studies [203, 204]. Other possible explanations are: physician underestimation of risk, misinterpretation of symptoms, and bias against referral for interventional treatment of cardiovascular disease in women [43]. In addition, in cardiovascular trials sometimes women who meet inclusion criteria might be less disposed than men to participate because of a greater perceived risk of harm and adverse events [205].

Differences in inflammatory marker levels and their impact on atherothrombotic risk relative incidence and expression of genetic polymorphisms affecting platelet responsiveness, and the role of hormones in mediating platelet effects need to be better understood in order to clarify the higher baseline levels of platelet reactivity observed in women. Achieving female representation in platelet-related research requires specific trial designs for genetic, *in vitro*, and clinical studies. Sex-specific treatment regimens targeted at optimizing safety and efficacy of antithrombotic therapy should be done based on the mechanistic keystones aforementioned in order to provide future directions for research.

Summary

The existence of sex differences in platelet and coagulation biology translates into gender-related differences in treatment options in a wide spectrum of cardiovascular disease manifestations [205]. Currently, the majority of clinical results concerning gender differences have been based on subgroup analyses without sufficient statistical power. There are just few comparative studies which have given some clues about sex-related differences in platelet function, even though the different response of women to antithrombotic therapies compared with men has been well known since long ago, including their enhanced bleeding tendency, even with appropriate dosing, and their less benefit in regard to the prevention of ischemic events. In general, the evidence shows a slower improvement of clinical outcomes among women than men, revealing the necessity to optimize therapy for prevention and treatment of ischemic coronary events and primary and secondary prevention of stroke in the setting of AF. The absence of specific recommendations on the optimal antithrombotic treatment for women highlights the necessity of dedicated trials to assess the efficacy of antithrombotic treatment strategies in women. Further investigations designed with caution are definitely needed in order to shed some light on all the knowledge shadows that could be affecting ominously women health care. Moreover, in order to draw appropriate conclusions which can be extrapolated to real life clinical practice, the study design of large randomized trials should take gender-related differences into account.

Disclosures Dominick J. Angiolillo (corresponding author) reports receiving: Received payment as an individual for: (a) Consulting fee or honorarium from Bristol Myers Squibb, Sanofi-Aventis, Eli Lilly, Daiichi Sankyo, The Medicines Company, AstraZeneca, Merck, Evolva, Abbott Vascular and PLx Pharma; (b) Participation in review activities from Johnson & Johnson, St. Jude, and Sunovion. Institutional payments for grants from Bristol Myers Squibb, Sanofi-Aventis, Glaxo Smith Kline, Otsuka, Eli Lilly, Daiichi Sankyo, The Medicines Company, AstraZeneca, Evolva; and has other financial relationships with Esther and King Biomedical Research Grant.

Ana Muñiz-Lozano: has no conflict of interest to report.
Fabiana Rollini: has no conflict of interest to report.
Francesco Franchi: has no conflict of interest to report.
Jung Rae Cho: has no conflict of interest to report.

Acknowledgements Ana Muñiz-Lozano is recipient of a training grant from the Spanish Society of Cardiology ("Beca de la Sección de Cardiopatía Isquémica para Formación e Investigación Post Residencia en el Extranjero" – Sociedad Española de Cardiología).

References

1. Kim C, Fahrenbruch CE, Menon V. Enrollment of women in National Heart, Lung, and Blood Institute-funded cardiovascular controlled trials fails to meet current federal mandates for inclusion. J Am Coll Cardiol. 2008;52:672–3.
2. Melloni C, Berger JS, Wang TY, et al. Representation of women in randomized clinical trials of cardiovascular disease prevention. Circ Cardiovasc Qual Outcomes. 2010;3:135–42.
3. Wolbrette D, Hementkumar P. Arrhythmias and women. Curr Opin Cardiol. 1999;14:36–43.
4. Makkar RR, Fromm BS, Steinmen RT, et al. Female gender as a risk factor for torsades de pointes associated with cardiovascular drugs. JAMA. 1993;270:2590–7.
5. Wang TY, Angiolillo DJ, Cushman M, et al. Platelet biology and response to antiplatelet therapy in women: implications for the development and use of antiplatelet pharmacotherapies for cardiovascular disease. J Am Coll Cardiol. 2012;59:891–900.
6. Capodanno D, Angiolillo DJ. Impact of race and gender on antithrombotic therapy. Thromb Haemost. 2010;104:471–84.
7. Potpara TS, Marinkovic JM, Polovina MM, et al. Gender-related differences in presentation, treatment and long-term outcome in patients with first-diagnosed atrial fibrillation and structurally normal heart: the Belgrade atrial fibrillation study. Int J Cardiol. 2012;161:39–44.
8. Rauch U. Gender differences in anticoagulation and antithrombotic therapy. Handb Exp Pharmacol. 2012;214:523–42.
9. Becker DM, Segal J, Vaidya D, et al. Sex differences in platelet reactivity and response to low-dose aspirin therapy. JAMA. 2006;295:1420–7.
10. Buchanan MR, Rischke JA, Butt R, et al. The sex-related differences in aspirin pharmacokinetics in rabbits and man and its relationship to antiplatelet effects. Thromb Res. 1983;29:125–39.
11. Ho PC, Triggs EJ, Bourne DW, et al. The effects of age and sex on the disposition of acetylsalicylic acid and its metabolites. Br J Clin Pharmacol. 1985;19:675–84.
12. The GUSTO Investigators. An international randomized trial comparing four thrombolytic strategies for acute myocardial infarction. N Engl J Med. 1993;329:673–82.
13. Antithrombotic Trialists' (ATT) Collaboration, Baigent C, Blackwell L, Collins R, et al. Aspirin in the primary and secondary prevention of vascular disease: collaborative meta-analysis of individual participant data from randomised trials. Lancet. 2009;373:1849–60.
14. Ferreiro JL, Sibbing D, Angiolillo DJ, et al. Platelet function testing and risk of bleeding complications. Thromb Haemost. 2010;103:1128–35.
15. Steinhubl SR, Berger PB, Mann 3rd JT, et al.; CREDO Investigators. Clopidogrel for the reduction of events during observation. Early and sustained dual oral antiplatelet therapy following percutaneous coronary intervention: a randomized controlled trial. JAMA. 2002;288:2411–20.
16. Berger JS, Bhatt DL, Cannon CP, et al. The relative efficacy and safety of clopidogrel in women and men. J Am Coll Cardiol. 2009;54:1935–45.
17. Wiviott SD, Braunwald E, McCabe CH, et al. Prasugrel versus clopidogrel in patients with acute coronary syndromes. N Engl J Med. 2007;357:2001–15.
18. Wallentin L, Becker RC, Budaj A, et al.; PLATO Investigators. Ticagrelor versus clopidogrel in patients with acute coronary syndromes. N Engl J Med. 2009;361:1045–57.
19. Coller BS, Peerschke EI, Scudder LE, et al. A murine monoclonal antibody that completely blocks the binding of fibrinogen to platelets produces a thrombasthenic-like state in normal platelets and binds to glycoproteins IIb and/or IIIa. J Clin Invest. 1983;72:325–38.

20. Cho L, Topol EJ, Balog C, et al. Clinical benefit of glycoprotein IIb/IIIa blockade with Abciximab is independent of gender: pooled analysis from EPIC, EPILOG and EPISTENT trials. Evaluation of 7E3 for the Prevention of Ischemic Complications. Evaluation in Percutaneous Transluminal Coronary Angioplasty to Improve Long- Term Outcome with Abciximab GP IIb/IIIa blockade. Evaluation of Platelet IIb/IIIa Inhibitor for Stent. J Am Coll Cardiol. 2000;36:381–6.

21. Fernandes LS, Tcheng JE, O'Shea JC, et al.; ESPRIT investigators. Is glycoprotein IIb/IIIa antagonism as effective in women as in men following percutaneous coronary intervention? Lessons from the ESPRIT study. J Am Coll Cardiol. 2002;40:1085–91.

22. Wiviott SD, Cannon CP, Morrow DA, et al. Differential expression of cardiac biomarkers by gender in patients with unstable angina/non-ST-elevation myocardial infarction: a TACTICS-TIMI 18 (Treat Angina with Aggrastat and determine Cost of Therapy with an Invasive or Conservative Strategy-Thrombolysis in Myocardial Infarction 18) substudy. Circulation. 2004;109:580–6.

23. Granger CB, Hirsch J, Califf RM, et al. Activated partial thromboplastin time and outcome after thrombolytic therapy for acute myocardial infarction: results from the GUSTO-I trial. Circulation. 1996;93:870–8.

24. FRagmin and Fast Revascularisation during InStability in Coronary artery disease Investigators. Long-term low-molecular-mass heparin in unstable coronary artery disease: FRISC II prospective randomised multicentre study. Lancet. 1999;354(9180):701–7.

25. Toss H, Wallentin L, Siegbahn A, et al. Influences of sex and smoking habits on anticoagulant activity in low-molecular-weight heparin treatment of unstable coronary artery disease. Am Heart J. 1999;137:72–8.

26. Cohen M, Antman EM, Gurfinkel EP, et al.; ESSENCE (Efficacy and Safety of Subcutaneous Enoxaparin in Non-Q-wave Coronary Events) and TIMI (Thrombolysis in Myocardial Infarction) 11B Investigators. Enoxaparin in unstable angina/non-ST-segment elevation myocardial infarction: treatment benefits in prespecified subgroups. J Thromb Thrombolysis. 2001;12:199–206.

27. Mega JL, Morrow DA, Ostör E, et al. Outcomes and optimal antithrombotic therapy in women undergoing fibrinolysis for ST-elevation myocardial infarction. Circulation. 2007;115:2822–8.

28. Fang MC, Singer DE, Chang Y, et al. Gender differences in the risk of ischemic stroke and peripheral embolism in atrial fibrillation: the AnTicoagulation and risk factors in atrial fibrillation (ATRIA) study. Circulation. 2005;112:1687–91.

29. Hughes M, Lip GY. Guideline development group for the NICE national clinical guideline for management of atrial fibrillation in primary and secondary care. QJM. 2007;100:599–607.

30. Chacko M, Lincoff AM, Wolski KE, et al. Ischemic and bleeding outcomes in women treated with bivalirudin during percutaneous coronary intervention: a subgroup analysis of the randomized evaluation in PCI linking angiomax to reduced clinical events (REPLACE)-2 trial. Am Heart J. 2006;151:1032.e1–7.

31. Manoukian SV, Feit F, Mehran R, et al. Impact of major bleeding on 30-day mortality and clinical outcomes in patients with acute coronary syndromes: an analysis from the ACUITY trial. J Am Coll Cardiol. 2007;49:1362–8.

32. Mehran R, Lansky AJ, Witzenbichler B, et al.; HORIZONS-AMI Trial Investigators. Bivalirudin in patients undergoing primary angioplasty for acute myocardial infarction (HORIZONSAMI):1-year results of a randomised controlled trial. Lancet. 2009;374:1149–59.

33. Connolly SJ, Ezekowitz MD, Yusuf S, et al.; The RE-LY Steering Committee and Investigators. Dabigatran versus warfarin in patients with atrial fibrillation. N Engl J Med. 2009;361:1139–51.

34. Yusuf S, Mehta SR, Chrolavicius S, et al. Comparison of fondaparinux and enoxaparin in acute coronary syndromes. N Engl J Med. 2006;354:1464–76.

35. Yusuf S, Mehta SR, Chrolavicius S, et al.; OASIS-6 Trial Group. Effects of fondaparinux on mortality and reinfarction in patients with acute ST-segment elevation myocardial infarction: the OASIS-6 randomized trial. JAMA. 2006;295:1519–30.

36. Oldgren J, Oldgren J, Wallentin L, et al.; OASIS-6 Investigators. Effects of fondaparinux in patients with ST-segment elevation acute myocardial infarction not receiving reperfusion treatment. Eur Heart J. 2008;29:315–23.

37. Woodfield SL, Lundergan CF, Reiner JS, et al. Gender and acute myocardial infarction: is there a different response to thrombolysis? J Am Coll Cardiol. 1997;291:35–42.

38. ISIS-2 (Second International Study of Infarct Survival) Collaborative Group. Randomised trial of intravenous streptokinase, oral aspirin, both, or neither among 17 187 cases of suspected acute myocardial infarction: ISIS-2. Lancet. 1988;2:349–60.

39. World Health Organization (WHO). Women's health: key facts. Fact Sheet no. 334. Basel: WHO, Nov 2009. http://www.who.int/mediacentre/factsheets/fs334/en/.

40. Xu J, Kochanek KD, Murphy SL, et al. Deaths: final data for 2007. Natl Vital Stat Rep. 2009;57:1–134.

41. Hall MJ, DeFrances CJ, Williams SN, et al. National hospital discharge survey: 2007 summary. Natl Health Stat Rep. 2010;29:1–20.

42. Blomkalns AL, Chen AY, Hochman JS, et al.; CRUSADE Investigators. Gender disparities in the diagnosis and treatment of non-ST-segment elevation acute coronary syndromes: large-scale observations from the CRUSADE (can rapid risk stratification of unstable angina patients suppress adverse outcomes with early implementation of the American College of Cardiology/American Heart Association Guidelines) national quality improvement initiative. J Am Coll Cardiol. 2005;45:832–7.

43. Kim ESH, Menon V. Status of women in cardiovascular clinical trials. Arterioscler Thromb Vasc Biol. 2009;29:279–83.

44. Chiaramonte GR, Friend R. Medical students' and residents' gender bias in the diagnosis, treatment, and interpretation of coronary heart disease symptoms. Health Psychol. 2006;25:255–66.

45. Van Spall HG, Toren A, Kiss A, et al. Eligibility criteria of randomized controlled trials published in high-impact general medical journals: a systematic sampling review. JAMA. 2007;297:1233–40.

46. Gurwitz JH, Col NF, Avorn J, et al. The exclusion of the elderly and women from clinical trials in acute myocardial infarction. JAMA. 1992;268:1417–22.

47. Rosamond W, Flegal K, Friday G, et al. Heart disease and stroke statistics-2007 update: a report from the American Heart Association Statistics Committee and Stroke Statistics Subcommittee. Circulation. 2007;115:e69–171.

48. National Heart, Lung, and Blood Institute (NHLBI). Incidence and prevalence: 2006 chart book on cardiovascular and lung diseases. Bethesda: NHLBI; 2006. Available at: http://www.nhlbi.nih.gov/resources/docs/06_ip_chtbk.pdf. Accessed 6 June 2011.

49. American Heart Association. Heart disease and stroke statistics-2011 update. Dallas: American Heart Association; 2011. Available at: http://circ.ahajournals.org/cgi/reprint/CIR.0b013e3182009701

50. American Heart Association. Women and cardiovascular disease: statistics. Dallas: American Heart Association; 2004. Available at: http://americanheart.org; http://www.heart.org/idc/groups/heart-public/%40wcm/%40sop/%40smd/documents/downloadable/ucm_319576.pdf

51. Chandra NC, Ziegelstein RC, Rogers WJ, et al. Observations of the treatment of women in the United States with myocardial infarction: a report from the National Registry of Myocardial Infarction- I. Arch Intern Med. 1998;158:981–8.

52. Gurbel PA, Becker RC, Mann KG, et al. Platelet function monitoring in patients with coronary artery disease. J Am Coll Cardiol. 2007;50:1822–34.

53. Johnson M, Ramey E, Ramwell PW. Sex and age differences in human platelet aggregation. Nature. 1975;253:355–7.

54. Faraday N, Goldschmidt-Clermont PJ, Bray PF. Sex differences in platelet GPIIb-IIIa activation. Thromb Haemost. 1997;77:748–54.

55. Kurrelmeyer K, Becker L, Becker D, et al. Platelet hyperreactivity in women from families with premature atherosclerosis. J Am Med Womens Assoc. 2003;58:272–7.

56. Snoep JD, Roest M, Barendrecht AD, et al. High platelet reactivity is associated with myocardial infarction in premenopausal women: a population-based case–control study. J Thromb Haemost. 2010;8:906–13.

57. Eidelman O, Jozwik C, Huang W, et al. Gender dependence for a subset of the low-abundance signaling proteome in human platelets. Hum Genomics Proteomics. 2010;2010:164906.

58. Hobson AR, Qureshi Z, Banks P, et al. Gender and responses to aspirin and clopidogrel: insights using short thrombelastography. Cardiovasc Ther. 2009;27:246–52.

59. Gurbel PA, Bliden KP, Cohen E, et al. Race and sex differences in thrombogenicity: risk of ischemic events following coronary stenting. Blood Coagul Fibrinolysis. 2008;19:268–75.

60. Badimon L, Storey RF, Vilahur G. Update on lipids, inflammation and atherothrombosis. Thromb Haemost. 2011;105 Suppl 1:S34–42.

61. Langer HF, Gawaz M. Platelet-vessel wall interactions in atherosclerotic disease. Thromb Haemost. 2008;99:480–6.

62. Ross R. Atherosclerosis—an inflammatory disease. N Engl J Med. 1999;340:115–26.

63. Libby P, Simon DI. Inflammation and thrombosis: the clot thickens. Circulation. 2001;103:1718–20.

64. Ridker PM, Hennekens CH, Buring JE, et al. C-reactive protein and other markers of inflammation in the prediction of cardiovascular disease in women. N Engl J Med. 2000;342:836–43.

65. Cushman M, Arnold AM, Psaty BM, et al. C-reactive protein and the 10-year incidence of coronary heart disease in older men and women: the cardiovascular health study. Circulation. 2005;112:25–31.

66. Buckley DI, Fu R, Freeman M, et al. C-reactive protein as a risk factor for coronary heart disease: a systematic review and meta-analyses for the U.S. preventive services task force. Ann Intern Med. 2009;151:483–95.

67. Margolis KL, Manson JE, Greenland P, et al.; Women's Health Initiative Research Group. Leukocyte count as a predictor of cardiovascular events and mortality in postmenopausal women: the Women's health initiative observational study. Arch Intern Med. 2005;165:500–8.

68. Ridker PM, Buring JE, Rifai N. Soluble P-selectin and the risk of future cardiovascular events. Circulation. 2001;103:491–5.

69. Muhlestein JB. Effect of antiplatelet therapy on inflammatory markers in atherothrombotic patients. Thromb Haemost. 2010;103:71–82.

70. Fisher M, Cushman M, Knappertz V, et al. An assessment of the joint associations of aspirin and statin use with C-reactive protein concentration. Am Heart J. 2008;156:106–11.

71. Quinn MJ, Bhatt DL, Zidar F, et al. Effect of clopidogrel pretreatment on inflammatory marker expression in patients undergoing percutaneous coronary intervention. Am J Cardiol. 2004;93:679–84.

72. Angiolillo DJ, Fernandez-Ortiz A, Bernardo E, et al. Clopidogrel withdrawal is associated with proinflammatory and prothrombotic effects in patients with diabetes and coronary artery disease. Diabetes. 2006;55:780–4.

73. Tarantino MD, Kunicki TJ, Nugent DJ. The estrogen receptor is present in human megakaryocytes. Ann N Y Acad Sci. 1994;714:293–6.

74. Khetawat G, Faraday N, Nealen ML, et al. Human megakaryocytes and platelets contain the estrogen receptor beta and androgen receptor (AR): testosterone regulates AR expression. Blood. 2000;95:2289–96.

75. Wu GJ, Lee JJ, Chou DS, et al. Inhibitory signaling of 17-estradiol in platelet activation: the pivotal role of cyclic AMP-mediated nitric oxide synthase activation. Eur J Pharmacol. 2010;649:140–9.

76. Jones SB, Bylund DB, Rieser CA, et al. α2-Adrenergic receptor binding in human platelets: alterations during the menstrual cycle. Clin Pharmacol Ther. 1983;34:90–6.

77. Yee DL, Sun CW, Bergeron AL, et al. Aggregometry detects platelet hyperreactivity in healthy individuals. Blood. 2005;106:2723–9.
78. Braunstein JB, Kershner DW, Bray P, et al. Interaction of hemostatic genetics with hormone therapy: new insights to explain arterial thrombosis in postmenopausal women. Chest. 2002;121:906–20.
79. Cushman M, Legault C, Barrett-Connor E, et al. Effect of postmenopausal hormones on inflammation-sensitive proteins: the Postmenopausal Estrogen/Progestin Interventions (PEPI) Study. Circulation. 1999;100:717–22.
80. Ridker PM, Hennekens CH, Rifai N, et al. Hormone replacement therapy and increased plasma concentration of C-reactive protein. Circulation. 1999;100:713–6.
81. Rossouw JE, Cushman M, Greenland P, et al. Inflammatory, lipid, thrombotic, and genetic markers of coronary heart disease risk in the women's health initiative trials of hormone therapy. Arch Intern Med. 2008;168:2245–53.
82. Weiss EJ, Bray PF, Tayback M, et al. A polymorphism of a platelet glycoprotein receptor as an inherited risk factor for coronary thrombosis. N Engl J Med. 1996;334:1090–4.
83. Zotz RB, Klein M, Dauben HP, et al. Prospective analysis after coronary-artery bypass grafting: platelet GP IIIa polymorphism (HPA-1b/PlA2) is a risk factor for bypass occlusion, myocardial infarction, and death. Thromb Haemost. 2000;83:404–7.
84. Bray PF. Platelet glycoprotein polymorphisms as risk factors for thrombosis. Curr Opin Hematol. 2000;7:284–9.
85. Bray PF, Howard TD, Vittinghoff E, et al. Effect of genetic variations in platelet glycoproteins Ibα and VI on the risk for coronary heart disease events in postmenopausal women taking hormone therapy. Blood. 2007;109:1862–9.
86. Eikelboom JW, Mehta SR, Anand SS, et al. Adverse impact of bleeding on prognosis in patients with acute coronary syndromes. Circulation. 2006;114:774–82.
87. Rao SV, Eikelboom JA, Granger CB, et al. Bleeding and blood transfusion issues in patients with non–ST-segment elevation acute coronary syndromes. Eur Heart J. 2007;28:1193–204.
88. Rao SV, O'Grady K, Pieper KS, et al. A comparison of the clinical impact of bleeding measured by two different classifications among patients with acute coronary syndromes. J Am Coll Cardiol. 2006;47:809–16.
89. Ridker PM, Cook NR, Lee IM, et al. A randomized trial of low-dose aspirin in the primary prevention of cardiovascular disease in women. N Engl J Med. 2005;352:1293–304.
90. Berger JS, Roncaglioni MC, Avanzini F, et al. Aspirin for the primary prevention of cardiovascular events in women and men: a sex-specific meta-analysis of randomized controlled trials. JAMA. 2006;295:306–13 (erratum in J Am Med Assoc 2006;295:2002).
91. Subherwal S, Bach RG, Chen AY, et al. Baseline risk of major bleeding in non-ST-segment-elevation myocardial infarction: the CRUSADE (can rapid risk stratification of unstable angina patients suppress ADverse outcomes with early implementation of the ACC/AHA guidelines) bleeding score. Circulation. 2009;119:1873–82.
92. Alexander KP, Chen AY, Newby LK, et al. Sex differences in major bleeding with glycoprotein IIb/IIIa inhibitors: results from the CRUSADE (can rapid risk stratification of unstable angina patients suppress ADverse outcomes with early implementation of the ACC/AHA guidelines) initiative. Circulation. 2006;114:1380–7.
93. Ahmed B, Piper WD, Malenka D, et al. Significantly improved vascular complications among women undergoing percutaneous coronary intervention: a report from the Northern New England Percutaneous Coronary Intervention Registry. Circ Cardiovasc Interv. 2009;2:423–9.
94. Moukarbel GV, Signorovitch JE, Pfeffer MA, et al. Gastrointestinal bleeding in high risk survivors of myocardial infarction: the VALIANT trial. Eur Heart J. 2009;30:2226–32.
95. Ahmed B, Lischke S, Holterman LA, et al. Angiographic predictors of vascular complications among women undergoing cardiac catheterization and intervention. J Invasive Cardiol. 2010;22:512–6.
96. Bowyer L, Brown MA, Jones M. Vascular reactivity in men and women of reproductive age. Am J Obstet Gynecol. 2001;185:88–96.

97. Angiolillo DJ, Fernández-Ortiz A, Bernardo E, et al. Platelet aggregation according to body mass index in patients undergoing coronary stenting: should clopidogrel loading-dose be weight adjusted? J Invasive Cardiol. 2004;16:169–74.

98. Alexander KP, Chen AY, Roe MT, et al. Excess dosing of antiplatelet and antithrombin agents in the treatment of non-ST-segment elevation acute coronary syndromes. JAMA. 2005;294:3108–16 (erratum in J Am Med Assoc 2006;295:628).

99. Iijima R, Ndrepepa G, Mehilli J, et al. Profile of bleeding and ischaemic complications with bivalirudin and unfractionated heparin after percutaneous coronary intervention. Eur Heart J. 2009;30:290–6.

100. Lansky AJ, Mehran R, Cristea E, et al. Impact of sex and antithrombins strategy on early and late clinical outcomes in patients with non-ST-elevation acute coronary syndromes (from the ACUITY trial). Am J Cardiol. 2009;103:1196–203.

101. Wang TY, Xiao L, Alexander KP, et al. Antiplatelet therapy use after discharge among acute myocardial infarction patients with in-hospital bleeding. Circulation. 2008;118:2139–45.

102. Campbell CL, Steinhubl SR, Hooper WC, et al. Bleeding events are associated with an increase in markers of inflammation in acute coronary syndromes: an ACUITY trial substudy. J Thromb Thrombolysis. 2011;31:139–45.

103. Dickstein K, Vardas PE, Auricchio A, et al. 2010 Focused Update of ESC Guidelines on device therapy in heart failure: an update of the 2008 ESC Guidelines for the diagnosis and treatment of acute and chronic heart failure and the 2007 ESC guidelines for cardiac and resynchronization therapy. Developed with the special contribution of the Heart Failure Association and the European Heart Rhythm Association. Eur Heart J. 2010;31:2677–87.

104. Schulman RJ, Beyth C, Kearon MN, et al.; American College of Chest Physicians. Hemorrhagic complications of anticoagulant and thrombolytic treatment: American College of Chest Physicians Evidence-Based Clinical Practice Guidelines (8th Edition). Chest. 2008;133:257S–98.

105. Pengo V, Legnani C, Noventa F, et al.; ISCOAT Study Group (Italian Study on Complications of Oral Anticoagulant Therapy). Oral anticoagulant therapy in patients with nonrheumatic atrial fibrillation and risk of bleeding. A Multicenter Inception Cohort Study. Thromb Haemost. 2001;85:418–22.

106. van der Meer FJ, Rosendaal FR, Vandenbroucke JP, et al. Bleeding complications in oral anticoagulant therapy. An analysis of risk factors. Arch Intern Med. 1993;153:1557–62.

107. Jick H, Slone D, Borda IT, et al. Efficacy and toxicity of heparin in relation to age and sex. N Engl J Med. 1968;279:284–6.

108. Patrono C, García Rodríguez LA, Landolfi R, et al. Low-dose aspirin for the prevention of atherothrombosis. N Engl J Med. 2005;353:2373–83.

109. The RISC Group. Risk of myocardial infarction and death during treatment with low dose aspirin and intravenous heparin in men with unstable coronary artery disease. Lancet. 1990;336:827–30.

110. Gum PA, Kottke-Marchant K, Poggio ED, et al. Profile and prevalence of aspirin resistance in patients with cardiovascular disease. Am J Cardiol. 2001;88:230–5.

111. Gum PA, Kottke-Marchant K, Welsh PA, et al. A prospective, blinded determination of the natural history of aspirin resistance among stable patients with cardiovascular disease. J Am Coll Cardiol. 2003;41:961–5.

112. Qayyum R, Becker DM, Yanek LR, et al. Platelet inhibition by aspirin 81 and 325 mg/day in men versus women without clinically apparent cardiovascular disease. Am J Cardiol. 2008;101:1359–63.

113. Eikelboom JW, Hankey GJ, Thom J, et al.; Clopidogrel for High Atherothrombotic Risk and Ischemic Stabilization, Management and Avoidance (CHARISMA) Investigators. Incomplete inhibition of thromboxane biosynthesis by acetylsalicylic acid: determinants and effect on cardiovascular risk. Circulation. 2008;118:1705–12.

114. Eikelboom JW, Hirsh J, Weitz JI, et al. Aspirin-resistant thromboxane biosynthesis and the risk of myocardial infarction, stroke, or cardiovascular death in patients at high risk for cardiovascular events. Circulation. 2002;105:1650–5.

115. Yerman T, Gan WQ, Sin DD, et al. The influence of gender on the effects of aspirin in preventing myocardial infarction. BMC Med. 2007;5:29.

116. Quinn MJ, Aronow HD, Califf RM, et al. Aspirin dose and six-month outcome after an acute coronary syndrome. J Am Coll Cardiol. 2004;43:972–8.

117. Peters RJ, Mehta SR, Fox KA, Trial Investigators CURE, et al. Effects of aspirin dose when used alone or in combination with clopidogrel in patients with acute coronary syndromes: observations from the Clopidogrel in Unstable angina to prevent Recurrent Events (CURE) study. Circulation. 2003;108:1682–7.

118. Steinhubl SR, Bhatt DL, Brennan DM, et al.; CHARISMA Investigators. Aspirin to prevent cardiovascular disease: the association of aspirin dose and clopidogrel with thrombosis and bleeding. Ann Intern Med. 2009;150:379–86.

119. Wolff T, Miller T, Ko S. Aspirin for the primary prevention of cardiovascular events: an update of the evidence for the U.S. Preventive Services Task Force. Ann Intern Med. 2009;150:405–10.

120. Goldstein LB, Adams R, Alberts MJ, et al.; American Heart Association, American Stroke Association Stroke Council. Primary prevention of ischemic stroke: a guideline from the American Heart Association/American Stroke Association Stroke Council. Circulation. 2006;113:e873–923 (erratum in Circulation 2006;114:e617).

121. Mosca L, Banka CL, Benjamin EJ, et al. Evidence-based guidelines for cardiovascular disease prevention in women: 2007 update. Circulation. 2007;115:1481–501.

122. Mosca L, Benjamin EJ, Berra K, et al. Effectiveness-based guidelines for the prevention of cardiovascular disease in women–2011 update: a guideline from the American Heart Association. Circulation. 2011;123:1243–62.

123. D'Agostino Sr RB, Vasan RS, Pencina MJ, et al. General cardiovascular risk profile for use in primary care: the Framingham Heart Study. Circulation. 2008;117:743–53.

124. Ridker PM, Buring JE, Rifai N, et al. Development and validation of improved algorithms for the assessment of global cardiovascular risk in women: the Reynolds Risk Score. JAMA. 2007;297:611–9.

125. Bertrand ME, Rupprecht HJ, Urban P, et al.; CLASSICS Investigators. Double-blind study of the safety of clopidogrel with and without a loading dose in combination with aspirin compared with ticlopidine in combination with aspirin after coronary stenting: the clopidogrel aspirin stent international cooperative study (CLASSICS). Circulation. 2000;102:624–9.

126. Jochmann N, Stangl K, Garbe E, et al. Female-specific aspects in the pharmacotherapy of chronic cardiovascular diseases. Eur Heart J. 2005;26:1585–95.

127. Serebruany VL, Steinhubl SR, Berger PB, et al. Variability in platelet responsiveness to clopidogrel among 544 individuals. J Am Coll Cardiol. 2005;45:246–51.

128. Price MJ. Monitoring platelet function to reduce the risk of ischemic and bleeding complications. Am J Cardiol. 2009;103(Suppl):35A–9.

129. Ferreiro JL, Angiolillo DJ. Clopidogrel response variability: current status and future directions. Thromb Haemost. 2009;102:7–14.

130. Yusuf S, Zhao F, Mehta SR, et al.; Clopidogrel in Unstable Angina to Prevent Recurrent Events Trial Investigators. Effects of clopidogrel in addition to aspirin in patients with acute coronary syndromes without ST-segment elevation. N Engl J Med. 2001;345:494–502.

131. Mehta SR, Yusuf S, Peters RJ, et al.; Clopidogrel in Unstable angina to prevent Recurrent Events trial (CURE) Investigators. Effects of pretreatment with clopidogrel and aspirin followed by long-term therapy in patients undergoing percutaneous coronary intervention: the PCI-CURE study. Lancet. 2001;358:527–33.

132. Sabatine MS, Cannon CP, Gibson CM, et al.; CLARITY-TIMI 28 Investigators. Addition of clopidogrel to aspirin and fibrinolytic therapy for myocardial infarction with ST-segment elevation. N Engl J Med. 2005;352:1179–89.

133. Chen ZM, Jiang LX, Chen YP, et al.; COMMIT (ClOpidogrel and Metoprolol in Myocardial Infarction Trial) collaborative group. Addition of clopidogrel to aspirin in 45,852 patients with acute myocardial infarction: randomised placebo-controlled trial. Lancet. 2005;366:1607–21.

134. Bhatt DL, Fox KA, Hacke W, et al.; CHARISMA Investigators. Clopidogrel and aspirin versus aspirin alone for the prevention of atherothrombotic events. N Engl J Med. 2006;354:1706–17.

135. Sibbing D, Koch W, Gebhard D, et al. Cytochrome 2C19*17 allelic variant, platelet aggregation, bleeding events, and stent thrombosis in clopidogrel-treated patients with coronary stent placement. Circulation. 2010;121:512–8.

136. Mega JL, Close SL, Wiviott SD, et al. Cytochrome p-450 polymorphisms and response to clopidogrel. N Engl J Med. 2009;360:354–62.

137. Angiolillo DJ, Suryadevara S, Capranzano P, et al. Prasugrel: a novel platelet ADP P2Y12 receptor antagonist. A review on its mechanism of action and clinical development. Expert Opin Pharmacother. 2008;9:2893–900.

138. Mega JL, Close SL, Wiviott SD, et al. Cytochrome P450 genetic polymorphisms and the response to prasugrel: relationship to pharmacokinetic, pharmacodynamic, and clinical outcomes. Circulation. 2009;119:2553–60.

139. Tardiff BE, Jennings LK, Harrington RA, et al.; PERIGEE Investigators. Pharmacodynamics and pharmacokinetics of eptifibatide in patients with acute coronary syndromes: prospective analysis from PURSUIT. Circulation. 2001;104:399–405.

140. Boersma E, Harrington RA, Moliterno DJ, et al. Platelet glycoprotein IIb/IIIa inhibitors in acute coronary syndromes: a meta-analysis of all major randomised clinical trials. Lancet. 2002;359:189–98.

141. Giugliano RP, White JA, Bode C, et al.; EARLY ACS Investigators. Early versus delayed, provisional eptifibatide in acute coronary syndromes. N Engl J Med. 2009;360:2176–90.

142. Hirsh J, Warkentin TE, Raschke R, et al. Heparin and low-molecular-weight heparin: mechanisms of action, pharmacokinetics, dosing considerations, monitoring, efficacy, and safety. Chest. 1998;114:489S–510.

143. Hochman JS, Wali AU, Gavrila D, et al. A new regimen for heparin use in acute coronary syndromes. Am Heart J. 1999;138:313–8.

144. Dose-ranging trial of enoxaparin for unstable angina: results of TIMI 11A. Thrombolysis in Myocardial Infarction 11A Investigators. J Am Coll Cardiol. 1997;29:1474–82.

145. Becker RC, Spencer FA, Gibson M, et al.; TIMI 11A Investigators. Influence of patient characteristics and renal function on factor Xa inhibition pharmacokinetics and pharmacodynamics after enoxaparin administration in non-ST-segment elevation acute coronary syndromes. Am Heart J. 2002;143:753–9.

146. Fragmin during Instability in Coronary Artery Disease (FRISC) Study Group. Low-molecular-weight heparin during instability in coronary artery disease. Lancet. 1996;347:561–8.

147. White HD, Kleiman NS, Mahaffey KW, et al. Efficacy and safety of enoxaparin compared with unfractionated heparin in high-risk patients with non-ST-segment elevation acute coronary syndrome undergoing percutaneous coronary intervention in the Superior Yield of the New Strategy of Enoxaparin, Revascularization and Glycoprotein IIb/IIIa Inhibitors (SYNERGY) trial. Am Heart J. 2006;152:1042–50.

148. Anderson JL, Adams CD, Antman EM, et al. 2012 ACCF/AHA focused update incorporated Into the ACCF/AHA 2007 guidelines for the management of patients With unstable angina/non-ST-elevation myocardial infarction: a report of the American College of Cardiology Foundation/American Heart Association Task Force on Practice Guidelines. J Am Coll Cardiol. 2013;61:e179–347.

149. Kushner FG, Hand M, Smith Jr SC, et al. 2009 focused updates: ACC/AHA guidelines for the management of patients with ST-elevation myocardial infarction (updating the 2004 guideline and 2007 focused update) and ACC/AHA/SCAI guidelines on percutaneous coronary intervention (updating the 2005 guideline and 2007 focused update) a report of the American College of Cardiology Foundation/American Heart Association Task Force on Practice Guidelines. J Am Coll Cardiol. 2009;54:2205–41.

150. Lincoff AM, Bittl JA, Harrington RA, et al.; REPLACE-2 Investigators. Bivalirudin and provisional glycoprotein IIb/IIIa blockade compared with heparin and planned glycoprotein

IIb/IIIa blockade during percutaneous coronary intervention: REPLACE-2 randomized trial. JAMA. 2003;289:853–63.

151. Lincoff AM, Kleiman NS, Kereiakes DJ, et al.; REPLACE-2 Investigators. Long-term efficacy of bivalirudin and provisional glycoprotein IIb/IIIa blockade vs heparin and planned glycoprotein IIb/IIIa blockade during percutaneous coronary revascularization: REPLACE-2 randomized trial. JAMA. 2004;292:696–703.

152. Stone GW, McLaurin BT, Cox DA, et al.; ACUITY Investigators. Bivalirudin for patients with acute coronary syndromes. N Engl J Med. 2006;355:2203–16.

153. Stone GW, White HD, Ohman EM, et al.; Acute Catheterization and Urgent Intervention Triage strategy (ACUITY) trial investigators. Bivalirudin in patients with acute coronary syndromes undergoing percutaneous coronary intervention: a subgroup analysis from the Acute Catheterization and Urgent Intervention Triage strategy (ACUITY) trial. Lancet. 2007;369:907–19.

154. Stone GW, Witzenbichler B, Guagliumi G, et al.; HORIZONS-AMI Trial Investigators. Bivalirudin during primary PCI in acute myocardial infarction. N Engl J Med. 2008;358:2218–30.

155. Grinfeld L, Belardi J, Lansky A, et al.. Impact of gender on the safety and effectiveness of bivalirudin in patients with acute myocardial infarction undergoing primary angioplasty. Abstract presented at: Annual meeting of the American College of Cardiology, Chicago; 2008.

156. Madsen JK, Chevalier B, Darius H, et al. Ischaemic events and bleeding in patients undergoing percutaneous coronary intervention with concomitant bivalirudin treatment. EuroIntervention. 2008;3:610–6.

157. Shammas NW, Allie D, Hall P, et al.; APPROVE Investigators. Predictors of in-hospital and 30-day complications of peripheral vascular interventions using bivalirudin as the primary anticoagulant: results from the APPROVE Registry. J Invasive Cardiol. 2005;17:356–9.

158. Roguin A, Steinberg BA, Watkins SP, et al. Safety of bivalirudin during percutaneous coronary interventions in patients with abnormal renal function. Int J Cardiovasc Intervent. 2005;7:88–92.

159. Blick SK, Orman JS, Wagstaff AJ, et al. Fondaparinux sodium: a review of its use in the management of acute coronary syndromes. Am J Cardiovasc Drugs. 2008;8:113–25.

160. Poli D, Antonucci E, Grifoni E, et al. Bleeding risk during oral anticoagulation in atrial fibrillation patients older than 80 years. J Am Coll Cardiol. 2009;54:999–1002.

161. Poli D, Antonucci E, Grifoni E, et al. Gender differences in stroke risk of atrial fibrillation patients on oral anticoagulant treatment. Thromb Haemost. 2009;101:938–42.

162. Friberg J, Scharling H, Gadsbøll N, et al.; Jensen Copenhagen City Heart Study. Comparison of the impact of atrial fibrillation on the risk of stroke and cardiovascular death in women versus men (The Copenhagen City Heart Study). Am J Cardiol. 2004;94:889–94.

163. Levy S, Maarek M, Coumel P, et al. Characterization of different subsets of atrial fibrillation in general practice in France. The ALFA study. Circulation. 1999;99:3028–35.

164. Ong L, Irvine J, Nolan R, et al. Gender differences and quality of life in atrial fibrillation: the mediating role of depression. J Psychosom Res. 2006;61:769–74.

165. Humphries KH, Kerr CR, Conolly SJ, et al. New-onset atrial fibrillation: sex differences in presentation, treatment, and outcome. Circulation. 2001;103:2365–70.

166. Rienstra M, Van Veldhuisen DJ, Hagens VE, et al. Gender-related differences in rhythm control treatment in persistent atrial fibrillation. Data of the rate control versus electrical cardioversion (RACE) study. J Am Coll Cardiol. 2005;46:1298–306.

167. Dagres N, Nieuwlaat R, Vardas PE, et al. Gender-related differences in presentation, treatment, and outcome of patients with atrial fibrillation in Europe. A report from the Euro Heart Survey on atrial fibrillation. J Am Coll Cardiol. 2007;49:572–7.

168. Benjamin J, Levy D, Vaziri S, et al. Independent risk factors for atrial fibrillation in a population-based cohort: the Framingham heart study. JAMA. 1994;271:840–4.

169. Hart R, Pearce L, McBride R, et al. Factors associated with ischemic stroke during aspirin therapy in atrial fibrillation: analysis of 2012 participants in the SPAF I–III clinical trials. Stroke. 1999;30:1223–9.

170. Wang TJ, Massaro JM, Levy D, et al. A risk score for predicting stroke or death in individuals with new-onset atrial fibrillation in the community. The Framingham Heart Study. JAMA. 2003;290:1049–56.
171. Stroke in Atrial Fibrillation Working Group. Independent predictors of stroke in atrial fibrillation: a systematic review. Neurology. 2007;69:546–54.
172. Gomberg-Maitland M, Wenger NK, et al. Anticoagulation in women with non-valvular atrial fibrillation in the stroke prevention using an oral thrombin inhibitor (SPORTIF) trials. Eur Heart J. 2006;27:1947–53.
173. Camm JA, Kirchof P, Lip GYH, et al. Guidelines for the management of atrial fibrillation. The Task Force for the Management of Atrial Fibrillation of the European Society of Cardiology (ESC). Eur Heart J. 2010;31:2369–429.
174. Benjamin EJ, Wolf PA, D'Agostino RB, et al. Impact of atrial fibrillation on the risk of death: the Framingham Heart Study. Circulation. 1998;98:946–52.
175. Michelena HI, Powell BD, Brady PA, et al. Gender in atrial fibrillation: ten years later. Gend Med. 2010;7:206–17.
176. Conway DS, Heeringa J, Van Der Kuip DA, et al. Atrial fibrillation and the prothrombotic state in the elderly: the Rotterdam Study. Stroke. 2003;34:413–7.
177. Wang TD, Chen WJ, Su SS, et al. Increased levels of tissue plasminogen activator antigen and factor VIII activity in nonvalvular atrial fibrillation: relation to predictors of thromboembolism. J Cardiovasc Electrophysiol. 2001;12:877–84.
178. Feinberg WM, Pearce LA, Hart RG, et al. Markers of thrombin and platelet activity in patients with atrial fibrillation: correlation with stroke among 1531 participants in the stroke prevention in atrial fibrillation III study. Stroke. 1999;30:2547–53.
179. Risk factors for stroke and efficacy of antithrombotic therapy in atrial fibrillation. Analysis of pooled data from five randomized controlled trials. Arch Intern Med. 1994;154:1449–57.
180. Garcia D, Regan S, Crowther M, et al. Warfarin maintenance dosing patterns in clinical practice. Chest. 2005;127:2049–56.
181. Lip GY, Andreotti F, Fauchier L, et al. (2011) Document reviewers: Collet JP, Rubboli A, Poli D, Camm J. Bleeding risk assessment and management in atrial fibrillation patients: a position document from the European Heart Rhythm Association, endorsed by the European Society of Cardiology Working Group on Thrombosis Europace 13:723–746.
182. Shen AY, Yao JF, Brar SS, et al. Racial/ethnic differences in the risk of intracranial hemorrhage among patients with atrial fibrillation. J Am Coll Cardiol. 2007;50:309–15.
183. Poli D, Antonucci E, Testa S, et al.; Palareti Italian Federation of Anticoagulation Clinics. Bleeding risk in very old patients on vitamin K antagonist treatment: results of a prospective collaborative study on elderly patients followed by Italian Centres for Anticoagulation. Circulation. 2011;124:824–9.
184. Connolly SJ, Eikelboom J, Joyner C, et al.; AVERROES Steering Committee and Investigators. Apixaban in patients with atrial fibrillation. N Engl J Med. 2011;364: 806–17.
185. Fibrinolytic Therapy Trialists' (FTT) Collaborative Group. Indications for fibrinolytic therapy in suspected acute myocardial infarction: collaborative overview of early mortality and major morbidity results from all randomised trials of more than 1000 patients. Lancet. 1994;343:311–22.
186. Gruppo Italiano per lo Studio Della Streptochinasi nell'Infarto Miocardico (GISSI). Effectiveness of intravenous thrombolytic treatment in acute myocardial infarction. Lancet. 1986;1:397–402.
187. Wilcox RG, von der Lippe G, Olsson CG, et al. Trial of tissue plasminogen activator for mortality reduction in acute myocardial infarction: Anglo-Scandinavian Study of Early Thrombolysis (ASSET). Lancet. 1988;2:525–30.
188. Moen EK, Asher CR, Miller DP, et al. Long-term follow-up of gender-specific outcomes after thrombolytic therapy for acute myocardial infarction from the GUSTO-I trial. Global Utilization of Streptokinase and Tissue Plasminogen Activator for Occluded Coronary Arteries. J Womens Health. 1997;6:285–93.

189. Lee KL, Woodlief LH, Topol EJ, et al. Predictors of 30-day mortality in the era of reperfusion for acute myocardial infarction. Circulation. 1995;91:1659–68.
190. White HD, Barbash GI, Modan M, et al. After correcting for worse baseline characteristics, women treated with thrombolytic therapy for acute myocardial infarction have the same mortality and morbidity as men except for a higher incidence of hemorrhagic stroke. The Investigators of the International Tissue Plasminogen Activator/Streptokinase Mortality Study. Circulation. 1993;88:2097–103.
191. Weaver WD, White HD, Wilcox RG, et al.; GUSTO-I Investigators. Comparisons of characteristics and outcomes among women and men with acute myocardial infarction treated with thrombolytic therapy. JAMA. 1996;275:777–82.
192. Nicolau JC, Auxiliadora Ferraz M, Nogueira PR, et al. The role of gender in the long-term prognosis of patients with myocardial infarction submitted to fibrinolytic treatment. Ann Epidemiol. 2004;14:17–23.
193. Van de Werf F, Barron HV, Armstrong PW, et al.; ASSENT-2 Investigators. Incidence and predictors of bleeding events after fibrinolytic therapy with fibrin-specific agents: a comparison of TNK-tPA and rt-PA. Eur Heart J. 2001;22:2253–61.
194. Berkowitz SD, Granger CB, Pieper KS, et al.; Global Utilization of Streptokinase and Tissue Plasminogen activator for Occluded coronary arteries (GUSTO) I Investigators Incidence and predictors of bleeding after contemporary thrombolytic therapy for myocardial infarction. Circulation. 1997;95:2508–16.
195. Topol EJ. Reperfusion therapy for acute myocardial infarction with fibrinolytic therapy or combination reduced fibrinolytic therapy and platelet glycoprotein IIb/IIIa inhibition: the GUSTO V randomised trial. Lancet. 2001;357:1905–14.
196. Reynolds HR, Farkouh ME, Lincoff AM, et al.; GUSTO V Investigators. Impact of female sex on death and bleeding after fibrinolytic treatment of myocardial infarction in GUSTO V. Arch Intern Med. 2007;167:2054–60.
197. Mudrick DW, Chen AY, Roe MT, et al. Changes in glycoprotein IIb/IIIa inhibitor excess dosing with site-specific safety feedback in the can rapid risk stratification of unstable angina patients suppress ADverse outcomes with early implementation of the ACC/AHA guidelines (CRUSADE) initiative. Am Heart J. 2010;160:1072–8.
198. Price MJ, Berger PB, Teirstein PS, et al.; GRAVITAS Investigators. Standard- vs high-dose clopidogrel based on platelet function testing after percutaneous coronary intervention: the GRAVITAS randomized trial. JAMA. 2011;305:1097–105.
199. Cuisset T, Frere C, Quilici J, et al. Glycoprotein IIb/IIIa inhibitors improve outcome after coronary stenting in clopidogrel nonresponders: a prospective, randomized study. JACC Cardiovasc Interv. 2008;1:649–53.
200. Jeong YH, Lee SW, Choi BR, et al. Randomized comparison of adjunctive cilostazol versus high maintenance dose clopidogrel in patients with high post-treatment platelet reactivity: results of the ACCEL-RESISTANCE (adjunctive cilostazol versus high maintenance dose clopidogrel in patients with clopidogrel resistance) randomized study. J Am Coll Cardiol. 2009;53:1101–9.
201. Han Y, Li Y, Wang S, et al. Cilostazol in addition to aspirin and clopidogrel improves long-term outcomes after percutaneous coronary intervention in patients with acute coronary syndromes: a randomized, controlled study. Am Heart J. 2009;157:733–9.
202. Faxon DP, Freedman JE. Facts and controversies of aspirin and clopidogrel therapy. Am Heart J. 2009;157:412–22.
203. Dauerman HL, Bhatt DL, Gretler DD, et al.; 2009 Platelet Colloquium Participants. Bridging the gap between clinical trials of antiplatelet therapies and clinical applications among elderly patients. Am Heart J. 2010;159:508–17.
204. Lee PY, Alexander KP, Hammill BG, et al. Representation of elderly persons and women in published randomized trials of acute coronary syndromes. JAMA. 2001;286:708–13.
205. Ding EL, Powe NR, Manson JE, et al. Sex differences in perceived risks, distrust, and willingness to participate in clinical trials: a randomized study of cardiovascular prevention trials. Arch Intern Med. 2007;167:905–12.

Chapter 16
Effects of Hormones and Hormone Therapy on Cardiovascular Health in Women

Renee M. Dallasen, Hanna Z. Mieszczanska, and Diane M. Hartmann

Cardiovascular disease (CVD) is the leading cause of mortality and morbidity in American women, causing approximately 250,000 women to die each year of ischemic heart disease, roughly six times more than the number of women who die from breast cancer [1]. When compared to age-matched men, the incidence of coronary heart disease (CHD) is much lower in younger women [2]. The Framingham population study showed that coronary artery disease usually manifests 10 years later in women than it does in men [3]. This lag was punctuated by the age of menopause and was suggestive of a protective effect of estrogen [4]. The potential protective effects of female hormones on the cardiovascular system have been a topic of great interest. Loss of this protection after menopause may be linked to the increased incidence of CHD in older women [2].

Despite these epidemiological observations, the Women's Health Initiative (WHI) has not confirmed a postmenopausal cardioprotective effect of estrogen [5]. In this chapter, mechanisms of vascular aging, the effects of menopause on cardiac risk factors, and the evidence for and against hormone therapy in postmenopausal women will be discussed.

Effects of Aging on Endothelial Function

Aging is associated with endothelial dysfunction, impaired angiogenesis, arterial stiffening and remodeling, and increased prevalence of atherosclerosis [6, 7]. Endothelial dysfunction is known to be the primary event in atherogenesis.

R.M. Dallasen, MD (✉) • D.M. Hartmann, MD
Department of Medicine and Department of Obstetrics and Gynecology,
University of Rochester Medical Center, Rochester, NY, USA
e-mail: renee_dallasen@urmc.rochester.edu

H.Z. Mieszczanska, MD
Division of Cardiology, University of Rochester Medical Center, Rochester, NY, USA

H.Z. Mieszczanska, G.P. Velarde (eds.),
Management of Cardiovascular Disease in Women,
DOI 10.1007/978-1-4471-5517-1_16, © Springer-Verlag London 2014

Dysfunctional endothelium has been associated with many cardiovascular risk factors including dyslipidemia, hypertension, smoking, diabetes mellitus, family history, and pre-stenotic coronary plaque [8]. Endothelial dysfunction can also be a manifestation of Syndrome X in the absence of medial coronary plaque [9, 10].

The endothelial tissue, the innermost layer of the vascular wall, regulates vascular homeostasis by maintaining a balance between vasodilation and vasoconstriction, inhibition and stimulation of smooth muscle proliferation and migration, and thrombogenesis and fibrinolysis. Vasodilation is caused by the release of nitric oxide (NO), prostacyclin, and bradykinin, whereas vasoconstriction depends on the release of endothelin and angiotensin II. Endothelial dependent vasodilation is impaired in menopausal women [11, 12]. Experimental studies have shown that estrogens modulate the response of vessels to various vasoactive substances, including angiotensin II, norepinephrine, and aldosterone, thereby preventing the same degree of vasoconstriction seen in men [13, 14].

While the mechanisms of vascular dysfunction in aging are numerous, decreased NO bioavailability is most reported. An increase in oxidative stress from toxic chemical environments, including abnormal lipid levels, diabetes, or increased shear stress from hypertension, can inactivate NO and thus compromise the endothelial vascular homeostasis [12]. Endothelial dysfunction is related to the loss of endogenous estrogen and serves as an independent predictor of future CVD events [6].

Effects of Female Hormones

Men have been known to develop coronary heart disease earlier in life than women. The incidence of CVD is much lower in premenopausal women but increases after menopause. For many years, estrogen has been thought to provide females with cardiovascular protection [15]. Twelve months of amenorrhea leading to permanent cessation of menses following the decline of ovarian function defines menopause. The median age of menopause is 51 years. Menopause is associated with decreased estradiol levels, which result in vasomotor symptoms, including hot flashes and night sweats. By considering both the direct and indirect effects of estrogen on the vasculature, one can begin to understand why a lack of estrogen may lead to endothelial dysfunction.

The direct effects of estrogen are thought to account for the majority of its cardio-protective effects and include prevention of atherosclerosis, facilitation of angiogenesis, and collateral vessel formation via the stimulation of endothelial cell proliferation and inhibition of vascular smooth muscle cell proliferation [16]. Estrogens are believed to be protective to coronary vessels by providing improved vascular tone. Additionally, estrogen can increase the production or the release of relaxing factors from the endothelium, thus improving endothelial function [17, 18].

Estrogen acts through its receptors to inhibit vascular smooth muscle cell proliferation and matrix deposition, thus preventing arterial intimal thickening [7, 19].

Table 16.1 Summary of the effects of estrogen

Direct effects	Indirect effects
Arterial vasodilatation	Lowers cholesterol
Improves vascular tone	Decreases insulin resistance
Inhibits smooth muscle proliferation	Inhibits platelet aggregation
Inhibits endothelial dysfunction	Improves fibrinolysis and activates coagulation
Facilitates angiogenesis	Exerts antioxidant effects

Progestogens can also cause vasodilation through increasing NOS and inducing cyclooxygenases [16].

In terms of indirect effects, estrogen affects the lipid profile, glucose and insulin metabolism, and the coagulation profile. In premenopausal women, estrogen has been shown to improve the lipid profile by reducing low-density lipoprotein (LDL) cholesterol, increasing high-density lipoprotein (HDL) cholesterol, and decreasing serum Lp (a) lipoprotein concentrations [18, 20]. The Framingham study, involving women between the ages of 29 and 62 followed longitudinally for 18 years, demonstrated a significant increase in cholesterol levels between premenopausal and postmenopausal exams. The increase occurred around the time of the menopausal transition, suggesting a causal effect [2]. Estrogen also exerts indirect effects on glucose and insulin metabolism by increasing pancreatic insulin secretion and decreasing insulin resistance [21].

In addition to its direct effects on cardiovascular function, estrogen indirectly affects both coagulation and fibrinolysis, exerting both pro-coagulant and fibrinolytic effects. Estrogen has been shown to decrease levels of fibrinogen, plasminogen activator inhibitor-1, antithrombin III, and protein S [16]. Platelet aggregation is inhibited by estrogen [21]. Despite these antithrombotic effects, estrogen has been associated with thromboembolic disease. Procoagulant effects of estrogen include increased levels of prothrombin, factors VII, X, and protein C [22]. The effects of estrogen are summarized in Table 16.1.

While estrogen exerts several favorable effects on the vasculature of young healthy individuals, aging limits its ability to confer these favorable effects. Atherosclerotic coronary arteries have fewer estrogen receptors than normal coronary arteries, and thus less NO release leads to unfavorable effects on the vasculature [7, 16]. The effects of hormone therapy on the vasculature are complex. Hormone therapy exerts both pro-inflammatory and anti-inflammatory effects in addition to both activating coagulation and improving fibrinolysis [17].

There is evidence to suggest pro-atherogenic effects of estrogen in atherosclerotic vessels, which can lead to plaque destabilization and CVD events. Estrogen induces matrix metalloproteinases, which can weaken the fibrous caps of plaques and thus lead to plaque destabilization and rupture. Unlike statins, estrogen cannot inhibit progression of atherosclerosis in the presence of advanced atherosclerotic lesions [6].

Table 16.2 Effects of menopause on cardiac risk factors

Cardiac risk factors after menopause	
Lipid profile	Increased total cholesterol level
	Decreased High Density Lipoprotein (HDL) cholesterol level
	Increased triglyceride level
Blood pressure	Increased prevalence of hypertension
Diabetes mellitus	Increased prevalence (insulin resistance increases)
Obesity* (e.g., BMI ≥30 kg/m^2)	Increased prevalence
Central obesity (waist circumference >35 in.)	Increased prevalence
	Body fat is redistributed into the abdomen, which can lead to impaired glucose tolerance
Metabolic syndrome	Increased prevalence

Adapted with permission from Shaw et al. [59]
*Obesity increasing in the last decade such that ~25 % of women are now obese with a body mass index (BMI) ≥30 kg/m^2. Additionally, women generally engage in less leisure-time physical activity and exhibit a greater functional decline in their postmenopausal years

Effects of Menopause on Cardiovascular Risk Factors

In addition to the increased risk of CVD, which comes with postmenopausal changes in sex hormone levels, menopause is also associated with a higher incidence of cardiac risk factors including diabetes, hypertension, obesity, dyslipidemia, and other co-morbidities. The lipid profile is adversely affected during menopause; total cholesterol, LDL, and triglycerides are increased while HDL is decreased. Insulin and glucose metabolism is impaired, as evidenced by increased insulin resistance in postmenopausal women. Postmenopausal women tend to have more abdominal obesity due to body fat redistribution, which is associated with alterations in the lipid profile and glucose metabolism. These women are predisposed to the metabolic syndrome, which can be defined as having central obesity, impaired fasting glucose, hyperlipidemia, and elevated blood pressure [21]. The pro-coagulant effects of estrogen can become predominant as fibrinogen, factor VII activity, antithrombin III, and plasminogen activator inhibitor-1 (PAI-1) are increased after menopause [21] (Table 16.2).

Evidence for the Association Between Menopause and CHD

The Framingham study provides supporting evidence for the association between postmenopausal status and CHD. An analysis of a cohort of 2,873 women followed for 24 years revealed the incidence of cardiovascular disease in age matched men under 60 years was twice that of same age women. Among postmenopausal women up to the age of 55 years, cardiovascular disease was twice that of premenopausal women, with 70 cardiovascular events occurring in postmenopausal women compared to 20 events in premenopausal women. When analyzing the risk of stroke, MI, and congestive heart failure (CHF), however, the number of events was smaller. Premenopausal and postmenopausal women experienced 9 and 39 events respectively, a difference that does not meet statistical significance [23]. In the Nurses Health study, a prospective cohort of 35,616 healthy, naturally postmenopausal women, a younger age at menopause was associated with a higher risk of CHD [24].

These adverse effects on the cardiovascular system may be seen sooner in women who smoke and thus undergo natural menopause at an earlier age [2]. Women who smoke typically reach menopause 2 years earlier than non-smokers [25].

Women with polycystic ovary syndrome (PCOS) are predisposed to CHD and may suffer from adverse cardiovascular events, given the associated endocrine and metabolic abnormalities such as insulin resistance, glucose intolerance, lipid abnormalities, hypertension, and increased levels of plasminogen activator inhibitor [26]. In premenopausal women with coronary risk factors undergoing coronary angiography for suspected myocardial ischemia, disruption of the ovulatory cycle characterized by hypoestrogenemia of hypothalamic origin, was also associated with angiographic coronary artery disease [27].

The risk of CHD differs in women undergoing menopause prematurely by bilateral oophorectomy. Several studies have shown increased CHD risk among females who underwent surgical menopause. Women who underwent bilateral oophorectomy and did not use estrogen replacement therapy were found to be at increased risk of CHD when compared to age-matched controls in the Nurses' Health Study (risk ratio 2.2) [28]. In a study by Rosenberg et al., the relative risk of developing a myocardial infarction increased with decreasing age at bilateral oophorectomy [29].

The Multi-ethnic Study of Atherosclerosis (MESA), a multicenter, longitudinal cohort study involving 3,213 men and 3,601 women, found that early menopause was a strong predictor of CHD and stroke (twofold increased risk), regardless of traditional CVD risk factors in the population-based sample of multiethnic US women [30].

Prevention and Treatment of CHD in Postmenopausal Women

Lifestyle modification with a focus on risk factor reduction should be the first step in the prevention of CHD [21]. Women should be encouraged to stop smoking. The risk of CHD is two to four times greater in women who smoke [2, 31]. Diet should be modified to include less saturated fat intake. Weight should be controlled through both diet and physical activity. In women with established hypertension, appropriate antihypertensive therapy should be given [21, 32].

In the past, hormone therapy (HT) was believed to be beneficial for women's hearts and was routinely prescribed for CHD prevention in the postmenopausal years. In the Postmenopausal Estrogen/Progestin Interventions (PEPI) trial, a randomized clinical trial published in 1995, postmenopausal women, ages 45–64 years, receiving either estrogen alone or in combination with a progestin, were observed to have a reduction in LDL, increased HDL levels, and lower fibrinogen levels. Unopposed estrogen has been most effective at increasing HDL cholesterol (HDL-C), however it is associated with endometrial hyperplasia, thus limiting its use to women without a uterus. A conjugated equine estrogen (CEE) with cyclic micronized progesterone (MP) used in women with a uterus still showed a favorable effect on HDL-C without the risk of endometrial hyperplasia [33]. To explain the risks and benefits of HT, the mechanisms of action should be considered.

HT Effects on the Cardiovascular System

HT decreases inflammatory markers and can lower levels of cell adhesion molecule E-selectin in menopausal women. Reduced inflammatory markers and adhesion molecules result in less collagen deposition and vascular remodeling, which can then retard or inhibit atheroma development [21, 34]. Some observational studies and the WHI estrogen therapy (ET) trial have suggested that long term HT is associated with less accumulation of coronary artery calcium and therefore slower development of atherosclerosis [35]. The recent Kronos Early Estrogen Prevention Study (KEEPS), a 4 year randomized, double blinded, placebo controlled clinical trial involving 727 healthy women aged 42–58 (mean age, 52) within 3 years of the onset of menopause, evaluated the effects of menopausal hormone therapy on subclinical atherosclerosis. Women received low dose oral or transdermal estrogen and cyclic monthly progesterone. A nonsignificant trend of less accumulation of coronary artery calcium was seen in the hormone therapy arm of the study. There was also no significant difference in the rate of progression of carotid intima media thickness between the treatment and placebo groups. However, the trial demonstrated very little progression of coronary calcium in these newly menopausal women in general, so the statistical power to see a significant difference over 4 years was very limited [36, 37].

HT Effects on Lipids and the Lipoprotein Profile

HT reduces total cholesterol levels by 5–10 % within 3 months of use [21]. Oral estrogen lowers LDL through the upregulation of apolipoprotein B_{100} receptors, especially in the liver. It also increases clearance of lipoproteins and chylomicron remnants from the circulation. HDL is increased by estrogen via a decrease in its catabolism by hepatic lipase. Androgenic progestins such as medroxyprogesterone acetate (MPA) can reverse the positive effects of estrogen on HDL [21]. While oral estrogen increases triglycerides, transdermal preparations decrease triglyceride production by avoiding first pass hepatic effect [38]. The results of KEEPS provide further evidence for the differing effects of HT depending on the route of administration. Due to its first pass liver metabolism, oral estrogen was associated with a significant reduction in LDL cholesterol and an increase in HDL cholesterol, triglyceride, and C-reactive protein levels. Transdermal estradiol, on the other hand, was associated with a neutral effect on lipids [36, 37].

HT Effects on the Metabolism of Glucose and Insulin

The effects on glucose and insulin metabolism may also depend on the preparation of estrogen. Oral 17-β estradiol has been shown to decrease insulin resistance while alkylated estrogens such as ethinyl estradiol and conjugated equine estrogens have been associated with a rise in insulin levels and impaired glucose tolerance. The effects of estrogen on glucose and insulin metabolism may be modified with the addition of a progestin. Strongly androgenic progestins have been associated with increased insulin resistance, whereas non-androgenic progestins have little adverse effect [21]. Transdermal estradiol was thought to have fairly neutral effects on glucose and insulin metabolism, however, in the recent Kronos Early Estrogen Prevention Study (KEEPS), there was an unexpected significant improvement in insulin resistance with transdermal estrogen, which was not seen with oral estrogen [36, 37].

HT Effects on the Coagulation System

HT has complex effects on the coagulation system, affecting both coagulation and fibrinolysis. Oral estrogen can increase thrombogenesis, which is usually seen around the time of initiation of HT. It is thought that initiation of estrogen therapy causes a transient imbalance between coagulation and fibrinolysis, favoring the procoagulant effects. This increased risk of thrombogenesis is reduced as the procoagulant and fibrinolytic effects come back into balance with each other. Transdermal administration of estrogen may avoid adverse pro-coagulant effects [21].

HT Effects on Blood Pressure

HT plays a complex role on blood pressure. With high doses of an oral contraceptive pill, there is risk of developing hypertension. Oral estrogen has been associated with increased plasma renin activity and plasma aldosterone [2]. On the other hand, the overall effects of HT on blood pressure are beneficial. Estrogen appears to elicit a reduction in resistance to blood flow and increase vessel elasticity, which may reduce the risk of coronary artery vasospasm or atherogenesis [21]. Recently, the KEEPS found no adverse effect on blood pressure, either systolic or diastolic, from either form of estrogen therapy [36, 37]. These findings were in contrast to the WHI findings with higher doses of estrogen.

Postmenopausal Hormone Therapy

Most women will live a third of their life after menopause, therefore it is important to be aware of the symptoms and available treatment options associated with estrogen loss [2]. Hormone therapy (HT) utilizes estrogen, with or without the addition of progestin. Estrogen can be given continuously in the form of tablets, skin patches, gels, subcutaneous implants, or intranasal sprays. Both natural estrogens and synthetic derivatives are available for HT. Systemic estrogen therapy (ET) has been proven to be the most effective treatment for vasomotor symptoms. Growing observational evidence is showing that transdermal ET may be associated with less risk of deep vein thrombosis, stroke, and MI [39, 40]. Transdermal preparations of estradiol also have the advantage of avoiding first pass hepatic effect, and thus may provide potential benefit to women with hypothyroidism or low libido. In women with a uterus, combination estrogen and progestin is necessary to avoid adverse effects of unopposed estrogen on the endometrium that can lead to endometrial cancer. Therefore, estrogen is typically combined with a progestin and is referred to as estrogen plus progestin therapy (EPT). Treatment may be cyclic, with daily estrogen and 12–14 days of progestin each month, or continuous-combined with both daily estrogen and low dose progestin [38].

Menopausal hormone therapy continues to have a clinical role in the management of vasomotor symptoms. For healthy women younger than 60 years and within 10 years of menopause, HT seems to be associated with low cardiovascular risk. If started on HT, women should use the lowest effective dose for the shortest duration of time to achieve treatment goals of relieving debilitating hot flashes and night sweats. Studies have shown that, for many women, low doses relieve vasomotor symptoms as effectively as standard doses. The need for continuing therapy should be assessed at least annually [38].

Contraindications of HT include breast or endometrial cancer, cardiovascular disease, thromboembolic disorders, and active liver or gallbladder disease. In women with contraindications to HT, alternatives to treat bothersome night sweats and hot flashes include lifestyle modifications (i.e. reducing body temperature, maintaining a healthy weight, smoking cessation, relaxation techniques, and acupuncture), non-prescription medications including vitamin E, soy products, and non-hormonal prescription medications, which include clonidine, paroxetine, venlafaxine, and gabapentin [38].

Primary and Secondary Prevention of Coronary Heart Disease

Given multiple potentially beneficial effects of estrogens on the cardiovascular system, there was a lot of expectation for the protective effects of postmenopausal hormone therapy for CVD prevention in women [17]. Due to the compelling evidence of cardioprotection by estrogen, the Coronary Drug Project, a randomized clinical trial funded in 1965 by the National Heart Institute, was designed to examine the benefits of estrogen in men who were at high risk of a heart attack [41]. Since optimal doses of estrogen for men were not known, men received a high dose of 2.5 mg of estrogen daily. Prevention of heart attacks was not seen, and the study was stopped early due to higher mortality among men receiving estrogen therapy.

Although the Coronary Drug Project had been terminated early, postmenopausal women in general practice continued to be treated with estrogen based on epidemiologic studies showing reduced rates of CHD among users of estrogen therapy [15].

Data from Observational Studies

Several observational studies involving postmenopausal women showed a lower risk of cardiovascular events and of all-cause mortality in women taking hormone therapy [15]. The Nurse's Health Study (NHS), the largest and longest prospective cohort study of women's health, showed a beneficial effect of menopausal hormone treatment (HT) on CVD events. The study began in 1976 and included 121,700 female nurses between the ages of 30 and 55 years. Participants were asked about postmenopausal hormone use and cardiovascular risk factors. After 20 years, the study suggested that women who took estrogen had a relative risk of death from CHD of 0.47 compared with non-users. Mortality due to stroke was also reduced with a relative risk of 0.68 [42]. A meta-analysis including observational studies conducted until 2000 revealed an overall benefit to using HT in terms of CVD mortality (relative risk [RR] 0.75) and coronary artery disease (CAD) incidence (RR 0.74). This benefit was not as obvious after adjusting for socioeconomic and major risk factors [6, 43].

Since HT was believed to be beneficial for women's cardiovascular health, several large, randomized clinical trials were conducted to "prove" the benefit of HT to any remaining physicians who were not prescribing it for that purpose. For this reason, it has been a surprise that the major randomized trials designed to prove the cardiac benefits of HT failed to do so.

Data from Randomized Controlled Trials

Randomized controlled trials were focused on delineating the effectiveness of hormone therapy on the prevention of cardiovascular disease. These trials did not occur until three decades after the Coronary Drug Project. Results from three large randomized clinical trials, which significantly influenced clinical care for women, were the Heart and Estrogen/Progestin Replacement Study (HERS) [44], the Estrogen Replacement and Atherosclerosis (ERA) trial [45], and the Women's Health Initiative (WHI) trial [5, 46].

Secondary Prevention

The HERS study [44], published in 1998, was the first large-scale randomized clinical outcome trial to evaluate the effects of HT on secondary prevention of CHD in 2,763 postmenopausal women. Participants, with a mean age of 66.7 years and documented existing coronary artery disease, were randomly assigned to take either placebo or combination hormone therapy (noncyclic conjugated equine estrogens [CEE] 0.625 mg+medroxyprogesterone acetate 2.5 mg) and followed for 4.1 years. There was no difference in the primary outcome of nonfatal myocardial infarction (MI) and coronary death between the hormone and placebo arms. A post-hoc time trend analysis of the data showed a significant time trend suggesting an excess of coronary events among hormone-treated women during the first year after the randomization (hazard ratio 1.52), with a trend toward fewer events at 3–5 years of follow up.

Given the decreased risk of coronary events at 3–5 years of follow-up in the HERS study, women were followed for an additional 2.7 years in an open-label, event surveillance study, HERS II. In HERS II, women remained on their original drug assignments. At the end of the study, hormone therapy failed to reveal a decreased risk of coronary events in women with established CHD, even after adjusting for potential confounders such as aspirin therapy, statin use, smoking, etc [47, 48].

The results from the Estrogen Replacement and Atherosclerosis (ERA) trial were reported in 2000. ERA was a randomized angiographic end-point trial comparing the effects of estrogen therapy (ET) and combination hormone therapy (HT) to placebo in postmenopausal women with pre-existing coronary artery disease. The trial also failed to show a benefit in women receiving ET and HT on the progression of atherosclerosis. This lack of benefit occurred despite the fact that women receiving HT in this study had a significant increase in HDL cholesterol and a decrease in LDL cholesterol [45].

The conclusion from these studies was that there was no long-term difference between women receiving HT and those receiving placebo and that postmenopausal hormone therapy should not be used for the sole purpose of secondary prevention of CHD in women with a history of established coronary artery disease [19, 49]. Since women enrolled in HERS and ERA had established coronary artery disease, the results of these studies may not directly apply to the use of hormone therapy in healthy postmenopausal women [50].

Primary Prevention

For many years, hormone therapy was thought to play a role in the primary prevention of CHD in "healthy" women. In order to study this hypothesis, a large, randomized trial, the Women's Health Initiative (WHI), was designed to compare HT with placebo in postmenopausal women [5]. The WHI included 16,608 healthy women, ages 50–79 years, with an intact uterus and no pre-existing coronary artery disease. Subjects were randomized to receive either conjugated equine estrogen (0.625 mg/day) with medroxyprogesterone acetate (2.5 mg/day) or placebo. The trial had several different arms, including an estrogen plus progestin arm (EPT) and an estrogen-only arm (ET) for women post hysterectomy (~10,739 women). In May 2002, after a mean follow up of 5.2 years, the study was stopped prematurely due to a 26 % increased risk of invasive breast cancer and excessive CVD events in the EPT group during the first year and nearly a 30 % increased risk of coronary events, mainly nonfatal myocardial infarctions. A 41 % increased risk of stroke and a doubled risk of venous thromboembolism was also seen [49]. Controversy erupted when investigators felt compelled to send letters to women participating in the trial stating that those in the EPT group had experienced an increased risk of breast cancer, heart attacks, strokes, and blood clots during the early portion of the trial. At the same time, however, investigators stated that only 1 % of study participants had experienced adverse events and that the data was very preliminary. They pointed out the early detriment seen with HT in the HERS trial disappeared after the first year.

The estrogen only arm of the study, however, showed no significant effect of HT on CVD risk. Overall CVD risk was estimated to be increased by eight cases per 10,000 women per year in the combined therapy group while the risk was estimated to be decreased by three cases per 10,000 women per year in the estrogen only group [35]. Women in the ET arm of the WHI also demonstrated no increased risk of breast cancer. The WHI trial was actually terminated early (in 2002) after finding a small but significant increase in cardiovascular events and other adverse outcomes in the hormone therapy group. The early termination of the WHI trial created much controversy regarding the role of HT and its effects on cardiovascular health in women. The trial changed the practice of prescribing HT for postmenopausal women. Many women had their hormone therapy discontinued at that time.

The aforementioned trials showed that menopausal hormone therapy did not prevent incidence or recurrence of CVD in women and increased their risk of stroke. Taken together, the cumulative data of HERS, ERA, and WHI supported the concept that HT should not be used in the prevention of cardiovascular disease and redirected focus on established preventative lifestyle and medical therapies such as smoking cessation, heart healthy diet, physical activity, weight management, as well as control of hypertension and hypercholesterolemia [47].

Additional Outcomes from Observational Studies and Clinical Trials

Stroke

The estrogen plus progestin arm (EPT) and estrogen arm (ET) in the WHI revealed an increased risk of ischemic stroke. This risk tended to be higher in those taking estrogen only. There were eight additional strokes per 10,000 women per year of EPT and 11 additional strokes per 10,000 women per year of ET. Stroke risk nearly doubled in the ET group of women within 10 years of menopause. The ET arm of the study was thus terminated 8 months early after nearly 7 years due to increased stroke risk (HR 1.39; estimated at an excess of 12 cases per 10,000 patient years) with 0.625 mg CEE. Lower stroke risk was seen in the combined group. Excess stroke risk dissipated after discontinuation of HT. Findings from the Nurses' Health Study were consistent with those of the WHI, indicating an increased risk of ischemic stroke with HT. However, results from observational studies have been inconsistent [35].

Venous Thromboembolism

In both observational and randomized controlled studies, the risk of venous thrombo-embolism (VTE) increased with oral HT in postmenopausal women. In the WHI, VTE risk emerged shortly after initiation of HT (during the first 1–2 years). The risk seemed to decrease with time. Analysis of the entire cohort demonstrated more cases of VTE in the combined therapy group than in the estrogen alone group. In women who started HT before age 60 years, VTE risk was lower than in those who initiated HT after 60 years. Initiation of HT with lower doses of estrogen and less androgenic progestins in younger women ages 50–59 or those within 10 years of menopause without underlying thromboembolic disease is associated with less risk of thrombo-sis. The rising incidence of venous thromboembolism with age can be explained, in part, by the fact that abnormal endovascular surfaces are more likely to give rise to intravascular clots. Also, estrogen has more favorable effects on healthy vasculature than atherosclerotic arteries [35, 51]. All three randomized controlled trials showed an increase in VTE and its associated complications including phlebitis and pulmo-nary emboli in patients taking HT. Thus, HT should be avoided in women who have had recent fractures, cancer, recent surgery, a history of blood clots, or any other fac-tor that predisposes them to the development of clotting abnormalities [38].

Diabetes Mellitus

In the combined therapy group of the WHI, women had a statistically significant 21 % reduction in the incidence of type 2 diabetes mellitus (T2DM). In the HERS study, a similar risk reduction was noted. Women receiving estrogen only in the WHI had a 12 % reduction in the incidence of T2DM. In the PEPI trial, fasting glucose levels were reduced in women receiving HT, however glucose levels after a 2 h oral glucose tolerance test were elevated [35].

Total Mortality

Total mortality was reduced by 30 % in both the EPT and ET groups in the WHI when initiated in women younger than 60. The risk reduction was statistically significant when the groups were combined.

Table 16.3 Clinical outcomes of WHI (estrogen + progestin)

Adverse event	Hazard ratio (HR)	Increased absolute risk per 10,000 women-years
CHD	1.29	7
Stroke	1.41	8
VTE	2.11	18
Breast cancer	1.26	8

Data collected from Writing Group for Women's Health Initiative Investigators. Rossouw et al. [5], Manson et al. [60], Chlebowski et al. [61]

CHD coronary heart disease, *VTE* venous thromboembolism

Ten fewer deaths per 10,000 women aged 50–59 years occurred whereas 16 additional deaths occurred in women aged 70–79 years [35].

The clinical outcomes of the WHI are summarized in Table 16.3.

Inconsistencies Between Observational and Randomized Trials of HT and CHD

Observational studies may be misleading because women who take postmenopausal hormones tend to have a better CHD profile and obtain more preventive care than non-users [44]. The discrepancy may also be due to differences between study populations and treatments. Most of the observational studies of HT enrolled relatively young and healthy postmenopausal women who started HT around the time of menopause for symptomatic relief [52, 53]. In contrast, subjects in HERS were older with coronary artery disease and were treated with estrogen plus progesterone. When the Nurses' Health Study (NHS) was compared to the WHI, significant differences were also found between involved groups. Women in the NHS were younger (55 years or younger) with less cardiovascular risk factors, and treatment had been started sooner after menopause. In contrast, women in the WHI were, on average, 63 years old when they began HT.

The Timing Hypothesis

Due to the small but significant increased risk of cardiovascular events and other adverse outcomes in the hormone therapy group of the WHI, the study was terminated early. Secondary analyses of the WHI indicate timing of initiation of HT may be responsible for the disparity in findings between observational and randomized controlled trials [17, 54]. Secondary analyses of clinical and observational studies have helped to resolve some of the disparate findings. A subgroup analysis of the NHS revealed loss of protective effects in older women [16], whereas a subgroup of women in the WHI, who were younger (50–59 years) or within only 10 years of menopause receiving estrogen only, did not appear to be at increased risk of cardiovascular events.

Table 16.4 Event risk by years since menopause for estrogen only (CEE)

Years since menopause	<10 years	10–19	≥20	
Event	HR	HR	HR	P value for trend
CHD	0.48	0.96	1.12	0.15
Stroke	2.24	1.47	1.2	0.24
Total mortality	0.65	0.93	1.16	0.42

Adapted from Rossouw et al. [54]

Abbreviations: *CEE* conjugated equine estrogens, *CHD* coronary heart disease, *HR* hazard ratio

Table 16.5 Event risk by years since menopause for combined HT (CEE+MPA)

Years since menopause	<10 years	10–19	≥20	Effectiveness-based guidelines for the prevention of cardiovascular disease in women–2011 update: a guideline from the American Heart Association
Event	HR	HR	HR	P value for trend
CHD	0.88	1.23	1.66	0.05
Stroke	1.58	1.12	1.35	0.87
Total mortality	0.81	1.03	1.11	0.93

Adapted from Rossouw et al. [54]

Abbreviations: *HT* hormone therapy, *CEE* conjugated equine estrogens, *MPA* medroxyprogesterone acetate, *CHD* coronary heart disease, *HR* hazard ratio

These women were also shown to have less coronary artery calcification compared to those taking placebo [6]. For women ages 50–59 in the estrogen only arm of the WHI, the hazard ratios for CHD and MI were 0.48 and 0.54 respectively, indicating that ET may reduce CHD risk when initiated in younger, recently menopausal women. When the ET and EPT trials were combined to investigate the effects of HT in relation to age and proximity to menopause, women who initiated HT more than 10 years beyond menopause were at increased risk of CHD. These sub-analyses suggest that the timing of initiation of hormone treatment in relation to the onset of menopause may influence the risk of CVD events. The WHI and HERS have shown that late starting of HT is either ineffective or harmful (Tables 16.4 and 16.5).

By beginning menopausal hormone therapy early in appropriate postmenopausal women, cardiovascular risk factors may be minimized. What the "timing hypothesis" implies is that a young healthy woman with significant vasomotor complaints close to menopausal transition may benefit from HT and avoid the risk of CVD given that she has normal vasculature [49].

The previously mentioned Kronos Early Estrogen Prevention Study (KEEPS) [37] found HT to be helpful in controlling symptoms in newly menopausal younger women (mean age 52). Since KEEPS was not large enough to investigate outcomes, the study focused on surrogate markers of atherosclerosis, changes in vascular biomarkers, cognitive function, mood, and quality of life. No significant difference between the treatment and placebo groups was found between the rates of atherosclerosis progression measured by carotid intima media thickness or coronary artery calcium. Although little progression of atherosclerosis was observed in these newly menopausal women, the study lacked sufficient statistical power to evaluate this question. Overall, the findings of this study showed several favorable effects of hormone therapy in newly menopausal women but stressed the need for individualized and

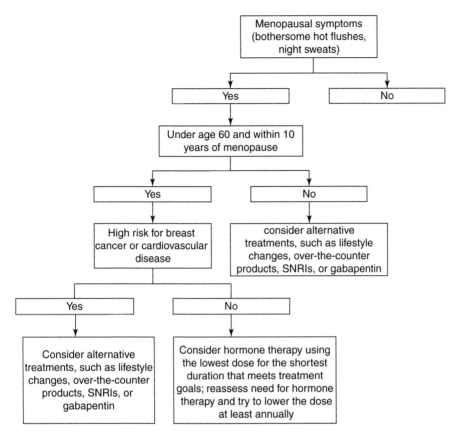

Fig. 16.1 Decision tree for patients with menopausal symptoms, including bothersome hot flushes and night sweats. *SNRI* serotonin–nore- pinephrine reuptake inhibitor (With permission from Shrifen [38]). *HT* hormone therapy

personalized care since oral and transdermal preparations of estrogen may have different effects and advantages depending on underlying cardiovascular risk factors, personal preferences, and priorities of treatment. Of note, transdermal estrogen has not been associated with increases in triglycerides or C-reactive protein, and, therefore, may be more beneficial than oral estrogen in obese postmenopausal women with the metabolic syndrome [36]. The results of KEEPS provided reassurance to recently menopausal women taking HT for short-term menopausal symptom relief.

If initiating HT, non-modifiable risk factors, such as family history and age, in addition to modifiable risk factors, including smoking, obesity, and a sedentary lifestyle, should be taken into account. Further support for the importance of evaluating women for cardiovascular risk factors prior to initiating HT is provided by a 2008 study published in the Journal of the American Heart Association that found that hot flashes were associated with subclinical cardiovascular disease as evidenced by lower flow mediated vasodilation and increased aortic calcification [55]. When prescribing HT, proper time of initiation, effective formulation, dose, route, regimen, and duration of HT should be established in order to avoid adverse effects (Fig. 16.1).

Conclusions

A lower incidence of CVD in premenopausal women compared to age-matched men may be explained by the protective role of sex hormones. The incidence becomes comparable or even higher in women than in men after 10 years of menopause, making CVD the primary cause of death in postmenopausal women, exceeding all cancer deaths combined [7]. Postmenopausal women undergo several hormonal, metabolic, and vascular changes that predispose them to an increase in heart disease. HT was used routinely in the past since it was thought to reduce the risk of cardiovascular disease in postmenopausal women. Despite all of the previously noted benefits of estrogen for CVD prevention in women, exogenous estrogen in postmenopausal women has shown to be, in fact, possibly harmful. Two studies in particular – the Heart and Estrogen/Progestin Replacement Study (HERS) and the Women's Health Initiative (WHI) – failed to prove the beneficial effects of hormone therapy in postmenopausal women (in either secondary or primary cardiovascular prevention). In response to the WHI, many women discontinued menopausal hormone therapy.

Physicians continue to recommend HT for vasomotor symptoms associated with menopause and their potential consequences such as diminished sleep quality, irritability, and difficulty concentrating. HT may also be used to prevent osteoporosis and improve genito-urinary symptoms in selected women after menopause. Treatment with HT must be individualized. A woman's risk of stroke, CHD, venous thromboembolism, and breast cancer should be considered. Since the WHI, a substantial amount of research has led to a greater understanding of the benefits and risks of HT. Evidence suggests that the timing of HT and the route of delivery may produce different effects. Depending on a woman's symptoms or underlying risk factors, one route of delivery may prove more advantageous than another [36]. Observational and clinical trials have revealed that if HT is given to healthy, young women around the time of the menopausal transition, there is less risk for CVD events. However, if HT is administered to women who are farther out from their menopausal transition, they are more likely to suffer from a cardiovascular adverse event. Therefore, women should be asked about their cardiac risk factors as well as their predispositions to thromboembolic disease if considering HT for debilitating menopausal symptoms. The lowest effective doses of estrogen for the shortest duration should be used for management of vasomotor symptoms.

Based on current American Heart Association (AHA) Effectiveness-Based Guidelines for the Prevention of Cardiovascular Disease in Women, hormone therapy should not be used for the prevention of CVD, or as primary therapy for lowering cholesterol in postmenopausal women. HT is also not recommended in postmenopausal women with coronary artery disease or smokers [56, 57]. However, a report by the International Menopause Society from 2008 ruled out early harm of HT on CHD in newly postmenopausal women [58]. Additional research is necessary to understand the effects of HT on individual women, with the consideration of the effects of genetics and lifestyle [35]. The early identification of women at high risk of CVD and the implementation of appropriate lifestyle modifications, or statin therapy if necessary, to reduce the risk are very important.

References

1. Go AS, Roger VL, Benjamin EJ, Berry JD, Borden WB, Bravata DM, Dai S, Ford ES, Fox CS, Franco S, Fullerton HJ, Gillespie C, Hailpern SM, Heit JA, Howard VJ, Huffman MD, Kissela BM, Kittner SJ, Lackland DT, Lichtman JH, Lisabeth LD, Magid D, Marcus GM, Marelli A, Matchar DB, McGuire DK, Mohler ER, Moy CS, Mussolino ME, Nichol G, Paynter NP, Schreiner PJ, Sorlie PD, Stein J, Turan TN, Virani SS, Wong ND, Woo D, Turner MB, American Heart Association Statistics Committee and Stroke Statistics Subcommittee. Heart disease and stroke statistics—2013 update: a report from the American Heart Association. Circulation. 2013;127:e6–245.
2. Edmunds E, Lip GY. Cardiovascular risk in women: the cardiologist's perspective. QJM. 2000;93(3):135–45.
3. Lerner DJ, Kannel WB. Patterns of coronary heart disease morbidity and mortality in the sexes: a 26-year follow-up of the Framingham population. Am Heart J. 1986;111(2):383–90.
4. Dougherty AH. Gender balance in cardiovascular research: importance to women's health. Tex Heart Inst J. 2011;38(2):148–50.
5. Rossouw JE, et al. Risks and benefits of estrogen plus progestin in healthy postmenopausal women: principal results from the Women's Health Initiative randomized controlled trial. JAMA. 2002;288(3):321–33.
6. Bechlioulis A, et al. Menopause and hormone therapy: from vascular endothelial function to cardiovascular disease. Hellenic J Cardiol. 2009;50(4):303–15.
7. Novella S, et al. Vascular aging in women: is estrogen the fountain of youth? Front Physiol. 2012;3:165.
8. Schachinger V, Britten MB, Zeiher AM. Prognostic impact of coronary vasodilator dysfunction on adverse long-term outcome of coronary heart disease. Circulation. 2000;101(16): 1899–906.
9. Erbel R, et al. Value of intracoronary ultrasound and Doppler in the differentiation of angiographically normal coronary arteries: a prospective study in patients with angina pectoris. Eur Heart J. 1996;17(6):880–9.
10. Vita JA, et al. Coronary vasomotor response to acetylcholine relates to risk factors for coronary artery disease. Circulation. 1990;81(2):491–7.
11. Sanada M, et al. Comparison of forearm endothelial function between premenopausal and postmenopausal women with or without hypercholesterolemia. Maturitas. 2003;44(4): 307–15.
12. Young J, Libby P. Atherosclerosis. In: Lilly L, editor. Pathophysiology of heart disease. Philadelphia, Baltimore, MD: Lippincott Williams & Wilkins; 2007. p. 118–40.
13. Kneale BJ, et al. Gender differences in sensitivity to adrenergic agonists of forearm resistance vasculature. J Am Coll Cardiol. 2000;36(4):1233–8.
14. Vitale C, et al. Gender differences in the cardiovascular effects of sex hormones. Fundam Clin Pharmacol. 2010;24(6):675–85.
15. Barrett-Connor E. Women and heart disease: neglected directions for future research. J Cardiovasc Transl Res. 2009;2(3):256–7.
16. Gungor F, Kalelioglu I, Turfanda A. Vascular effects of estrogen and progestins and risk of coronary artery disease: importance of timing of estrogen treatment. Angiology. 2009;60(3):308–17.
17. Vaccarino V, et al. Ischaemic heart disease in women: are there sex differences in pathophysiology and risk factors? Position paper from the working group on coronary pathophysiology and microcirculation of the European Society of Cardiology. Cardiovasc Res. 2011; 90(1):9–17.
18. Mendelsohn ME, Karas RH. The protective effects of estrogen on the cardiovascular system. N Engl J Med. 1999;340(23):1801–11.
19. Booth EA, Lucchesi BR. Estrogen-mediated protection in myocardial ischemia-reperfusion injury. Cardiovasc Toxicol. 2008;8(3):101–13.

20. Mendelsohn ME. Protective effects of estrogen on the cardiovascular system. Am J Cardiol. 2002;89(12A):12E–7; discussion 17E–18E.
21. Stevenson JC. Menopausal hormone therapy. In: Women & heart disease. Abingdon, Oxon, United Kingdom: Taylor & Francis; 2005. p. 375–90.
22. Wenger NK. Menopausal hormone therapy. In: Shaw LJ, Redberg RF, editors. Contemporary cardiology: coronary disease in women: evidence-based diagnosis and treatment. Totowa: Humana Press Inc; 2004.
23. Gordon T, et al. Menopause and coronary heart disease. The Framingham Study. Ann Intern Med. 1978;89(2):157–61.
24. Hu FB, et al. Age at natural menopause and risk of cardiovascular disease. Arch Intern Med. 1999;159(10):1061–6.
25. McKinlay SM, Bifano NL, McKinlay JB. Smoking and age at menopause in women. Ann Intern Med. 1985;103(3):350–6.
26. Lakhani K, Hardiman P. Polycystic ovary syndrome. In: Wenger N, Collins P, editors. Women & heart disease. Abingdon, Oxon, United Kingdom: Taylor & Francis; 2005. p. 391–9.
27. Bairey Merz CN, et al. Hypoestrogenemia of hypothalamic origin and coronary artery disease in premenopausal women: a report from the NHLBI-sponsored WISE study. J Am Coll Cardiol. 2003;41(3):413–9.
28. Colditz GA, et al. Menopause and the risk of coronary heart disease in women. N Engl J Med. 1987;316(18):1105–10.
29. Rosenberg L, et al. Early menopause and the risk of myocardial infarction. Am J Obstet Gynecol. 1981;139(1):47–51.
30. Wellons M, et al. Early menopause predicts future coronary heart disease and stroke: the Multi-Ethnic Study of Atherosclerosis. Menopause. 2012;19(10):1081–7.
31. U.S. Department of Health and Human Services. Reducing the Health Consequences of Smoking: 25 Years of Progress. A Report of the Surgeon General. U.S. Department of Health and Human Services, Public Health Service, Centers for Disease Control, Center for Chronic Disease Prevention and Health Promotion, Office on Smoking and Health. DHHS Publication No. (CDC) 1989;89–8411.
32. Gorodeski GI. Update on cardiovascular disease in post-menopausal women. Best Pract Res Clin Obstet Gynaecol. 2002;16(3):329–55.
33. Effects of estrogen or estrogen/progestin regimens on heart disease risk factors in postmenopausal women. The Postmenopausal Estrogen/Progestin Interventions (PEPI) Trial. The Writing Group for the PEPI Trial. JAMA. 1995;273(3):199–208.
34. Hofbauer LC, Khosla S, Schoppet M. Estrogen therapy and coronary-artery calcification. N Engl J Med. 2007;357(12):1253–4; author reply 1254.
35. North American Menopause Society. Hormone therapy position statement of: the North American Menopause Society. Menopause. 2012;19(3):257–71.
36. Manson JE. The kronos early estrogen prevention study by charlotte barker. Womens Health (Lond Engl). 2013;9(1):9–11.
37. Harman SM, et al. KEEPS: the kronos early estrogen prevention study. Climacteric. 2005;8(1):3–12.
38. Shifren JL, Schiff I. Role of hormone therapy in the management of menopause. Obstet Gynecol. 2010;115(4):839–55.
39. Scarabin PY, Oger E, Plu-Bureau G. Differential association of oral and transdermal oestrogen-replacement therapy with venous thromboembolism risk. Lancet. 2003;362(9382):428–32.
40. Canonico M, et al. Hormone replacement therapy and risk of venous thromboembolism in postmenopausal women: systematic review and meta-analysis. BMJ. 2008;336(7655):1227–31.
41. The Coronary Drug Project. Findings leading to discontinuation of the 2.5-mg day estrogen group. The coronary Drug Project Research Group. JAMA. 1973;226(6):652–7.
42. Grodstein F, et al. Postmenopausal hormone therapy and mortality. N Engl J Med. 1997;336(25):1769–75.

43. Humphrey LL, Chan BK, Sox HC. Postmenopausal hormone replacement therapy and the primary prevention of cardiovascular disease. Ann Intern Med. 2002;137(4): 273–84.
44. Hulley S, et al. Randomized trial of estrogen plus progestin for secondary prevention of coronary heart disease in postmenopausal women. Heart and Estrogen/progestin Replacement Study (HERS) Research Group. JAMA. 1998;280(7):605–13.
45. Herrington DM, et al. The estrogen replacement and atherosclerosis (ERA) study: study design and baseline characteristics of the cohort. Control Clin Trials. 2000;21(3):257–85.
46. Anderson GL, et al. Effects of conjugated equine estrogen in postmenopausal women with hysterectomy: the Women's Health Initiative randomized controlled trial. JAMA. 2004; 291(14):1701–12.
47. Wenger NK. Women and coronary heart disease: a century after Herrick: understudied, underdiagnosed, and undertreated. Circulation. 2012;126(5):604–11.
48. Grady D, et al. Cardiovascular disease outcomes during 6.8 years of hormone therapy: Heart and Estrogen/progestin Replacement Study follow-up (HERS II). JAMA. 2002;288(1): 49–57.
49. Choi SD, et al. The timing hypothesis remains a valid explanation of differential cardioprotective effects of menopausal hormone treatment. Menopause. 2011;18(2):230–6.
50. Abramson BL. Postmenopausal hormone replacement therapy and the prevention of cardiovascular disease: a review. J Cardiovasc Risk. 2002;9(6):309–14.
51. Rossouw JE, et al. Lessons learned from the Women's Health Initiative trials of menopausal hormone therapy. Obstet Gynecol. 2013;121(1):172–6.
52. Maclaran K, Stevenson JC. Primary prevention of cardiovascular disease with HRT. Womens Health (Lond Engl). 2012;8(1):63–74.
53. Rossouw JE. Coronary heart disease in menopausal women: implications of primary and secondary prevention trials of hormones. Maturitas. 2005;51(1):51–63.
54. Rossouw JE, et al. Postmenopausal hormone therapy and risk of cardiovascular disease by age and years since menopause. JAMA. 2007;297(13):1465–77.
55. Thurston RC, et al. Hot flashes and subclinical cardiovascular disease: findings from the Study of Women's Health Across the Nation Heart Study. Circulation. 2008;118(12):1234–40.
56. Mosca L, et al. Effectiveness-based guidelines for the prevention of cardiovascular disease in women–2011 update: a guideline from the American Heart Association. Circulation. 2011; 123(11):1243–62.
57. LaCroix AZ, et al. Health outcomes after stopping conjugated equine estrogens among postmenopausal women with prior hysterectomy: a randomized controlled trial. JAMA. 2011;305(13):1305–14.
58. Pines A, et al. HRT in the early menopause: scientific evidence and common perceptions. Climacteric. 2008;11(4):267–72.
59. Shaw JL, Bairey Merz CN, Pepine CJ, et al. Insights from the NHLBI-sponsored women's ischemia syndrome evaluation (WISE) study: part I: gender differences in traditional and novel risk factors, symptom evaluation, and gender optimized diagnostic strategies. J Am Coll Cardiol. 2006;47:4S–20.
60. Manson JE, et al. Estrogen plus progestin and the risk of coronary heart disease. N Engl J Med. 2003;349:523–34.
61. Chlebowski RT, et al. Influence of estrogen plus progestin on breast cancer and mammography in healthy postmenopausal women: the Women's Health Initiative Randomized Trial. JAMA. 2003;289:3243–53.

Chapter 17
Gender Considerations in Peripheral Vascular Disease

Lydia R. Engwenyu, Wassim Jawad, Ambar Patel, and Luis A. Guzman

Introduction

Peripheral vascular disease (PVD) encompasses disease processes in the vascular bed outside of the coronary circulation. The focus of this chapter is on the diagnosis and management of these diseases with an emphasis on the gender based differences. We mainly discuss arterial disease where the most common pathology involves atherosclerotic disease. The chapter outline the disease process in three major territories: Carotid Artery Atherosclerotic Disease, Abdominal Aortic Aneurysms, and Lower Extremity Atherosclerotic Ischemic Disease. In addition to being commonly encountered, these diseases are discussed because they are considered coronary artery disease equivalents and included as such in the Framingham risk calculation. Even though the clinical consequences of atherosclerosis vary according to the territory involved, mortality is highly related to coexisting coronary involvement. Cardiac death represents 70 % of the overall mortality of patients with peripheral vascular disease [1]. The involvement of multiple vascular beds appears to be an expression of more advanced atherosclerotic disease process associated with a worse prognosis. The understanding of this process is critical for the development of preventive strategies and institution of appropriate treatment. A significant amount of patients carrying these conditions remain undiagnosed for many years. This is true for both genders. However, women are more likely to suffer from undiagnosed peripheral vascular disease. Increased awareness and dedicated research in this area can help overcome gender-based misconceptions to both

L.R. Engwenyu, MD • W. Jawad, MD • A. Patel, MD • L.A. Guzman, MD (✉)
Division of Cardiology, Department of Cardiovascular Medicine,
University of Florida College of Medicine-Jacksonville,
655 West 8th Street, Jacksonville, FL 32092, USA
e-mail: luis.guzman@jax.ufl.edu

H.Z. Mieszczanska, G.P. Velarde (eds.),
Management of Cardiovascular Disease in Women,
DOI 10.1007/978-1-4471-5517-1_17, © Springer-Verlag London 2014

prevent peripheral vascular disease in women and help clinicians and patients more effectively address these diseases when manifested. In addition, a major goal in combating these diseases should be the primary prevention of atherosclerotic disease (discussed elsewhere).

Carotid Artery Stenosis

Clinical Scenarios

1. A 60 year old woman with a history of DM and a strong family history of coronary artery disease presents to your outpatient clinic to establish care. She has no complaints at the time of the appointment. You take a detailed history which raises no specific concerns and proceed to the physical examination. On physical exam, you notice a right sided carotid bruit. Your patient says that she has not been told about this before. How should this woman be managed?
2. A 76 year old woman with a history of HTN and dyslipidemia is admitted to the hospital because of dull left arm pain and SOB for the past 6 h. She recently retired and had previously been active with volunteer work in her community. Her CXR is negative for an acute cardiopulmonary process. Cardiac biomarkers are negative but her symptoms are recognized as angina and she undergoes a left sided cardiac catheterization procedure revealing significant three vessel coronary artery disease. Cardiothoracic surgery is contacted for coronary artery bypass grafting. As part of the preoperative work-up, a carotid Doppler is ordered and the result returns with an 80 % stenosis of the right internal carotid artery. How should this woman be managed?

Prevalence/Incidence, Morbidity/Mortality Associated with the Disease

Each year, about 700,000 people experience a new (500,000) or recurrent (200,000) stroke, and the great majority are ischemic events [2]. Cerebral ischemic events differ from acute coronary events in that they are more likely related to embolic phenomenon. Stroke is a leading cause of death in the United States and the personal and financial consequences of a stroke can be debilitating.

Carotid artery stenosis has been implicated with approximately 20–25 % of ischemic strokes [3]. When carotid artery stenosis is detected, management should consist of both medical management and secondary prevention interventions. Decisions for invasive interventions are based on stenosis severity, symptoms, and the perceived risks and benefits of the procedure in which there does appear to be a difference between men and women. Risk stratification based on plaque characteristics, identified by various imaging modalities, is under investigation and may be included in future guidelines.

Smoking and advanced age are the two strong risk factors associated with the development of carotid atherosclerosis. The disease is more common in women than men after the age of 75 and more women are expected to be affected with increasing life expectancies. Smoking is a modifiable risk factor and smoking cessation should be emphasized especially if the presence of carotid stenosis is known. Hypertension is also a strong risk factor in patients with stroke. Similar to atherosclerotic disease in the coronary arteries, diabetes, and dyslipidemia are also risk factors for carotid artery disease.

Carotid atherosclerotic disease, along with being a risk factor for stroke, is strongly correlated with severe coronary artery disease (CAD) [4]. Approximately 50–60 % of patients with carotid disease have severe CAD. Additionally, increased carotid intimal media thickness has been associated with increased risk of MI [5]. The secondary prevention measures have the dual impact of carotid plaque stabilization and prevention of acute coronary syndrome.

Screening: History/Symptoms, Physical Examination, Imaging Studies

History taking should include a detailed investigation of neurologic symptoms. Classifying symptomatic vs. asymptomatic carotid stenosis is important because treatment strategies can differ, especially for women. Unilateral symptoms of weakness or numbness, difficulty with speech, and visual symptoms including amaurosis fugax are clues for cerebral embolization. Symptoms of retinal artery and ophthalmic artery occlusion are considered stroke equivalents. It is important to mention that syncope or near syncope is not considered a symptom associated with carotid artery stenosis and it is a rare manifestation of carotid disease.

Physical exam should include auscultation for a carotid bruit. This can help localize the lesion, however the absence of a bruit does not rule out significant carotid stenosis [6]. A fundoscopic exam can detect retinal artery embolization. Cardiac auscultation can help to identify a potential abnormal rhythm such as atrial fibrillation which may be the source of embolization. Even if carotid artery disease is suspected, it is important to rule out other possible co-existing etiologies for stroke.

Duplex Ultrasound: first line test, noninvasive, cost effective, ideal for following patients over time.

Peak systolic velocity ratios are obtained comparing the internal carotid artery (ICA) and the common carotid artery (CCA). ICA/CCA of less than 2 means there is not a significant stenosis. ICA/CCA of greater than 4 suggests a severe stenosis. In general, higher peak systolic velocities are indicative of higher amounts of stenosis. Table 17.1 shows the ultrasound measurements and degree of lumen occupied by plaque, with the corresponding percent stenosis [7].

Table 17.1 Doppler ultrasound in the evaluation of internal carotid artery stenosis

Degree of stenosis (%)	ICA PSV (cm/s)	Plaque estimate (%)	ICA/CCA PSV ratio	Diagnostic accuracy (%)
Normal	<125	None	<2.0	
<50	<125	<50	<2.0	90
50–69	125–230	≥50	2.0–4.0	40
≥70	>230	≥50	>4.0	90
Near occlusion	High, low or undetectable	Visible	Variable	

CCA common carotid artery, *ICA* internal carotid artery, *PSV* peak systolic velocity

CT angiography (CTA): equal to carotid Doppler, more costly, recommended to visualize other parts of the vasculature and surrounding tissues if a systemic process or local compression is suspected. CT may be advantageous in providing enhanced visualization. The disadvantage is the need for contrast injection and it cannot be performed at the bedside.

MRI: considered equal to Doppler and CTA, most costly, has the benefit of further delineating characteristics of carotid plaques that have been associated with prognostic implications.

Carotid Angiography: gold standard for assessment of carotid atherosclerosis and allows for assessment of collateral circulation that is known to be associated with reduced stroke risk. Requires the use of contrast (significantly less than CTA), and carries a small risk of stroke, not present with other modalities.

Treatment Options

Medical Management

Treatment goals should include secondary prevention measures in accordance with ACC/AHA guidelines [8]. This includes aggressive blood pressure control, dyslipidemia management, smoking cessation, and the addition of an antiplatelet agent [8]. There is not consistent evidence regarding which agent is the best antihypertensive to prevent stroke. ACE inhibitors and diuretics are accepted first line medications. Regardless of the agent chosen, benefit is seen when the patient's blood pressure is reduced to goal [8]. Strict blood pressure control with a goal blood pressure of less than 130/80 is recommended. Lipid management with a statin is recommended with a goal of LDL less than 100 and most cardiologists recommending a LDL goal of less than 70 both to prevent progression of the plaque and for stabilization [8]. There is some evidence of improved outcomes if the statin is started prior to any planned intervention [9]. Control of diabetes is not known to change outcomes in large vessel disease, but the general consensus is that there should be a goal hemoglobin a1c value of less than 7. Low dose aspirin and/or another antiplatelet medication should be started and continued indefinitely as long as there are no contraindications. The presence of more than one vascular territory affected means that a patient has a higher relative risk of dying from a cardiac cause and should affect a clinicians approach to the patient.

Carotid Endartectomy (CEA)

Carotid endartectomy is currently considered the standard of care for prevention of CVA in patients with significant stenoses regardless of symptoms. It has proven usefulness in prevention in combination with medical therapy as compared to medical management alone. Evidence from the North American Symptomatic Carotid Endarterectomy Trial (NASCET) showed sustained benefit in the reduction of stroke or death in symptomatic patients treated with CEA as opposed to medical therapy alone. The benefit was more significant according to the degree of stenosis (70–99 % stenosis – 9 % vs. 26 % (P<0.001) at 26 months. 50–69 % stenosis – 15.7 % vs. 22.2 % (p=0.045) at 5 years. <50 % stenosis – No benefit) [10]. The Asymptomatic Carotid artery stenosis (ACAS) demonstrated this benefit in asymptomatic patients with carotid stenosis of 60 % percent or more [11]. However, the data from these trials were derived from mostly male patients with extrapolations of the benefit for women obtained from subgroup analysis. There is evidence that symptomatic women derive less benefit than men from CEA and there is not clear evidence that women with asymptomatic carotid disease even benefit from the procedure [11, 12]. A discussion of CEA in women should include a standard discussion of risks including risk of MI, stroke, or death along with other surgical risks including cranial nerve palsies and wound complications. It should be clear that the quoted benefits of the procedure are based on data mainly from men and that the benefit is known to be lower in women. Surgeons keep track of procedural outcomes and it may be possible to see the outcomes specifically for women to obtain a more accurate assessment of risk according to gender.

Carotid Artery Stenting (CAS)

Carotid Artery Angioplasty with stent placement is a percutaneous procedure that has evolved into an accepted alternative to CEA in both symptomatic and asymptomatic patients with carotid disease. It has the potential positive attributes of minimal invasiveness, shorter post procedural recovery, and shorter hospital stay. Several randomized studies comparing CEA and CAS have been conducted and summarized in Table 17.2. The largest study using a more contemporary approach and with adequate follow up is the Carotid Revascularization Endarterectomy vs. Stenting Trial (CREST) trial. It compared the outcomes of carotid-artery stenting with those of carotid endarterectomy among patients with symptomatic or asymptomatic extracranial carotid stenosis. The primary end point of the study, myocardial infarction, stroke or death was similar and no statistically significant difference between the two alternative revascularization modalities [13]. Although, there was

Table 17.2 Summary of clinical trials comparing carotid artery stenting (CAS) and carotid endarterctomy (CEA)

Trial	No. of patients	Type of study	Study arm	Outcome (stroke, MI or death)
CAVATAS [14]	504	Randomized	CAS vs. CEA	No difference
SAPPHIRE [15]	98	Randomized	CAS vs. CEA	16.8 % vs. 16.5 % (p=0.95)
EVA-3S [16]	527	Randomized	CAS vs. CEA	9.6 % vs. 3.9 % at 30 days (RR 2.5; 95 % CI 1.2–5.1)
				11.7 % vs. 6.1 % at 6 months
SPACE [17]	1,214	Randomized	CAS vs. CEA	9.5 % vs. 8.8 % at 2 years (HR 1.10; 95 % 0.75–1.61)
CREST [13]	1,321	Randomized	CAS vs. CEA	6.7 % vs. 5.4 % at 180 days (HR 1.26; 95 % CI 0.81–1.96)
ICSS [18]	1,710	Randomized	CAS vs. CEA	8.5 % vs. 5.2 % at 120 days (HR 1.69; 95 % CI 1.16–2.45)

CAVATAS carotid and vertebral artery transluminal angioplasty study, *SAPPHIRE* stenting and angioplasty with protection in patients at high risk for endarterectomy, *EVA-3S* endarterectomy vs. angioplasty in patients with symptomatic severe carotid stenosis, *SPACE* stent-protected angioplasty vs. carotid endarterectomy, *CREST* carotid revascularization endarterectomy versus stenting trial, *ICSS* international carotid stenting study, *MT* medical therapy

no statistically significant difference in outcomes between men and women, there was a trend towards worse outcomes for women. CEA seemed to be better for older patients (defined as above75). CAS is preferred in certain groups that are known to have worse surgical outcomes including those with previous neck surgery or radiation, prior CEA, and younger patients. CAS does carry a higher risk of minor stroke than CEA. However, CEA carries a higher risk of myocardial infarction [13].

Clinical Scenarios Revisited

1. The woman in scenario 1 should have risk factors addressed at this appointment. This includes smoking cessation if applicable, blood pressure control with a goal of 130/80 (ACE-I in the absence of a contraindication is preferred because of DM), lipid management, and blood glucose management as a standard of care. Carotid Doppler should be ordered to evaluate the bruit heard on physical exam. This patient may or may not have significant carotid disease. If significant disease is found, then medical management is indicated with low dose aspirin. The woman can be classified as having asymptomatic carotid stenosis. Further interventions, either CEA or CAS risk and benefits should be discussed with the patient. Even though the data remains controversial, the fact the patient is 60 years of age, will probable benefit more with carotid revascularization. Whereas for older patients, mainly women, the benefit of revascularization is less clear.

2. The woman in scenario 2 should also be evaluated in more detail to determine if she has symptoms of stroke or TIA. This patient represents a complicated situation in which it is necessary to perform both a carotid intervention and CABG. There is no recommendation for routine carotid screening prior to CABG in asymptomatic patients. However, the presence of significant disease is associated with an increased risk of stroke during coronary surgery. Conversely, the risk of MI during a carotid intervention is also increased if associated advanced CAD. There is no clear answer regarding which procedure to perform first. It is accepted that the symptomatic territory should be approached first. If she is considered to be symptomatic, this may prompt clinicians to pursue carotid intervention sooner after bypass surgery. If asymptomatic, the coronary revascularization should be performed. The asymptomatic carotid disease should be addressed at a later time. Even though proposed by some high volume institutions, significant controversy remains, regarding the combined approach of both territories within the same setting.

Abdominal Aortic Aneurysms

Clinical Scenarios

3. A 72 y/o woman with a past medical history of hypertension and dyslipidemia is involved in a motor vehicle collision. She is transported to the nearest hospital where she is evaluated by CT scans, not found to have any major traumatic injuries, and deemed safe for discharge. However, the CT scan of the abdomen reveals an abdominal aortic aneurysm that is 4.9 cm in diameter. How should this woman be managed?
4. A 65 y/o woman with a history of hypertension and long time smoking presents to your outpatient clinic for an appointment. She mentions that her older brother's physician ordered an imaging test for an abdominal aortic aneurysm and he was found to have a large 7 cm aneurysm. He is scheduled for surgical repair next week. She is concerned that she may also have one and asks if she can have a test done to find out. How should this woman be managed?

Prevalence/Incidence, Morbidity/Mortality Associated with the Disease

Abdominal aortic aneurysms (AAAs) account for 15,000 deaths yearly and are the 10th leading cause of death in the United States [19]. They are more common in men, but are associated with rupture more frequently in women [20]. In fact, although the ratio of the prevalence of AAA is 9:1 with more men being affected,

Table 17.3 Risk factors for abdominal aortic aneurysms

Risk factor	Comments
Smoking	Risk increases with duration of smoking; smoking also increases risk of aneurysm expansion and rupture
Male gender	Men are 5–10 times more likely than women to have an abdominal aneurysm
Age	Typically appearing after age 45 in men age 65 in women
Family history of abdominal aneurysm	Confers a twofold increased risk of abdominal aneurysm
Hypertension	Treat hypertension effectively in patients with abdominal aortic aneurysm
Hyperlipidemia	Statin therapy to treat hyperlipidemia is reasonable
Atherosclerosis	There is an association of atherosclerosis and abdominal aneurysms

women account for 40 % of all deaths from AAA. The risk factors for AAA are age, hypertension, dyslipidemia, and smoking (Table 17.3). Unlike other atherosclerotic disease, diabetes seems to have a protective role [20]. There is also a genetic component with those with a first degree relative with an AAA have a high prevalence of disease [21].

Screening: History/Symptoms, Physical Examination, Imaging Studies

Most AAAs are not identified by complaints and most often recognized by imaging done for other reasons. Patient may complain of abdominal pain that radiates to the back as the aneurysm compresses surrounding structures. Clinicians should ask about these symptoms. On gentle examination of the abdomen, a pulsatile mass may be found. This is easier to identify in non-obese patients. There may also be evidence of an abdominal bruit or signs of symptoms of embolic phenomenon distal to the AAA or atherosclerotic disease in the abdominal or iliac arteries. If an AAA is suspected based on history or physical exam findings, further imaging studies should be pursued. The use of imaging for screening in women at risk but without symptoms is controversial. The USPHF recommends screening for men above the age of 65 with a history of smoking but there is no recommendation for women [22]. Thus, when clinicians determine that screening is warranted there will be variations in insurance coverage of screening in asymptomatic women. It is reasonable to screen women with a long time history of smoking and several societies recommend that women with a family history of AAA be screened as well [23]. However, this topic remains controversial.

A diameter of 3 cm is considered to be indicative of an aneurysm. However, this value is based on male patients that are known to have larger diameters of their aorta. Thus, the determination of what constitutes an aneurysm in women is not clear but is likely below the accepted 3 cm cut off. A definition of 50 % larger than the normal diameter of the aorta has been recommended for use, especially for women, to better classify who has an aneurysm [24].

Imaging studies allows for assessment of the size of the aneurysm which is necessary to determine the risks of rupture and determine the possible benefit of an invention. Same modalities are also used to follow the aneurysm over time to determine the rate of growth. Aneurysms should be followed yearly at 3 cm, every 6 months between 4 to 5 cm, and every 3 to 6 months at 5 cm. In addition to size, the location of the AAA can be determined by imaging and this allows for preoperative planning.

Abdominal Ultrasound: ideal method to screen for abdominal aortic aneurysms in asymptomatic patients.

It does not involve radiation exposure and is accurate in determining the size of aneurysms.

Good for following the AAA over time due to lack of ionizing radiation involved in the study. The disadvantage of the study is that it cannot provide accurate visualization of branch vessels necessary for preoperative planning.

CT scan: it is the most accurate imaging modality for determining the size of the aneurysm and

It is helpful for preoperative planning by allowing for visualization of surrounding structures and branch vessels.

Disadvantage: ionizing radiation and the need for contrast which is not ideal if a patient has renal failure.

It is not ideal for frequent testing needed to track aneurysm changes over time.

MRI: considered an accurate modality and avoids the need for contrast.

Disadvantage: time consuming and costly. It is also not the best technique for treatment planning.

As CT, It is not ideal for frequent testing needed to track aneurysm changes over time.

Treatment Options

The medical management of AAA includes aggressive management of risk factors including dyslipidemia and hypertension. The preferred class of medications for treating hypertension in patients with AAA is B-blockers. By reducing pulse pressure, they can decrease the progression of AAA and decrease the risk of rupture [25].

Table 17.4 shows the annual risk of rupture according to aneurysm size [26]. Guidelines recommend intervention when an AAA is 5.5 cm in size or if a patient is symptomatic [27]. However, these guidelines were developed based on data from men. Based on data demonstrating a high risk of rupture in women at lower diameters, certain societies have recommended that surgery or endovascular repair should be offered to women at diameters of 5 cm or with symptoms [28]. Although AAAs are less prevalent among women, they are more prone to rupture and tend to rupture at smaller aortic

Table 17.4 Annual risk of abdominal aortic aneurysm rupture according to aneurysm diameter

Diameter of abdominal aortic aneurysm (cm)	Annual risk of rupture (%)
<4.0	0.3
4.0–4.9	1.5
5.0–5.9	6.5
6.0–6.9	10
>7.0	33

diameters compared with men. Even though elective repair of asymptomatic AAAs is recommended when the diameter reaches 5.5 cm, many experts lower the threshold to 4.5 to 5.0 cm, especially among patients of a smaller body size, women, or those with a family history of rupture [29, 30].

Surgical Open Repair or AAA

Surgery to repair an AAA involves placement of a graft in the diseased aorta. It is the older of the two options for repair of AAA. Although it is more invasive, it is also considered more durable with less need for repeat procedure. It is considered major surgery and preoperative assessment needs to include cardiac preoperative assessment. This is especially important due to the high coexistence of AAAs and severe coronary artery disease [31].

Percutaneous Endovascular Repair of AAA (EVAR)

Endovascular repair involves graft placement intravascularly using, most commonly, the femoral artery as an access point. The femoral artery can be accessed percutaneously or by surgical cutdown. Endovascular repair has the major advantage of being associated with decreased perioperative mortality [29]. It is a procedure that is done by vascular surgeons, some trained interventional cardiologists, and interventional radiologists. It accounts for half of all AAA repairs done in the United States. The disadvantages are the risk of conversion to an open procedure, the use of contrast that may result in renal complications, and the potential to develop an endoleak. An endoleak describes a situation in which there is persistent blood flow into the aneurysmal sac after the procedure. It can require correction with another procedure. For this reason, patients with endovascular repair should have a close follow up.

Thus, as shown by UK EVAR trial investigator group (Fig. 17.1), EVAR offers no clear long term advantage over open repair among those who are good candidates for either procedure [26, 29]. Consequently, the choice of which approach to take for aortic repair should be individualized for each patient and based on age, comorbidities, patient preference, and aortic anatomy. For those with increased surgical risk due to comorbidities, endovascular repair appears to be the first treatment choice [28].

Kaplan-Meier Estimates for Total Survival and Aneurysm-Related Survival During 8 Years fo Follow-Up

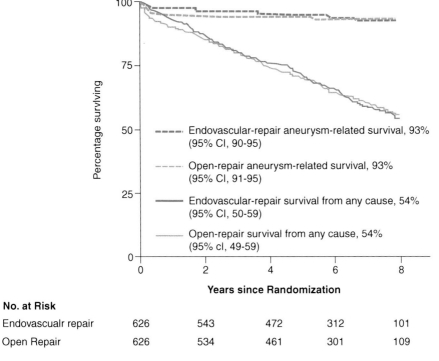

No. at Risk					
Endovascualr repair	626	543	472	312	101
Open Repair	626	534	461	301	109

Fig. 17.1 Kaplan-Meier estimates for total survival and aneurysm-related survival during 8 years of follow-up (Reprinted with permission from EVAR Trial Investigators [29]). Among patients randomly assigned to either endovascular repair or open repair of an abdominal aortic aneurysm, an early benefit with respect to aneurysm-related mortality in the endovascular-repair group was lost by the end of the study, at least partially because of fatal endograft ruptures (adjusted hazard ratio with endovascular repair, 0.92; 95 % confidence interval [CI], 0.57–1.49; p=0.73). By the end of 8 years of follow-up, there was no significant difference between the two groups in the risk of death from any cause (adjusted hazard ratio, 1.03; 95 % CI, 0.86–1.23; p=0.72)

Clinical Scenarios Revisited

3. This woman's AAA was found incidentally and she has no symptoms. However, the size of the aneurysm is concerning. There are no guidelines for the need for surgical or endovascular repair in asymptomatic women but it is known that women have a higher risk of rupture at lower diameters. Elective repair for AAA should be considered in women starting at diameters of 4.5 cm and a discussion of this option should take place. If the woman declines repair the AAA should be followed every 3–6 months with imaging. Continue efforts at risk factor modification by addressing hypertension and dyslipidemia and ensure she does not smoke. A B-blocker should be added to her regimen because of some evidence that it may prevent progression.

4. There are no clear guidelines regarding AAA screening in women. If this patient was a man, the guidelines would recommend a onetime screening. This woman is more at risk for AAA because she is a smoker and because she has a first degree relative with an AAA. It is advisable to offer this woman screening. It may not be covered by certain insurance plans and this should be communicated to her prior to ordering studies. Aside from screening, ensure good blood pressure control and strongly encourage smoking cessation.

Lower Extremity Peripheral Arterial Disease (LE PAD)

Clinical Scenarios

5. A 57 year old woman is referred to your clinic with ongoing leg cramps. They are not always associated with exertion and never occur at rest. She is a 35 pack-year smoker with hypertension and hyperlipidemia. She has never been diagnosed with coronary artery disease, nor does she have angina symptoms. Resting ankle-brachial index is 0.92. She is comfortable on exam, with a blood pressure of 161/74 and heart rate of 84. There are no ulcers, and pedal pulses are 1+ bilaterally. She is only on HCTZ 25 mg daily and simvastatin 20 mg daily. How should she be managed?
6. A 63 year old woman with non-insulin dependent diabetes mellitus, hypertension and hyperlipidemia is referred to the ER with worsening right lower extremity pain over the past week, which is now occurring at rest. She has a known history of lower extremity peripheral arterial disease with prior stenting of the right popliteal artery. She has no muscle weakness on that side, but has mild sensory loss in her toes. How should this patient be managed?

The 2011Focused update of the 2005 guidelines by the ACCF/AHA centered on lower extremity peripheral arterial disease (LE PAD) and abdominal aortic disease, but did not make any gender distinctions. This is likely because the diagnosis and management of PAD in women are the same as in men [32]. However, there are several important differences with regard to risk and outcomes.

Risk Factors

Diabetes is a major risk factor, seen in 12–20 % of patients with LE PAD. It can increase risk two to four-fold. According to the Framingham Heart Study, women with diabetes were noted to have an 8.6 fold increase in risk, while men had a 3.5 fold increase [33]. This risk increases incrementally with increasing severity and duration of diabetes. The risk of critical limb ischemia is also noted to be greater in diabetics overall. The mortality of diabetic patients with critical limb ischemia is double and the risk of amputation is four fold higher as compare with similar patients without diabetes [32]. Hypertension is also associated with LE PAD, but is more highly associated with cerebrovascular disease and coronary artery disease. It has been noted that hypertensive men are 2.5 times more likely to develop LE PAD, while women are 4 times more likely [32]. Smoking is and continues to be the leading risk factor in developing LE PAD. It is 2–3 times more likely to cause LE PAD than it is to cause coronary artery disease (CAD). Furthermore, 80 % of patients with LE PAD are smokers, and there is a clear dose dependent increase in risk. This risk seems to be the same in women as it is in men [32]. The other major risk factors of note, including hyperlipidemia, homocysteinemia, and elevated CRP did not highlight significant gender-specific differences in risk.

Symptoms

Intermittent claudication is the main symptom noted in patients with LE PAD, and is the main symptom healthcare providers try to elicit during their evaluation. The symptoms of chronic PAD progress rather slowly over time. Thus, after 5–10 years, more than 70 % of patients report either no change or improvement in their symptoms, while 20–30 % have progressive symptoms [34]. In the Framingham Heart Study, there was a cohort of 2,336 men and 2,873 women, aged 28–62, who were followed every 2 years since 1978 [34]. The annual incidence increased with age and prevalence of risk factors, and intermittent claudication was twice as prevalent in men. The combination of male sex, and smoking resulted in a 1.5 fold increase in risk of developing intermittent claudication [32]. However, asymptomatic LE PAD is the most common presentation of LE PAD. In asymptomatic patients, the diagnosis rests on the clinicians degree of suspicion and often times the physical exam. Physical exam findings of LE PAD include loss of hair growth, coolness of the extremities, reduced or absent pulses on palpation, and non-healing ulcers. Criqui et al. used four non-invasive tests in addition to symptoms (segmental blood pressures, Doppler derived flow velocities, post-occlusive reactive hyperemia and pulse re-appearance half time), and showed that only 20 % of patients with objective evidence of LE PAD actually had symptoms. In that study, 2.2 % of men and 1.7 % of women had claudication [35]. The Rotterdam Study also set out to further define the age and sex specific prevalence of LE PAD and intermittent claudication using 7,715 subjects (60 % men, 40 % women) aged 55 and older. LE PAD was prevalent in 19.1 % of patients, yet claudication in only 1.6 %, most of these being men [36]. More importantly, whether or not a patient had symptoms did not seem to affect outcomes in either population [32].

Even though it has been shown that claudication is associated with greater rate of functional decline, the degree of impairment and rate of functional decline is greater in women. Furthermore, it was observed that women who smoked developed LE PAD as much as 20 years sooner than men who smoked (10 years versus 30 years respectively) [36–38].

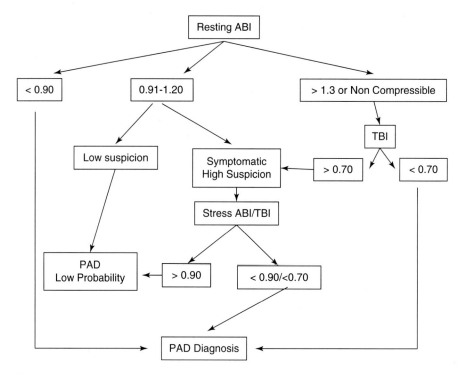

Fig. 17.2 ABI and clinical suspicion of PAD

Risk of Cardiovascular Events

Patients with LE PAD are known to be at increased risk of myocardial infarction (MI), stroke and cardiovascular related death. There is a 20–60 % increase in risk of MI, a 2 to 6-fold increase in risk of death from coronary heart disease, and a 40 % increase in risk of stroke [32]. In the ARIC study, men with LE PAD were 4–5 times more likely to have a stroke/TIA than men without LE PAD. It suggested that in women, however, this difference was not significant [39, 40]. The Health ABC study later on, however, has subsequently shown that not only do women have a higher prevalence of subclinical PAD; they also have a higher incidence of stroke than men [41].

Diagnosis of LE PAD

The diagnosis of LE PAD is dependent on the practitioner's degree of suspicion based on symptoms, risk factors and careful physical exam. If LE PAD is suspected, by non-invasive testing in the form of ankle-brachial index (ABI) or toe-brachial index (TBI) measurement should be pursued. The following flowchart provides an overview of the approach to diagnosing LE PAD and how to interpret the results of ABI/TBI's (Fig. 17.2) [42].

Management Options

Treatment Management

The initial approach to treating patients with LE PAD is aggressively managing all modifiable risk factors, including smoking cessation, diabetes, hyperlipidemia and blood pressure control. Statin therapy with LDL goal <100 mg/dL carries a Class I indication [32]. Goal blood pressure in non-diabetics is less than 135/85 mmHg (130/80 in diabetics) [32] ref. Beta-blockers are not contraindicated in LE PAD patients and may be used. ACE inhibitors are also useful especially in patients with increased cardiovascular risk. Maintaining a hemoglobin A1c less than 7 % is of utmost importance, as are regular diabetic foot examinations. Aspirin (typically 75–325 mg daily) is the antiplatelet of choice in patients with confirmed LE PAD [32] ref. These have been shown to decrease risk of cardiovascular events such as myocardial infarction and stroke. Clopidogrel 75 mg daily is an acceptable alternative to aspirin [43]. Cilostazol is the drug of choice in management of symptomatic LE PAD and is shown to be effective in improving walking distance [32]. Pentoxifylline is an alternative to cilostazol; however its benefits are not as well established. Exercise program is the most effective and class 1A recommendation for symptomatic patient with well-established improvement in walking capacity as well as decrease cardiovascular mortality [32].

Invasive Management

Invasive measures are reserved predominantly for patients that have disabling symptoms or critical limb ischemia [32]. Various classification schemes (namely the Rutherford and Fontaine categories of limb ischemia) exist in grading degree of symptoms, and are very useful decision aides in the type of intervention pursued (Table 17.5) [44].

Patients with lifestyle-limiting symptoms can be considered for percutaneous interventions such as balloon angioplasty, stenting and/or atherectomy procedures. More complex disease may warrant surgery interventions in the form of bypass. Patients with acute limb ischemia may be candidates for catheter based thrombolysis. Suitable candidates for this approach are those whose symptoms have been less than 14 days duration [32].

Clinical Scenarios Revisited

5. The woman in this case has fairly atypical claudication symptoms; however given her risk factors, an exercise ABI is warranted. Further management of her case is based on management of her modifiable risk factors, namely her blood pressure and lipids. If her exercise ABI does in fact confirm that she has LE PAD, she will also require antiplatelet therapy with aspirin and probably may benefit from a walking program.

Table 17.5 Clinical classification of LE PAD

Classification	Stage	Clinical description
Fontaine	I	Asymptomatic
	IIa	Mild claudication
	IIb	Moderate to severe claudication
	III	Rest pain
	IV	Ulcer and gangrene
Rutherford	0	Asymptomatic
	I	Mild claudication
	II	Moderate claudication
	III	Severe claudication
	IV	Rest pain
	V	Minor tissue loss
	VI	Major tissue loss or gangrene

6. This patient has acute limb ischemia and Rutherford category IV symptoms of ischemic rest pain without evidence of tissue injury. Given the chronology of her symptoms (<14 days), she is a suitable candidate for catheter based evaluation and if confirmed local intra-arterial thrombolysis. She should have emergent specialist consultation to save her from potential limb loss.

Summary

Peripheral vascular disease represents the disease processes in the vascular bed outside of the coronary circulation. Even though the clinical consequences of atherosclerosis vary according to the territory involved, mortality is highly related to coexisting coronary involvement. Disease awareness to implement adequate primary and secondary prevention strategies that target both PVD and CAD are major goals to improve long term outcomes in this population. Significant advances in diagnostic modalities, medications, and procedural interventions for PVD have been developed, however, a significant proportion of patients with PVD remain undiagnosed for many years. Even though PVD affect both genders, the majority of the information is dominated by studies of the disease process in men. Several gender based differences have been described and discussed along this chapter. These include differences in the prevalence of the disease in the different affected territories, age, clinical presentation, associated conditions, and disease progression as well as differences in the response to treatment modalities. Knowledge and understanding of these gender-related differences are key to properly diagnose and treat both men and women with peripheral vascular disease.

References

1. Fowkes FG, Housley E, Cawood EH, Macintyre CC, Ruckley CV, Prescott RJ. Edinburgh artery study: prevalence of asymptomatic and symptomatic peripheral arterial disease in the general population. Int J Epidemiol. 1991;20(2):384–92.

2. Thom T, Haase N, Rosamond W, Howard VJ, Rumsfeld J, Manolio T, Zheng ZJ, Flegal K, O'Donnell C, Kittner S, et al. Heart disease and stroke statistics – 2006 update: a report from the American Heart Association Statistics Committee and Stroke Statistics Subcommittee. Circulation. 2006;113(6):e85–151.
3. Sacco RL. Clinical practice. Extracranial carotid stenosis. N Engl J Med. 2001;345(15): 1113–8.
4. Golomb BA, Dang TT, Criqui MH. Peripheral arterial disease: morbidity and mortality implications. Circulation. 2006;114(7):688–99.
5. Lorenz MW, Markus HS, Bots ML, Rosvall M, Sitzer M. Prediction of clinical cardiovascular events with carotid intima-media thickness: a systematic review and meta-analysis. Circulation. 2007;115(4):459–67.
6. McColgan P, Bentley P, McCarron M, Sharma P. Evaluation of the clinical utility of a carotid bruit. QJM. 2012;105(12):1171–7.
7. Grant EG, Benson CB, Moneta GL, Alexandrov AV, Baker JD, Bluth EI, Carroll BA, Eliasziw M, Gocke J, Hertzberg BS, et al. Carotid artery stenosis: gray-scale and Doppler US diagnosis – Society of Radiologists in Ultrasound Consensus Conference. Radiology. 2003;229(2): 340–6.
8. Smith Jr SC, Benjamin EJ, Bonow RO, Braun LT, Creager MA, Franklin BA, Gibbons RJ, Grundy SM, Hiratzka LF, Jones DW, et al. AHA/ACCF secondary prevention and risk reduction therapy for patients with coronary and other atherosclerotic vascular disease: 2011 update: a guideline from the American Heart Association and American College of Cardiology Foundation Endorsed by the World Heart Federation and the Preventive Cardiovascular Nurses Association. J Am Coll Cardiol. 2011;58(23):2432–46.
9. Puato M, Faggin E, Rattazzi M, Zambon A, Cipollone F, Grego F, Ganassin L, Plebani M, Mezzetti A, Pauletto P. Atorvastatin reduces macrophage accumulation in atherosclerotic plaques: a comparison of a nonstatin-based regimen in patients undergoing carotid endarterectomy. Stroke. 2010;41(6):1163–8.
10. North American Symptomatic Carotid Endarterectomy Trial Collaborators. Beneficial effect of carotid endarterectomy in symptomatic patients with high-grade carotid stenosis. N Engl J Med. 1991;325(7):445–53.
11. Endarterectomy for asymptomatic carotid artery stenosis. Executive Committee for the Asymptomatic Carotid Atherosclerosis Study. JAMA. 1995;273(18):1421–8.
12. Schneider JR, Droste JS, Golan JF. Carotid endarterectomy in women versus men: patient characteristics and outcomes. J Vasc Surg. 1997;25(5):890–6; discussion 897–8.
13. Brott TG, Hobson 2nd RW, Howard G, Roubin GS, Clark WM, Brooks W, Mackey A, Hill MD, Leimgruber PP, Sheffet AJ, et al. Stenting versus endarterectomy for treatment of carotid-artery stenosis. N Engl J Med. 2010;363(1):11–23.
14. Ederle J, Bonati LH, Dobson J, Featherstone RL, Gaines PA, Beard JD, Venables GS, Markus HS, Clifton A, Sandercock P, et al. Endovascular treatment with angioplasty or stenting versus endarterectomy in patients with carotid artery stenosis in the carotid and vertebral artery transluminal angioplasty study (CAVATAS): long-term follow-up of a randomised trial. Lancet Neurol. 2009;8(10):898–907.
15. Gurm HS, Yadav JS, Fayad P, Katzen BT, Mishkel GJ, Bajwa TK, Ansel G, Strickman NE, Wang H, Cohen SA, et al. Long-term results of carotid stenting versus endarterectomy in high-risk patients. N Engl J Med. 2008;358(15):1572–9.
16. Mas JL, Trinquart L, Leys D, Albucher JF, Rousseau H, Viguier A, Bossavy JP, Denis B, Piquet P, Garnier P, et al. Endarterectomy Versus Angioplasty in Patients with Symptomatic Severe Carotid Stenosis (EVA-3S) trial: results up to 4 years from a randomised, multicentre trial. Lancet Neurol. 2008;7(10):885–92.
17. Eckstein HH, Ringleb P, Allenberg JR, Berger J, Fraedrich G, Hacke W, Hennerici M, Stingele R, Fiehler J, Zeumer H, et al. Results of the Stent-Protected Angioplasty versus Carotid Endarterectomy (SPACE) study to treat symptomatic stenoses at 2 years: a multinational, prospective, randomised trial. Lancet Neurol. 2008;7(10):893–902.
18. International Carotid Stenting Study Investigators, Ederle J, Dobson J, Featherstone RL, Bonati LH, van der Worp HB, de Borst GJ, Lo TH, Gaines P, Dorman PJ, et al. Carotid artery

stenting compared with endarterectomy in patients with symptomatic carotid stenosis (International Carotid Stenting Study): an interim analysis of a randomised controlled trial. Lancet. 2010;375(9719):985–97.

19. McPhee JT, Hill JS, Eslami MH. The impact of gender on presentation, therapy, and mortality of abdominal aortic aneurysm in the United States, 2001-2004. J Vasc Surg. 2007;45(5): 891–9.

20. Shantikumar S, Ajjan R, Porter KE, Scott DJ. Diabetes and the abdominal aortic aneurysm. Eur J Vasc Endovasc Surg. 2010;39(2):200–7.

21. Larsson E, Granath F, Swedenborg J, Hultgren R. A population-based case-control study of the familial risk of abdominal aortic aneurysm. J Vasc Surg. 2009;49(1):47–50; discussion 51.

22. Ferket BS, Grootenboer N, Colkesen EB, Visser JJ, van Sambeek MR, Spronk S, Steyerberg EW, Hunink MG. Systematic review of guidelines on abdominal aortic aneurysm screening. J Vasc Surg. 2012;55(5):1296–304.

23. Kent KC, Zwolak RM, Jaff MR, Hollenbeck ST, Thompson RW, Schermerhorn ML, Sicard GA, Riles TS, Cronenwett JL, Society for Vascular Surgery, et al. Screening for abdominal aortic aneurysm: a consensus statement. J Vasc Surg. 2004;39(1):267–9.

24. Hager A, Kaemmerer H, Rapp-Bernhardt U, Blucher S, Rapp K, Bernhardt TM, Galanski M, Hess J. Diameters of the thoracic aorta throughout life as measured with helical computed tomography. J Thorac Cardiovasc Surg. 2002;123(6):1060–6.

25. Gadowski GR, Pilcher DB, Ricci MA. Abdominal aortic aneurysm expansion rate: effect of size and beta-adrenergic blockade. J Vasc Surg. 1994;19(4):727–31.

26. Brown LC, Powell JT. Risk factors for aneurysm rupture in patients kept under ultrasound surveillance. UK Small Aneurysm Trial Participants. Ann Surg. 1999;230(3):289–96.

27. Brewster DC, Cronenwett JL, Hallett Jr JW, Johnston KW, Krupski WC, Matsumura JS, Joint Council of the American Association for Vascular Surgery and Society for Vascular Surgery. Guidelines for the treatment of abdominal aortic aneurysms. Report of a subcommittee of the Joint Council of the American Association for Vascular Surgery and Society for Vascular Surgery. J Vasc Surg. 2003;37(5):1106–17.

28. Norman PE, Powell JT. Abdominal aortic aneurysm: the prognosis in women is worse than in men. Circulation. 2007;115(22):2865–9.

29. United Kingdom EVAR Trial Investigators, Greenhalgh RM, Brown LC, Powell JT, Thompson SG, Epstein D, Sculpher MJ. Endovascular versus open repair of abdominal aortic aneurysm. N Engl J Med. 2010;362(20):1863–71.

30. Coady MA, Ikonomidis JS, Cheung AT, Matsumoto AH, Dake MD, Chaikof EL, Cambria RP, Mora-Mangano CT, Sundt TM, Sellke FW, et al. Surgical management of descending thoracic aortic disease: open and endovascular approaches: a scientific statement from the American Heart Association. Circulation. 2010;121(25):2780–804.

31. Madaric J, Vulev I, Bartunek J, Mistrik A, Verhamme K, De Bruyne B, Riecansky I. Frequency of abdominal aortic aneurysm in patients >60 years of age with coronary artery disease. Am J Cardiol. 2005;96(9):1214–6.

32. Rooke TW, Hirsch AT, Misra S, Sidawy AN, Beckman JA, Findeiss LK, Golzarian J, Gornik HL, Halperin JL, Jaff MR, et al. 2011 ACCF/AHA focused update of the guideline for the management of patients with peripheral artery disease (updating the 2005 guideline): a report of the American College of Cardiology Foundation/American Heart Association Task Force on Practice Guidelines. J Am Coll Cardiol. 2011;58(19):2020–45.

33. Kannel WB, McGee DL. Update on some epidemiologic features of intermittent claudication: the Framingham study. J Am Geriatr Soc. 1985;33(1):13–8.

34. Kannel WB, Skinner Jr JJ, Schwartz MJ, Shurtleff D. Intermittent claudication. Incidence in the Framingham study. Circulation. 1970;41(5):875–83.

35. Hooi JD, Stoffers HE, Kester AD, Rinkens PE, Kaiser V, van Ree JW, Knottnerus JA. Risk factors and cardiovascular diseases associated with asymptomatic peripheral arterial occlusive disease. The Limburg PAOD Study. Peripheral arterial occlusive disease. Scand J Prim Health Care. 1998;16(3):177–82.

36. Murabito JM, Evans JC, Nieto K, Larson MG, Levy D, Wilson PW. Prevalence and clinical correlates of peripheral arterial disease in the Framingham offspring study. Am Heart J. 2002;143(6):961–5.
37. Criqui MH, Fronek A, Barrett-Connor E, Klauber MR, Gabriel S, Goodman D. The prevalence of peripheral arterial disease in a defined population. Circulation. 1985;71(3):510–5.
38. Meijer WT, Hoes AW, Rutgers D, Bots ML, Hofman A, Grobbee DE. Peripheral arterial disease in the elderly: the Rotterdam study. Arterioscler Thromb Vasc Biol. 1998;18(2):185–92.
39. Sigvant B, Wiberg-Hedman K, Bergqvist D, Rolandsson O, Wahlberg E. Risk factor profiles and use of cardiovascular drug prevention in women and men with peripheral arterial disease. Eur J Cardiovasc Prev Rehabil. 2009;16(1):39–46.
40. Zheng ZJ, Sharrett AR, Chambless LE, Rosamond WD, Nieto FJ, Sheps DS, Dobs A, Evans GW, Heiss G. Associations of ankle-brachial index with clinical coronary heart disease, stroke and preclinical carotid and popliteal atherosclerosis: the Atherosclerosis Risk in Communities (ARIC) study. Atherosclerosis. 1997;131(1):115–25.
41. Hiramoto JS, Katz R, Ix JH, Wassel C, Rodondi N, Windham BG, Harris T, Koster A, Satterfield S, Newman A, et al. Sex differences in the prevalence and clinical outcomes of subclinical peripheral artery disease in the health, aging, and body composition (health ABC) study. Vascular. March 19, 2013 [Epub ahead of print].
42. Lyden SP, Joseph D. The clinical presentation of peripheral arterial disease and guidance for early recognition. Cleve Clin J Med. 2006;73 Suppl 4:S15–21.
43. Cannon CP, Investigators CAPRIE. Effectiveness of clopidogrel versus aspirin in preventing acute myocardial infarction in patients with symptomatic atherothrombosis (CAPRIE trial). Am J Cardiol. 2002;90(7):760–2.
44. Rutherford RB. Standards for evaluating results of interventional therapy for peripheral vascular disease. Circulation. 1991;83(2 Suppl):I6–11.

Chapter 18
A Holistic Integrative Medicine Approach to Cardiovascular Disease

Mimi Guarneri

Introduction

Integrative Medicine by definition is a bridge between conventional Western Medicine and other global healing traditions. The term Holistic refers to treating the whole person: mind, body, emotions and spirit. Holistic Integrative Medicine is not synonymous with Alternative or Complementary Medicine; rather, Holistic Integrative Medicine makes use of the best of conventional medicine combined with techniques from other global healing traditions to prevent and treat chronic disease.

Holistic Integrative Medicine is not about the substitution of a supplement for a drug. Rather, it is about treating all of the risk factors for cardiovascular disease (CVD) and getting to their underlying causes. These risk factors are multi-factorial and may include sedentary lifestyle, hypertension, diabetes, dyslipidemia, tobacco use and central obesity. The psychological risks linked to CVD have been well-described and include stress, anxiety, depression and social isolation.

According to Women Heart, 8.6 million women worldwide die from heart disease each year, accounting for a third of all deaths in women. Three million women die from stroke each year. Stroke accounts for more deaths among women than men (11 % vs. 8.4 %), with additional risk for CVD unique to women related to oral contraceptive use in combination with tobacco.

Research points to an infinite number of insults with only a few responses which lead to atherosclerosis. These include inflammation, oxidative stress and immune dysfunction. Although genetics account for approximately 20 % of cardiovascular risk, 70–90 % of chronic disease is related to an individual's lifestyle and environment. It is this intimate interaction between our genes and the environment that determines health or disease. Although we are born with a certain genetic code,

M. Guarneri, MD, FACC
UCSD School of Medicine, Scripps Center for Integrative Medicine, La Jolla, CA, USA
e-mail: mguarnerimd@gmail.com

H.Z. Mieszczanska, G.P. Velarde (eds.),
Management of Cardiovascular Disease in Women,
DOI 10.1007/978-1-4471-5517-1_18, © Springer-Verlag London 2014

we turn genes on and off by how we live our lives. This is our greatest opportunity for understanding the key steps to the prevention of cardiovascular disease. No field lends itself better to this integration than cardiology, which utilizes the best of technology and mandates the need for aggressive lifestyle change.

While conventional medicine excels at acute care, Holistic Integrative Medicine offers expertise in nutrition, nutraceuticals, exercise and mind-body interventions that are pivotal to CVD treatment and prevention.

Food Is Medicine

From Hippocrates we have learned that food is medicine. Today we also know that food is information. For example, our food choices turn on genes that lead to the formation of anti or pro-inflammatory cytokines. The largest prospective study to look at the benefits of monounsaturated fats and a modified Mediterranean diet is the Lyon Heart study.

This study randomized patients with known CVD to a modified Mediterranean diet or the American Heart Association (AHA) step 1 diet [1]. The modified Mediterranean diet is anti-inflammatory and includes a high consumption of fresh fruits and vegetables; the use of whole-grains rather than refined carbohydrates; low to moderate amounts of dairy, fish and poultry; low amounts of red meat; minimal amounts of processed foods and a low to moderate consumption of wine. The primary monounsaturated fat is alpha-linolenic acid (ALA) enriched canola oil. The experimental group experienced 60 % fewer cardiovascular events and 80 % fewer late diagnoses of cancer. This was further supported in the Indo-Mediterranean Heart study where the Indo-Mediterranean diet group experienced 49 % fewer cardiovascular events, 62 % fewer sudden deaths and 51 % fewer non-fatal myocardial infarctions in comparison to the National Cholesterol Education Program (NCEP) diet group [2]. Both of these diets are high in omega-3 content and are anti-inflammatory. Diets high in saturated fat and refined sugar reduce endothelium–dependent relaxation and increase inflammatory markers such as interleukin-18 and tumor necrosis factor.

The Omni Heart Randomized Trial evaluated the effect of protein, monounsaturated fat and carbohydrate intake on blood pressure and serum lipids [3]. In this study a high carbohydrate (58 %) diet was compared to a protein-modified diet (25 %) and a high monounsaturated fat diet (37 %). Compared with baseline, the 10-year Framingham risk was lowered in each group by 16–21 %. Both the protein and unsaturated fat diets demonstrated greater risk reduction than the high-carbohydrate diet. In addition, the higher-protein diet demonstrated the greatest LDL and blood pressure reductions. These patients were encouraged to have two-thirds of their protein from plant sources such as legumes, grains, nuts and seeds.

Hu and Willet reviewed 147 epidemiological and dietary intervention studies and concluded these nutrition principles for prevention of CVD [4]:

1. Increase consumption of omega-3 fatty acids from fish, fish oil supplement, and plant sources.
2. Substitute non-hydrogenated unsaturated fats for saturated and trans fats.
3. Consume a diet high in fruits, vegetables, nuts, and whole grains, and low in sugar and refined grain products.

Based on the research, nutrition recommendations include:

- low glycemic index carbohydrates
- organic fruits and vegetables, especially green leafy vegetables
- whole grains: quinoa, rye, barley, buckwheat, oats
- high-quality fats: avocado, nuts, nut butters, seeds, extra virgin olive oil (first or cold pressed)
- omega-3 s from fish such as salmon, herring, mackerel or sardines, or from flaxseed
- plant-based protein (nuts, beans and legumes) along with lean meats
- free-range organic eggs
- fiber (should be slowly increased with the goal being 25–35 g/day)
- foods high in antioxidants
- less dairy (many people have lactose intolerance)
- anti-inflammatory spices like turmeric, cinnamon, oregano and ginger
- functional foods: almonds, chocolate, tea, soy, miso, tempeh
- viscous fibers: eggplant, oats, and psyllium
- tea and chocolate to reduce free radicals (due to high concentration of flavonoids)

In addition, we recommend five cups of green tea daily to reduce cardiovascular mortality as well as to lower cholesterol [5]. Flavonoids, especially those found in green tea, have been shown to have antithrombotic effects [6]. Consumption of black tea is associated with a reduction in acute myocardial infarction [7] and improved endothelial relaxation [8].

Hypertension

Hypertension affects at least 50 million Americans and results from an interaction between genes and the environment. Although the incidence increases with age and is more prevalent among certain ethnic groups such as African Americans, 95 % of what we label Essential Hypertension is lifestyle-related and therefore preventable. Since the release of the 2003 JNC VII report, pre-hypertension is now defined as a blood pressure of 120–130 mmHg systolic and 80–89 mmHg diastolic. Although JNC VII recommends lifestyle change for treating individuals with hypertension and pre-hypertension, their recommendations are limited and do not take supplements, mind-body interventions and vegan/vegetarian diets into consideration [9]. This is unfortunate, since meta-analyses demonstrate that a mean reduction in diastolic blood pressure of 5–6 mmHg is associated with 20–25 % less coronary disease and 35–40 % less stroke [10].

Nutrition Considerations for Hypertension

Our modern-day diet is responsible for a number of nutrition-related diseases. Research has demonstrated that vegetarians have less hypertension and coronary artery disease than non-vegetarians. Vegetarian diets are higher in potassium, fiber and complex carbohydrates. Vegetarians consume more calcium, magnesium, vitamin C and essential fatty acids. In addition, the vegetarian diet contains less saturated fat.

The potassium-to-sodium ratio is one of the keys to the vegetarian diet being associated with less hypertension. The ideal potassium-to-sodium ratio is 5:1. In the typical American diet, this ratio is frequently 1:2. Americans consume more than 5,000 mg of sodium per day. Just eating more fruits and vegetables helps to shift this ratio.

Potassium increases naturesis, improves insulin sensitivity and decreases sensitivity to Angiotensin II and catecholamines. The recommended dietary intake for potassium in hypertensive patients is 4.7 g/day with less than 1,500 mg of sodium. It is important to remind patients that dairy such as cottage cheese may contain high amounts of sodium. Potassium supplementation in foods or through the use of salt substitutes should be monitored closely and reduced in patients with renal impairment and those taking potassium-sparing medications.

The DASH trial was a multicenter, 11-week study that evaluated diet patterns on blood pressure. A total of 459 subjects were divided into three categories: increased fruits and vegetables, control, and a combination diet rich in fruits and vegetables and low in dairy and saturated fat. The combination diet led to a mean blood pressure reduction of −11.4 mmHg SBP and −5.5 DBP [11]. Additional dietary factors that affect blood pressure and are easy to implement include decreasing alcohol consumption, increasing fiber, and adding soy and olive oil. In the Shanghai Women's Health Study soy protein intake was inversely related to SBP and DBP [12]. Similarly, a meta-analysis of fiber in 25 randomized controlled trials demonstrated significant reductions in blood pressure [13].

Many foods act as natural anti-hypertensive compounds. Foods high in magnesium, such as green leafy vegetables, not only have high fiber but the magnesium competes with sodium for binding sites on vascular smooth muscle cells. In essence, magnesium acts as a calcium channel blocker. Chelated forms of magnesium at 500–1,000 mg/day are well-tolerated. As with potassium, magnesium should be used with caution or avoided in patients with known renal impairment.

Selected Supplements for Cardiovascular Disease

Omega-3 Fatty Acids

Double-blind studies have demonstrated that flax and/or fish oil supplementation is effective in decreasing blood pressure. EPA and DHA competitively inhibit the potent vasoconstrictor thromboxane A2. A meta-analysis of 32 trials demonstrated a 3.4 mmHg drop in systolic and a 2.0 mmHg drop in diastolic blood pressure on consuming 5.6 g/day of fish oil [14].

Coenzyme Q10

Coenzyme Q10 levels have been found to be reduced in patients with hypertension and congestive heart failure. A series of eight small studies has demonstrated average systolic blood pressure decreases of 16 mmHg and average diastolic blood pressure decreases of 10 mmHg [15].

The current recommended dose is 60–120 mg taken with food. CoQ10 levels can be measured and higher doses may be indicated. Patients taking coumadin should be monitored as it has been reported that CoQ10 can decrease coumadin levels. Side effects include nausea, anorexia, and diarrhea and epigastric discomfort.

Q-SYMBIO is now the largest trial to date of CoQ10 in heart failure in the modern era. Mortensen presented results from 420 patients with class III or IV HF who were randomized to CoQ10 three times daily or placebo. After 2 years there was a significant reduction in the incidence of major adverse cardiovascular events in the CoQ10 group: 14 % (29 patients) in the CoQ10 group versus 25 % (55 patients) in the placebo group (hazard ratio 2.0, CI 1.3–3.2, p=0.003). Mortensen also reported a significant reduction in overall mortality: 9 % (18 patients) in the CoQ10 group versus 17 % (18 patients) in the placebo group (HR 2.1, CI 1.2–3.8, p=0.01) There were also significant reductions in cardiovascular mortality (p=0.02) and HF hospitalizations (p=0.05) [16].

Magnesium

An inverse correlation exists between magnesium levels and blood pressure. In the Nurses Heart Study and Honolulu Heart Study low magnesium correlated with hypertension [17, 18]. Women taking 300 mg/day had less hypertension than those on less than 200 mg/day. I recommend chelated magnesium at 250 mg twice per day. Patients are advised to monitor their bowel habits as magnesium can cause soft stool. Adverse side effects include diarrhea and renal stones. As with potassium, magnesium should be monitored closely or avoided in patients with renal insufficiency.

Potassium

As noted above, improving the potassium to sodium ratio is a key to improving blood pressure. A meta-analysis of 19 studies has demonstrated a significant reduction in blood pressure in patients taking oral potassium; −8.2 SBP, −4.5 DBP [19]. Potassium is best taken in food and in salt substitutes. Potassium should be avoided in patients with renal insufficiency and those on potassium-sparing medications.

Vitamin C

One of the many effects of vitamin C is that it induces a sodium diuresis. There is an inverse correlation between vitamin C level and blood pressure. In a study of elderly patients with refractory hypertension, 600 mg of vitamin C lowered the blood pressure 20/16 mmHg. Those with the lowest ascorbate levels had the best response [20].

Vitamin D

Vitamin D levels are also inversely related to blood pressure. Levels lower than 30 ng/ml result in elevations of the plasma renin angiotensin system. In a study of 148 women with low vitamin D3 levels, the administration of 800 IU of D3 and 1,200 mg of calcium reduced SBP 9.3 % [21]. The same effect was not noted with calcium alone.

Aged Garlic Extract

In a randomized placebo-controlled trial with 50 patients, 900 mg of aged garlic extract with 2.4 mg of S-allylcysteine daily for 12 weeks reduced SBP 10 mmHg in patients with hypertension [22]. Four cloves of garlic are required to decrease blood pressure. This contains approximately 10,000 mcg of allicin.

Aged garlic extract has also been found to slow vascular calcification. Sixty individuals were randomized to a daily capsule of placebo vs. Aged Garlic Extract-S inclusive of aged garlic-extract (250 mg) plus vitamin-B12 (100 μg), folic acid (300 μg), vitamin B6 (12.5 mg) and L-arginine (100 mg). Participants underwent coronary artery calcium (CAC) scoring and wEAT(white adipose tissue) and bEAT(brown adipose tissue) measurements at baseline and 12 months. CAC progression was defined as an annual increase in CAC>15 % from baseline to 12 months. There was a strong correlation between increase in wEAT and CAC ($r^2=0.54$, p=0.0001). At 1 year, the risks of CAC progression and increased wEAT and homocysteine were significantly lower in AGE-S to placebo (p<0.05). In addition, bEAT was higher in AGE-S as compared to placebo (p<0.05). Maximum beneficial effect of AGE-S was noted with an increase in bEAT/wEAT ratio, and lack of progression of homocysteine and CAC. The authors concluded AGE-S is associated with increase in bEAT/wEAT ratio, reduction of homocysteine and lack of progression of CAC [23].

Tea, Coffee and Cocoa

Black tea and green tea have been shown to decrease blood pressure in humans. Dark chocolate (100 g) and cocoa are high in polyphenols. A meta-analysis of 297 hypertensive patients given cocoa for 2 weeks had a 4.5/2.5 mmHg drop in blood pressure [24]. Likewise, polyphenols, chlorogenic acid (CGAs) and di-hydrocaffeic acids decrease blood pressure. CGAs are found in coffee bean extract. At 140 mg/day, green coffee bean extract has been shown to decrease SBP and DBP [25].

However, the results on coffee are conflicting. Coffee contains other compounds such as hydroxyhydroquinone, which antagonizes the beneficial effect of CGA. In addition, it is important to note that slow metabolizers of caffeine have a much higher risk of developing hypertension than fast metabolizers. In this group, caffeine should be reduced or avoided.

Vitamin E and Antioxidants

The Nurses' Health Study, which was observational in design, reported a 34 % reduction in cardiovascular events in subjects taking vitamin E supplementation [26]. Since that initial observation, multiple studies have attempted to evaluate vitamin E in the primary and secondary prevention of cardiovascular disease. In the primary prevention project, 4,495 patients were followed for 3.6 years on 300 IU of vitamin E supplementation without demonstrating improvement in cardiovascular morbidity [27]. Multiple secondary prevention studies, including HOPE [28] and GISSI-P (GISSI-Prevenzione Investigators 1999), failed to demonstrate benefit from vitamin E supplementation.

HATS compared treatment regimens of lipid-modifying therapy and antioxidant-vitamin therapy, alone and together [29]. The 3-year, double-blind trial included 160 patients with coronary disease, low levels of HDL-C and normal levels of LDL-C. Patients were assigned to one of four treatment regimens: simvastatin (10–20 mg/day) plus niacin (2–4 g/day); antioxidants; simvastatin (10–20 mg/day) plus niacin (2–4 g/day) plus antioxidants; or placebo. The primary end points were angiographic evidence of change in coronary stenosis and the occurrence of a first cardiovascular event (fatal/nonfatal MI, stroke or revascularization). The average stenosis progressed with placebo (3.9 %), antioxidants (1.8 %) and simvastatin plus niacin plus antioxidants (0.7 %). There was a 0.4 % regression with simvastatin plus niacin alone (p<0.001). In conclusion, the combination of simvastatin plus niacin greatly reduced the rate of major coronary events (60–90 %) and substantially slowed progression of coronary atherosclerosis in patients with low HDL-C. While HATS further supported the use of niacin for raising HDL and reducing plaque formation in combination with statin therapy, no further advantage was seen in the group receiving antioxidants and combination statin-niacin therapy. These studies did not attempt to assess the inflammatory and oxidative state of subjects prior to initiation and following therapy.

In a randomized double-blind placebo-controlled trial, subjects were given 1,600 IU of RRR-alpha tocopherol versus placebo and followed for 6 months [30]. Subjects taking the vitamin E had a statistically significant reduction in hs-CRP, urinary F2 isoprostanes, monocyte superoxide anion, and tumor necrosis factor release, compared with baseline and placebo. Despite this reduction in oxidative and inflammatory markers, no change was seen in carotid intimal-medial thickness. Multiple trial design concerns have been raised to explain the inconsistency of the observational and randomized study data [31]. These include:

• Not using the right type of supplement formulation
• Not using the correct dosage
• Not using a complex antioxidant mixture
• Not choosing the right study population
• Not looking at functional biomarkers

One of the important variables missing from all of these studies is nutritional status. Until biomarkers and nutritional status are included with these research variables, it is premature to conclude that antioxidants offer no benefit in cardiovascular disease prevention.

Heavy Metal Toxicity and Cardiovascular Disease

Mercury and cadmium toxicity should be evaluated in any patient with hypertension, coronary heart disease, cerebral vascular disease, cerebrovascular accident, or other vascular disease. The overall vascular effects of mercury include increased oxidative stress and inflammation, reduced oxidative defense, thrombosis, vascular smooth muscle dysfunction, endothelial dysfunction, dyslipidemia, and immune and mitochondrial dysfunction [32]. The clinical consequences of mercury toxicity include hypertension, coronary heart disease, myocardial infarction, cardiac arrhythmias, reduced heart rate variability, increased carotid intima-media thickness and carotid artery obstruction, cerebrovascular accident, generalized atherosclerosis, and renal dysfunction, insufficiency, and proteinuria.

Cadmium has less cardiovascular effect, but as it accumulates in the kidney and is associated with proteinuria and renal dysfunction leading to hypertension [33]. Mercury, cadmium and other heavy metals will decrease COMT, thereby affecting the metabolism of epinephrine, norepinephrine and dopamine. As a result, hypertension may be the first clue to heavy metal toxicity. Routine blood screening may not reveal the total body burden of heavy metals. Challenge testing with chelating agents such as DMSA and DMPS should be considered in patients suspected of having heavy metal toxicity.

Chelation for CAD

A multicenter NHLBI and NCCAM study was conducted to access whether EDTA chelation therapy reduced cardiovascular events in patients with cardiovascular disease (TACT).

The study was a double-blind, placebo-controlled, randomized trial enrolling 1,708 patients aged 50 years or older who had experienced a myocardial infarction (MI) at least 6 weeks prior and had serum creatinine levels of 2.0 mg/dL or less [34]. Participants were recruited at 134 US and Canadian sites. Patients were randomized to receive 40 infusions of a 500-mL chelation solution (3 g of disodium EDTA, 7 g of ascorbate, B vitamins, electrolytes, procaine, and heparin) (n=839) vs. placebo (n=869) and an oral vitamin-mineral regimen vs. an oral placebo. Infusions were administered weekly for 30 weeks, followed by 10 infusions 2–8 weeks apart. Fifteen percent discontinued infusions (n=38 [16 %] in the chelation group and n=41 [15 %] in the placebo group) because of adverse events. The primary end point was a composite of total mortality, recurrent MI, stroke, coronary revascularization, or hospitalization for angina. Qualifying previous MIs occurred a median of 4.6 years before enrollment. The primary end point occurred in 222 (26 %) of the chelation group and 261 (30 %) of the placebo group (hazard ratio [HR], 0.82 [95 % CI, 0.69–0.99]; P=.035). There was no effect on total mortality (chelation: 87 deaths [10 %]; placebo, 93 deaths [11 %]; (P=.64). The study was not powered for this comparison. The effect of EDTA chelation on the components of the primary end point other than death was of similar magnitude as its overall effect (MI: chelation, 6 %; placebo, 8 %; HR, 0.77 [95 % CI, 0.54–1.11]; stroke: chelation, 1.2 %; placebo, 1.5 %; HR, 0.77 [95 % CI, 0.34–1.76]; coronary revascularization: chelation, 15 %; placebo, 18 %; HR, 0.81 [95 % CI, 0.64–1.02]; hospitalization for angina: chelation, 1.6 %; placebo, 2.1 %; HR, 0.72 [95 % CI, 0.35–1.47]). The authors concluded that among stable patients with a history of MI, use of an intravenous chelation regimen with disodium EDTA, compared with placebo, modestly reduced the risk of adverse cardiovascular outcomes, many of which were revascularization procedures.

Physical and Psychological Resiliency

Research has shown that the physical deterioration associated with aging is related to stress and a sedentary lifestyle. For example, chronic stress leads to overproduction of cortisol, which is associated with an increased risk for central obesity, diabetes, hypertension, osteoporosis, infection and sarcopenia. All of these conditions are more prevalent as we age.

The role of stress in the development of CVD has been well described in the literature. Although stress may at times be an adaptive response to ensure survival, stress hormones (most notably epinephrine, cortisol and aldosterone) are associated with impaired glucose metabolism, weight gain, arrhythmia, hypertension, hyperlipidemia, inflammation and coronary spasm. In addition, stress can adversely affect autonomic and vascular tone, immune function, coagulation and the perception of pain.

A stress response may have multiple triggers. These include psychological triggers such as frustration, anger and anxiety. Other triggers may be environmental and include chemical/toxin exposure, infection and allergens. Physiological triggers of a stress reaction may include pain or insomnia. In addition, negative emotional states such as sadness, hopelessness and depression are independent risk factors for cardiovascular disease. At a minimum, all patients should be screened for perceived stress, hostility, depression and social isolation. Low social economic status, which is associated with health disparities and adverse childhood events, are additional potent risk factors that affect health and should be addressed as well.

The European Cardiovascular Disease Guidelines recommend a short assessment of psychosocial risk in clinical practice [35]. These include:

1. **Depression**: Do you feel down, depressed and hopeless? Have you lost interest and pleasure in life?
2. **Social Isolation**: Are you living alone? Do you lack a close friend or confidant? Do you lack any person to help you in case of illness?
3. **Work and Family Stress**: Do you have enough control over how to meet the demands at work? Is your reward appropriate for your effort? Do you have serious problems with your spouse?
4. **Hostility**: Do you frequently feel angry over little things? If someone annoys you, do you regularly let your partner know? Do you often feel annoyed about habits that others have?
5. **Low Socio-Economic Status**: Are you a manual worker? What is your highest educational degree?

Enhancing Resiliency

Exercise and stress management have remarkable health benefits. These benefits affect not only the physical body but the emotional and mental body as well. Weight loss is frequently the result of a consistent exercise program. A review of 11 weight loss studies concluded that the average SBP and DBP reduction per kilogram of weight loss was 1.6 and 1.1 mmHg, respectively [36]. On average, 60 min of mild exercise three times per week is associated with a SBP reduction of 11 mmHg and a DBP reduction of 6 mmHg [37].

Regular exercise and stress management:

1. Improves insulin sensitivity
2. Increases vitality and energy
3. Improves sleep

4. Decreases tension and stress
5. Improves mood and depression
6. Lowers blood sugar and triglycerides
7. Lowers LDL cholesterol
8. Improves diabetes
9. Lowers blood pressure
10. Improves basal metabolic rate
11. Improves heart rate variability

In addition to exercise, many techniques are available that can enhance resiliency. These include proper sleep, exercise, guided imagery, laughter, meditation, yoga and deep breathing. A recent secondary cardiovascular prevention study was conducted to assess the impact of Transcendental Meditation [38]. In this study, 201 black men and women with coronary heart disease were randomized to the TM program or health education. The primary end point was the composite of all-cause mortality, myocardial infarction, or stroke. Secondary end points included the composite of cardiovascular mortality, revascularizations, and cardiovascular hospitalizations; blood pressure; psychosocial stress factors; and lifestyle behaviors. During an average follow-up of 5.4 years, there was a 48 % risk reduction in the primary end point in the TM group (hazard ratio, 0.52; 95 % confidence interval, 0.29–0.92; P=0.025). The TM group also showed a 24 % risk reduction in the secondary end point (hazard ratio, 0.76; 95 % confidence interval, 0.51–0.1.13; P=0.17). There were reductions of 4.9 mmHg in systolic blood pressure (95 % confidence interval −8.3 to −1.5 mmHg; P=0.01) and anger expression (P<0.05 for all scales). Adherence was associated with survival.

In addition, spiritual practices such as contemplative prayer, forgiveness and service are important keys to finding inner peace. Since the stress response is frequently related to an individual's perception of an event, it is important to practice an attitude of gratitude. In addition, it is important to practice effective communication with friends, family and co-workers, manage time efficiently and develop fun leisure activities.

General Recommendations for Cardiovascular Health

1. Sodium <1,500 mg based on Dash II
2. Potassium 4 g (avoid in patients with renal insufficiency)
3. Potassium/Sodium Ration >3:1
4. Magnesium 500–1,000 mg/day
5. Zinc 50 mg (must factor in zinc/copper ratio)
6. Potassium-containing foods (broccoli, spinach, pumpkin, squash and bananas)
7. Garlic 4 fresh cloves per day or aged 600 mg BID
8. Omega 3 fatty acids 2–3 g
9. Omega 9 fatty acids (olives or olive oil)
10. Omega 3:6 ratio 1.1–1.2 (can be measured)

11. Protein 25–30 % of calories
12. Complex Carbohydrates and Fiber 40 % of Calories
13. Protein 1.5–1.8 g/kg
14. Body Mass Index <25
15. Alcohol restriction
16. Caffeine restriction or elimination depending on genetic polymorphism
17. Exercise: aerobic (20 min); resistance training (40 min)
18. Specific foods to consider: dark chocolate(100 g), pomegranate juice (8 oz), steel cut oats or oat bran, green leafy vegetables, celery, lycopene
19. Meditation
20. Gratefulness
21. Appreciation
22. Forgiveness

Conclusion

We have all the tools and evidence-based research to prevent cardiovascular disease. Health is more than the absence of disease. Health is a cohesive balance of body, mind and spirit. Our patients need to enhance their soil through lifestyle change.

There are many paths to healing and not everyone requires the same prescription. Good medicine requires spending time with our patients, developing their trust and partnering with them as we lead them on a healing journey. The word doctor means teacher. As teachers, our role is to guide our patients in healthy nutrition choices, physical activity including cardiac rehabilitation, and techniques to transform how they response to stress and tension.

References

1. de Lorgeril M, Salen P, Martin JL, Monjaud I, Delaye J, Mamelle N. Mediterranean diet, traditional risk factors, and the rate of cardiovascular complications after myocardial infarction: final report of the Lyon Diet Heart Study. Circulation. 1999;99:779–85.
2. Singh RB, Dubnov G, Niaz MA, et al. Effect of an Indo-Mediterranean diet on progression of coronary artery disease in high risk patients (Indo-Mediterranean Diet Heart Study): a randomised single-blind trial. Lancet. 2002;360:1455–61.
3. Appel JL, Sacks F. Effects of protein, monosaturated fat, and carbohydrate intake on blood pressure and serum lipids. JAMA. 2005;294:2455–64.
4. Hu FB, Willett WC. Optimal diets for prevention of coronary heart disease. JAMA. 2002;288:2569–78.
5. Kuriyama S, et al. Green tea consumption and mortality due to cardiovascular disease, cancer, and all causes in Japan: the Ohsaki study. JAMA. 2006;296(10):1255–65.
6. Son DJ, et al. Antiplatelet effect of green tea catechins: a possible mechanism through arachidonic acid pathway. Prostaglandins Leukot Essent Fatty Acids. 2004;71(1):25–31.

7. Geleijnse J, et al. Inverse assoc of tea and flavonoid intakes with incident myocardial infarction: the Rotterdam Study. Am J Clin Nutr. 2002;75(5):880–6.
8. Duffy S, et al. Short and long term black tea consumption reverses endothelial dysfunction in patients with coronary artery disease. Circulation. 2001;104(2):151–6.
9. Chobanian AV, et al. The seventh report of The Joint Committee on Prevention, Detection, Evaluation and Treatment of High Blood Pressure. The JNC 7 Report. JAMA. 2003;289:2560–71.
10. Collins R, et al. Short term reductions in blood pressure. Lancet. 1990;335:827–38.
11. Appel LJ, et al. A clinical trial of the effects of dietary patterns on blood pressure. DASH Collaborative Research Group. N Engl J Med. 1997;336:1117–24.
12. Yang G, et al. Longitudinal study of soy food intake and blood pressure among middle-aged and elderly Chinese women. Am J Clin Nutr. 2005;81:1012–7.
13. Whelton SP, et al. Effect of dietary fiber intake on blood pressure: a meta-analysis of randomized, controlled clinical trials. J Hypertens. 2005;23:475–81.
14. Morris MC, et al. Does fish Oil lower blood pressure? A meta-analysis of controlled trials. Circulation. 1993;88:523–33.
15. Rosenfeldt F, et al. Systematic review of effect of coenzyme Q10 in physical exercise, hypertension and heart failure. Biofactors. 2003;18:91–100.
16. Mortensen SA. Heart failure 2013 congress in Lisbon, Portugal. 2013.
17. Ascherio A, et al. A prospective study of nutritional factors and hypertension among US men. Circulation. 1992;86:1475–84.
18. Witteman JCM, et al. A prospective study of nutritional factors and hypertension among US women. Circulation. 1989;80:1320–7.
19. Cappuccio FP, et al. Does potassium supplementation lower blood pressure? J Hypertens. 1991;9:465–73.
20. Sato K, et al. Effects of ascorbic acid on ambulatory blood pressure in elderly patients with refractory hypertension. Arzneimittelforschung. 2006;56(7):535–40.
21. Pfeifer M, et al. Effects of short term vitamin D3 and calcium supplementation and parathyroid hormone levels in elderly women. J Clin Endocrinol Metab. 2001;86:1633–7.
22. Reid K, et al. Aged Garlic extract lowers blood pressure in patients with treated but uncontrolled hypertension. Maturitas. 2010;67(2):144–50.
23. Ahmadi N, Nabavi V, Hajsadeghi F, Zeb I, Flores F, Ebrahimi R, Budoff M. Aged garlic extract with supplement is associated with increase in brown adipose, decrease in white adipose tissue and predict lack of progression in coronary atherosclerosis. Int J Cardiol. 2013;168(3):2310–4.
24. Desch S, et al. Effect of cocoa products on blood pressure: systematic review and meta-analysis. Am J Hypertension. 2010;23(1):97–103.
25. Taubert D, et al. Effect of coca and tea intake on blood pressure. Arch Intern Med. 2007;167(7):626–34.
26. Lopez-Garcia E, et al. Consumption of (n-3) fatty acids is related to plasma biomarkers of inflammation and endothelial activation in women. J Nutr. 2004;134(7):1806–11.
27. Sacco M, et al., PPP Collaborative Group. Primary prevention of cardiovascular events with low-dose aspirin and vitamin E in type 2 diabetic patients: results of the Primary Prevention Project (PPP) trial. Diabetes Care. 2003;26(12):3264–72.
28. Yusuf S, et al. Effects of an angiotensin-converting-enzyme inhibitor, ramipril, on cardiovascular events in high-risk patients. The Heart Outcomes Prevention Evaluation Study Investigators. N Engl J Med. 2000;342(3):145–53.
29. Brown BG, Zhao XQ, Chait A, et al. Simvastatin and niacin, antioxidant vitamins, or the combination for the prevention of coronary disease. N Engl J Med. 2001;354(22):1583–92.
30. Devaraj S, Tang R, Adams-Huet B, et al. Effect of high-dose alpha-tocopherol supplementation on biomarkers of oxidative stress and inflammation and carotid atherosclerosis in patients with coronary artery disease. Am J Clin Nutr. 2007;86(5):1392–8.
31. Blumberg J, Frei B. Why clinical trials of vitamin E and cardiovascular diseases may be fatally flawed. Free Radic Biol Med. 2007;43:1374–6.

32. Houston M. Role of mercury toxicity in hypertension, cardiovascular disease, and stroke. J Clin Hypertens (Greenwich). 2011;13(8):621–7.
33. Houston M. The role of mercury and cadmium heavy metals in vascular disease, hypertension, coronary heart disease, and myocardial infarction. Altern Ther Health Med. 2007;13(2): S128–33.
34. Lamas GA, Goertz C, Boineau R, Mark DB, Rozema T, Nahin RL, Lindblad L, Lewis EF, Drisko J, Lee KL, TACT Investigators. Effect of disodium EDTA chelation regimen on cardio-vascular events in patients with previous myocardial infarction: the TACT randomized trial. JAMA. 2013;309(12):1241–50.
35. Perk J et al. European Guidelines on Cardiovascular Disease Prevention in Clinical Practice. European Heart Journal. 2012;33(13):1635–701.
36. Stamler J. Epidemiologic findings on body mass and blood pressure in adults. Ann Epidemiol. 1991;1:347–62.
37. Arakawa K. Effects of exercise on hypertension and associated complications. Hypertens Res. 1999;19(Suppl):S87–91.
38. Schneider RH, Grim CE, Rainforth MV, Kotchen T, Nidich SI, Gaylord-King C, Salerno JW, Kotchen JM, Alexander CN. Stress reduction in the secondary prevention of cardiovascular dis-ease: randomized, controlled trial of transcendental meditation and health education in Blacks. Circ Cardiovasc Qual Outcomes. 2012;5(6):750–8. doi:10.1161/CIRCOUTCOMES.112.967406. Epub 2012 Nov 13.

Chapter 19
The Impact of Stress, Depression, and Other Psychosocial Factors on Women's Cardiovascular Health

Katherine S. Dodd and Malgorzata Relja

With the evolutionary transition of female roles as the number of women in the modern workplace has exponentially increased over time, women today find themselves in a historically unique, complex and challenging environment. As they attempt to balance family and career commitments, pressures and expectations, unique stresses and strains impact their psychosocial experiences and cardiovascular health.

More so than men, it is a struggle for women to maintain their own health as they divide their focus and efforts on their multiple obligations [1]. In our current demanding world, there is a balancing act every day for the many women who have to work full time, often juggling professional careers while at the same time continuing to care for their families and aging parents. As women become preoccupied by their roles as mothers, wives and care providers, activities such as attending their own doctor's appointments, exercising, and preparing healthy meals may be intentionally or unintentionally sacrificed or postponed.

Unfortunately, many women fail to recognize the importance of their own health, forgetting that caring properly for themselves will also allow them to excel in their many roles. The immense responsibilities placed on women in our society are overwhelming and often lead to stress and depression, which in turn, negatively affects their cardiovascular health. In fact, atypical chest pain and palpitations in women is often stress related. Depression causes mental and physical strain and is typically accompanied by an unhealthy diet lacking nutrients, failure to exercise, and poor

K.S. Dodd, DO, MPH (✉)
Department of Medicine, University of Rochester Medical Center,
601 Elmwood Avenue, Box MED, Rochester, NY 14642, USA
e-mail: katherine_dodd@urmc.rochester.edu

M. Relja, MD, DABPN
Horizon Health Mental Health Center,
65 Brunswick St, 3rd Floor, Fredericton, NB E3B 1G5, Canada

H.Z. Mieszczanska, G.P. Velarde (eds.),
Management of Cardiovascular Disease in Women,
DOI 10.1007/978-1-4471-5517-1_19, © Springer-Verlag London 2014

stress management techniques. In a depressed state, women are unable to optimally care for others, but also themselves. The perception of stress by women varies greatly and it is what makes some women more prone to depression and causes them to succumb to the consequences of stress. In this chapter, we will be discussing the pathophysiologic effects of stress and the psychosocial risk factors such as depression and anxiety that impact a woman's health. Our hope is that healthcare professionals will become more adept at identifying and treating depression along with other biopsychosocial stressors, so women may achieve their goal of having a healthy family, career, and life [1].

Stress

Women encounter a wide variety of psychological and socioeconomic risk factors which influence their likelihood to develop heart disease. One of these major risk factors is stress, in part, because the stress women experience is very different than that of their male counterparts. To understand this better, it is helpful to define stress, describe different kinds of stress, and illustrate the impact it has on a women's cardiovascular health. Stress can be acute or chronic. Acute stress is transient and is typically associated with anticipation of an upcoming event or may be a reflection of a recent experience which induced worry. This short-term, fleeting type of stress manifests as anger, anxiety, depression, palpitations, high blood pressure, headache, muscle spasm, or gastrointestinal symptoms. Acute stress is easy to recognize and therefore has a better chance of being treated. Although it is short lived, it can have a more profound impact on health when it is frequently encountered and episodic. Acute episodic stress is demonstrated most clearly by the quintessential "type A" personality who tends to take on more responsibility that he or she can manage comfortably. The idea that a "type A" personality is a predisposing factor for poor cardiovascular health was a theory proposed in the 1950s by two cardiologists [2].

Although chronic stress can appear similar to acute stress, it is the lengthy duration of the stress that causes a greater impact on health than acute stress. Also, since it persists longer, the stress experience can grow and intensify over time, ultimately leading to a permanent poor health outcome. Chronic stress is much more difficult to manage as well because it is ingrained and habitual, and not as easily recognized. It is stimulated by situations that are unrelentingly demanding, often causing maladaptive behaviors, which can be harmful to health. Some research suggests that chronic stress can negatively effect blood glucose levels in addition to cardiovascular health [3]. Stress can be positive or negative. Examples of positive stressors include marriage, admission to graduate school, or participating in a scholarly or athletic competition. Negative stressors include the death of a family member, losing a job, financial troubles and divorce. Both positive and negative stress impacts cardiovascular health.

Psychosocial Risk Factors

There is increasing evidence that psychological stress can influence the onset and clinical course of ischemic heart disease, especially in women. The conclusions of the INTERHEART study pointed towards significant increased risk of myocardial infarction associated with exposure to both individual and multiple psychosocial risk factors such as traumatic life events, depression, perceived loss of control and elevated stress levels in the workplace or at home (adjusted odds ratio of 2.6 in men and 3.5 in women) [4].

Women face a variety of unique psychosocial stressors that impact their health. One of these stressors is employment, and the characteristics of work can impact a woman's cardiovascular health [5]. Currently, there are many more women in the workforce than in previous generations, so women have had to take on the new role of breadwinner or career woman, while still maintaining their more established roles as mother or caregiver. The demands of continuing education or establishing oneself in a career are overwhelming for many women. Another difficulty for women in the workforce is returning to work after a shortened maternity leave. Work poses its own set of challenges for women, in the sense that it is often a place of high demand, yet limited control [6]. There is an economic burden associated with work which men are not faced with as much as women. The employment status of a woman also appears to play a role in her risk of developing heart disease. There is some evidence that women employed outside of their home are actually at lower risk of coronary heart disease than women whose primary role is homemaker. On the other hand stress and work overload seems to be a greater problem for full time employed women, particularly in families with small children. In sum, prevention of workplace stress may decrease the incidence of heart disease among women [7].

Outside of the workforce, the role of woman as caregiver has expanded to not only that of a caretaker of children, but also of ill spouse and/or parents. It is not uncommon to come across a mother who is struggling to meet the needs of her young children while simultaneously trying to care for another family member. Interestingly, one study demonstrated that among cardiac rehabilitation participants, women were more likely than men to miss scheduled sessions, likely due to their multiple other responsibilities, and the tendency of a woman to put others before themself [8]. Research has suggested that higher levels of caregiver burden for ill spouses increase the risk of the development of coronary heart disease in women [9]. Women who tend to be caretakers often neglect their health and make their families the priority. This leads to poor nutrition, obesity, lack of exercise, chronic fatigue, poor coping including smoking, alcohol and drug abuse. Although it has consistently been found that employment does not correlate with negative health consequences, women in most industrialized countries tend to have more health-related problems than their male counterparts. Some of the most common health issues cited by women include somatic and musculoskeletal complaints, absenteeism from work, use of medical drugs and visits to doctors [8].

Minority women and women of low socioeconomic status are especially at risk for cardiovascular disease [10]. The rate of decline of mortality due to cardiovascular disease is significantly less for black women than for white women. According to the U.S. Department of Health and Human Services Office on Minority Health, African American men and women are 30 % more likely to die from heart disease than white men. Minorities are also more likely to have co-morbidities that typically go hand-in-hand with cardiovascular disease. For example, roughly 35 % of blacks have hypertension compared to 24 % of whites. Mexican Americans are several times more likely than whites to be overweight and obese. This is important as high blood pressure and obesity are two of the leading risk factors for heart disease. Premature death is also higher for Hispanics, Asian and Pacific Islanders, and American Indians or Alaska Natives when compared to whites [11]. In women with already established cardiovascular disease, low socioeconomic status predicts a poorer prognosis. In women without cardiovascular disease, having a low socioeconomic status places a woman at much higher risk of eventually developing it. Both level of education and access to healthcare affect a woman's heart health as well [11].

Pathophysiologic Effects of Stress

Psychosocial stress is a proven risk factor for cardiovascular disease in both patients with established CVD and healthy individuals [12]. It is also associated with adverse health behaviors. Utilizing various measures in the assessment of psychosocial stress, a direct correlation can be shown both in terms of higher prevalence and clustering of traditional cardiovascular risk factors. For example, risk factors such as increased blood pressure, cardiac reactivity, blood cholesterol, and cigarette smoking, in addition to poor diet and exercise habits, are correlated with Type A behavior personality [13]. There also appears to be an association between psychosocial stress and endothelial dysfunction, as resulting catecholamine and blood pressure surges may result in intimal damage, inflammatory-induced free radicals blocking nitric oxide synthesis, and increased endothelial reactivity triggered by activated platelets [14]. The pathophysiologic effects of stress on women are many (see Fig. 19.1). For example, stress causes an enhanced sympathetic response leading to elevated blood pressure, fast heart rate, and in the end, remodelling of the heart. Alterations in autonomic function, as measured by heart rate variability, have been associated with prothrombotic changes in women with ischemic heart disease [15, 16].

There is a long established association between acute cardiovascular events such as myocardial infarction and unstable angina occurring in a circadian rhythm which is correlated with the rhythm of sympathetic nervous system activity [17]. Mental stress has been shown to increase heart rate, blood pressure, and myocardial oxygen demand. These effects are mediated at least in part by catecholamine secretion. Another study also has shown a link between psychosocial stress and plaque rupture in the setting of increased sympathetic nervous system activity with surges in heart rate, blood pressure, as well as weakening of the collagenous plaque cap from

PATHOPYSIOLOGIC EFFECTS OF STRESS RESPONSE

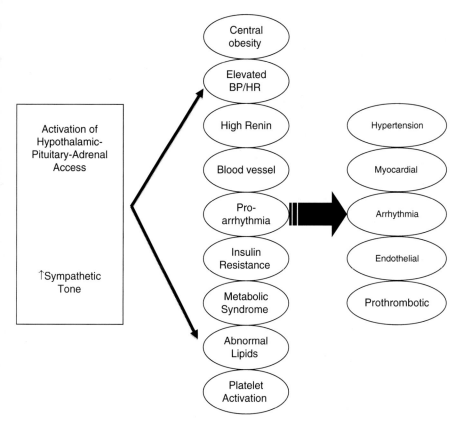

Fig. 19.1 Pathophysiologic mechanisms of stress on the development of atherosclerosis. Stress activates the hypothalamic-pituitary-adrenal axis and the sympathetic nervous system and depresses the parasympathetic nervous system. This results in numerous adverse effects peripherally which promote a heightened physiologic response and increase the risk of cardiovascular related events (Adapted with permission from Rozanski et al. [15], figure 7)

inflammatory processes, all of which may contribute to plaque instability [18]. Anger and other forms of mental stress were specified as triggers for myocardial infarction in a study that examined the behaviors leading up to left ventricular dysfunction and blood pressure elevation in coronary patients [19]. In addition to hemodynamic effects, mental stress also has been shown to increase platelet aggregability as well as coagulation [20].

The literature has demonstrated that during periods of stress that affect a whole population, the numbers of people presenting with heart attacks is increased. For example, the rate of admission for acute myocardial infarction increased significantly on the day England lost to Argentina in the 1998 World Cup [21]. Similarly, on the day of the Los Angeles Earthquake in 1994, there was a large increase in the number of sudden cardiac deaths from cardiac causes related to atherosclerotic cardiovascular disease [22]. Studies have also shown that women under a greater degree of stress have higher cortisol levels, which in turn, may influence eating behavior and lead to weight gain. High cortisol levels have been shown to accelerate aging, increase abdominal fat accumulation, and impair immune function [23]. It is clear that insulin resistance and diabetes brought on as a result of abdominal obesity, which may be the result of blunted sex hormones and hypercortisolemia, are particularly important cardiovascular risk factors in women [15].

There is a growing body of literature on the influence of stress on telomeres. A telomere is a repetitive sequence of nucleotides at the end of a chromosome which protects the chromosome from deterioration. As telomeres shorten, important genomic information is lost. Interestingly, one recent study demonstrated that there is a stress related shortening of telomeres in the cells of women taking care of chronically ill children and among women who were formerly abused [24, 25]. In contrast, exercise and meditation have been found to reduce stress, and some small studies have demonstrated that these two beneficial activities actually prevent shortening of telomeres [26]. Shorter telomeres are associated with many age related diseases and predict an increased incidence and poorer prognosis for cardiovascular disease. So called "resiliency factors" dampen the effects of stress on the heart. For example, regular exercise, consumption of fruits and vegetables, abstaining from alcohol and tobacco, significantly decrease a woman's risk of developing heart disease [27]. Waist circumference has also been shown to correlate with future cardiovascular events in women [28]. Multiple studies support evidence that diets consisting mainly of fruits and vegetables offer significant protection against coronary heart disease, reduce levels of circulating inflammatory agents, and decrease insulin resistance [29–31]. Although behavior modifications are extremely effective, pharmacologic agents may also be used adjunctively to control co-morbidities associated with poor cardiovascular health, such as high blood pressure and diabetes.

Studies point to a link between acute psychological stress leading to acute MI and sudden cardiac death in certain susceptible individuals. Although gender differences in this link are not clear, there are cardiovascular conditions that are almost exclusive to women. The most notable example of this is Takotsubo cardiomyopathy. In this specific cardiomyopathy, sudden, unexpected emotional or physical stress causes a reversible cardiomyopathy with markedly elevated levels of plasma catecholamines [32]. The left ventricular chamber is predominantly affected with transient hypokinesis, akinesis, or dyskinesis of the apical and mid segments; regional wall motion abnormalities may extend beyond a single epicardial vascular distribution in the absence of obstructive coronary disease or angiographic evidence of acute plaque rupture. The prognosis of patients with Takotsubo cardiomyopathy is generally favorable and systolic function may recover with hemodynamic and pharmacologic support [33]. Takotsubo cardiomyopathy occurs predominantly in postmenopausal, older women, which is in concordance with the fact that the great majority of women who have established heart disease are older [34].

Depression and Anxiety

As stated already in this chapter, women encounter specific stressors and are vulnerable to certain illnesses which ultimately contribute to their risk of cardiovascular disease. In particular, women are more likely than men to experience depression, anxiety, and abuse, which in turn, influences their heart health. Studies have shown that women are twice as likely to suffer from major depression during their lifetime as men [1]. In addition, this condition leads to many negative lifestyle choices, including sedentary behavior and smoking, as well as a failure to adhere to medical treatment. As a result, women with depression may have as much as a 50 % increased risk of experiencing adverse cardiac events [35].

The immense responsibilities placed on women in our society often lead to excess stress which may trigger depression. Depressed mood and social isolation are associated with damaging health behaviors such as cigarette smoking, poor diet and lack of exercise which are well known risk factors for coronary heart disease (CHD). Also, studies have demonstrated that depression makes women less compliant in taking their cardiovascular medications [36]. It is important that all women with heart disease are evaluated for depressive symptoms so they can be referred for treatment if necessary [27]. Roughly one in every eight woman can expect to develop clinical depression during their lifetime [37], with several factors unique to women, including developmental, reproductive, hormonal, genetic, and biological differences (e.g. premenstrual syndrome, childbirth, infertility and menopause) all contributing to its development. Approximately 10–15 % of all new mothers experience postpartum depression [38]. There is also a strong relationship between eating disorders (anorexia and bulimia nervosa) and depression in women. Research shows that one out of three people with the condition also suffer from some form of substance abuse or dependence [38].

Unfortunately, depression in women is misdiagnosed approximately 30–50 % of the time and fewer than half of the women suffering from it actually seek care [39]. However, clinical depression is a treatable illness which can be managed successfully with medication, psychotherapy or a combination of both. According to a Mental Health America survey on public attitudes and beliefs about clinical depression: More than one-half of women believe it is "normal" for a woman to be depressed during menopause and that treatment is not necessary [38]. More than one-half of women believe it is a "normal part of aging" and that it is normal for a mother to feel depressed for at least 2 weeks after giving birth [38]. More than one-half of women cited denial as a barrier to treatment while 41 % of women surveyed cited embarrassment or shame as barriers to treatment. In general, over one-half of the women said they think they "know" more about depression than men do [38].

Depression and the other unique psychosocial risk factors mentioned already in this chapter make women more prone to develop heart disease [40]. Both in cases with and without known cardiovascular disease, clinical evidence points to depression as a significant and independent predictor of morbidity and mortality in such individuals. In fact, heart disease is the leading cause of death among American women [41]. It is also important to realize the outcomes of women with heart disease are worse than in men. For example, women are more likely to die from a heart attack than men and 1-year mortality after a heart attack is greater in women [42]. The INTERHEART study was undertaken to determine risk factors for acute myocardial infarction stratified by different populations. Specifically, it investigated the association of psychosocial risk factors with risk of acute myocardial infarction (MI) in 11,119 cases and 13,648 controls from 52 countries [4]. One of the most significant findings of the INTERHEART study was the correlation between stress and the risk of MI. Episodic stress in the workplace or at home increased MI risk by 45 %, while sustained permanent stress increased risk by 117 % [4]. It also demonstrated that smoking, high cholesterol, diabetes, obesity, diet, high blood pressure, physical inactivity, alcohol consumption, and psychosocial factors account for over 90 % of the risk of heart attack [4]. Additional studies support the direct dose response between weight and high blood pressure, which is an important risk factor for cardiovascular disease [43]. It has been shown that by getting just moderate exercise, like walking daily, a woman can lower her risk of heart disease by 50 % [44, 45]. In addition, when designing treatment plans for women with established heart disease, some consideration must be taken into account of the different psychosocial roles that they may be involved in, such as being caretakers of children, aging sick parents, and older ill spouses, in addition to their work responsibilities, and the sometime overlapping nature of these responsibilities [46].

Often times, it is believed that health conditions that lead to an increased risk of heart disease are more prevalent among men. However, among Americans, the prevalence of diabetes is roughly the same in both men and women [47]. The same misconception may be said for elevated blood pressure, but according to national statistics, the same number of American women have hypertension as their male counterparts [48]. Among Americans over the age of 60, the percentage of women living in the United States with obesity is slightly greater than number of men who are obese [49]. Therefore, there are a great proportion of American women with serious co-morbidities such as high blood pressure, obesity, and diabetes which ultimately places them at a higher risk for sub-optimal heart health.

Although genetic factors play a large role in the state of health of an individual, there are many other controllable factors that women can modify to positively influence their state of health. For example, women can adopt a holistic approach and address different parts of health – mind, body, and soul. One easily modifiable risk factor to reduce a woman's chances of developing cardiovascular disease is cessation of smoking. An article from the American Journal of Public Health which looked at trends in mortality in U.S. women demonstrated that mortality disparities widened in review of recent data, in part, because of causes of death for which smoking is a major risk factor [50]. One of the major risk factors influencing death from heart disease is smoking. Therefore, by tirelessly encouraging smoking cessation, healthcare providers can hope to reduce the rates of cardiovascular disease among their female patients [27]. Adhering to a Mediterranean or low fat diet has also been shown to positively influence heart health [31, 51, 52]. Health interventions that target the common co-morbidities women have, such as high blood pressure or obesity, should also be initiated for secondary prevention.

Fig. 19.2 Six reasons that promote interest in the evaluation and management of psychosocial stress in cardiac practice (Adapted with permission from Rozanski et al. [15], figure 7)

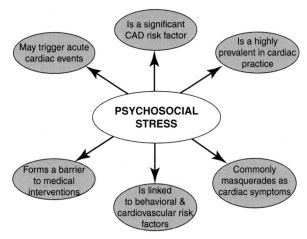

Summary

The link between ischemic heart disease in women and psychosocial factors is gaining more and more support as a result of accumulating clinical evidence. Research suggests there to be a strong link between psychosocial stress and all recognized mechanisms underlying cardiac events (clustering of traditional cardiovascular risk factors, endothelial dysfunction, myocardial ischemia, plaque rupture, thrombosis, and malignant arrhythmias). General acceptance of psychosocial stress as a nontraditional risk factor is becoming more widespread [12]. Further, there is increasingly greater interest in targeting the evaluation and management of psychosocial stress in cardiac practice because psychosocial stressors have such an immense impact on cardiovascular health in women (Fig. 19.2).

It is clear that women are not only affected by psychosocial factors such as depression, but that the typical contemporary woman who is balancing career and family responsibilities experiences a unique kind of stress that might be described as female role overload. It is especially important to utilize current evidence to both identify those women who are at increased risk of coronary heart disease (CHD) as a result of depression or stress (associated with multiple roles, including responsibilities at work, home, caregiving responsibilities, lack of personal time, sleep deprivation, fatigue, etc.), and to create interventions that take these psychological factors into consideration in treatment options for both those with CHD and those at risk. It is important to keep in mind that adherence to treatment and prevention recommendations in women may be affected by these same female role overload factors.

We want to emphasize the importance of an early and a multidisciplinary approach to keep women healthy in order to prevent deleterious consequences in the future. It is of great importance for healthcare providers to identify which populations they should focus their attention on to promote cardiovascular health. For example, effort should be placed on identifying woman who are depressed [53]. We know that women are much more likely than men to suffer from depression and anxiety. We also know that women face a challenging set of both acute and chronic, negative and positive stressors over the span of their lifetime which ultimately shapes their heart health. Research has shown that at risk women over 45 years of age who are informed about their condition are more likely to be motivated to modify their cardiovascular risk factors [54]. Steps to ameliorate the effects of stress on a woman's health should be taken by women and their healthcare providers for primary prevention. Integrative medicine and a holistic cardiac care approach in women must be employed. A recent study evaluating a holistic cardiac rehabilitation program in reducing biopsychosocial risk factors among patients with coronary heart disease demonstrated a reduction in perceived stress, depression, and cholesterol levels among patients cared for using a holistic approach [55]. In the future, it will be essential to focus on assisting women to increase their social support, address their spirituality, treat their depression, reduce the hostility they encounter at work, and boost their overall health status and life satisfaction.

Healthcare providers should have a heightened awareness of depression in women and try to recognize subclinical depression so that it can be treated appropriately. They should provide education and support to encourage cessation of smoking. Incentives to adopt healthier lifestyles including a dedicated exercise regimen, healthy diet, and mechanisms to alleviate stress should also be emphasized. There is an increased need for awareness of cardiovascular disease as a major public health issue for women [56, 57]. Further, emphasis should be placed on primary prevention of cardiovascular disease in women given the number of women it affects. The importance of behavioral factors has been included in the latest ESC guidelines for CVD prevention [58], but a more gender-specific approach for cardiology patients will be needed in the education and training of healthcare providers.

References

1. Low CA, Thurston RC, Matthews KA. Psychosocial factors in the development of heart disease in women: current research and future directions. Psychosom Med. 2010;72(9):842–54.
2. Friedman HS, Booth-Kewley S. Personality, type A behavior, and coronary heart disease: the role of emotional expression. J Pers Soc Psychol. 1987;53(4):783–92.
3. Marcovecchio ML, Chiarelli F. The effects of acute and chronic stress on diabetes control. Sci Signal. 2012;5(247):pt10.
4. Rosengren A, Hawken S, Ounpuu S, et al. Association of psychosocial risk factors with risk of acute myocardial infarction in 11119 cases and 13648 controls from 52 countries (the INTERHEART study): case–control study. Lancet. 2004;364(9438):953–62.
5. Chikani V, Reding D, Gunderson P, McCarty CA. Psychosocial work characteristics predict cardiovascular disease risk factors and health functioning in rural women: the Wisconsin Rural Women's Health Study. J Rural Health. 2005;21(4):295–302.
6. Kivimaki M, Kawachi I. Need for more individual-level meta-analyses in social epidemiology: example of job strain and coronary heart disease. Am J Epidemiol. 2013;177(1):1–2.
7. Kivimaki M, Nyberg ST, Batty GD, et al. Job strain as a risk factor for coronary heart disease: a collaborative meta-analysis of individual participant data. Lancet. 2012;380(9852): 1491–7.

8. Schuster PM, Waldron J. Gender differences in cardiac rehabilitation patients. Rehabil Nurs. 1991;16(5):248–53.
9. Lee S, Colditz GA, Berkman LF, Kawachi I. Caregiving and risk of coronary heart disease in U.S. women: a prospective study. Am J Prev Med. 2003;24(2):113–9.
10. Sperlich S, Arnhold-Kerri S, Geyer S. What accounts for depressive symptoms among mothers? The impact of socioeconomic status, family structure and psychosocial stress. Int J Public Health. 2011;56(4):385–96.
11. U.S. Department of Health and Human Services Office on Minority Health. http://minorityhealth.hhs.gov/templates/browse.aspx?lvl=1&lvlID=2.
12. Bairey Merz CN, Dwyer J, Nordstrom CK, Walton KG, Salerno JW, Schneider RH. Psychosocial stress and cardiovascular disease: pathophysiological links. Behav Med. 2002;27(4):141–7.
13. Williams Jr RB, Barefoot JC, Haney TL, et al. Type A behavior and angiographically documented coronary atherosclerosis in a sample of 2,289 patients. Psychosom Med. 1988; 50(2):139–52.
14. Glasser SP, Selwyn AP, Ganz P. Atherosclerosis: risk factors and the vascular endothelium. Am Heart J. 1996;131(2):379–84.
15. Rozanski A, Blumenthal JA, Davidson KW, Saab PG, Kubzansky L. The epidemiology, pathophysiology, and management of psychosocial risk factors in cardiac practice: the emerging field of behavioral cardiology. J Am Coll Cardiol. 2005;45(5):637–51.
16. Maas AH, van der Schouw YT, Regitz-Zagrosek V, et al. Red alert for women's heart: the urgent need for more research and knowledge on cardiovascular disease in women: proceedings of the workshop held in Brussels on gender differences in cardiovascular disease, 29 September 2010. Eur Heart J. 2011;32(11):1362–8.
17. Muller JE, Stone PH, Turi ZG, et al. Circadian variation in the frequency of onset of acute myocardial infarction. N Engl J Med. 1985;313(21):1315–22.
18. Mittleman MA, Maclure M, Sherwood JB, et al. Triggering of acute myocardial infarction onset by episodes of anger. Determinants of Myocardial Infarction Onset Study Investigators. Circulation. 1995;92(7):1720–5.
19. Bairey CN, Krantz DS, Rozanski A. Mental stress as an acute trigger of ischemic left ventricular dysfunction and blood pressure elevation in coronary artery disease. Am J Cardiol. 1990;66(16):28G–31.
20. Levine SP, Towell BL, Suarez AM, Knieriem LK, Harris MM, George JN. Platelet activation and secretion associated with emotional stress. Circulation. 1985;71(6):1129–34.
21. Carroll D, Ebrahim S, Tilling K, Macleod J, Smith GD. Admissions for myocardial infarction and World Cup football: database survey. BMJ. 2002;325(7378):1439–42.
22. Rosenman KD. Sudden cardiac death triggered by an earthquake. N Engl J Med. 1996; 334(25):1673.
23. Rozanski A, Blumenthal JA, Kaplan J. Impact of psychological factors on the pathogenesis of cardiovascular disease and implications for therapy. Circulation. 1999;99(16):2192–217.
24. Epel ES, Blackburn EH, Lin J, et al. Accelerated telomere shortening in response to life stress. Proc Natl Acad Sci U S A. 2004;101(49):17312–5.
25. Humphreys J, Epel ES, Cooper BA, Lin J, Blackburn EH, Lee KA. Telomere shortening in formerly abused and never abused women. Biol Res Nurs. 2012;14(2):115–23.
26. Jacobs TL, Epel ES, Lin J, et al. Intensive meditation training, immune cell telomerase activity, and psychological mediators. Psychoneuroendocrinology. 2011;36(5):664–81.
27. Mosca L, Appel LJ, Benjamin EJ, et al. Evidence-based guidelines for cardiovascular disease prevention in women. J Am Coll Cardiol. 2004;43(5):900–21.
28. Mosca L, Edelman D, Mochari H, Christian AH, Paultre F, Pollin I. Waist circumference predicts cardiometabolic and global Framingham risk among women screened during National Woman's Heart Day. J Womens Health (Larchmt). 2006;15(1):24–34.
29. Esposito K, Marfella R, Ciotola M, et al. Effect of a mediterranean-style diet on endothelial dysfunction and markers of vascular inflammation in the metabolic syndrome: a randomized trial. JAMA. 2004;292(12):1440–6.

30. Hu FB, Willett WC. Optimal diets for prevention of coronary heart disease. JAMA. 2002;288(20):2569–78.
31. Knoops KT, de Groot LC, Kromhout D, et al. Mediterranean diet, lifestyle factors, and 10-year mortality in elderly European men and women: the HALE project. JAMA. 2004;292(12): 1433–9.
32. Liang JJ, Cha YM, Oh JK, Prasad A. Sudden cardiac death: an increasingly recognized presentation of apical ballooning syndrome (Takotsubo cardiomyopathy). Heart Lung. 2013;42(4): 270–2.
33. Akashi YJ, Goldstein DS, Barbaro G, Ueyama T. Takotsubo cardiomyopathy: a new form of acute, reversible heart failure. Circulation. 2008;118(25):2754–62.
34. Sy F, Basraon J, Zheng H, Singh M, Richina J, Ambrose JA. Frequency of Takotsubo cardiomyopathy in postmenopausal women presenting with an acute coronary syndrome. Am J Cardiol. 2013;112(4):479–82.
35. Vaccarino V, Badimon L, Corti R, et al. Ischaemic heart disease in women: are there sex differences in pathophysiology and risk factors? Position paper from the working group on coronary pathophysiology and microcirculation of the European Society of Cardiology. Cardiovasc Res. 2011;90(1):9–17.
36. Bane C, Hughes CM, McElnay JC. The impact of depressive symptoms and psychosocial factors on medication adherence in cardiovascular disease. Patient Educ Couns. 2006;60(2): 187–93.
37. National Institute of Mental Health. http://www.nimh.nih.gov/statistics/1mdd_adult.shtml. Statistics on women and depression.
38. Mental Health America. http://www.nmha.org/index.cfm?objectid=C7DF952E-1372-4D20-C8A3DDCD5459D07BDEPRESSIONINWOMEN.
39. Blehar MC, Keita GP. Women and depression: a millennial perspective. J Affect Disord. 2003;74(1):1–4.
40. Wenger NK. Coronary heart disease in men and women: does 1 size fit all? No! Clin Cardiol. 2011;34(11):663–7.
41. Minino AM, Murphy SL, Xu J, Kochanek KD. Deaths: final data for 2008. Natl Vital Stat Rep. 2011;59(10):1–126.
42. Wenger NK. An update on coronary heart disease in women. Int J Fertil Womens Med. 1998;43(2):84–90.
43. Stevens VJ, Obarzanek E, Cook NR, et al. Long-term weight loss and changes in blood pressure: results of the Trials of Hypertension Prevention, phase II. Ann Intern Med. 2001;134(1):1–11.
44. Blair SN, Kohl 3rd HW, Paffenbarger Jr RS, Clark DG, Cooper KH, Gibbons LW. Physical fitness and all-cause mortality. A prospective study of healthy men and women. JAMA. 1989;262(17):2395–401.
45. Thompson PD, Buchner D, Pina IL, et al. Exercise and physical activity in the prevention and treatment of atherosclerotic cardiovascular disease: a statement from the Council on Clinical Cardiology (Subcommittee on Exercise, Rehabilitation, and Prevention) and the Council on Nutrition, Physical Activity, and Metabolism (Subcommittee on Physical Activity). Circulation. 2003;107(24):3109–16.
46. Wenger NK, Speroff L, Packard B. Cardiovascular health and disease in women. N Engl J Med. 1993;329(4):247–56.
47. National Center for Health Statistics. Health, United States, 2012: With Special Feature on Emergency Care. Hyattsville. 2013.
48. Yoon SS, Burt V, Louis T, Carroll MD. Hypertension among adults in the United States, 2009–2010. NCHS Data Brief. 2012;107:1–8.
49. Ogden CL, Carroll MD, Kit BK, Flegal KM. Prevalence of obesity in the United States, 2009–2010. NCHS Data Brief. 2012;82:1–8.
50. Montez JK, Zajacova A. Trends in mortality risk by education level and cause of death among US White women from 1986 to 2006. Am J Public Health. 2013;103(3):473–9.

51. Fuentes F, Lopez-Miranda J, Sanchez E, et al. Mediterranean and low-fat diets improve endothelial function in hypercholesterolemic men. Ann Intern Med. 2001;134(12):1115–9.
52. Joshipura KJ, Hu FB, Manson JE, et al. The effect of fruit and vegetable intake on risk for coronary heart disease. Ann Intern Med. 2001;134(12):1106–14.
53. Cyranowski JM, Schott LL, Kravitz HM, et al. Psychosocial features associated with lifetime comorbidity of major depression and anxiety disorders among a community sample of mid-life women: the SWAN mental health study. Depress Anxiety. 2012;29(12):1050–7.
54. Galbraith EM, Mehta PK, Veledar E, Vaccarino V, Wenger NK. Women and heart disease: knowledge, worry, and motivation. J Womens Health (Larchmt). 2011;20(10):1529–34.
55. Kreikebaum S, Guarneri E, Talavera G, Madanat H, Smith T. Evaluation of a holistic cardiac rehabilitation in the reduction of biopsychosocial risk factors among patients with coronary heart disease. Psychol Health Med. 2011;16(3):276–90.
56. Wenger NK. Addressing coronary heart disease risk in women. Cleve Clin J Med. 1998;65(9):464–9.
57. Wenger NK. The female heart is vulnerable to cardiovascular disease: emerging prevention evidence for women must inform emerging prevention strategies for women. Circ Cardiovasc Qual Outcomes. 2010;3(2):118–9.
58. Perk J, De Backer G, Gohlke H, et al. European Guidelines on cardiovascular disease prevention in clinical practice (version 2012). The Fifth Joint Task Force of the European Society of Cardiology and Other Societies on Cardiovascular Disease Prevention in Clinical Practice (constituted by representatives of nine societies and by invited experts). Eur Heart J. 2012;33(13):1635–701.

Chapter 20
Pharmacotherapy Considerations in Cardiovascular Disease in Women: Therapeutic Implications for Cardiovascular Disease

Justin Tinsley, Gladys P. Velarde, and Marci DeLosSantos

Introduction

Cardiovascular disease (CVD) claims almost as many women's lives as the next five diseases states in combination [1]. Furthermore, women who sustain a myocardial infarction (MI) have higher morbidity and mortality compared with men. Typically the higher risk is within the first 30 days of MI however some studies have shown the higher risk in women to be present for up to 1 year [2]. Due to the higher risk of morbidity and mortality it is imperative that clinicians treat women with effective and evidence based therapeutic regimens. Based on guidelines, patients with heart disease should be prescribed a myriad of medications from anti-hypertensives, lipid lowering medications, anticoagulants and/or anti-arrhythmics. Due to lack of therapeutic studies in special populations and or misunderstanding of the available data, women and elderly patients are less likely to receive these vital medications, even when coronary artery disease is documented or after myocardial infarction [3]. The limited therapeutic interventional studies performed in women have contributed to some of the confusion, but the studies available suggest that women benefit as much or more than men in some instances.

The question remains whether or not these medications work similarly in both genders.

Published trials have revealed differences in efficacy and adverse drug effects in a number of major cardiovascular medications. In general, women experience greater risk of adverse reactions to medications compared to men [4]. This has been

J. Tinsley, PharmD • M. DeLosSantos, PharmD, BCPS (AQ Card)
Department of Pharmacy, University of Florida Health – Jacksonville, Jacksonville, FL, USA

G.P. Velarde, MD, FACC (✉)
Division of Cardiology, University of Florida College of Medicine-Jacksonville,
ACC Building 5th Floor, 655 West 8th Street, Jacksonville, FL 32209, USA
e-mail: gladys.velarde@jax.ufl.edu

H.Z. Mieszczanska, G.P. Velarde (eds.), 427
Management of Cardiovascular Disease in Women,
DOI 10.1007/978-1-4471-5517-1_20, © Springer-Verlag London 2014

consistently been reported for ACE inhibitors, thrombolytic therapy, digoxin, and QT prolonging medications.

Knowledge of gender related physiological, pharmacokinetics, and pharmacodynamics differences of the most important treatment modalities for coronary disease is critical and may have significant impact on the clinical response and outcomes seen in women compared to men [5]. This chapter will review some of the biological differences in pharmacokinetics and pharmacodynamics seen in women, specifically as it relates to some of the most common medications used to treat coronary disease.

Limitations in Assessing Differences in Drug Effect

Several factors need to be taken into account when analyzing differences in drug effects between men and women (Table 20.1). In general non-biological and biological factors account for the majority of the differences. A non-biological factor is the process of drug development which does not include diverse populations which are seen in every day practice. The drug development process typically begins with young male animal models of a well selected-genetic background which are kept in a pathogen free environment that precludes interaction of drug effects with an activated immune system. Furthermore, phase 1 and phase 2 trials include mostly young men preventing systemic development of adequate doses for the elderly and women in particular. Well described biological differences exist in pharmacokinetics and pharmacodynamics between men and women that clearly impact the efficacy and adverse effects of medications [6].

When reviewing the existing literature, it is evident that women are underrepresented in clinical trials as stated previously, the reasons for this are multifactorial and beyond the scope of this discussion [7]. Recently, the National institutes of Health has committed to a strategic plan to ensure more women are enrolled in clinical studies. The goals for women's research for 2020 include "increasing sex

Table 20.1 Factors contributing to gender differences in drug effects [8]

Non-biological	Biological
Drug development process	**Pharmacokinetics**
Mainly done in young male animals of well selected genetic background	Body composition
	Weight
Reductionist approach	Absorption
Clinical phase 1 and 2 trials mainly include young men	Drug distribution
	Metabolic enzymes
	Routes of excretion
	Pharmacodynamics
	Gender differences in:
	Blood flow to different organs
	Ion channel composition in different organs

Table 20.2 Women Health 2020 goals [8]

Office of Research on Women's Health 2020 goals
National Institutes of Health
U.S. Department of Health & Human Services:
Increase sex differences research in basic science studies
Incorporate findings of sex/gender differences in the design and application of new technologies, medical devices, and therapeutic drugs
Actualize personalized prevention, diagnostics, and therapeutics for girls and women
Create strategic alliances and partnerships to maximize the domestic and global impact of Women's Health Research
Develop and implement new communication and social networking technologies to increase understanding and appreciation of Women's Health and Wellness Research
Employ innovative strategies to build a well-trained, diverse, and vigorous Women's Health Research Workforce

Physiologic gender differences: Adapted from: http://orwh.od.nih.gov/research/strategicplan/index.asp

difference research in basic science studies" as well as "incorporating findings of sex/gender differences in the design and application of new technologies, medical devices, and therapeutic drugs (Table 20.2)" [8]. With the completion of these goals, we hope to gain more knowledge regarding adequate dosing and efficacy of major therapeutic interventions.

A number of physiologic differences exist between men and women that in part explain differences in drug effect. Gender differences have been found in regard to blood flow to different organ systems in human and animal models. Males have been shown to have more blood flow to the kidneys and muscle tissue whereas women have more blood flow distributed to adipose tissue and liver. In regards to the heart women have been shown to have a 5 % of blood flow distribution versus 4 % for men but this difference accentuates with pregnancy [9]. Women also have been noted to have higher heart rates at rest, shorter sinus recovery time and longer corrected QT intervals compared with men [5]. Differences in gender hormones may explain some of these findings, but the precise mechanism is not well understood.

These physiological differences between men and women can affect how a medication is absorbed, metabolized and ultimately excreted from the body which describes the processes of pharmacokinetics and pharmacodynamics that will be review below.

Pharmacokinetics in Women

Pharmacokinetics describes what happens to a drug after it has been administered. This includes drug absorption, distribution and elimination or excretion [10, 11]. The goal of any therapeutic agent is to enhance efficacy and minimize toxicity

[10, 11]. Therefore pharmacokinetics allows us to safely manage medications by predicting the concentrations in the body and maintaining appropriate therapeutic efficacy.

In order for a medication to reach its site of action, the medication needs to be absorbed. Medication absorption is affected by many different factors including route. Differences in drug route could play a role in the amount of drug that is allowed into the body and the length of time in which a drug takes to reach its desired target organ or receptor. The oral route is much slower compared to other routes such as intravenous or sublingual. For example, consider the use of nitroglycerin for a patient that is experiencing angina. At the first sign of chest pain sublingual nitroglycerin may be given to ensure continued and appropriate blood flow to the heart. By applying the medication under the tongue rather than digesting the tablet orally we allow for quicker response of nitric oxide release therefore faster onset of action and greater efficacy. Oral nitrate tablets have shown much slower time to effect.

Absorption times can be affected by other factors other than route. When comparing absorption rates, women have longer gastrointestinal transit times compared with men, approximately 91.7 h in women and 44.8 h in men and therefore bioavailability of a medication may be greater in women [12–14]. Women also appear to have less gastric acidity therefore absorption of certain medications may be altered. Due to the difference in acidity, there will be decrease absorption for weak acids and increase absorption for weak bases in women [15]. Additionally, women have a smaller body surface and less cardiac output compared to men which may decrease absorption of some medications as well [15]. Once a medication is absorbed, it needs to travel to its site of action. The concept of a medication getting to its site of action is volume of distribution. Factors that affect volume of distribution are protein binding, molecular size of medications, and whether a medication is lipophilic or hydrophilic. In general, no differences have been found between men and women in regards to protein binding [15]. However it has been shown that volume of distribution is decreased in women compare to men. This decrease is thought to be secondary to women having lower total body water, lower intra- and extracellular water, and lower total blood volume. Therefore there will be higher concentrations of water soluble medications in females and potentially an increase in a woman's clinical response to a water soluble medication [15, 16]. An example of this is atenolol which has been shown to have better blood pressure lowering effects compared to men secondary to the lower volume of distribution [10]. Furthermore, women have a higher percentage of body fat in relationship to total body weight compared to men [17]. In general, body weight increases from young adulthood to the age of 60. After 60, the overall body size decreases and fat in women increases [18]. Therefore, lipid soluble medications, such as benzodiazepines, could distribute to more areas of the body and thereby increasing the effect of the medication in women [12, 16].

After a medication is distributed it is metabolized to allow it to exert its effect. The main site of metabolism is the liver via the cytochrome 450 systems; however other sites of metabolism include the lungs, kidneys, skin, and gastrointestinal tract [13]. There is conflicting information about gender differences in drug metabolism.

Table 20.3 Pathway/rate of metabolism (not all inclusive) from: (1) Jochmann et al. [5]. (2) Soldin et al. [13]. (3) Stephen et al. [14] (4) Schwartz [18]

CYP1A2	CYP2C9	CYP2C19	CYP2D6	CYP3A4
M>F/M=F	**M=F**	**M=F**	**M>F**	**M<F**
Clomipramine	Ibuprofen	Diazepam	Codeine	Alprazolam
Acetaminophen	Warfarin	Omeprazole	Flecainide	Atorvastatin
Clozapine	Fluvastatin	Citalopram	Fluoxetine	Diltiazem
Olanzapine	Glipizide	Irbesartan	Metoprolol	Lovastatin
Theophylline	Losartan	Celecoxib	Mexiletine	Quinidine
Clopidogrel	Phenytoin		Propranolol	Verapamil
Propranolol	Torsemide		Haloperidol	Simvastatin
				Amiodarone
				Amlodipine

Even though there is large variation in metabolism of medications, most gender related differences appear to be eliminated by controlling for height, weight, surface area, and body composition [13]. One study by Bebia et al. indicates that the CYP1A system showed decrease clearance of up to 10–20 % in women compared to men. However, another study showed no difference in clearance [5]. Given the conflicting findings, it is postulated that other environmental factors may explain the difference seen in this system. Factors such as diet, smoking, and alcohol use indeed seem to play a role. Furthermore, no consistent gender-related difference in clearance in regards to CYP2C pathway has been shown. The CYP2D6 system has been shown to manifest slower clearance in women compared to men and therefore it has been suggested that the dose of medications that are metabolized through this pathway may need to be reduced by 10–20 %. The CYP3A system was shown by Wolbold et al. to have 15–35 % faster clearance in women suggesting that medications metabolized by this enzyme such as verapamil, nifedipine, and amlodipine may need higher dosing [5, 13, 14, 18]. Table 20.3 summarizes these findings.

Once the medication has been used by the body, it needs to be removed. Excretion is final route by which drug metabolites are removed from the body and is primarily handled by the kidneys [13]. The primary technique by which excretion is measured is called clearance. Clearance is defined as a hypothetical volume of distribution of the unmetabolized drug which is cleared per unit of time (ml/min or ml/h) by any pathway of drug removal (renal, hepatic (or) other pathway of elimination) [19]. It has well been established that renal clearance decreases with age. Similarly, several drug trials have shown that women have lower clearance at all ages compared to men [13]. Werner and colleagues also demonstrated that women have less elimination of certain loop diuretics, torsemide specifically, thus leading to higher adverse reactions (ADRs) in women compared to men [20]. For example in a German Pharmacovigilance Project, 66 % of hospitalizations due to torasemide ADRs occurred in women [20]. It is thus critically important to consider women's decreased renal clearance when prescribing medications that are primarily eliminated by the kidney, especially if a toxic metabolite is formed when the medication is metabolized.

Table 20.4 Metabolism during pregnancy

Metabolism	First trimester	Second trimester	Third trimester
CYP 1A2	Dec 33 %	Dec 50 %	Dec 60 %
CYP 2A6	–	Inc 54 %	Inc 54 %
CYP 2A9	No change	No change	Inc 20 %
CYP 2C19	–	Dec 50 %	Dec 50 %
CYP 2D6	–	–	Inc 50 %
CYP 3A4	–	–	Inc 50 – 100 %
Renal	Inc 20–65 %	Inc 20–65 %	Inc 20–65 %

Adapted from: Anderson and Carr [21]

Pharmacokinetic Changes During Pregnancy

Pharmacokinetic studies have shown metabolism of medications via the cytochrome P450 system are altered during pregnancy as summarized in Table 20.4 [21]. As pregnancy progresses, metabolism progressively decreases through the 1A2 pathway. In the third trimester 1A2 and 2C19 activity decreases, 60 and 50 % respectively. However 2A6 increases 54 %, 2A9 increases 20 %, 2D6 increase 50 %, and 3A4 increases 50–100 %. In addition renal metabolism increases 20–65 % in each trimester [21].

A review by Anderson and Carr in the late 1980s and early 1990s estimated that approximately 12 % of women had hypertension during pregnancy [21]. It is expected that this number has increased significantly and therefore the amount of medications used to treat hypertension has also increased. The primary medication used to treat hypertension is methyldopa due to its decreased risk on the fetus (pregnancy category B) [22]. Other treatments which are used less frequency are clonidine, hydralazine, beta blockers and calcium channel blockers [17]. Since atenolol, furosemide and methyldopa are greater than 90, 60–90 and 50 % renally eliminated respectively, we would anticipate that there would be less effect on blood pressure with higher renal clearance as the pregnancy progresses. Nevertheless given decreased fetal risk, methyldopa is favored for BP control during pregnancy. Furthermore, diltiazem and nifedipine are mainly metabolized by CYP 3A4 and metoprolol is mainly metabolized by 2D6, therefore these medications may have less effect of blood pressure during the third trimester since the 3A4 and 2D6 pathways have increased activity during the third trimester [21].

Role of Genetic Polymorphism

Genetic Polymorphism may modify drug response. In the cardiovascular field, this has been associated with the metabolism of beta blockers and calcium channel blockers and response to ACE inhibitors. Some cardiovascular phenotypes are

Table 20.5 Gender differences in drug effects of some common medications (not inclusive)

Adverse effects	Trend towards benefit	Require dose adaptation
Digoxin (^ mortality) in women with heart failure	Calcium channel blockers – amlodipine	BB – metoprolol
QT prolonging drugs (^ Torsades)	Ramipril	CCB – verapamil
ACE I (^ cough)	Eplerenone	

associated with autosomal gene polymorphisms that have been shown to manifest gender differences in drug response [23]. Examples of these are shown in Table 20.5. Genes located in the X chromosome are also good candidates to account for some gender differences. Carrel and Willard among others have extensively studied how mutations in these genes or functionally related polymorphisms might be better compensated in women [24]. For example genes for Angiotensin Converting Enzyme −2 (ACE-2) and angiotensin II receptor (ATR2) are located in the X chromosome [25]. The AT2R has been shown to modulate left ventricular hypertrophy in women with HCM independently of the circulating RAS but this has not been shown in men. Studies have suggested that LV mass in women is in part regulated by number of specific alleles of the AT2R gene [26]. In Transgenic mice models a more severe cardiovascular phenotype was seen in male rather than female animals and this correlated to earlier development of and faster progression to heart failure [27]. Interestingly, a variety of factors and complex interactions ranging from diet, sex hormonal influences, removal of ovaries and administration of exogenous estrogen, or age, seem to change gene expression adding to the complexity of the pathways that lead to gender differences in drug responses [28].

Role of Sex Hormones

Estrogens and progestins interacts with a large number of cardiovascular drugs possibly by inhibiting CYP enzymes or increasing drug glucuronidation [5]. Menstrual cycle, pregnancy, and menopause can modify this interaction due to variation of levels of estrogen and other hormones, alterations in total body water due to renal plasma flow variations and changes in glomerular filtration during these specific periods for women. For example, it has been reported that menstruation, pregnancy and, ovariectomy can modulate CYP2D6 activity [29]. The clinical relevance of these changes is not clear. Interactions with exogenous hormone therapy such as hormone replacement therapy (HRT) and oral contraceptives must also be taken into account. Estrogens seem to interfere with the synthesis of Angiotensinogen in the liver and also with the expression of Angiotensin I receptor (ATR-1) in the myocardium [30]. On the other hand estrogens appear to increase the expression of AT2R in the myocardium. In the cardiovascular system, progesterones appear to have a partially synergistic and/ or antagonistic relationship with estrogens [31]. In some animal models (ovariectomized rabbits), progesterone was seen to exert a direct inhibitory effect on the atheroprotective action of estrogen [31], while in other models (ischemic rats) progesterone has been shown to have cardioprotective effects but only in female ischemic rats. These findings suggest complex interactions with endogenous estrogen.

Gender differences in drug metabolism can in part be explained by the dismorphic expression of CYP450 and other liver-expressed genes (females predominantly express CYP3A4). This expression is in part regulated by GH (Growth Hormone) release by the pituitary gland which shows significant gender difference in its pattern of release [32]

Pharmacodynamics in Women

Pharmacodynamics describes the principle of drug action and its resulting effect at its target site, i.e. receptor or membrane [10]. This concept is often used to examine overall maximum effect of a drug and/or the sensitivity of the target area to the drug concentration [11]. Current literature regarding differences of pharmacodynamics between men and women is limited. Most pharmacodynamic data deals primarily with the elderly. Despite the lack of pharmacodynamic studies in women we can hypothesize that there may be differences in drug response due to gender by evaluating adverse drug reports.

Currently, the Food and Drug Administration (FDA) holds a database in which patients and providers can voluntarily document adverse events. The reporting system is known as FAERS (FDA Adverse Event Reporting System) which allows the FDA to monitor medication and report post-marketing data to the public [33]. A study by Moore et al. examined adverse event data from FAERS between 1998 and 2005. In their analysis they found that more women had adverse events (55.5 %) compared to men (45.5 %) and the adverse effects were more serious in women [15]. When age was closely examined patients between 45 and 64 years old had 33.7 % of the events which accounted for 22.2 % of the total population. Individuals that were greater than or equal to 65 years old were found to have 33.6 % of the adverse events but only accounted for 12.6 % of the total population. Of the cardiovascular drugs that totaled 500, more adverse events in any year were reported in women. HMG-CoA reductase inhibitors (statins) were associated with the most issues. Cerivastatin, which was later withdrawn from the market, was found to have 1,573 events [34]. Furthermore, out of 10 medications that were withdrawn from market during 1997 and 2000, 8 were withdrawn secondary to greater adverse effects in women [15]. In general women have a 1.5- to 1.7-fold greater risk of developing an adverse drug reaction. The reasons for this increased risk are not entirely clear but include gender-related differences in pharmacokinetics already discussed, immunological and hormonal factors as well as differences in the use of medications by women compared with men, polypharmacy and increasing age.

Gender Differences Within Specific Medication Classes and Medications

Beta Blockers

Gender-specific differences in the pharmacokinetics of beta-blockers lead to greater drug exposure in women [35]. The pharmacokinetics differences can be due to lower volume of distribution and slower clearance. Furthermore, pharmacodynamic differences may be secondary to estrogen deficiency in older women which can modulate the up regulation of beta receptors therefore more receptors to exert its effect [5]. Hormone supplementation with estrogens and progestins can prevent such upregulation [36]. Since sex hormones can modulate the regulation of beta adrenergic receptors in the heart and vessels, gender specific differences in the pharmacodynamics of beta receptor blockers are to be expected [5]. Gender differences have been described for response to cardio selective and non-selective beta blockers. Men have greater clearance of both selective and non-selective beta blockers leading to faster clearance of these drugs compared to women [35]. Higher beta-blocker plasma levels in women translates into a more pronounced decrease in heart rate and systolic blood pressure than men [35].

Women have been a minority in heart failure clinical trials testing beta-blockers, representing 20–30 % in the first major trials [37]. Two major trials, the MERIT Heart Failure study and the COPERNICUS trial, failed to find a beneficial effect on mortality in women [38, 39]. In a detailed gender-specific *post-hoc* analysis for the CIBIS II study, women profited significantly from treatment with bisoprolol which had a greater unadjusted effect on all-cause mortality in women than in men [40]. Pooling of mortality results from MERIT Heart Failure, CIBIS II and COPERNICUS showed survival benefits in both women and men [41] (Fig. 20.1). The lack of evidence in some large beta-blocker studies is therefore probably due to the under representation of women in these trials.

Findings of beta-blocker therapy in secondary prevention after myocardial infarction have revealed conflicting findings with respect to gender specific differences. However, most of these studies have not included sufficient number of women to enable definitive conclusions [42]. A meta-analysis of more than 5,000 patients (1,121 women) investigating effect of metoprolol post myocardial infarction showed that reduction of cardiovascular death was comparable in women and men [43]. Similarly, the ISIS-I and ISIS-II trials demonstrated that improved survival in women receiving beta blockers and aspirin was comparable to that in men [44, 45].

In summary, beta blockers are effective for women in ischemic heart disease and heart failure, though data is not as extensive and as solid as it is for men. Caution should be exercised in dosing beta-blockers in women as they tend to be poor metabolizers leading to higher plasma concentration of these drugs compared to men.

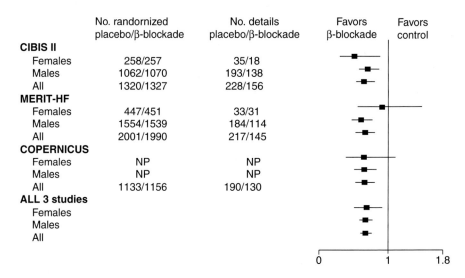

	No. randomized placebo/β-blockade	No. details placebo/β-blockade	Favors β-blockade	Favors control
CIBIS II				
Females	258/257	35/18		
Males	1062/1070	193/138		
All	1320/1327	228/156		
MERIT-HF				
Females	447/451	33/31		
Males	1554/1539	184/114		
All	2001/1990	217/145		
COPERNICUS				
Females	NP	NP		
Males	NP	NP		
All	1133/1156	190/130		
ALL 3 studies				
Females				
Males				
All				

Fig. 20.1 Relative risk ratios and 95 % confidence intervals for total mortality in women and men, in studies evaluating the impact of B-blockade in heart failure (Adapted with permission from Jochmann et al. [5])

ACE Inhibitors and ARBs

The Renin-Angiotensin System (RAS) is a key regulator of blood pressure Endogenous RAS activity differs between men and women [46]. Gender differences may also be seen with medications that work against the RAS. Estrogens increase angiotensin II (Ang II) plasma levels, leading to a decrease of angiotensin converting enzyme (ACE) and renin activity via negative feedback. Therefore estrogens net effect is to decrease the activity of the RAS, leading to less effect when using angiotensin converting enzyme inhibitors (ACE-I) or angiotensin receptor blockers (ARB) [46]. Subsequently, premenopausal women show lower ACE activity than post-menopausal women but this difference is abolished in woman taking exogenous estrogen [47].

ACE-I (and more recently ARBs) have been part of evidence-based therapy for heart failure and hypertension for decades. Several multicenter studies, e.g. CONSENSUS I, SAVE, and SOLVD, have shown a much smaller mortality reduction in women compared to men. However it is now recognized that these findings were likely due to the small percentage of women included in those trials [48]. Later trials, including a meta-analysis of more than 7,000 patients in 1995, have shown comparable benefits in women and men [49]. However, on the basis of the small proportion of women included in ACE-I studies, data for women are less advantageous than for men and the question of less benefit from this therapy based on gender remains unanswered. Although animal models have shown gender differences in response to Ang II even during endogenous blockade of the ACE system, this has not been consistently seen in human studies [47].

Relevant gender-specific pharmacokinetic differences have not been described for ACE-I captopril or lisinopril, however, higher plasma levels have been seen to occur in women than in men with fixed doses of ramipril [50, 51]. Furthermore, there have not been any clinical differences in the effects of ACEI and ARBs between women and men despite higher concentrations in women. In regards to adverse effects, there is a 1.5 to 2 fold higher chance women will experience a cough when compared to men, however there is no difference in the incidence of angioedema or urticarial between the two [51]. Genetic polymorphisms in the bradykinin receptors seem to be associated with ACE-I induced cough [52].

Although clinical data has not shown major gender differences concerning the effects of angiotensin receptor blockers (ARBs), experimental data suggest sex-specific differences in response to RAS activation. Ang II, the main effector of RAS, acts via two main receptors, with AT1-R causing primarily vasoconstriction and with AT2-R causing vasodilation [53, 54]. In the rat model, Sampson and colleagues demonstrated that chronic AT2-R blockade caused a greater hypotensive effect in female compared to male rats [55]. Similarly, other investigators hypothesized that female sex shifts balance of RAS towards primarily vasodilation through observations of decreased expression of AT1-R and up-regulation of AT2-R expression with estrogens as well as increased expression of AT1-R in ovariectomized rodents [56]. This enhanced vasodilator pathway of the RAS may be one mechanism for the apparent cardiovascular protection seen in premenopausal females. Major clinical trials have investigated the effects of AT1-R blockers in hypertension, heart failure, and after myocardial infarction, and a clear therapeutic role against cardiovascular disease has been seen. These studies did not determine gender specific differences but with the exception of LIFE (Losartan Intervention for Endpoint Reduction in Hypertension), which enrolled 54 % women, have included significantly fewer women than men [57–59]. No gender differences in benefits or adverse reactions has been noted with ARBs.

In summary, ACE-I and ARBs are effective in the treatment of hypertension, ischemic heart disease and heart failure. Though data is not as robust as seen in men, especially for heart failure with systolic dysfunction, pooled analysis does suggest a benefit. Women do have a higher adverse profile when it comes to ACE-I associated cough and this should be kept in mind.

Aldosterone Antagonists

Aldosterone represents another important component of the RAS and a prime therapeutic target.

Aldosterone is a potent vasoconstrictor and its antagonism at its receptor site has proven beneficial in the management of severe systolic heart failure. There have not been any gender specific studies between men and women in regards to aldosterone antagonists [5]. Clinical studies have not demonstrated gender-specific differences in neither RALES (Randomized Aldactone Evaluation Study) nor EPHESUS

(Eplerenone Post-Acute Myocardial Infarction Heart Failure Efficacy and Survival Study) trials though the latter showed a trend towards a greater benefit for women treated with eplerenone for all-cause mortality compared with men at 30 days. These results were not further assessed at 4 months. In both studies the enrollment of women was shy of 30 % [60, 61].

Digoxin

Digoxin is an example of a medication where careful consideration of pharmacokinetic properties is needed prior to prescribing the medication [7]. Digoxin is used to help treat symptoms associated with heart failure and help control heart rate in patients with atrial fibrillation. Digoxin works by inhibiting sodium-potassium pumps leading to increase in intracellular calcium and ultimately improving myocardial muscle contraction [9]. In 1997, the Digitalis Investigation Group (DIG) reported the results of a randomized trial evaluating the efficacy of digoxin therapy for patients with heart failure [62]. Although no mortality benefit was seen with digoxin therapy in this landmark trial, digoxin did decrease risk of hospitalization for heart failure. Thereafter, several national and international guidelines strongly endorsed the use of digoxin for these patients.

However in a post hoc subgroup analysis, digoxin was associated with a significantly higher risk of death among women taking digoxin compared with those taking placebo, an effect that was not observed in men [63]. Potential explanations for the unexpected results included dose-related effects, as well as an interaction with hormone replacement therapy [64]. Despite lower administered digoxin doses, women demonstrated higher serum levels than did men suggesting gender specific differences in cellular sodium and calcium handling that could explain the different effects of glycosides in women and men. Greater toxicity in women has been shown to be in part due to lower sodium concentrations and fewer Na-K ATPase pumps which allows for greater concentrations in women. Some studies have demonstrated lower Na+ concentrations and fewer Na-K ATPase pumps in erythrocytes, skeletal muscle and potentially in cardiomyocytes [65]. Additional retrospective analysis of the DIG trial revealed the significant importance of digitalis levels for both genders as higher serum digoxin concentrations were associated with increased crude all-cause mortality in men as well, whereas lower levels were associated with a better prognosis [66]. In the absence of definitive evidence, doses should now be used that lead to plasma levels below 0.8 ng/ml.

Although digoxin has fallen out of favor due to the DIG trial findings, it is still being used and recommended in several national and international cardiovascular guidelines. Due to its narrow therapeutic window, appropriate monitoring is essential to prevent toxicity (Table 20.5). It is important to mention that obtaining a blood level of digoxin only estimates the amount of digoxin at the receptors in the cardiac tissues where the drug produces its effect [10]. These data reinforce the possibilities of gender-related effects and underscore the need to perform gender-specific analysis and to include sufficient numbers of women in clinical trials.

In summary, the effect of digoxin therapy differs between men and women. Digoxin therapy is associated with an increased risk of death among women with heart failure and depressed left ventricular systolic function at relatively lower levels when compared to men (and in men at increasing doses). In absence of definite evidence, plasma levels should be monitored to be kept below 0.8 ng/ml if this medication is used.

Calcium Channel Blockers

Gender specific differences in pharmacokinetics have been described for some calcium channel blockers [67–69]. Differences in hepatic metabolism and gut absorption account for most of the differences seen with verapamil – a non-dihydropyridine [70]. Gender differences in the CYP3A and or the P-glycoprotein (P-gp) in the gut and liver lead to a lower concentration and higher clearance of verapamil in women compared to men [70, 71]. Differences have been seen in terms of route of administration as well. Women demonstrate a faster clearance of intravenous verapamil [68]. In women, slower clearance was observed after a single initial oral dose but faster clearance after steady state was achieved relative to men [68]. Verapamil clearance is also decreased in elderly woman showing greater effect on blood pressure and heart rate since higher concentrations are present [72].

Amlodipine, a long acting dihydropyridine calcium channel blocker, has been extensively studied in the CV literature. In contrast to verapamil, it has high bioavailability, is metabolized by several CYP pathways, not considered a P-gp substrate, and has low rates of first pass hepatic metabolism [73]. Some investigators have shown a more potent diastolic blood pressure reduction effect in women relative to men with amlodipine, however this has not been consistently shown in the literature [73]. Similarly, these investigators have reported a higher incidence of edema in women which has been confirmed in other studies [73, 74].

It has not been determined whether the pharmacokinetic differences among calcium channel blockers have relevant clinical impact. The major hypertension trials with calcium channel blockers have included comparable number of women participants and in many cases more. These have not revealed evidence for gender-specific differences in outcomes.

In summary, CCBs are effective medications in the treatment of HTN where most of the gender specific data comes from. Verapamil and nifedipine are metabolized faster in women leading to lower concentrations except in elderly women where adjusted dosing may be needed to avoid supratherapeutic ranges. Women are more susceptible to lower extremity edema with amlodipine than men. No difference in gender-specific outcomes has been revealed.

Aspirin

Gender-specific differences in pharmacokinetics of aspirin have been known for decades. Slower clearance and greater bioavailability of aspirin in women, in turn with significant prolongation of half-life is well known [75]. However, this difference is not significant in women taken oral contraceptives since metabolism is faster under hormonal influences [76]. Some in vitro observations relative to effects of aspirin on thrombocyte aggregation and testosterone and estradiol influences on aspirin-induced inhibition of platelet aggregation have questionable clinical relevance.

For secondary prevention, benefits of aspirin for men and women are well documented with reductions of myocardial infarction, stroke, and CV death by 25 % in both genders [77]. Similarly, aspirin's value in acute myocardial infarction therapy is also well established for both genders [44].

For primary prevention, the benefit is less clear in women. The Women's Health Study showed that aspirin reduced the risk of stroke by about 24 % and did not influence their risk of MI or mortality. In the subgroup of older women (>65 years), aspirin was effective in the primary prevention of CV events and mostly driven by stroke benefit [78]. These findings suggest gender related differences that may go beyond pharmacokinetics but that remains unclear. For a more in depth analysis of gender related differences in aspirin and platelet biology please refer to the antithrombotic issues chapter in women in this text.

Anti-arrhythmics

Gender specific differences in myocardial repolarization have been known for some time [79].

Several explanations have been proposed but no definite mechanism has been elucidated. The role of sex steroids is supported by the fact that in childhood QT time is of equal length in both genders and it appears to shorten in young men with elevated androgen levels. Similarly the incidence of acquired long QT syndrome is higher in women than in men [80]. A number of medications including anti-arrhythmics, psychotropic drugs, antifungals and some antibiotics can induce this syndrome (see Fig. 20.2). Class I and III anti-arrhythmics potentially associated with prolongation of QT interval, more often lead to torsades de pointes tachycardia in women [81]. Another potential explanation for this phenomenon includes hormonal influences, smaller volumes of distribution which results in greater concentrations and ion channel modifications leading to more side effects and higher risk of pro-arrhythmias in women compared with men [81, 82].

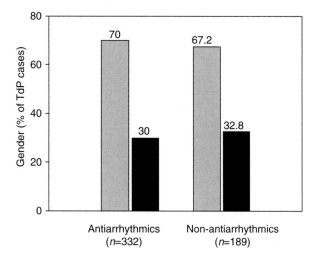

Fig. 20.2 Relationship between female (*grey bars*) and male (*black bars*) genders and *torsades de pointe* tachycardia for anti-arrhythmic and non-anti-arrhythmic medications in a database search (Adapted with permission from Jochmann et al. [5])

Statins

Only slight gender specific differences in statins pharmacokinetics is appreciated. Mostly all statins (with exception of pravastatin and rosuvastatin – CYP independent) are metabolized by CYP 3A4 (CYP2C9 for fluvastatin) therefore drug interactions with substances also metabolized via CYP3A4 have to be considered [83–85]. In general, plasma concentrations of statins appear to be higher in women however these are considered to be non-significant as no major dose adjustment has been recommended. Nonetheless, when it comes to adverse drug reactions, women (especially older and thin) appear to have more side effects [34]. This may be secondary to pharmacodynamics differences and needs to be taken into consideration.

Studies with statins have revealed a similar reduction in cardiovascular events for women and men in major primary and secondary prevention trials (4S, CARE, TNT, PROVE IT). Though the percentage of women in these studies was about 25 % on average, a major meta-analysis showed comparable benefits (Fig. 20.3) [86]. Despite beneficial effects seen in both primary and secondary prevention of CVD for both genders, statins continue to be underutilized in women compared to in men

Diuretics

Many sources of evidence have shown that women experience more frequently adverse drug reactions associated with diuretics. These are not fully explained by

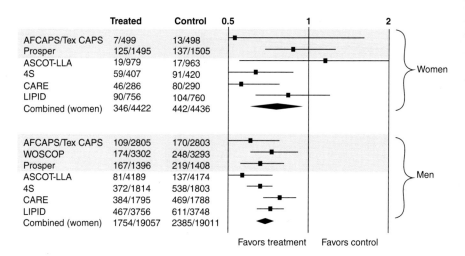

	Treated	Control	0.5	1	2	

Fig. 20.3 Relative risk ratios and 95 % confidence intervals for major coronary events in women and men in outcome studies, in evaluation of the impact of statins on major coronary events. *Grey bars* indicate primary prevention studies. WOSCOP included only men (Adapted with permission from Jochmann et al. [5])

prescription habits with a known tendency of providers to prescribe diuretics to women for edema. Animal studies support the notion that gender-specific differences of adverse and therapeutic effects of diuretics may exist. Werner et al. studied the impact of genetic polymorphism in the pharmacokinetics of torsemide and identified gender as a potential explanation for the increase in adverse side effects seen in women [20].

Very limited data regarding gender-specific differences is available for thiazide diuretics. In several animal models, all diuretics appear to cause a more effective diuresis, natriuresis, and kaliuresis in females rather than male animals (rats especially) [87]. Similarly, adverse effects like hyponatremia and hypokalemia occur more frequently in women than in men taking diuretics and both of these electrolyte disturbances can potentially cause severe arrhythmias. Though this suspicion has not been confirmed in clinical trials, this potential danger needs to be considered when prescribing diuretics for women, especially in those with concomitant therapy that may lead to further alterations (digoxin, QT prolonging drugs, etc.).

Summary

Gender specific differences exist between men and women in terms of pharmacokinetics and pharmacodynamics for many important cardiovascular drugs though clinical consequences in the majority of cases are not that dissimilar. Pharmacokinetic differences for women include higher concentrations of medication due to lower body weight, smaller volumes of distribution, larger free fractions of medication being available to exert its effect, and decreased clearance. Secondly, pharmacodynamic differences such as number of receptors and greater affinities of receptors have been shown to increase sensitivity. In part due to these differences, women have been shown to experience more adverse drug reactions. Other influencing factors, from complex ones such as genetic polymorphisms to hormonal influences at cellular and receptor levels, to more simple ones such as patient compliance and inappropriate dosing of a medication also may contribute to adverse reactions in a female patient.

Despite some of the differences seen in pharmacokinetics and pharmacodynamics for some CV drugs, gender-specific analyses is still lacking for many drugs in this class. Similarly despite some pertinent pharmacokinetic gender observations, women continue to be underrepresented in drug clinical trials so we have not yet been able to thoroughly study the impact of these differences in clinical outcomes. Most current treatment guidelines do not differentiate between treatment for men and women with conditions such as myocardial infarction, heart failure, hypertension and in general, cardiovascular disease as the primary and secondary prognostic significance of these cardiovascular therapeutic strategies show only slight differences between the genders in data available to date. Despite current guidelines, women continue to be under treated when it comes to CV preventive therapeutic strategies.

Further gender specific research needs to be conducted to better determine differences in pharmacokinetics and pharmacodynamics and whether these differences will result in a significant clinical difference in our ever growing female population.

References

1. Finks SW. Cardiovascular disease in women. In: Richardson MM, editor in chief. Pharmacotherapy self-assessment program. 7th ed. Lanexa: American College of Clinical Pharmacy. p. 179–201; 2010.
2. Bonarjee V, Rosengren A, Snapinn S, James M, Dickstein K. Sex-based short- and long-term survival in patients following complicated myocardial infarction. Eur Heart J. 2006;27(18): 2177–83.
3. Dey S, Flather MD, Devlin G, et al. Sex-related differences in the presentation, treatment and outcomes among patients with acute coronary syndromes: the Global Registry of Acute Coronary Events. Heart. 2009;95:20–6.
4. Martin RM, Biswas PN, Freemantle SN, Pearce GL, Mann RD. Age and sex distribution of suspected adverse drug reactions to newly marketed drugs in general practice in England: analysis of 48 cohort studies. Br J Clin Pharmacol. 1998;46:505–11.
5. Jochmann N, Stangl K, Garbe E, Baumann G, Stangl V. Female-specific aspects in the pharmacotherapy of chronic cardiovascular diseases. Eur Heart J. 2005;26:1585–95.
6. Raz L, Miller VM. Considerations of sex and gender differences in preclinical and clinical trials. In: Regitz-Zagrosek V, editor. Sex and gender differences in pharmacology. Heidelberg: Springer; 2012.
7. Harris D, Douglas P. Enrollment of Women in Cardiovascular Clinical Trials Funded by the National Heart, Lung, and Blood Institute. N Engl J Med. 2000;343:475–80.

8. National Institutes of Health Web site. http://orwh.od.nih.gov/research/strategicplan/index. asp. Accessed 1 Feb 2013.

9. Williams LR, Leggett RW. Reference values for resting blood flow to organs of man. Clin Physiol Meas. 1989;10(3):187–217.

10. Dipiro JT, Spruill WJ, Wade WE, et al. Concepts in clinical pharmacokinetics. 5th ed. Bethesda: American Society of Health-System Pharmacists; 2010. p. 1–18.

11. Katzung BG. Lange's: basic & clinical pharmacology. 8th ed. New York: McGraw-Hill; 2001. p. 35–50.

12. Schwartz JB. The influence of sex on pharmacokinetics. Clin Pharmacokinet. 2003;42(2):107–21.

13. Soldin OP, Chung SH, Mattison DR. Sex differences in drug disposition. J Biomed Biotechnol. 2011;1–14.

14. Stephen AM, Wiggins HS, Englyst HN, et al. The effect of age, sex and level of intake of dietary fibre from wheat on large-bowel function in thirty healthy subjects. Br J Nutr. 1986;56:349–61.

15. Soldin OP, Mattison DR. Sex differences in pharmacokinetics and pharmacodynamics. Clin Pharmacokinet. 2009;48(3):143–7.

16. Wooten JM. Pharmacotherapy considerations in elderly adults. South Med J. 2012;105(8): 437–45.

17. Bebia Z, Buch SC, Wilson JW, et al. Bioequivalence revisited: influence of age and sex on CYP enzymes. Clin Pharmacol Ther. 2004;76(6):618–27.

18. Schwartz JB. The current state of knowledge on age, sex, and their interactions on clinical pharmacology. Clin Pharmacol Ther. 2007;82(1):87–95.

19. Ritschel WA, Kearns GL. Handbook of basic pharmacokinetics. 5th ed. Washington, D.C.: American Pharmaceutical Association; 1999. p. 3.

20. Werner U, Werner D, Heinbüchner S, et al. Gender is an important determinant of the disposition of the loop diuretic torasemide. J Clin Pharmacol. 2010;50(2):160–8.

21. Anderson GD, Carr DB. Effect of pregnancy on the pharmacokinetics of antihypertensive drugs. Clin Pharmacokinet. 2009;48(3):159–68.

22. Micromedex® 2.0 Web site. http://www.thomsonhc.com/micromedex2/librarian. Accessed 1 Feb 2013.

23. Tomalik-Scharte D, Lazar A, Fuhr U, et al. The clinical role of genetic polymorphisms in drug-metabolizing enzymes. Pharmacogenomics J. 2008;8:4–15.

24. Carrel L, Willar HF. X-inactivation profile reveals extensive variability in x-linked gene expression in females. Nature. 2005;434:400–4.

25. Tipnis SR, Hooper NM, Hyde R, et al. A human homolog of angiotensin-converting enzyme. Cloning and functional expression as a captopril-intensive carboxypeptidase. J Biol Chem. 2000;275:33238–43.

26. Denium J, van Gool JM, Koflard MJ, ten Cate FJ. Angiotensin II type 2 receptors and cardiac hypertrophy in women with hypertrophic cardiomyopathy. Hypertension. 2001;38:1278–81.

27. Leinwand LA. Sex is a potent modifier of the cardiovascular system. J Clin Invest. 2003; 112:302–7.

28. Xin HB, Senbonmatsu T, Cheng DS, et al. Oestrogen protects FKBP12.6 null mice from cardiac hypertrophy. Nature. 2002;416:334–8.

29. Isoherranen N, Thummel KE. Drug metabolism and transport during pregnancy: how does drug disposition change during pregnancy and what are the mechanisms that cause such changes? Drug Metab Dispos. 2013;41(2):256–62.

30. Regitz-Zagrosek V, Lehmkuhl E, Lehmkuhl HB, Hetzer R. Gender aspects in heart failure. Pathophysiology and medical therapy. Arch Mal Coeur Vaiss. 2004;97:899–908.

31. Edwards DP. Regulation of signal transduction pathways by estrogen and progesterone. Annu Rev Physiol. 2005;67:335–76.

32. Waxman DJ, Holloway MG. Sex differences in the expression of hepatic drug metabolizing enzymes. Mol Pharmacol. 2009;76:215–28.

33. U.S. Food and Drug Administration Website. http://www.fda.gov/Drugs/GuidanceCompliance RegulatoryInformation/Survellance/AdverseDrugEffects/default.htm. Accessed 31 Jan 2013.

34. Moore TJ, Cohen MR, Furberg CD. Serious adverse drug events reported to the Food and Drug Administration, 1998–2005. Arch Intern Med. 2007;167(16):1752–9.

35. Luzier AB, Killian A, Wilton JH, Wilson MF, Forrest A, Kazierad DJ. Gender-related effects on metoprolol pharmacokinetics and pharmacodynamics in healthy volunteers. Clin Pharmacol Ther. 1999;66:594–601.
36. Thawornkaiwong A, Preawnim S, Wattanapermpool J. Upregulation of b-1-adrenergic receptors in ovariectomized rat hearts. Life Sci. 2003;72:1813–24.
37. Walle T, Byinton RP, Furberg CD, McIntyre KM, Vonkonas PS. Biologic determinants of propranolol disposition: results from 1308 patients in the Beta-Blocker Heart Attack Trial. Clin Pharmacol Ther. 1985;38:509–18.
38. MERIT-HF Study Group. Effect of metoprolol CR/XL in chronic heart failure: Metoprolol CR/XL Randomised Intervention Trial in Congestive Heart Failure (MERIT-HF). Lancet. 1999;353:2001–7.
39. Carvedilol Prospective Randomized Cumulative Survival (COPERNICUS) Study Group. Effect of carvedilol on the morbidity of patients with severe chronic heart failure: results of the carvedilol prospective randomized cumulative survival (COPERNICUS) study. Circulation. 2002;106:2194–9.
40. Tabassome S, Mary-Krause M, Funck-Brentano C, Jaillon P, on behalf of the CIBIS II Investigators. Sex differences in the prognosis of congestive heart failure: results from the Cardiac Insufficiency Bisoprolol Study (CIBIS II). Circulation. 2001;103:375–80.
41. Ghali JK, Pina IL, Gottlieb SS, Deedwania PC, Wikstrand JC. Metoprolol CR/XL in female patients with heart failure: analysis of the experience in metoprolol extended-release randomized intervention trial in heart failure (MERIT-HF). Circulation. 2002;105:1585–91.
42. The beta-Blocker Heart Attack Trial (BHAT). A randomized trial of propranolol in patients with acute myocardial infarction. JAMA. 1982;247:1707–14.
43. Olsson G, Wikstrand J, Warnold I, Manger Cats V, McBoyle D, Herlitz J, Hialmarson A, Sonneblick EH. Metoprolol-induced reduction in postinfarction mortality: Pooled results from five double-blind randomized trials. Eur Heart J. 1992;13:28–32.
44. Infarct Survival Collaborative Group. Randomised trial of intravenous atenolol amount 16,027 cases of suspected acute myocardial infarction: ISIS-1. Lancet. 1986;2(8498):57–66.
45. Infarct Survival Collaborative Group. Randomised trial of intravenous streptokinase, oral aspirin, both, or neither among 17,187 cases of suspected acute myocardial infarction: ISIS-2. Lancet. 1988;2(8607):57–66.
46. Fischer M, Baessler A, Schunkert H. Renin angiotensin system and gender differences in the cardiovascular system. Cardiovasc Res. 2002;53:672–7.
47. Schunkert H, Danser AH, Hense HW, Derkx FH, Kurzinger S, Riegger GA. Effects of estrogen replacement therapy on the renin-angiotensin system in postmenopausal women. Circulation. 1997;95:39–45.
48. Regitz-Zagosek V. Therapeutic implications of the gender-specific aspects of cardiovascular disease. Nat Rev Drug Discov. 2006;5:425–38.
49. Garg R, Yusuf S. Overview of randomized trials of angiotensin-converting enzyme inhibitors on mortality and morbidity in patients with heart failure. Collaborative Group on ACE Inhibitor Trials. JAMA. 1995;273:1450–6.
50. Saenz-Campos D, Bayes MC, Masana E, Martin S, Barbanoj M, Jane F. Sex-related pharmacokinetic and pharmacodynamic variations of lisinopril. Methods Find Exp Clin Pharmacol. 1996;18:533–8.
51. Mackay FJ, Pearce GL, Mann RD. Cough and angiotensin II receptor antagonists: cause or confounding? Br J Clin Pharmacol. 1999;47:111–4.
52. Mas S, Gasso P, Alvarez S, Ortiz J, Sotoca JM, Francino A, Carne X, Laguente A. Pharmacogenetic predictors of angiotensin-converting enzyme inhibitor-induced cough: The role of ACE, ABO, and BDKRB2 genes. Pharmacogenet Genomics. 2011;21:531–8.
53. Berry C, Touyz R, Dominiczak AF, Webb RC, Johns DG. Angiotensin receptors: signaling, vascular pathophysiology, and interactions with ceramide. Am J Physiol Heart Circ Physiol. 2001;281:H2337–65.
54. You D, Loufrani L, Baron C, Levy BI, Widdop RE, Henrion D. High blood pressure reduction reverses angiotensin II type 2 receptor-mediated vasoconstriction into vasodilation in spontaneously hypertensive rats. Circulation. 2005;111:1006–11.

55. Sampson AK, Moritz KM, Jones ES, Flower RL, Widdop RE, Denton KM. Enhanced angiotensin II type 2 receptor mechanisms mediate decreases in arterial pressure attributable to chronic low-dose angiotensin II in female rats. Hypertension. 2008;52:666–71.
56. Nickenig G, Baumer AT, Grohe C, Kahlert S, Strehlow K, Rosenkranz S, Stablein A, Beckers F, Smits JF, Daemen MJ, et al. Estrogen modulates AT1 receptor gene expression in vitro and in vivo. Circulation. 1998;97:2197–201.
57. Gleiter CH, Mo'rike KE. Clinical pharmacokinetics of candesartan. Clin Pharmacokinet. 2002;41:7–17.
58. Israili ZH. Clinical pharmacokinetics of angiotensin II (AT1) receptor blockers in hypertension. J Hum Hypertens. 2000;14:73–86.
59. Vachharajani NN, Shyu WC, Smith RA, Greene DS. The effects of age and gender on the pharmacokinetics of irbesartan. Br J Clin Pharmacol. 1998;46:611–3.
60. Pitt B, Zannad F, Remme WJ, Cody R, Castaigne A, Perez A, Palensky J, Wittes J. The effect of spironolactone in morbidity and mortality in patients with severe heart failure. N Engl J Med. 1999;341:709–17.
61. Pitt B, Remme W, Zannad F, Neaton J, Martinez F, Roniker B, Bittman R, Hurley S, Kleiman J, Gatlin M, Eplerenone Post-Acute Myocardial Infarction Heart Failure Efficacy and Survival Study Investigators. Eplerenone, a selective aldosterone blocker in patients with left ventricular dysfunction after myocardial infarction. N Engl J Med. 2003;348:1309–21.
62. The Digitalis Investigation Group. The effect of digoxin on mortality and morbidity in patients with heart failure. N Engl J Med. 1997;336:525–33.
63. Rathore S, Wang Y, Krumholz H. Sex differences in the effect of digoxin for the treatment of heart failure. N Engl J Med. 2002;347(18):1403–10.
64. Furberg CD, Vittinghoff E, Davidson M, Herrington DM, Simon JA, Wenger NK, Hulley S. Subgroup interactions in the Heart and Estrogen/Progestin Replacement Study: lessons learned. Circulation. 2002;105:917–22.
65. Green HJ, Duscha BD, Sullivan MJ, Ketyian SJ, Kraus WE. Normal skeletal muscle Na(þ)-K(þ) pump concentration in patients with chronic heart failure. Muscle Nerve. 2001;24:69–76.
66. Rathore SS, Curtis JP, Wang Y, Bristow MR, Krumholz H. Association of serum digoxin concentration and outcomes in patients with heart failure. JAMA. 2003;289:871–8.
67. Kang D, Verotta D, Krecic-Shepard ME, Modi NB, Gupta SK, Schwartz JB. Population analyses of sustained-release verapamil in patients: effects of sex, race, and smoking. Clin Pharmacol Ther. 2003;73:31–40.
68. Krecic-Shepard ME, Barnas CR, Slimko J, Schwartz JB. Faster clearance of sustained release verapamil in men versus women: continuing observations on sex-specific differences after oral administration of verapamil. Clin Pharmacol Ther. 2000;68:286–92.
69. Krecic-Shepard ME, Park K, Barnas C, Slimko J, Kerwin DR, Schwartz JB. Race and sex influence clearance of nifedipine: results of a population study. Clin Pharmacol Ther. 2000;68:130–42.
70. Gupta SK, Atkinson L, Tu T, Longstreth JA. Age and gender related changes in stereoselective pharmacokinetics and pharmacodynamics of verapamil and norverapamil. Br J Clin Pharmacol. 1995;40:325–31.
71. Ueno K, Sato H. Sex-related differences in pharmacokinetics and pharmacodynamics of antihypertensive drugs. Hypertens Res. 2012;35:245–50.
72. Schwartz JB, Capili H, Daugherty J. Aging of women alters s-verapamil pharmacokinetics and pharmacodynamics. Clin Pharmacol Ther. 1994;55:509–17.
73. Kloner RA, Sowers JR, DiBona GF, Gaffney M, Wein M. Sex- and age-related antihypertensive effects of amlodipine. The Amlodipine Cardiovascular Community Trial Study Group. Am J Cardiol. 1996;77:713–22.
74. Greenblatt DJ, Harmatz JS, von Moltke LL, Wright CE, Shader RI. Age and gender effects on the pharmacokinetics and pharmacodynamics of triazolam, a cytochrome P450 3A substrate. Clin Pharmacol Ther. 2004;76:467–79.
75. Ho PC, Triggs EJ, Bourne DW, Heazlewood VJ. The effect of age and sex on the disposition of acetylsalicyl acid and its metabolites. Br J Clin Pharmacol. 1985;19:675–84.

76. Miners JO, Grugrinovich N, Whitehead AG, Robson RA, Birkett DJ. Influence of gender and oral contraceptive steroids on the metabolism of salicylic acid and acetylsalicylic acid. Br J Clin Pharmacol. 1986;22:135–42.
77. Antithrombotic Trialists Collaboration. Collaborative meta-analysis of randomised trials of antiplatelet therapy for prevention of death, myocardial infarction, and stroke in high risk patients. BMJ. 2002;324:71–86.
78. Ridker PM, Cook NR, Lee I-M, Gordon D, Gaziano JM, Manson JE, Hennekens CH, Buring JE. A randomized trial of low-dose aspirin in the primary prevention of cardiovascular disease in women. N Engl J Med. 2005;352:1293–304.
79. Bazett HC. An analysis of the time-relations of electrocardiograms. Heart. 1920;7:353–70.
80. Rautaharju PM, Zhou SH, Wong S, Calhoun HP, Berenson GS, Prineas R, Davignon A. Sex differences in the evolution of the electrocardiographic QT interval with age. Can J Cardiol. 1992;8:690–5.
81. Drici MD, Clement N. Is gender a risk factor for adverse drug reactions? The example of drug-induced long QT syndrome. Drug Saf. 2001;24:575–85.
82. Legato M. Gender and the heart: sex-specific differences in normal anatomy and physiology. J Gend Specif Med. 2000;3:15–8.
83. Gibson DM, Bron NJ, Richens A, Hounslow NJ, Sedman AJ, Whitfield LR. Effect of age and gender on pharmacokinetics of atorvastatin in humans. J Clin Pharmacol. 1996;36:242–6.
84. Cheng H, Rogers JD, Sweany AE, Dobrinska MR, Stein EA, Tate AC, Amin RD, Quan H. Influence of age and gender on the plasma profiles of 3-hydroxy-3-methylglutaryl-coenzyme A (HMG-CoA) reductase inhibitory activity following multiple doses of lovastatin and simvastatin. Pharm Res. 1992;9:1629–33.
85. Martin PD, Dane AL, Nwose OM, Schneck DW, Warwick MJ. No effect of age or gender on the pharmacokinetics of rosuvastatin: a new HMG-CoA reductase inhibitor. J Clin Pharmacol. 2002;42:1116–21.
86. Cheung BMY, Lauder IJ, Lau C-P, Kumana CR. Meta-analysis of large randomized controlled trials to evaluate the impact of statins on cardiovascular outcomes. Br J Clin Pharmacol. 2004;57:640–51.
87. Brandoni A, Villar SR, Torres AM. Gender-related differences in the pharmacodynamics of furosemide in rats. Pharmacology. 2004;70:107–12.

Index

A

Abramov, D., 142

ACC/AHA. *See* American College of Cardiology/American Heart Association (ACC/AHA)

ACE. *See* Angiotensin converting enzyme (ACE)

ACHD. *See* Adult congenital heart disease (ACHD)

ACS. *See* Acute coronary syndromes (ACS)

Acute aortic regurgitation, 200

Acute coronary syndromes (ACS)
  diagnosis, 114
  gender differences, management, 114–115
  invasive therapy (*see* Invasive therapy, ACS)
  maternal mortality, 312
  pathophysiology, 114

Acute myocardial infarction (AMI), 312

ADA. *See* American Diabetes Association (ADA)

Adenosine diphosphate P2Y12 receptor antagonists, 334–336

ADP P2Y12. *See* Adenosine diphosphate P2Y12 receptor antagonists

ADRs. *See* Adverse reactions (ADRs)

Adult congenital heart disease (ACHD)
  cardiac surgery, 248
  diagnosis, 237–238
  hormone therapy, 247
  lifestyle, 247
  morbidty, 239–240
  mortality, 238–239
  pregnancy, 241–246
  reproductive health counseling, 240–241

Adult treatment panel (ATP), 277

Adverse reactions (ADRs), 431

AF. *See* Atrial fibrillation (AF)

Aguila, A., 175–213

AHA. *See* American Heart Association (AHA)

American College of Cardiology/American Heart Association (ACC/AHA), 156, 160, 161

American Diabetes Association (ADA), 272

American Heart Association (AHA)
  gender differences, cardiac risk factors, 30
  recommendations, modifiable risk factors, 22–24

Ames, M., 257

AMI. *See* Acute myocardial infarction (AMI)

Anderson, G.D., 432

Angiolillo, D.J., 321–346

Angiotensin converting enzyme (ACE)
  ACE-I studies, 436, 437
  inhibitors and ARBs, 94–95, 254

Angiotensin receptor blockers (ARBs)
  and ACE inhibitors, 94–95, 436–437
  definition, 159–160

Anticoagulant therapy
  direct thrombin inhibitors, 122–125
  LMWF, 122
  UFH, 122

Antiplatelet therapy
  adenosine diphosphate P2Y12 receptor antagonists, 334–336
  aspirin, 94, 119, 331–334
  GP IIb/IIIa inhibitors, 121
  GP IIb/IIIa receptor, 336–337
  P2Y12 receptor inhibitors, 119–121

H.Z. Mieszczanska, G.P. Velarde (eds.),
Management of Cardiovascular Disease in Women,
DOI 10.1007/978-1-4471-5517-1, © Springer-Verlag London 2014

Printed by Publishers' Graphics LLC